Rheumatoid Arthritis: Symptoms, Diagnosis and Treatment

Rheumatoid Arthritis: Symptoms, Diagnosis and Treatment

Editor: Mary Kellar

FA
FOSTER
ACADEMICS

www.fosteracademics.com

www.fosteracademics.com

FOSTER ACADEMICS

Cataloging-in-Publication Data

Rheumatoid arthritis : symptoms, diagnosis and treatment / edited by Mary Kellar.
p. cm.
Includes bibliographical references and index.
ISBN 978-1-63242-567-6
1. Rheumatoid arthritis. 2. Rheumatoid arthritis--Diagnosis.
3. Rheumatoid arthritis--Treatment. I. Kellar, Mary.
RC933 .R44 2018
616.722--dc23

Foster Academics,
118-35 Queens Blvd., Suite 400,
Forest Hills, NY 11375, USA

ISBN 978-1-63242-567-6 (Hardback)

Printed and bound in China.

Contents

Preface

Rheumatoid arthritis is a disorder that affects the joints. It is an autoimmune disorder. Low red blood cell count and inflammation of the lungs and around the heart are common conditions associated with this disorder. The treatment of rheumatoid arthritis aims to facilitate the everyday functioning of the patient along with minimizing the pain. Some of the diverse topics covered in this book address the varied aspects that fall under the diagnosis and treatment of rheumatoid arthritis. It will serve as a reference to a broad spectrum of readers.

Various studies have approached the subject by analyzing it with a single perspective, but the present book provides diverse methodologies and techniques to address this field. This book contains theories and applications needed for understanding the subject from different perspectives. The aim is to keep the readers informed about the progresses in the field; therefore, the contributions were carefully examined to compile novel researches by specialists from across the globe.

Indeed, the job of the editor is the most crucial and challenging in compiling all chapters into a single book. In the end, I would extend my sincere thanks to the chapter authors for their profound work. I am also thankful for the support provided by my family and colleagues during the compilation of this book.

Editor

1

Impact of Rheumatoid Arthritis Disease Activity Test on Clinical Practice

John W. Peabody[1,2]*, Vibeke Strand[3], Riti Shimkhada[2,4], Rachel Lee[2], David Chernoff[5]

1 Departments of Epidemiology & Biostatistics and Medicine, University of California San Francisco, San Francisco, California, United States of America, **2** QURE Healthcare, San Rafael, California, United States of America, **3** Division of Immunology/Rheumatology, Stanford University, Stanford, California, United States of America, **4** Department of Health Policy and Management, University of California Los Angeles, Los Angeles, California, United States of America, **5** Crescendo Bioscience, South San Francisco, California, United States of America

Abstract

Background: Variability exists in the assessment of disease activity in rheumatoid arthritis (RA) patients that may affect quality of care.

Objectives: To measure the impact on quality of care of a Multi-Biomarker Disease Activity (MBDA) test that quantitatively assesses RA disease activity.

Methods: Board-certified rheumatologists without prior experience with the MBDA test (N = 81) were randomized into an intervention or control group as part of a longitudinal randomized-control study. All physicians were asked to care for three simulated RA patients, using Clinical Performance and Value (CPV™) vignettes, in a before and after design. CPV™ vignettes have been validated to assess the quality of clinical practice and identify variation in care. The vignettes covered all domains of a regular patient visit; scores were determined as a percentage of explicit predefined criteria completed. Three vignettes, representing typical RA cases, were administered each round. In the first round, no physician received information about the MBDA test. In the second round, only physicians in the intervention group were given educational materials about the test and hypothetical test results for each of the simulated patients. The outcome measures were the overall quality of care, disease assessment and treatment.

Results: The overall quality scores in the intervention group improved by 3 percent ($p = 0.02$) post-intervention compared with baseline, versus no change in the control group. The greatest benefit in the intervention group was to the quality of disease activity assessment and treatment decisions, which improved by 12 percent ($p < 0.01$) compared with no significant change in the control group. The intervention was associated with more appropriate use of biologic and/or combination DMARDs in the co-morbidity case type ($p < 0.01$).

Conclusions: Based on these results, use of the MBDA test improved the assessment and treatment decisions for simulated cases of RA and may prove useful for rheumatologists in clinical practice.

Editor: Oliver Frey, University Hospital Jena, Germany

Funding: Funding for this study was provided by Crescendo Bioscience, Inc., South San Francisco, California (http://www.crescendobio.com/). The funders were informed and contributed to study design, had no role in data collection or analysis, and agreed to the decision to publish and contributed to preparation of the manuscript.

Competing Interests: VS and DC are paid consultants of Crescendo Biosciences. QURE Healthcare was contracted by Crescendo to conduct this study and analysis. Crescendo Bioscience, Inc. was the commercial funder.

* E-mail: jpeabody@qurehealthcare.com

Introduction

Rheumatoid arthritis (RA) is a chronic, systemic inflammatory disorder that affects approximately 1.5 million people in the United States.[1] Unlike disease areas such as cardiology that have extensive research and appropriate use criteria, evidence-based medicine for RA diagnosis, evaluation and treatment are based on largely subjective criteria.[2,3] Until 2010, the classification criteria for RA had not changed in 23 years.[4] Recent treatment guidelines direct rheumatologists to treat RA promptly and aggressively, aiming for remission as a therapeutic target.[5,6] Nevertheless, early recognition of signs and symptoms and timely referral to rheumatologists remain challenging; appropriate use of non-biologic and biologic disease-modifying anti-rheumatic drugs (DMARDs) significantly improves outcomes but requires close monitoring of disease activity, including laboratory evaluations and imaging that is often difficult to achieve.[3,7] A number of composite tools are available for assessing disease activity in RA, of which 6 have been recommended by the American College of Rheumatology (ACR).[8] They are infrequently used in practice and have limitations, including reliance on subjective measures with frequent discordance between physician and patient assessments.[9] Patient global assessment and its contribution to the ACR/European League Against Rheumatism remission criteria are affected by non-inflammatory factors.[10] Moreover, individual variability in therapeutic responses and lack of objective biomarkers for identification of active disease can lead to variability in patient care that may affect the management of RA [11–15].

New technology and diagnostic tools have been shown to lower variability in clinical areas such as cardiology, radiology and oncology, [16] but so far this effect has not been demonstrated in rheumatology. Reducing the variability in rheumatologic assessments and treatment decisions would be beneficial in RA not only because it would lead to higher quality for the patient but it could lower aggregate health care costs. [17,18] By objectively quantifying disease activity in RA, physicians may be better equipped to allocate resources accurately, avoid ordering unnecessary tests, and change therapy effectively [19].

A multi-biomarker disease activity (MBDA) blood test (Vectra DA™; Crescendo Bioscience, Inc., South San Francisco, CA) is currently available in the U.S. to assess disease activity in adult patients with RA. The test is done by taking serum prepared from patient peripheral blood and sending it to a central laboratory for automated, multiplexed measurement of 12 protein biomarkers that play key roles in the underlying pathophysiology of RA. The MBDA test is based on an algorithm that uses the concentrations of the 12 biomarkers to generate a score that represents the level of RA disease activity on a scale of 1 (lowest activity) to 100 (greatest)[20,21] and, in studies of analytical validation, the test is precise and reproducible.[20] The MBDA test was developed to correlate with the 28-joint Disease Activity Score (DAS28) and has been clinically validated by correlations with DAS28 and other disease activity measures in independent RA cohorts, with thresholds established for low, moderate and high disease activity.[22,23] Other studies show that the MBDA test tracks responses to treatment with biologic and non-biologic DMARDs,[22,23] and may potentially be an indicator of progressive joint damage in patients with RA.[24] The MBDA test is not validated for diagnosing RA.

There are currently no blood tests that are specific for RA. The two clinical laboratory tests most closely associated with RA, rheumatoid factor and anti-citrullinated protein antibody tests, are for diagnosis and prognosis. The only blood tests that are routinely used to assess disease activity in RA are the erythrocyte sedimentation rate (ESR) and C-reactive protein (CRP). Both have limitations, as their values are in the normal range in up to half of patients with active disease, and they are often discordant with each other.[25,26] Roles for the MBDA test in RA patient management include situations where clinical evaluations and laboratory test results provide a mixed picture of disease activity, or assessment is confounded by symptoms from diseases other than RA. The MBDA test is well suited to being studied with case simulations because, as an objective test, the inclusion of a hypothetical MBDA score in a case simulation is sufficient to duplicate its real-life inclusion in the clinical decision-making process. Thus to evaluate the potential clinical utility of the MBDA test, we used simulated cases of RA patients and hypothetical MBDA scores to evaluate clinical practice by rheumatologists before and after exposure to the MBDA test.

Methods

Overview

This is a longitudinal randomized controlled study of practicing rheumatologists from across the U.S. with no prior experience with the MBDA test. In a "before and after" design, rheumatologists were asked to care for simulated patients with RA, using Clinical Performance and Value (CPV™) vignettes via web-based interactive sessions. Physicians completed the vignettes at baseline (3 cases pre-intervention, Round 1) and again 12 weeks later (3 cases post-intervention, Round 2). In Round 1, none of the rheumatologists received any information about the MBDA test and none of the vignettes included MBDA scores. In Round 2, rheumatologists who were randomized to the intervention group were introduced to the MBDA test and provided with a hypothetical test result for each Round 2 vignette, whereas MBDA test information and results were not made available to physicians randomized to the control group. This study was conducted in accordance with the ethical standards of the institutional review board (IRB), approved by the Essex IRB, Lebanon, NJ. Participants provided written consent to participate, and Essex IRB approved the consent form.

The Intervention

The intervention group received hypothetical MBDA scores, on a scale from 1 to 100, for each patient in the Round 2 vignettes. As is true for the actual MBDA test, lower scores indicated less disease activity and higher scores generally indicated a need to initiate or change therapy. Prior to receiving hypothetical MBDA scores rheumatologists in the intervention group were provided with information about the MBDA test and offered a variety of educational modalities, including emailed materials, mailed materials, access to a podcast, invitation to a live webinar and/or access to the Principal Investigator of the study and the Chief Medical Officer of Crescendo Bioscience for answers to specific questions.

Eligibility and Selection of Physicians

Eligibility for participation in the study was assessed using a physician questionnaire. Physicians had to be (1) board-certified rheumatologists, (2) English-speaking, (3) practicing in a community/non-academic based setting, (4) in practice with >200 RA patients in their care, (5) accessible by Internet, and (6) inexperienced with the MBDA test. From a nationally representative list of 2600 eligible rheumatologists, 81 physicians were selected for participation in this study (Figure 1). These physicians were randomized into one of two arms: 37 in the intervention arm, and 44 in the control arm. Only one physician was lost to follow-up between baseline and post-intervention assessments.

Clinical Performance and Value™ vignettes

The quality of clinical performance was measured at baseline (Round 1) and after 12-weeks (Round 2) using Clinical Performance and Value (CPV™) vignettes. CPV™ vignettes have been demonstrated to be a validated means for assessing differences in clinical practice and inherent variation in care independent of case mix.[27–29] The vignettes used in this study simulated clinical encounters involving patients with RA. In each vignette, the rheumatologists provided open-ended responses regarding clinical care. Responses were scored in 5 domains: taking a medical history, performing a physical examination, ordering appropriate laboratory and imaging tests, assessing disease activity and physical function, and prescribing treatment. Scoring criteria were derived from a literature review and expert opinion to generate an explicit evidence base. Scores for the completed vignettes were the percentage of physician answers that matched these evidence-based criteria.

Three types of CPV™ vignettes, representing typical cases seen by practicing rheumatologists, were prepared to evaluate the impact of the MBDA test result on patient management. Four vignettes were prepared for each type. Type A vignettes comprised

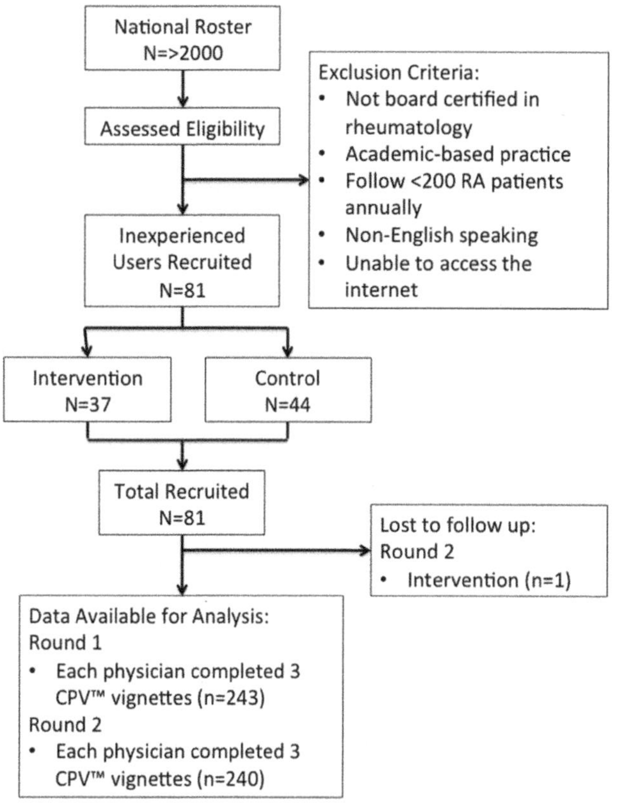

Figure 1. Flow diagram of sample selection.

RA cases insufficiently controlled with treatment and requiring addition of or increase in dosage of a non-biologic DMARD; Type B vignettes included RA cases who received inadequate treatment judged to require addition of a non-biologic or biologic DMARD; and Type C vignettes described cases of adequate treatment for RA but worsening symptoms due to one of four co-morbidities (depression, fibromyalgia, adenocarcinoma metastatic to bone and osteoarthritis). All physicians completed 2 randomly assigned cases for each of the 3 case types, one at baseline and one 12 weeks later or after the intervention, for a total of 6 vignettes per physician. Physicians were surveyed at the end of each round after completing 3 cases and asked what percentage of their cases the vignettes represented. On average the 3 case types in this study represented 62% to 80% of the types of patients that the rheumatologists in this study saw in their practices.

Analysis

Our primary hypothesis was that the MBDA test would improve quality of care. Quality was measured by the CPV™ vignettes. We used the overall quality score and in subsequent analyses determined that the disease activity assessment and treatment quality domain scores were the domains most affected by introduction of the MBDA test, as might be expected. As a corollary, we further hypothesized that quality effects would occur across all vignette case types (Types A, B, and C). Secondary outcomes included appropriate use of non-biologic or biologic DMARDs or combinations, number of imaging tests ordered, number of laboratory tests ordered, and use of other resources (which included use of office visits).

We used multivariate regression modeling to compare outcomes in Round 2 versus Round 1 in the intervention and the control groups. For the primary outcomes _ overall CPV™ quality scores and scores for the combined disease assessment and treatment domains–we used linear regression models of continuous data. Regression coefficients in the model included dummy variables for (1) intervention versus control groups, which captured whether the intervention group was significantly different from controls at baseline, (2) intervention group scores at Round 2 versus baseline, which captured changes over time in the intervention group, (3) control scores at Round 2 versus baseline, which captured changes over time in the control group, and (4) physician characteristics identified *a priori* as potential confounders: age, gender, years of rheumatology practice, number of days worked per week, practice location, single or multispecialty practice, employed by a health system, use/employ mid-level practitioners in office, on-site phlebotomy, number of patients seen per week and number of RA patients, and insurance coverage of patients (percent under Medicaid and percent under Medicare). We also included the interaction between facility variables: mid-level practitioners and multi-specialty facility.

For the secondary outcome, appropriate use of biologic or combination DMARDs, we used logistic regression controlling for the same variables as described above. We used a Poisson distribution for the number of imaging tests ordered, number of laboratory tests ordered, and use of resources. Regression models of the secondary outcomes controlled for the same co-variates described above for the primary outcomes. All analyses were conducted using STATA 12.0.

Results

There were no significant differences in physician characteristics between the intervention and control groups at baseline, with the exception of a difference in mid-level providers at the facility (Table 1). Quality scores, measured by CPV™ overall and disease activity assessment and treatment domain scores, differed significantly at baseline between the three case types, which reflected the different clinical scenarios completed by rheumatologists (Table 2). Type C cases, which presented patients with potentially confounding co-morbidities, resulted in the lowest baseline scores.

When we evaluated the impact of introducing the MBDA test into clinical practice on disease assessment and treatment quality scores, rheumatologists in the intervention group improved their quality scores by 12 percentage points for the 3 case types combined, after adjustment for the other covariates ($p<0.001$). This improvement was also significant for each of the 3 case types individually. The regression results, using combined CPV™ disease activity assessment and treatment domain scores, for all cases and disaggregated, are shown in Table 3. As expected, in the control group, no statistically significant improvements in treatment decisions were evident between Rounds 1 and 2.

When we looked at the impact on the overall quality scores, there was also a statistically significant improvement in the intervention group compared with controls following use of the MBDA test (Table 4). Physicians in the intervention group improved their scores by 3 percentage points overall in the 3 case types combined, after adjustment for the other covariates. These effects did not differ by case type (regression analysis results not shown). In the control group there were no significant improvements between Rounds 1 and 2.

Analysis of covariates controlled for in the quality models revealed some associations: employment in a health system resulted in a score that was greater by 8 percentage points for the combined disease activity assessment and treatment domain, and by 4 percentage points for the overall score. Analysis of overall

Table 1. Baseline Characteristics of Intervention and Control group physicians, All Case types.

	Intervention (n = 37)	Control (n = 44)	p-value
Number of rheumatology cases seen ≥30 per week	48.65	62.79	0.21
% of Medicare patients	40.03	38.63	0.61
% of Medicaid patients	7.86	7.51	0.88
On-site Phlebotomy	78.38	74.42	0.68
Employed by a system	21.62	20.93	0.94
Male	75.68	67.44	0.42
Practice at least 5/days per week	70.27	58.14	0.27
Age	49.70	48.95	0.74
Facility is multi-specialty	48.65	55.81	0.53
Facility has midlevel providers	35.14	6.98	<0.001

scores revealed they decreased slightly (by 0.26 percentage point) with each percent increase in the portion of Medicaid patients in a practice. Outcome scores for rheumatologists employed by a health care system and for those working in multi-specialty practices were significantly greater, by 4 and 3 percentage points respectively. For disease activity assessment and treatment quality outcomes, the effect of working in a multi-specialty practice was similar (3 percentage points) and an even greater effect (8 percentage points) was observed for rheumatologists working in a health care system (Table 3).

Analysis of the secondary endpoints revealed that in the intervention group there was significant improvement in the appropriate use of biologic or combination DMARDs in patients with co-morbidities; however, this association was only evident in case Type C, for which no change in RA therapy was appropriate, and not the others ($p = 0.008$). The significant marginal effects for the MBDA test here indicated that rheumatologists in the intervention group were 10 percentage points more likely to appropriately use biologic or combination DMARDS compared with baseline. There was no significant change in the likelihood of correctly using biologics in the other two case types or in the control group over time. There was also no observable impact of use of the MBDA test in the models examining imaging, laboratory use, and referrals (combined resource use), either for case types combined or individually.

Discussion

This study examined the impact of introducing an MBDA test on the quality of clinical practice for simulated patients with RA. Findings indicate that having knowledge of and access to the MBDA test result translated into better assessment and treatment decision-making by rheumatologists, evidenced by improved patient vignette scores in the intervention group compared with controls. These results, observed in a randomized controlled design, support the findings of earlier studies indicating that offering physicians a quantitative measure of disease activity improves their practice and may lead to better clinical outcomes.[19,30] In RA in particular, the lack of more objective measures of disease activity can make it difficult for physicians to make the most appropriate treatment decisions. The effect of the MBDA test intervention here indicates that by using a fully objective indicator of disease activity, rheumatologists may be able to more effectively assess and treat a variety of typical RA cases.

Poor quality and clinical variation are a challenge in general practice and specialty care.[31] New technology, however, is often not considered in discussions about how to improve practice

Table 2. Baseline Mean CPV Overall and Disease Assessment and Treatment Quality Scores for All Study Physicians.

	Mean	Standard deviation	p-value (Relative to Type C)
Overall CPV Score			
All Types	60.36	12.11	n/a
CPV Type A	61.97	12.48	<0.001
CPV Type B	62.01	11.69	<0.001
CPV Type C	57.09	11.58	n/a
CPV Disease Assessment and Treatment Domain Score			
All Types	54.01	21.71	n/a
CPV Type A	61.73	21.98	<0.001
CPV Type B	53.25	20.88	0.03
CPV Type C	47.04	19.86	n/a

CPV indicates Clinical Performance and Value.

Table 3. Multiple Linear Regression Models of CPV Disease Assessment and Treatment Scores by Case Type for All Cases and for Each Case Type.

	All Case Types		Type A		Type B		Type C	
	Coef	p-value	Coef	p-value	coef	p-value	coef	p-value
MBDA test Intervention at Round 2 compared with Baseline	12.49	<0.001	13.06	0.01	11.56	0.02	14.23	<0.001
Control at Round 2 compared with Baseline	3.02	0.24	0.06	0.99	1.55	0.73	7.64	0.08
MBDA test Intervention compared with control at Baseline	−4.68	0.09	−6.24	0.22	−6.15	0.22	−1.87	0.70
Number of rheum cases seen ≥30 per week	1.55	0.48	2.77	0.49	−0.03	0.99	2.79	0.47
% of Medicare patients	0.04	0.67	0.02	0.89	0.16	0.30	−0.09	0.55
% of Medicaid patients	−0.23	0.03	−0.35	0.08	−0.14	0.45	−0.30	0.11
On-site Phlebotomy	−5.19	0.03	−4.16	0.33	−9.19	0.03	−3.05	0.46
Employed by a system	7.82	<0.001	12.66	<0.001	2.53	0.54	7.43	0.07
Male	0.62	0.79	0.56	0.89	4.00	0.32	−1.87	0.64
Practice at least 5 days per week	−1.05	0.62	−1.22	0.75	−3.01	0.42	1.71	0.65
Age	−0.16	0.14	−0.27	0.17	−0.04	0.86	−0.12	0.52
Facility is multi-specialty	3.37	0.13	5.81	0.15	0.21	0.96	4.54	0.25
Facility has midlevel providers	0.36	0.93	8.10	0.29	−1.89	0.81	−5.51	0.46
Facility has midlevel providers and is multi-specialty	−6.65	0.20	−12.07	0.20	−3.37	0.72	−3.65	0.69
Constant	66.05	<0.001	76.32	<0.001	60.37	<0.001	58.94	<0.001

CPV indicates Clinical Performance and Value; MBDA, multi-biomarker disease activity.

Table 4. Multiple Linear Regression Model of Overall CPV scores for all Case Types.

	Coef	p-value
MBDA test Intervention at Round 2 compared to Baseline	3.51	0.02
Control at Round 2 compared to Baseline	1.97	0.17
MBDA test Intervention compared to control at Baseline	−0.36	0.82
Number of rheum cases seen>=30 per week	1.06	0.40
% of Medicare patients	−0.05	0.31
% of Medicaid patients	−0.26	<0.001
On-site Phlebotomy	−3.65	0.01
Employed by a system	4.39	<0.001
Male	−0.17	0.89
Practice at least 5/days per week	−1.97	0.10
Age	−.0001	.999
Facility is multi-specialty	3.36	0.01
Facility has midlevel providers	−0.84	0.73
Facility has midlevel providers and is multi-specialty	−5.91	0.05
Constant	66.57	<0.001

CPV indicates Clinical Performance and Value; MBDA, multi-biomarker disease activity.

where, increasingly, the health care conversation has turned to new payment models, performance incentives and care reorganization. However, advances in technology that provide physicians with information that cannot be derived from the physical exam or from a non-specific laboratory test, such as ESR or CRP, may help with decisions of whether to maintain or alter treatment. In this study the MBDA test led to significant improvement in quality for the combined domain of clinical assessment and treatment, where benefit is the most plausible, compared with the other domains that were evaluated–taking a medical history, performing a physical examination, and ordering appropriate laboratory and imaging tests. Thus, introduction of the MBDA test helped eliminate clinical and therapeutic ambiguity, resulted in better treatment decisions and improved quality of care for the RA cases represented in the vignettes.

These results further indicate that the MBDA test was particularly useful in those cases where there was an underlying co-morbidity, evident by the significant estimate of effects of the intervention on disease assessment and treatment domain quality scores in the type C vignettes where there was significant improvement in the appropriate use of biologic or combination DMARDs. The MBDA test thus appears to have helped rheumatologists distinguish between symptoms of RA and a co-morbid condition, and thereby avoid changing RA therapy when the new complaint was due to a different disease.

There are limitations to this study. First, our sample size was relatively small and thus likely limited our statistical power for the secondary outcomes. Second, because the control group received neither MBDA training, nor MBDA test results, the study did not directly address the independent effect of training alone. It seems likely, however, that little or no effect should have resulted from training independent of the MBDA test result. The study did not analyze the long-term impact of use of the MBDA test on physician practice and resulting improvements in patient outcomes; a third round of vignette administration could demonstrate whether the improvements observed were sustained beyond the limited study period. In addition, the MBDA test potentially may be used for long-term disease tracking, and this assessment of its use at a single time point, may not fully assess its impact on routine practice. Future studies could be designed to overcome these limitations by using a larger sample and longer time frame. Future work might also include additional case types, patient outcomes linked to the two groups of rheumatologists, sampling of academic practices and more analysis on resource utilization. Importantly, although the MBDA test results used in this study were designed to represent a real-world test, these results were hypothetical and might differ from those obtained for actual patients.

The methodology used in this study may prove particularly helpful to others wanting to demonstrate clinical effectiveness. Traditional clinical effectiveness trials are costly, confounded by case mix variation among different sites, and typically exceed the budgets of entrepreneurs, potentially stifling innovation. [32] By comparison, we used six CPV™ vignettes, expressly written for this study in RA, representing three of the most common types of RA cases: patients inadequately treated with non-biologic DMARDs, patients inadequately treated with a non-biologic DMARD in combination with another non-biologic or a biologic DMARD, and patients with co-morbidities. The case simulations used in this study have been rigorously validated against standardized patients in two large studies and shown to match actual practice.[28,29] Moreover, research using this evaluation technology has shown that higher quality vignette scores reflect better patient care.[27,33,34]

Expanding physician knowledge about critical details of the patient's disease not only facilitates clinical decision-making but may also optimize resource allocation by matching the best treatment to the individual patient type. It is not clear what impact this will have on costs. In RA, better precision in assessing disease activity may result in more appropriate use of non-biologic and/or biologic DMARDs, thereby reducing cost and risk of significant adverse effects that may be associated with biologic DMARDs. In other cases, better precision in assessing disease activity may indicate an earlier need for biologic DMARDs, which in turn can improve long-term outcomes, including lowering costs.

In spite of the limitations, this study shows that the availability of an MBDA test in clinical practice may impact decision-making and improve quality of care for patients with RA. Novel technologies for assisting physicians to assess RA disease activity and more appropriately treat patients should be similarly evaluated for gauging the impact on clinical care.

Acknowledgments

The authors thank Jhiedon Florentino, Dr. Czarina Acelajado, Jenifer Tiu for helpful comments.

Author Contributions

Conceived and designed the experiments: JP DC. Analyzed the data: JP RS RL VS. Wrote the paper: JP RS VS RL DC.

References

1. Sacks JJ, Luo YH, Helmick CG (2010) Prevalence of specific types of arthritis and other rheumatic conditions in the ambulatory health care system in the United States, 2001-2005. Arthritis Care Res (Hoboken) 62:460–4.
2. Fuster V, Ryden LE, Asinger RW, Cannom DS, Crijns HJ, et al. (2001) ACC/AHA/ESC Guidelines for the Management of Patients With Atrial Fibrillation: Executive Summary A Report of the American College of Cardiology/American Heart Association Task Force on Practice Guidelines and the European Society of Cardiology Committee for Practice Guidelines and Policy Conferences (Committee to Develop Guidelines for the Management of Patients With Atrial Fibrillation) Developed in Collaboration With the North American Society of Pacing and Electrophysiology. Circulation 104:2118–50.
3. Majithia V, Geraci SA (2007) Rheumatoid arthritis: diagnosis and management. Am J Med 120:936–9.
4. Aletaha D, Neogi T, Silman AJ, Funovits J, Felson DT, et al. (2010) Rheumatoid arthritis classification criteria: an American College of Rheumatology/European League Against Rheumatism collaborative initiative. Arthritis Rheum 62:2569–81.
5. Smolen JS, Aletaha D, Bijlsma JW, Breedveld FC, Boumpas D, et al. (2010) Treating rheumatoid arthritis to target: recommendations of an international task force. Ann Rheum Dis 69:631–637.
6. Smolen JS, Landewe R, Breedveld FC, Dougados M, Gaujoux-Viala C, et al. (2010) EULAR recommendations for the management of rheumatoid arthritis with synthetic and biological disease-modifying antirheumatic drugs. Ann Rheum Dis 69: 964–75.
7. Singh JA, Furst DE, Bharat A, Curtis JR, Kavanaugh AF, et al. (2012) Update of the 2008 American College of Rheumatology recommendations for the use of disease-modifying antirheumatic drugs and biologic agents in the treatment of rheumatoid arthritis. Arthritis Care Res 64:625–639.
8. Anderson J, Caplan L, Yazdany J, Robbins ML, Neogi T, et al. (2012) Rheumatoid arthritis disease activity measures: American College of Rheumatology recommendations for use in clinical practice. Arthritis Care Res 64:640–7.
9. Studenic P, Rader H, Smolen JS, Aletaha D (2012) Arthritis Rheum Discrepancies between patients and physicians in their perceptions of rheumatoid arthritis disease activity. Arthritis Rheum 64:2814–23.
10. Masri KR, Shaver KS, Shadouri SH (2012) Validity and reliability problems with patient global as a component of the ACR/EULAR remission criteria as used in clinical practice. J Rheumatol.39:1139–45.
11. Beresniak A, Russell AS, Haraoui B, Bessette L, Bombardier C, et al. (2007) Advantages and limitations of utility assessment methods in rheumatoid arthritis. J Rheumatol 34:2193–200.
12. Bykerk VP, Schieir O, Akhavan P, Hazlewood GS, Cheng CK, et al. (2011) Emerging Issues in Pharmacological Management of Rheumatoid Arthritis: Results of a National Needs Assessment Survey Identifying Practice Variations for the Development of Canadian Rheumatology Association Clinical Practice Recommendations. J Rheumatol 39:1555–8.
13. Lacaille D, Anis AH, Guh DP, Esdaile JM (2005) Gaps in care for rheumatoid arthritis: a population study. Arthritis Rheum 53:241–8.
14. MacLean CH, Louie R, Leake B, McCaffrey DF, Paulus HE, et al. (2000) Quality of care for patients with rheumatoid arthritis. JAMA 284:984–92.
15. Peabody JW, Strand V, Chernoff D, Ta HM (2012) Evaluation of Clinical Performance and Variation Among Three Types of Patients with Rheumatoid Arthritis: Opportunities to Raise Quality and Lower Costs. ISPOR 17th Annual International Meeting; Washington D.C.
16. Jiang Y, Nishikawa RM, Schmidt RA, Toledano AY, Doi K (2001) Potential of computer-aided diagnosis to reduce variability in radiologists' interpretations of mammograms depicting microcalcifications. Radiology 220:787–94.
17. Butcher L (2009) Health plans and providers struggle to fix payment system. Manag Care 18:30–3.
18. Panella M, Marchisio S, Di Stanislao F (2003) Reducing clinical variations with clinical pathways: do pathways work? Int J Qual Health Care 15:509–21.
19. Farheen K, Agarwal SK (2011)Assessment of disease activity and treatment outcomes in rheumatoid arthritis. J Manag Care Pharm 17:S09–13.
20. Eastman PS, Manning WC, Qureshi F, Haney D, Cavet G, et al. (2012) Characterization of a multiplex, 12-biomarker test for rheumatoid arthritis. J Pharm Biomed Anal 70:415–424.
21. Zhao X, Qureshi F, Eastman PS, Manning WC, Alexander C, et al. (2012) Pre-analytical effects of blood sampling and handling in quantitative immunoassays for rheumatoid arthritis. J Immunol Methods 30;72–80.
22. Bakker MF, Cavet G, Jacobs JW, Bijlsma JW, Haney DJ, et al. (2012) Performance of a multi-biomarker score measuring rheumatoid arthritis disease activity in the CAMERA tight control study. Ann Rheum Dis 71:1692–1697.
23. Curtis JR, van der Helm-van Mil AH, Knevel R, Huizinga TW, Haney DJ, et al. (2012) Validation of a novel multi-biomarker test to assess rheumatoid arthritis disease activity. Arthritis Care Res 64:1794–803.
24. van der Helm-van Mil AH, Knevel R, Cavet G, Huizinga TW, Haney DJ (2012) An evaluation of molecular and clinical remission in rheumatoid arthritis by assessing radiographic progression. Rheumatology: in press.
25. Graf J, Scherzer R, Grunfeld C, Imboden J (2009) Levels of C-reactive protein associated with high and very high cardiovascular risk are prevalent in patients with rheumatoid arthritis. PLoS One 4:e6242.
26. Wolfe F (2009) The many myths of erythrocyte sedimentation rate and C-reactive protein. J Rheumatol 36:1568–69.

27. Dresselhaus TR, Peabody JW, Luck J, Bertenthal D (2004) An evaluation of vignettes for predicting variation in the quality of preventive care. J Gen Intern Med 19:1013–8.
28. Peabody JW, Luck J, Glassman P, Dresselhaus TR, Lee M (2000) Comparison of vignettes, standardized patients, and chart abstraction: a prospective validation study of 3 methods for measuring quality. JAMA 283:1715–22.
29. Peabody JW, Luck J, Glassman P, Jain S, Hansen J, et al (2004) Measuring the quality of physician practice by using clinical vignettes: a prospective validation study. Ann Intern Med 141:771–80.
30. Fox MG, Stephens T, Jarjour WN, Anderson MW, Kimpel DL (2012) Contrast-enhanced magnetic resonance imaging positively impacts the management of some patients with rheumatoid arthritis or suspected RA. J Clin Rheumatol. 18:15–22.
31. Wennberg DE (1998) Variation in the delivery of health care: the stakes are high. Ann Intern Med 128:866–8.
32. Luce BR, Kramer JM, Goodman SN, Connor JT, Tunis S, et al. (2009) Rethinking randomized clinical trials for comparative effectiveness research: the need for transformational change. Ann Intern Med 151:206–9.
33. Peabody JW, Liu A (2007) A cross-national comparison of the quality of clinical care using vignettes. Health Policy Plan 22:294–302.
34. Solon O, Woo K, Quimbo SA, Shimkhada R, Florentino J, et al. (2009) A novel method for measuring health care system performance: experience from QIDS in the Philippines. Health Policy Plan 24:167–74.

2

Angiopoietin-Like 4 Is Over-Expressed in Rheumatoid Arthritis Patients: Association with Pathological Bone Resorption

Catherine Swales[1], Nicholas A. Athanasou[2], Helen J. Knowles[1]*

1 Botnar Research Centre, Nuffield Department of Orthopaedics Rheumatology and Musculoskeletal Sciences, University of Oxford, Oxford, United Kingdom, **2** Pathology Department, Nuffield Orthopaedic Centre, University of Oxford, Oxford, United Kingdom

Abstract

Introduction: Osteoclasts are responsible for the bone loss associated with rheumatoid arthritis (RA). The secreted adipokine angiopoietin-like 4 (ANGPTL4) specifically increases osteoclast-mediated bone resorption. We have investigated expression of ANGPTL4 and its regulatory transcription factor, hypoxia-inducible factor-1 alpha (HIF-1α), in osteoclasts and other cells within rheumatoid synovium. We have also examined whether circulating levels of ANGPTL4 differ in RA patients compared with that in normal controls or patients with osteoarthritis (OA).

Results: Immunohistochemical analysis revealed that bone-apposing osteoclasts within the rheumatoid synovium express both ANGPTL4 and HIF-1α. ANGPTL4 was also strongly expressed in synovial lining cells, endothelial cells, stromal cells, CD68+ macrophages and plasma cells within RA synovium. Little ANGPTL4 was evident in normal synovial tissue. This reflected the over-expression of HIF-1α in rheumatoid versus normal synovial tissue. The concentration of ANGPTL4 was higher in both the serum and the synovial fluid of RA patients than in patients with OA or normal controls. High serum ANGPTL4 associated with elevated levels of the serum marker of bone resorption, receptor activator for nuclear factor κB ligand (RANKL).

Conclusions: Over-expression of ANGPTL4 in multiple cell types within the rheumatoid synovium potentially provides a local pool of ANGPTL4 to stimulate osteoclast-mediated bone resorption in RA. Additionally, correlation of high serum ANGPTL4 with circulating RANKL suggests that ANGPTL4 may represent a novel marker for bone destruction in RA.

Editor: Luc Malaval, Université Jean Monnet, France

Funding: This work was supported by an Arthritis Research UK grant to HJK, grant number MP/19200 (www.arthritisresearchuk.org). Additional support was received from the Oxford National Institute for Health Research (NIHR) Biomedical Research Unit. The funders had no role in study design, data collection and analysis, decision to publish, or preparation of the manuscript.

Competing Interests: The authors have declared that no competing interests exist.

* Email: helen.knowles@ndorms.ox.ac.uk

Introduction

Rheumatoid arthritis (RA) is a chronic inflammatory disease characterised by erosion of articular cartilage and subchondral bone, leading to joint destruction, pain and loss of function. Bone loss in RA, comprising both juxta-articular bone erosions and systemic osteoporosis, is associated with progressive disability and is predictive of poor prognosis [1,2]. Both types of bone loss are mediated by osteoclasts [3,4], multinucleated cells specialised to carry out lacunar bone resorption. Inhibition of osteoclast activity effectively inhibits both the formation of new focal bone erosions and systemic bone loss [5,6].

In contrast to normal synovial tissue the rheumatoid synovium is hypoxic. Low tissue oxygen levels are also a poor prognostic indicator in RA [7,8]. Synovial lining cells, endothelial cells, fibroblasts, lymphocytes, plasma cells and CD68+ macrophages within the RA synovium express the hypoxia-inducible transcription factor, HIF [9–11]. HIF is a heterodimer comprising a hypoxia-inducible alpha subunit and a constitutively expressed beta subunit. Hypoxic accumulation and activation of HIF-alpha allows transcription of genes involved in processes including angiogenesis, inflammation, apoptosis and regulation of immune function [12].

HIF has not been described in osteoclasts in RA, although HIF-1α-positive osteoclasts are present in other osteoclast-rich pathologies such as the primary bone tumour Giant Cell Tumour of Bone [13]. Transient hypoxia increases osteoclast formation [14,15] by stimulating the fusion and differentiation of circulating CD14+ mononuclear precursors or synovial macrophages in the presence of macrophage-colony stimulating factor (M-CSF) and RANKL [16,17]. Hypoxia also causes increased bone resorption, via a HIF-1α-dependent mechanism to enhance osteoclast activity by increasing production of ATP under hypoxic conditions [14,18].

Angiopoietin-like 4 (ANGPTL4) is a HIF-1α-inducible pro-angiogenic adipokine [19,20]. It is over-expressed in the hypoxic, perinecrotic regions of solid tumours [19] and induced by hypoxia in multiple cell types including endothelial cells [19], articular chondrocytes [21], osteoclasts, osteoblasts [13] and fibroblast-like RA synoviocytes [22]. We have previously demonstrated that ANGPTL4 directly stimulates osteoclast activity and promotes bone resorption *in vitro* via a mechanism independent of RANKL [13].

This study investigates the over-expression of both ANGPTL4 and HIF-1α in RA, with specific reference to their expression in osteoclasts. We also assess correlations between the serum concentration of ANGPTL4 and markers of pathological bone resorption in RA.

Materials and Methods

Patients

RA patients were recruited through the rheumatology clinics at the Nuffield Orthopaedic Centre and serum samples were stored at −80°C until analysis. Synovial fluid was aspirated from the knee joints of patients with RA and non-inflammatory OA as previously described [23], OA being defined as non-inflammatory when neutrophils comprised <25% of the total synovial fluid cell population sampled. Serum from OA and injury repair patients and all formalin-fixed, paraffin-embedded tissue sections were obtained from the Oxford Musculoskeletal BioBank. RA was defined according to the 1987 American College of Rheumatology criteria and OA was diagnosed on clinical, radiographic and histologic criteria. Samples and/or data obtained were collected with informed written donor consent in full compliance with national and institutional ethical requirements, the United Kingdom Human Tissue Act and the Declaration of Helsinki. This study was approved under Oxford Musculoskeletal BioBank ethics (HTA Licence 12217, Oxfordshire Research Ethics Committee C, 09/H0606/11). RA and OA synovial fluid samples were collected with approval of the Oxford Central University Research Ethics Committee, 06/Q1606/139.

Immunohistochemistry and immunofluorescence

Wax-embedded samples of rheumatoid synovial tissue were sectioned and H&E stained. Antigen retrieval of deparaffinised sections was performed by microwaving in 1 mM EDTA (pH 8). Sections were exposed to anti-ANGPTL4 (H-200; Santa Cruz Biotechnology), anti-cathepsin K (clone 182-12G5, Calbiochem), anti-CD20 (clone L26; Dako), anti-CD68 (clone KP1; Dako), anti-HIF-1α (clone 54; BD Biosciences) or a serum control. For standard immunohistochemistry, staining was visualized with the VECTASTAIN Elite ABC Kit (Vector Laboratories). For immunofluorescence, secondary antibodies were DyLight 488 or 594 conjugates (Thermo Scientific). Image acquisition was performed using a Zeiss AxioImager MI microscope, AxioCam HRC camera and AxioVision software.

Osteoclasts in tissue sections were considered as large, multinucleated cells containing >3 nuclei; a widely accepted identification criterion in RA [23–26]. Osteoclast identification was additionally confirmed by staining for cathepsin K; an enzyme expressed at high levels in osteoclasts [27,28] and a validated osteoclast marker in RA [29,30].

Cell culture

Peripheral blood mononuclear cells were isolated from the blood of patients with RA using Histopaque (Sigma). CD14+ monocytes were selected (AutoMACS cell separator; Miltenyi Biotech), seeded into α-MEM (without ribonucleosides/deoxyribonucleosides, containing 10% FBS, 2 mM L-glutamine, 50 IU/ml penicillin and 50 μg/ml streptomycin sulphate) and differentiated into osteoclasts by supplementing with M-CSF (25 ng/ml) and RANKL (50 ng/ml) every 3–4 days for 12–16 days. Hypoxic exposure was at 2% O_2, 5% CO_2, balance N_2 for 24 h (MiniGalaxy incubator, RS Biotech).

Real-time PCR

Total RNA was extracted in TRI reagent (Sigma), treated with DNase I and reverse-transcribed (SuperScript VILO cDNA Synthesis Kit, Invitrogen). Real-time PCR was performed using Express SYBR GreenER qPCR Supermix Universal (Invitrogen) and predesigned intron-spanning QuantiTect primers (Qiagen) on a RotorGene RG-3000 (Corbett Research UK). Comparative quantification was performed, with target gene expression normalized to β-actin (ACTB).

ELISAs

Serum was analysed from 19 RA patients (age 62.1±13.7, 21.1% male, 78.9% female; clinical and serological characteristics are described in Table 1) and age- and sex-matched OA patients (n = 30; age 61.8±8.1, 20% male, 80% female) and normal controls (n = 30 surgical injury repair patients; age 61.0±7.8, 20% male, 80% female). Synovial fluid from a separate cohort of 8 RA patients and 7 non-inflammatory OA patients was digested with 2 mg/ml hyaluronidase prior to assay [23]. ANGPTL4 (R&D Systems), C-reactive protein (CRP) (Invitrogen) and RANKL (Peprotech) were assayed according to the manufacturer's instructions.

Statistics

For experiments with 2 conditions a Wilcoxon matched-pairs or Mann-Whitney test was used as appropriate. Statistics for serum data were performed using the Pearson correlation coefficient or Fisher's exact test. Results were calculated in GraphPad Prism 6 and considered significant at $p<0.05$.

Results

ANGPTL4 is strongly expressed by osteoclasts in RA

Rheumatoid synovial sections were screened for the presence of multi-nucleated cells (>3 nuclei) morphologically characteristic of osteoclasts. Numerous synovial osteoclasts were identified in 3/8 cases. In each instance, immunohistochemical analysis of the hyperplastic synovial tissue (Figure 1A) and synovium-bone interface (Figure 1B) revealed strong expression of ANGPTL4 in multi-nucleated cells that were confirmed as osteoclasts by double staining with cathepsin K (Figure 1C). Although other synovial cells were also ANGPTL4-positive, over 95% of osteoclasts expressed ANGPTL4 more strongly than the surrounding synovial cells in any given section. Scattered osteoclasts present in OA synovial sections were smaller (fewer nuclei) than those in RA and did not express immuno-detectable ANGPTL4 as revealed by either immunohistochemistry or immunofluorescence (Figure 1D).

RA osteoclasts express HIF-1α protein

Cytoplasmic expression of HIF-1α was observed in 22–50% of osteoclasts in any given rheumatoid synovial tissue section (Figure 2A). Where resorbing osteoclasts were visible at the synovium-bone interface, co-localised expression of HIF-1α and ANGPTL4 was also evident (Figure 2B). Osteoclasts derived from the circulating CD14+ monocytes of RA patients exhibited increased expression of ANGPTL4 mRNA following exposure to hypoxia (Figure 2C; mean induction 5.5-fold, range 1.7- to 17.2-fold). Expression of other HIF target genes was also increased (e.g. SLC2A1; mean induction 3.0-fold, range 1.2- to 5.6-fold).

Table 1. Clinical characteristics of RA patients in serum cohort.

Patient no.	Sex (M/F)	Age (yrs)	Seropositive (Y/N)	DAS score	CRP (μg/ml)
R1	F	70	Y	3.52	9.15
R2	F	72	Y	1.4	5.26
R3	F	87	Y	2.71	1.17
R4	F	67	Y	2.9	10.97
R5	F	45	Y	4.5	5.48
R6	F	69	N	2.14	2.39
R7	F	73	Y	2.88	0.42
R8	M	64	-	2.5	0.5
R9	M	40	Y	7.35	13.46
R10	F	48	Y	3.5	0.31
R11	F	59	Y	2.03	4.24
R12	F	34	Y	6.2	36.67
R13	F	66	Y	2	8.12
R14	F	44	N	3.32	0.79
R15	M	63	-	1.81	1.35
R16	M	76	Y	1.4	1.68
R17	F	65	Y	3.05	15.0
R18	F	70	-	-	4.36
R19	F	68	Y	4.1	8.7

DAS = disease activity score. CRP = C-reactive protein.

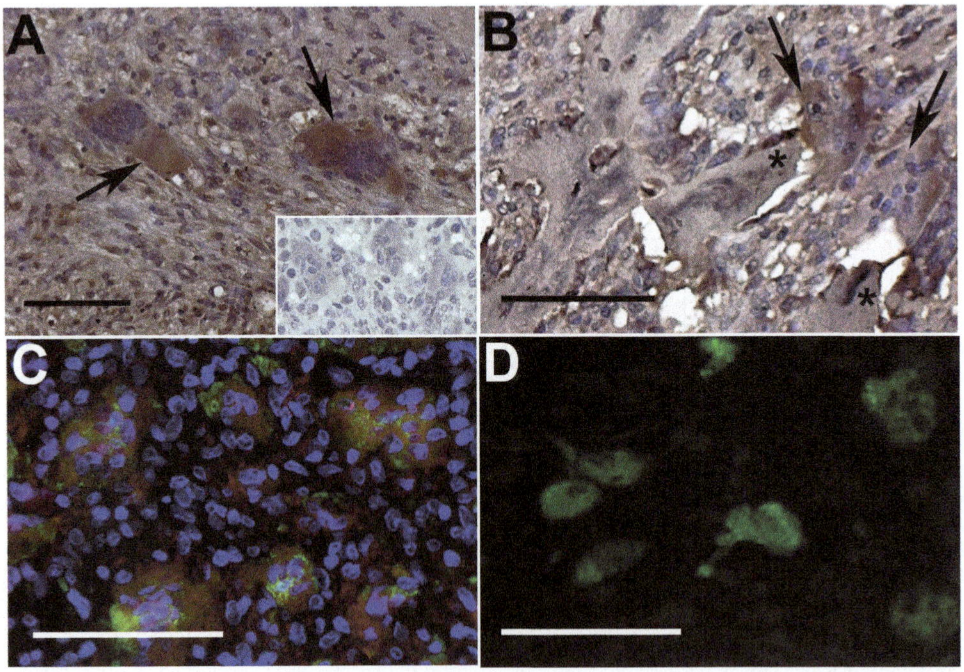

Figure 1. ANGPTL4 is expressed by osteoclasts in RA. (A) ANGPTL4 is strongly expressed by osteoclasts (arrows) in the RA synovium. Inset: Representative isotype control image. (B) Resorbing osteoclasts adjacent to bone (starred) express ANGPTL4. (C) ANGPTL4 (red) expression co-localises with cathepsin K-positive (green) osteoclasts. Representative images from n = 3 cases. (D) Cathepsin K-positive (green) osteoclasts in the OA synovium do not express detectable ANGPTL4 (red). All scale bars represent 100 μM.

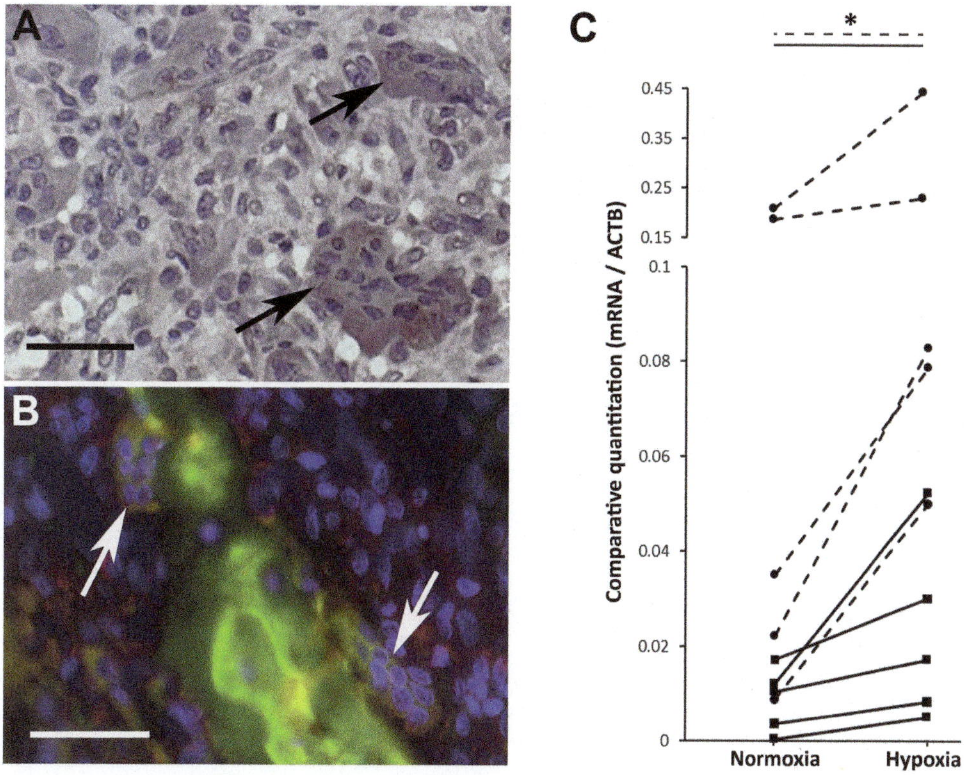

Figure 2. HIF-1α is expressed by osteoclasts in RA. (A) HIF-1α expression by osteoclasts in the RA synovium (arrows). Representative image from n = 3 cases. (B) HIF-1α (green) and ANGPTL4 (red) expression co-localises in 2 bone-apposing osteoclasts (arrows). All scale bars represent 100 μM. (C) ANGPTL4 (solid lines) and SLC2A1 (Glut-1; dashed lines) mRNA expression in monocyte-derived osteoclasts from RA patients following 24 h exposure to normoxia or hypoxia (2% O_2). Hypoxic fold-change in mRNA expression; *, $p<0.05$.

ANGPTL4 is over-expressed in synovial tissue in RA

As ANGPTL4 reactivity was observed in the synoviocytes adjacent to osteoclasts, we also studied ANGPTL4 expression in 5 additional osteoclast-negative cases of RA. ANGPTL4 was strongly expressed by the synovial lining cells, endothelial cells and stromal fibroblasts within RA synovial tissue (Figure 3A), compared with general low-level expression in normal synovium (Figure 3B). The expression pattern of ANGPTL4 was similar to that for HIF-1α in RA synovial sections (Figure 3C). HIF-1α was rarely detected in normal synovium (Figure 3D).

ANGPTL4 was also strongly expressed in the immediate vicinity of lymphoid aggregates in RA, in cells morphologically characteristic of macrophages and plasma cells (Figure 3E). Immunofluorescence confirmed that ANGPTL4 was not expressed by B cells (Figure 3F) or T cells (data not shown), but was expressed by CD68-positive macrophages (Figure 3G).

Both ANGPTL4 (Figure 3H, left panel) and HIF-1α (Figure 3H, right panel) were over-expressed in OA synovial tissue in comparison with the normal synovium, although not to the same degree (number of positive cells per field of view) as in RA synovial tissue.

ANGPTL4 is elevated in the serum and synovial fluid of RA patients

Given the striking over-expression of ANGPTL4 by multiple cell types within RA synovial tissue, we next assessed whether concentrations of secreted ANGPTL4 were also elevated in RA synovial fluid. ANGPTL4 was measured in synovial fluid aspirated from the knee joints of patients with RA and non-inflammatory OA controls. The ANGPTL4 concentration was significantly higher in the clarified synovial fluid of the RA population (Figure 4A).

Due to low patient numbers in the synovial fluid cohort, we expanded the study to look at serum concentrations of ANGPTL4. ANGPTL4 levels were significantly higher in the serum of patients with RA than in either OA patients or normal controls (Figure 4B). Within the RA population, serum ANGPTL4 positively correlated with age ($r = 0.460$, $p<0.048$).

The RA cohort comprised 2 sub-groups based on the serum level of ANGPTL4; 'low ANGPTL4' (≤170 ng/ml, serum ANGPTL4 within the normal range) and 'high ANGPTL4' (> 170 ng/ml; serum ANGPTL4 more than 10% above normal range). We therefore considered whether having 'high' serum ANGPTL4 might be indicative of disease severity. No significant difference was found between 'high' and 'low' groups with respect to age, DAS score or CRP.

Given the stimulatory effect of ANGPTL4 on osteoclast activity, we also assessed possible correlations with the circulating marker of bone erosion, RANKL. Considering all patient groups, serum concentrations of RANKL ranged from 0–392.7 ng/ml, with most individuals having undetectable serum RANKL. To prevent skewing of the analysis by high value data points in a small sample size, we assessed this data according to whether patients exhibited detectable circulating RANKL (RANKL-positive or RANKL-negative). 85.7% of 'high ANGPTL4' RA patients were RANKL-positive, compared with only 16.7% of 'low ANGPTL4' RA patients ($p<0.05$) and 20.0% of controls ($p<0.01$) (Figure 4C).

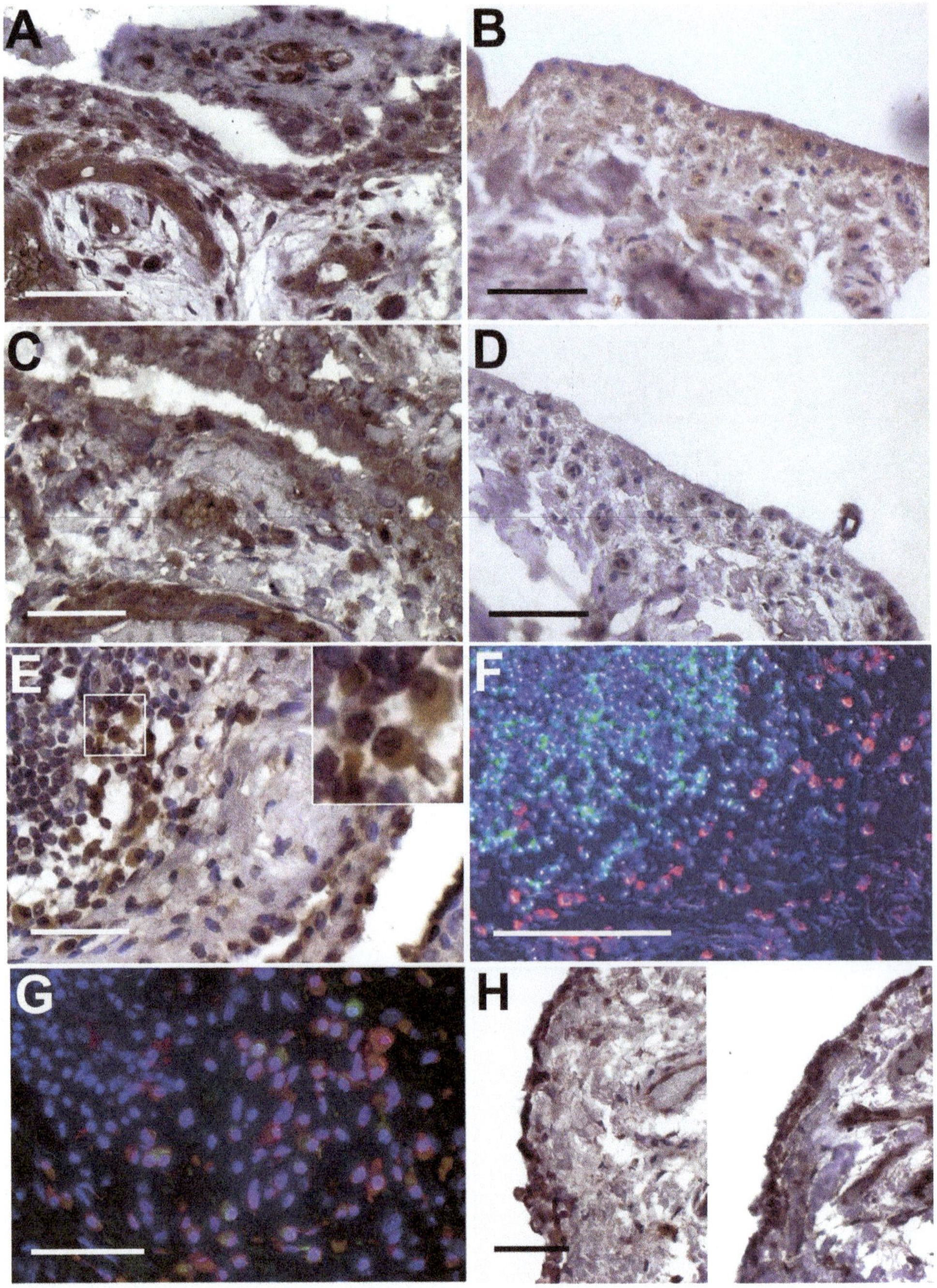

Figure 3. ANGPTL4 and HIF-1α are expressed in RA synovial tissue. (A) The RA synovium is strongly positive for ANGPTL4, as are adjacent blood vessels and surrounding stromal cells; (B) normal synovium shows weak, heterogeneous expression of ANGPTL4. (C) RA synovium is strongly positive for HIF-1α, as are adjacent blood vessels; (D) normal synovium generally does not express HIF-1α. (E) Synovial lining cells and stromal cells adjacent to lymphoid aggregates express ANGPTL4. Inset: ANGPTL4-positive plasma cells. (F) ANGPTL4 (red) is not expressed by B cells (CD20, green). (G) ANGPTL4 (red) is expressed by CD68-positive (green) macrophages adjacent to a lymphoid aggregate. (H) The OA synovium expresses elevated levels of both ANGPTL4 (left panel) and HIF-1α (right panel) compared with the normal synovium. Scale bars (A–F, H) represent 100 μM, scale bar (G) represents 50 μM.

Discussion

Inhibition of osteoclast-mediated bone resorption is a crucial component of targeted strategies to alleviate bone destruction in RA. ANGPTL4, a hypoxia-induced adipokine, has previously been shown to stimulate osteoclast activity *in vitro*. This study demonstrates increased expression of ANGPTL4 within rheumatoid synovial tissue, as well as increased secretion of ANGPTL4 into the synovial fluid and serum of patients with RA.

This is the first description of ANGPTL4 expression in RA synovial tissue. We have previously reported that ANGPTL4 functions in a paracrine manner to stimulate osteoclast activity and induce bone resorption [13]. This effect was independent of RANKL, as ANGPTL4 prevented both loss of osteoclast viability

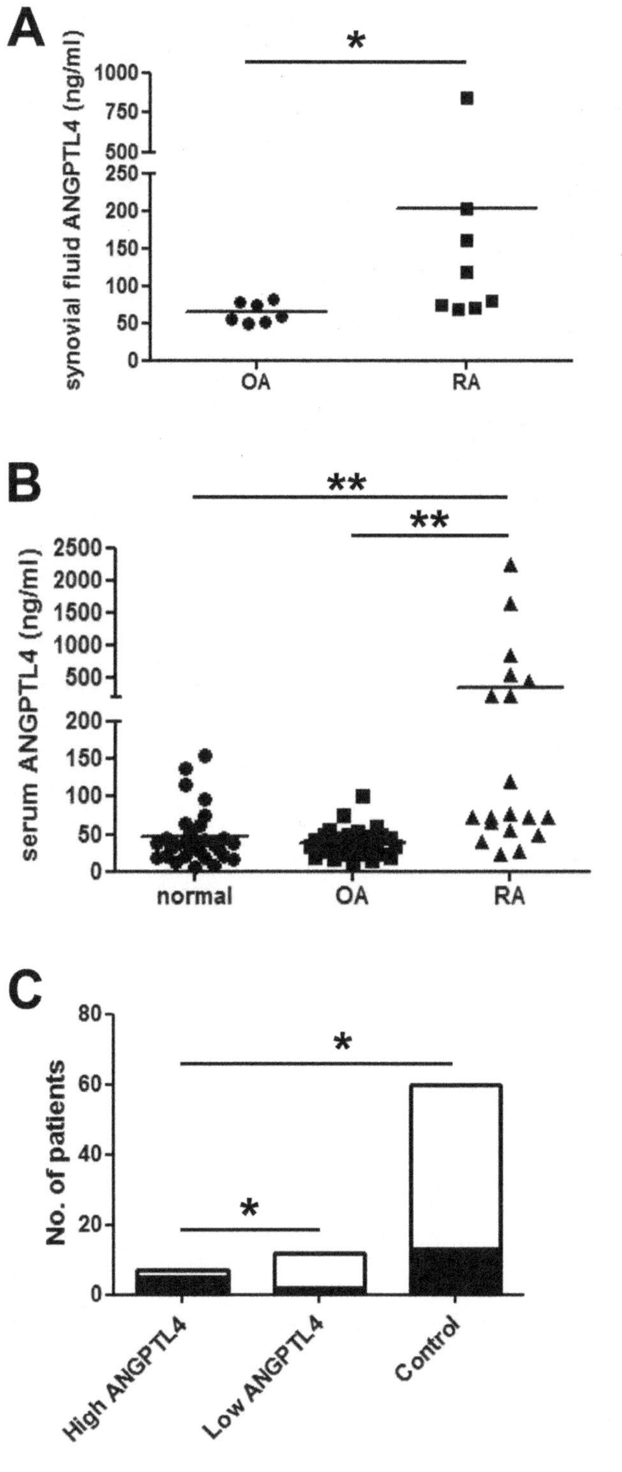

Figure 4. Serum and synovial fluid ANGPTL4 concentrations are elevated in RA. (A) Synovial fluid from RA patients contains more ANGPTL4 (203.3±264.8 ng/ml, range 68.7–847.3 ng/ml) than that from patients with non-inflammatory OA (64.4±13.6 ng/ml, range 50.4–82.2 ng/ml). *, $p<0.05$. (B) Serum from RA patients contains more ANGPTL4 (363.4±138.7 ng/ml, range 24.0–2235.0) than that from OA patients (39.0±3.4 ng/ml, range 11.9–100.5 ng/ml) or normal controls (45.8±6.7 ng/ml, range 6.5–154.7 ng/ml). **, $p<0.01$. (C) Serum from 'high ANGPTL4' RA patients is more likely to have detectable RANKL (black shading; RANKL-positive) than either serum from 'low ANGPTL4' RA patients or controls. White shading; RANKL-negative. *, $p<0.05$.

and loss of bone resorption following RANKL inhibition with the soluble decoy receptor osteoprotegerin [13]. Expression of ANGPTL4 in bone-apposing resorbing osteoclasts, as well as strong expression in other cells of the rheumatoid synovium, could generate an environment that supports and promotes bone erosion. This makes it potentially attractive as a secondary target, outside the RANKL/RANK pathway, for strategies to specifically prevent osteolytic bone disease in RA [5].

ANGPTL4 also has the potential to contribute to cartilage matrix destruction. Multi-nucleated cells resorbing cartilage in RA have an osteoclast-like phenotype and human monocyte-derived osteoclasts are capable of cartilage matrix resorption *in vitro* [24]. RA articular chondrocytes over-express ANGPTL4 which, when induced by hypoxia *in vitro*, stimulates production of the matrix metalloproteinases MMP-1 and MMP-3 [21]. ANGPTL4 might therefore induce both bone and cartilage erosion in RA, via effects on MMP production and osteoclast activation, to increase joint destruction.

It is interesting to consider whether the 3 out of 8 RA cases seen to contain numerous osteoclasts is a typical ratio. While it is consistent with what we have previously observed [23], it is not possible to tell from the literature whether this is a typical proportion. Although many papers measure expression and/or secretion of osteoclast-associated factors, very few actually show pictures of osteoclasts in human RA and we have found no mention of the frequency with which osteoclast-rich RA occurs. Furthermore, due to the flattening of some osteoclasts if the synovium pulls away from the bone during tissue processing, clear images cannot always be obtained. However, regardless of the proportion of cases where osteoclasts can be observed by immunohistochemistry, osteoclast-mediated bone erosion is a common and characteristic feature of RA.

This is also the first description of HIF-1α expression in RA osteoclasts. HIF-1α stimulates increased osteoclast-mediated bone resorption under hypoxic conditions [14]. HIF-1α also controls the over-expression of VEGF-A by large osteoclasts containing >10 nuclei, as found in RA, versus small osteoclasts containing 2–5 nuclei, as found in OA [31]. As ANGPTL4 is also a HIF target gene, this observation might explain why we only detected ANGPTL4 expression in RA-, but not OA-, associated osteoclasts. Promotion of pathological bone resorption in RA might be a crucial component of the mechanism by which HIF drives disease progression [32].

Co-localisation of HIF-1α and ANGPTL4 in bone-apposing osteoclasts supports our previous *in vitro* observations that ANGPTL4 is induced by HIF-1α in human osteoclasts [13]. However, not all ANGPTL4-positive osteoclasts expressed HIF-1α. This might be due to cytokine-mediated effects on gene expression. In fibroblast-like synoviocytes from RA, for example, TNFα induced expression of HIF-1α but not ANGPTL4, whereas IL-4 induced ANGPTL4 but not HIF [22]. ANGPTL4 is additionally regulated by the PPAR family of transcription factors [33], which might influence expression patterns. All other cell types within the RA synovium that we found to express ANGPTL4 also expressed HIF-1α, both in this study and as reported previously [9,12]. ANGPTL4 has been confirmed as a HIF target gene in human RA fibroblast-like synoviocytes *in vitro* [22].

ANGPTL4 mRNA and protein levels have previously been reported to increase in the early stages of murine collagen-induced arthritis, where expression was specific to the stromal fibroblast-like cells adjacent to blood vessels, suggestive of a role in angiogenesis [34] as reported in cancer [19,20]. Human RA fibroblast-like synoviocytes exposed to hypoxia *in vitro* also exhibited increased ANGPTL4 mRNA and protein expression [22]. As well as confirming ANGPTL4 expression in RA synovial fibroblasts *in situ*, we have observed cytoplasmic expression of ANGPTL4 in many other cell types including, but not restricted to, CD68+ macrophages, plasma cells, endothelial cells and osteoclasts within the hyperplastic synovium. Such wide-spread induction could rapidly provide a large local pool of pro-angiogenic ANGPTL4 to also stimulate blood vessel formation in RA.

The concentration range of serum ANGPTL4 in our normal controls and patients with OA (11.9–154.7 ng/ml) agrees with the 2–158 ng/ml previously reported in the normal population [35]. Distinct sub-groups of 'low ANGPTL4' and 'high ANGPTL4' RA patients were apparent, having serum ANGPTL4 either within the normal range or at least 10% above this range (217.3–2235.0 ng/ml). If clinically or radiologically relevant information could be found to correlate with 'high ANGPTL4', serum level of ANGPTL4 may prove a useful prognostic or diagnostic tool.

In agreement with our hypothesis that ANGPTL4 contributes to bone erosions in RA, 'high ANGPTL4' patients were significantly more likely to have detectable concentrations of serum RANKL. Circulating RANKL has recently been described to correlate with the level of erosive damage in RA, as well as being a prognostic factor for the progression of this structural damage, as assessed by radiography over a 3 year period [36]. While we did not have sufficient numbers in the current study to replicate this data for ANGPTL4, the only two non-erosive patients in our study population exhibited two of the three lowest serum concentrations of ANGPTL4. Although a larger study cohort is required, with matched serum, synovial tissue/fluid and radiological data, it is interesting to speculate that ANGPTL4 might represent not only a serum marker of either progression of joint damage or response to treatment, but also a potential therapeutic target.

In summary ANGPTL4 is over-expressed in osteoclasts and other cells within the rheumatoid synovium, in the synovial fluid and in the serum of patients with RA. High serum ANGPTL4 in RA correlates with high circulating levels of RANKL. As ANGPTL4 stimulates osteoclast resorption activity *in vitro*, it may therefore mediate osteolytic erosion of bone and cartilage in RA, thereby contributing to joint destruction in addition to its established pro-angiogenic role [22,34]. This suggests ANGPTL4 both as a possible target for therapies to treat several different aspects of the disease, as well as a novel marker for bone destruction in RA.

Acknowledgments

The authors would like to thank Dr David Mahoney for the synovial fluid samples.

Author Contributions

Conceived and designed the experiments: CS NAA HJK. Performed the experiments: HJK. Analyzed the data: CS NAA HJK. Contributed reagents/materials/analysis tools: CS NAA HJK. Contributed to the writing of the manuscript: CS HJK. Approved the final version of the manuscript: CS NAA HJK.

References

1. Kaarela K (1985) Prognostic factors and diagnostic criteria in early rheumatoid arthritis. Scand J Rheumatol 57: 1–54.
2. Gough AK, Lilley J, Eyre S, Holder RL, Emery P (1994) Generalised bone loss in patients with early rheumatoid arthritis. Lancet 344: 23–27.
3. Bromley M, Woolley DE (1984) Chondroclasts and osteoclasts at subchondral sites of erosion in the rheumatoid joint. Arthritis Rheum 27: 968–975.
4. Gough A, Sambrook P, Devlin J, Huissoon A, Njeh C, et al. (1998) Osteoclastic activation is the principal mechanism leading to secondary osteoporosis in rheumatoid arthritis. J Rheumatol 25: 1282–1289.
5. Tanaka S (2013) Regulation of bone destruction in rheumatoid arthritis through RANKL-RANK pathways. World J Orthop 4: 1–6.
6. Cohen SB, Dore RK, Lane NE, Ory PA, Peterfy CG, et al. (2008) Denosumab treatment effects on structural damage, bone mineral density, and bone turnover in rheumatoid arthritis: a twelve-month, multicenter, randomized, double-blind, placebo-controlled, phase II clinical trial. Arthritis Rheum 58: 1299–1309.
7. Treuhaft PS, McCarty DJ (1971) Synovial fluid pH, lactate, oxygen and carbon dioxide partial pressure in various joint diseases. Arthritis Rheum 14: 475–484.
8. Sivakumar B, Akhavani MA, Winlove CP, Taylor PC, Paleolog EM, et al. (2008) Synovial hypoxia as a cause of tendon rupture in rheumatoid arthritis. J Hand Surg 33: 49–58.
9. Giatromanolaki A, Sivridis E, Maltezos E, Athanasou N, Papazoglou D, et al. (2003) Upregulated hypoxia inducible factor-1alpha and -2alpha pathway in rheumatoid arthritis and osteoarthritis. Arthritis Res Ther 5: R193–201.
10. Hashimoto A, Tarner IH, Bohle RM, Gaumann A, Manetti M, et al. (2007) Analysis of vascular gene expression in arthritic synovium by laser-mediated microdissection. Arthritis Rheum 56: 1094–1105.
11. Hollander AP, Corke KP, Freemont AJ, Lewis CE (2001) Expression of hypoxia-inducible factor 1alpha by macrophages in the rheumatoid synovium: implications for targeting of therapeutic genes to the inflamed joint. Arthritis Rheum 44: 1540–1544.
12. Gaber T, Dziurla R, Tripmacher R, Burmester GR, Buttgereit F (2005) Hypoxia inducible factor (HIF) in rheumatology: low O2! See what HIF can do! Ann Rheum Dis 64: 971–980.
13. Knowles HJ, Cleton-Jansen AM, Korsching E, Athanasou NA (2010) Hypoxia-inducible factor regulates osteoclast-mediated bone resorption: role of angiopoietin-like 4. FASEB J 24: 4648–4659.
14. Knowles HJ, Athanasou NA (2009) Acute hypoxia and osteoclast activity: a balance between enhanced resorption and increased apoptosis. J Pathol 218: 256–264.
15. Arnett TR, Gibbons DC, Utting JC, Orriss IR, Hoebertz A, et al. (2003) Hypoxia is a major stimulator of osteoclast formation and bone resorption. J Cell Physiol 196: 2–8.
16. Fujikawa Y, Sabokbar A, Neale S, Athanasou NA (1996) Human osteoclast formation and bone resorption by monocytes and synovial macrophages in rheumatoid arthritis. Ann Rheum Dis 55: 816–822.
17. Yasuda H, Shima N, Nakagawa N, Yamaguchi K, Kinosaki M, et al. (1998) Osteoclast differentiation factor is a ligand for osteoprotegerin/osteoclastogenesis-inhibitory factor and is identical to TRANCE/RANKL. Proc Natl Acad Sci USA 95: 3597–3602.
18. Morten KJ, Badder L, Knowles HJ (2013) Differential regulation of HIF-mediated pathways increases mitochondrial metabolism and ATP production in hypoxic osteoclasts. J Pathol 229: 755–764.
19. Le Jan S, Amy C, Cazes A, Monnot C, Lamande N, et al. (2003) Angiopoietin-like 4 is a proangiogenic factor produced during ischemia and in conventional renal cell carcinoma. Am J Pathol 162: 1521–1528.
20. Zhang H, Wong CC, Wei H, Gilkes DM, Korangath P, et al. (2012) HIF-1-dependent expression of angiopoietin-like 4 and L1CAM mediates vascular metastasis of hypoxic breast cancer cells to the lungs. Oncogene 31: 1757–1770.
21. Murata M, Yudo K, Nakamura H, Chiba J, Okamoto K, Suematsu N, et al. (2009) Hypoxia upregulates the expression of angiopoietin-like-4 in human articular chondrocytes: role of angiopoietin-like-4 in the expression of matrix metalloproteinases and cartilage degradation. J Orthop Res 27: 50–57.
22. Larsen H, Muz B, Khong TL, Feldmann M, Paleolog EM (2012) Differential effects of Th1 versus Th2 cytokines in combination with hypoxia on HIFs and angiogenesis in RA. Arth Res Ther 14: R180.
23. Mahoney DJ, Swales C, Athanasou NA, Bombardieri M, Pitzalis C, et al. (2011) TSG-6 inhibits osteoclast activity via an autocrine mechanism and is functionally synergistic with osteoprotegerin. Arthritis Rheum 63: 1034–1043.
24. Knowles HJ, Moskovsky L, Thompson MS, Grunhen J, Cheng X, et al. (2012) Chondroclasts are mature osteoclasts which are capable of cartilage matrix resorption. Virchows Arch 461: 205–210.
25. Oshita K, Yamaoka K, Udagawa N, Fukuyo S, Sonomoto K, et al. (2011) Human mesenchymal stem cells inhibit osteoclastogenesis through osteoprotegerin production. Arthritis Rheum 63: 1658–1667.
26. Kim YG, Lee CK, Oh JS, Kim SH, Kim KA, Yoo B (2010) Effect of interleukin-32gamma on differentiation of osteoclasts from CD14+ monocytes. Arthritis Rheum 62: 515–523.
27. Troen BR (2003) Molecular mechanisms underlying osteoclast formation and activation. Exp Gerontol 38: 605–614.
28. Corisdeo S, Gyda M, Zaidi M, Moonga BS, Troen BR (2001) New insights into the regulation of cathepsin K gene expression by osteoprotegerin ligand. Biochem Biophys Res Commun 285: 335–339.
29. Hummel KM, Petrow PK, Franz JK, Muller-Ladner U, Aicher WK, et al. (1998) Cysteine proteinase cathepsin K mRNA is expressed in synovium of

patients with rheumatoid arthritis and is detected at sites of synovial bone destruction. J Rheumatol 25: 1887–1894.

30. Gravallese EM, Manning C, Tsay A, Naito A, Pan C, et al. (2000) Synovial tissue in rheumatoid arthritis is a source of osteoclast differentiation factor. Arthritis Rheum 43: 250–258.
31. Trebec-Reynolds DP, Voronov I, Heersche JN, Manolson MF (2010) VEGF-A expression in osteoclasts is regulated by NF-kappaB induction of HIF-1alpha. J Cell Biochem 110: 343–351.
32. Zhao X, Yue Y, Cheng W, Li J, Hu Y, et al. (2013) Hypoxia-inducible factor: a potential therapeutic target for rheumatoid arthritis. Curr Drug Targets 14: 700–707.
33. Mandard S, Zandbergen F, Tan NS, Escher P, Patsouris D, et al. (2004) The direct peroxisome proliferator-activated receptor target fasting-induced adipose factor (FIAF/PGAR/ANGPTL4) is present in blood plasma as a truncated protein that is increased by fenofibrate treatment. J Biol Chem 279: 34411–34420.
34. Hermann LM, Pinkerton M, Jennings K, Yang L, Grom A, et al. (2005) Angiopoietin-like-4 is a potential angiogenic mediator in arthritis. Clin Immunol 115: 93–101.
35. Robciuc MR, Tahvanainen E, Jauhiainen M, Ehnholm C (2009) Quantitation of serum angiopoietin-like proteins 3 and 4 in a Finnish population sample. J Lipid Res 51: 824–831.
36. Lanfant-Weybel K, Michot C, Daveau R, Milliez PY, Auquit-Auckbur I, et al. (2012) Synovium CD20 expression is a potential new predictor of bone erosion progression in very-early arthritis treated by sequential DMARDs monotherapy - a pilot study from the VErA cohort. Joint Bone Spine 79: 574–580.

3

Rheumatoid Arthritis and the Risk of Bipolar Disorder: A Nationwide Population-Based Study

Chih-Chao Hsu[1]¶, San-Chi Chen[2]¶, Chia-Jen Liu[2,3], Ti Lu[1], Cheng-Che Shen[4], Yu-Wen Hu[3,5], Chiu-Mei Yeh[6], Pan-Ming Chen[7], Tzeng-Ji Chen[6,8], Li-Yu Hu[1,3]*

1 Department of Psychiatry, Kaohsiung Veterans General Hospital, Kaohsiung, Taiwan, **2** Division of Hematology and Oncology, Department of Medicine, Taipei Veterans General Hospital, Taipei, Taiwan, **3** Institute of Public Health & School of Medicine, National Yang-Ming University, Taipei, Taiwan, **4** Department of Psychiatry, Chiayi Branch, Taichung Veterans General Hospital, Chiayi, Taiwan, **5** Cancer Center, Taipei Veterans General Hospital, Taipei, Taiwan, **6** Department of Family Medicine, Taipei Veterans General Hospital, Taipei, Taiwan, **7** Department of Psychiatry, Yuanshan Branch, Taipei Veterans General Hospital, Yilan, Taiwan, **8** School of Medicine, National Yang-Ming University, Taipei, Taiwan

Abstract

Background: Studies have suggested that chronic inflammation plays an essential role in the pathophysiology of both rheumatoid arthritis (RA) and bipolar disorder. The most common clinical features associated with RA are anxiety and depression. The risk of bipolar disorder among patients with RA has not been characterized adequately.

Objective: To determine the association between RA and the subsequent development of bipolar disorder and examine the risk factors for bipolar disorder among patients with RA.

Methods: We identified patients who were diagnosed with RA in the Taiwan National Health Insurance Research Database. A comparison cohort was created by matching patients without RA with those with RA according to age, sex, and comorbidities. The occurrence of bipolar disorder was evaluated in both cohorts.

Results: The RA cohort consisted of 2,570 patients, and the comparison cohort consisted of 2,570 matched control patients without RA. The incidence of bipolar disorder (incidence rate ratio = 2.13, 95% confidence interval [CI] = 1.12–4.24, $P = .013$) was higher among patients with RA than among control patients. Multivariate, matched regression models revealed that asthma (hazard ratio [HR] = 2.76, 95% CI 1.27–5.96, $P = .010$), liver cirrhosis (HR = 3.81, 95% CI = 1.04–14.02, $P = .044$), and alcohol use disorders (HR = 5.29, 95% CI = 1.71–16.37, $P = .004$) were independent risk factors for the development of bipolar disorder among patients with RA.

Conclusion: RA might increase the incidence of bipolar disorder development. Based on our data, we suggest that, following RA diagnosis, greater attention be focused on women with asthma, liver cirrhosis, and alcohol use disorder. Prospective clinical studies of the relationship between RA and bipolar disorder are warranted.

Editor: Anil Kumar, University of Missouri-Kansas City, United States of America

Funding: This study was supported by a grant from Taipei Veterans General Hospital (V103B-022 and V103E10-001). The funders had no role in study design, data collection and analysis, decision to publish, or preparation of the manuscript.

Competing Interests: The authors have declared that no competing interests exist.

* Email: chrishuly@gmail.com

¶ These authors contributed equally to this work.

Introduction

Rheumatoid arthritis (RA), an autoimmune disease, impairs patient health and has wider implications regarding health policy and costs. RA primarily affects the joints, but can also affect the entire body, causing systemic symptoms [1]. Several studies have compared patients with RA and healthy controls and have demonstrated that the mechanism involved in the pathogenesis of RA symptoms is related to chronic inflammation and associated with various cytokines [2].

Interest has grown in the psychiatric aspects of autoimmune diseases characterized by chronic inflammation, which might induce psychiatric illnesses through neuroinflammation and neurotransmitter abnormalities. Autoimmune diseases have been proved to be associated with psychiatric disorders, particularly schizophrenia, major depressive disorder, and bipolar disorder [3]. Studies have identified an association between RA and psychiatric disorders, particularly depressive disorder and schizophrenia [4–6]. However, the existence of this association remains uncertain. Moreover, few studies have investigated the association between RA and bipolar disorder.

Studies have shown that numerous cytokines circulating in plasma might impair the function of the blood-brain barrier [7],

Table 1. Baseline characteristics of patients with rheumatoid arthritis (RA) and the matched cohort.

Characteristics	Patients with RA n = 2,570 (%)		Matched cohort n = 2,570 (%)		*p* value
Median age, years (interquartile range)	51(41–60)		51(41–60)		
Age, years					
≥50	1,358	52.8	1,358	52.8	1.000
<50	1,212	47.2	1,212	47.2	
Sex					
Male	639	24.9	639	24.9	1.000
Female	1,931	75.1	1,931	75.1	
Comorbidities					
Hypertension	790	30.7	793	30.9	1.000
Dyslipidemia	739	28.8	739	28.8	0.157
COPD	582	22.6	583	22.7	0.973
Diabetes mellitus	497	19.3	497	19.3	1.000
Asthma	408	15.9	406	15.8	0.939
Chronic kidney disease	329	12.8	329	12.8	0.235
Cerebrovascular disease	310	12.1	309	12.1	1.000
Alcohol use disorder	65	2.5	53	2.1	<0.001
Liver cirrhosis	64	2.5	47	1.8	0.103
Malignancies	58	2.3	46	2.1	0.264
Coronary artery disease	27	1.1	24	0.9	0.928
Median follow-up years (interquartile range)	6.1(3.4–8.6)		6.1(3.4–8.6)		0.673

COPD, chronic obstructive pulmonary disease.

indicating that peripheral inflammation is associated with the upregulation of central nervous system (CNS) inflammation. Several studies have shown that chronic inflammation plays a vital role in the pathophysiology of common mental disorders [8], including bipolar disorder [9]. Therefore, we hypothesized that a history of RA increases the risk of the subsequent onset of bipolar disorder.

To test our hypothesis, we designed a nationwide population-based study to investigate the incidence of bipolar disorder among patients with RA.

Patients and Methods

Data Sources

The Taiwan National Health Insurance (NHI) program offers comprehensive, universal health insurance to all residents of Taiwan. The NHI program covers more than 96% of the residents of Taiwan and is contracted with 99% of all hospitals and clinics in Taiwan [10]. The program provides coverage for outpatient, inpatient, emergency, and traditional Chinese medicine services as well as prescription drugs. Multiple NHI databases, including NHI enrollment files, claims data, and a prescription drug registry, are managed and publicly released by the National Health Research Institutes (NHRI) of Taiwan. The Institutional Review Board of Taipei Veterans General Hospital approved this study (2013-03-035AC). Written consent from the study patients was not obtained because the NHI dataset consists of deidentified secondary data used for research purposes; the Institutional Review Board of Taipei Veterans General Hospital issued a formal written waiver for the need for consent. The National Health Insurance Research Database (NHIRD) is publicly released by the NHRI for research purposes only. Although confidentiality is guaranteed according to the data regulations of the NHRI, studies using this database still must be approved by the ethics committee. Detailed information on data requests is provided on the NHRI Web site (http://nhird.nhri.org.tw). Comments, problems, or requests regarding data application can be sent to the following NHRI email address: nhird@nhri.org.tw.

Study Design and Patients

We conducted a retrospective cohort study of patients who were newly diagnosed with RA between January 1, 2000, and December 31, 2010. We identified RA cases in the Taiwan National Health Insurance Research Database (NHIRD) based on International Classification of Diseases, Ninth Revision, Clinical Modification (ICD-9-CM) Code 714.0 and included only patients with RA who received a catastrophic illness certificate. The NHI program has specified 30 categories of catastrophic illness (e.g., cancers, hemophilia, autoimmune diseases including RA, and chronic renal failure). Eligible patients can apply for catastrophic illness certificates, and if approved, they are exempted from copayment of related medical costs. In this study, we relied on physicians' ability to make accurate diagnoses. However, RA diagnosis involves multiple criteria and ruling out diseases with RA-like symptoms. The possibility that RA diagnoses were misclassified was a concern. The issuance of certificates is validated based on a careful review of medical records, laboratory studies, and imaging studies conducted by at least 2 specialists. Therefore, we included only patients with RA who received a catastrophic illness certificate to ensure that RA diagnoses were valid. Several studies that have examined the epidemiology of systemic autoimmune diseases, particularly RA, by using the NHIRD have been published [11,12].

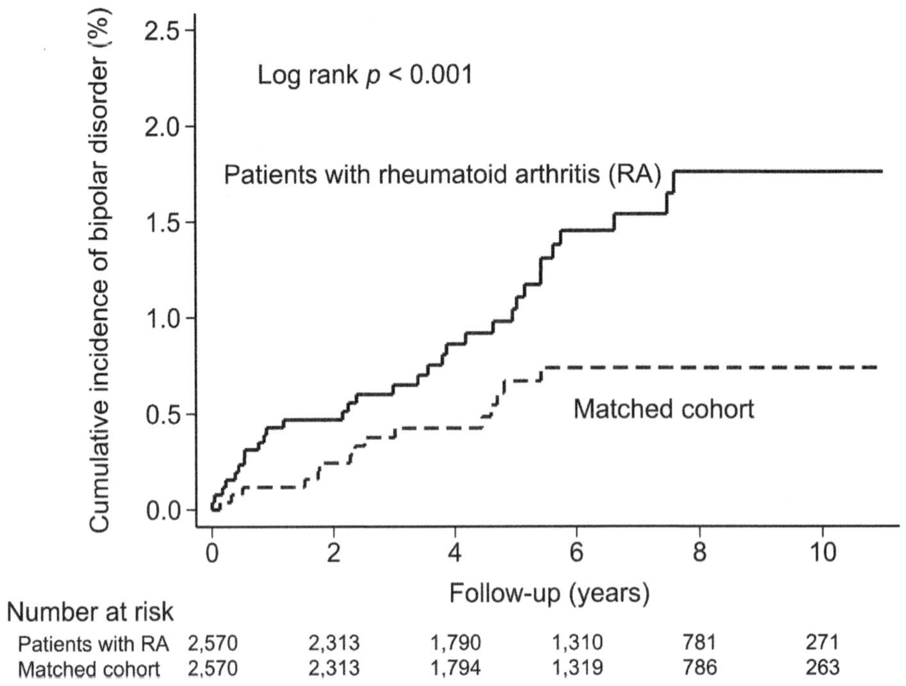

Figure 1. Cumulative incidence of bipolar disorder among patients with rheumatoid arthritis (RA) and the matched cohort.

Patients with bipolar disorder between January 1, 2000 and December 31, 2010 were identified based on the ICD-9-CM codes for bipolar disorder (296.0X, 296.1X, 296.4X, 296.5X, 296.6X, 296.7X, 296.80, or 296.89). However, to ensure that the bipolar disorder diagnoses in the database were reliable, we collected data on prescriptions of psychotropic agents for these patients. The role of medication in bipolar disorder treatment is firmly established. Therefore, we excluded patients who were diagnosed with bipolar disorder (according to ICD-9-CM codes) but did not receive any medication. We collected information on the use of drugs approved by the Food and Drug Administration of Taiwan for treating one (or more) phases of bipolar disorder, including acute mania/mixed episodes, bipolar depression, and bipolar maintenance. In addition to mood stabilizers, atypical antipsychotics such as aripiprazole, olanzapine, quetiapine, risperidone, and ziprasidone were included. These drugs were classified according to the World Health Organization Anatomical Therapeutic Chemical classification. Only patients who were prescribed these drugs for at least one month were included in our study. Furthermore, patients with mood disorders resulting from a general medical condition (ICD-9-CM Code 293.83) and patients with a history of mood disorders before the enrollment date were excluded from our study.

For each patient with RA in the NHIRD, one patient without RA matched according to age, sex, comorbidities [13], and enrollment date was selected. Although numerous studies have identified several comorbidities as risk factors for RA, based on the inflammation hypothesis proposed in this study, other inflammation-associated comorbidities were considered potential confounders. The exclusion criteria applied to the case cohort were applied to the matched comparison cohort. Both the patients with RA and comparison patients were followed until the development of bipolar disorder, death, or the end of the study period.

Statistical Analysis

The diagnosis of bipolar disorder served as the primary dependent variable. We calculated the bipolar disorder incidence rates (per 10 000 person-y) and the incidence rate ratios (IRRs). The study groups were compared using the χ^2 test for categorical variables. The Kaplan-Meier method was used to estimate the cumulative incidence of bipolar disorders, and a Cox proportional hazard model was used to identify risk factors for bipolar disorder in patients with RA. The qualifying criterion for inclusion in the multivariate analysis was a result in the univariate analysis with a P value of less than .1. The Perl programming language (Version 5.12.2) was used to extract data from the databases. Microsoft SQL Server 2005 (Microsoft Corp., Redmond, WA, USA) was used for data linkage, processing, and control sampling. The SPSS, Version 19.0 for Windows (IBM, Armonk, NY, USA) and the SAS, Version 9.2 (SAS Institute, Cary, NC, USA) computer software programs were used to perform all statistical analyses. Comparison results with a P value less than .05 were considered statistically significant.

Results

Patient Characteristics

Table 1 shows demographic and comorbidity data on the patients with RA and control patients. The median age of the patients was 51 years (interquartile range =41–60 y). The majority of patients in both cohorts were women (75.1%). Diabetes mellitus, chronic obstructive pulmonary disease, asthma, liver cirrhosis, alcohol use disorder, malignancy, chronic kidney disease, cerebral vascular disease, dyslipidemia, hypertension, and coronary artery disease were the most common comorbidities. No statistically significant differences were observed in baseline comorbidity data between the study groups.

Table 2. Incidence of bipolar disorder among patients with rheumatoid arthritis (RA) and the matched cohort.

	Patients with RA		Matched cohort			
	No. of bipolar disorder	Per 10,000 person-years	No. of bipolar disorder	Per 10,000 person-years	Risk ratio (95% CI)	*p* value
Total	32	20.7	15	9.7	2.13(1.12–4.24)	0.013
Age						
≥50	14	18.5	7	9.3	1.99(0.75–5.84)	0.136
<50	18	22.8	8	10.1	2.26(0.93–6.00)	0.051
Sex						
Male	5	13.0	3	7.8	1.67(0.33–10.76)	0.505
Female	27	23.2	12	10.3	2.25(1.10–4.87)	0.017
Follow-up						
0–1 y	11	43.1	3	11.7	3.67(0.97–20.50)	0.035
1–5 y	12	14.6	11	13.4	1.09(0.44–2.73)	0.839
≥5 y	9	19.0	1	2.1	8.99(1.25–394.20)	0.012

CI, confidence interval.

Incidence of Bipolar Disorder

The cumulative incidence rates of bipolar disorder are shown in Figure 1. As shown in Table 2, the risk of developing bipolar disorder was significantly higher among patients with RA than among patients in the matched cohort (IRR = 2.13; 95% confidence interval [CI] = 1.12–4.24; *P* = .013). After stratifying patients according to age and sex, we observed that patients with RA under 50 years old exhibited an increased incidence of subsequent bipolar disorder (IRR = 2.26; 95% CI = 0.93–6.00; *P* = .051), even when no obvious statistical difference was observed. Moreover, women with RA exhibited a higher risk of developing subsequent bipolar disorder than did men (IRR = 2.25; 95% CI = 1.10–4.87; *P* = .017). Furthermore, we stratified patients according to follow-up duration and observed that the risk of subsequent bipolar disorder was significantly higher in the first year (IRR = 3.67; 95% CI = 0.97–20.5; *P* = .035) and more than 5 years (IRR = 8.99; 95% CI = 1.25–394.20; *P* = .012) after RA diagnosis. Overall, our study indicated that the incidence of the development of bipolar disorder following RA diagnosis was 20.7 per 10 000 person-years.

Risks Factors for Bipolar Disorder Among Patients with Rheumatoid Arthritis

The results of the univariate and multivariate analyses revealed that asthma (hazard ratio [HR] = 2.76; 95% CI = 1.27–5.96; *P* = .010), liver cirrhosis (HR = 3.81; 95% CI = 1.04–14.02; *P* = .044), alcohol use disorders (HR = 5.29; 95% CI = 1.71–16.37; *P* = .004), and substance abuse (HR = 37.42; 95% CI = 10.31–135.82; *P* < .001) were independent risk factors for the development of bipolar disorder among patients with RA (Table 3).

Discussion

This is the first population-based study to examine RA as a risk factor for bipolar disorder by using a matched cohort and a maximal follow-up period of 10 years. The major finding of our study was the discovery of a higher incidence of subsequent bipolar disorder among patients with RA. Furthermore, women with RA had a higher risk of developing subsequent bipolar disorder than did men, and asthma, liver cirrhosis, and alcohol use disorder are potential risk factors for developing bipolar disorder.

This study revealed that patients with RA were at a higher risk of subsequent bipolar disorder. We hypothesized that this risk is linked to the mechanisms of immune dysfunction. Bipolar disorder development after RA might result from the inflammatory process activated by RA. In 2012, Lampa et al [14] investigated the influence of peripheral chronic joint inflammatory disease in RA on CNS inflammation and revealed that the chronic peripheral inflammatory process activated by RA might cause the upregulation of CNS inflammation. Studies have evidenced that chronic and mild inflammation in the periphery are key contributors to the pathophysiology of CNS inflammation in bipolar disorder [15,16] and that dysregulation of the inflammatory process in the brain triggers and exacerbates atherosclerosis, hypertension, diabetes, obesity, and hyperthyroidism [17–20]. Animal models have indicated that peripheral cytokines reach the brain through various mechanisms, including a leaky brain barrier, active transport, activation of endothelial cells, and binding to cytokine receptors [21]. In short, cytokines created through infectious and inflammatory processes play a vital role in mediating the cross-talk between the immune system and the brain and are therefore possible contributors to the development of several psychiatric diseases, including bipolar disorder [22,23].

Table 3. Risk factors for bipolar disorder among patients with rheumatoid arthritis.

Variables	Univariate analysis		Multivariate analysis[a]	
	HR (95% CI)	*p* value	HR (95% CI)	*p* value
Age ≥50 years	1.28(0.63–2.57)	0.493		
Female	1.77(0.68–4.58)	0.243		
Comorbidities				
Hypertension	1.17(0.55–2.48)	0.680		
Dyslipidemia	0.66(0.27–1.60)	0.356		
COPD	1.79(0.85–3.79)	0.127		
Diabetes mellitus	1.26(0.55–2.92)	0.587		
Asthma	3.12(1.50–6.48)	0.002	2.76(1.27–5.96)	0.010
Chronic kidney disease	0.50(0.12–2.09)	0.340		
Cerebrovascular disease	1.91(0.79–4.65)	0.153		
Alcohol use disorder	9.87(3.78–25.80)	<0.001	5.29(1.71–16.37)	0.004
Liver cirrhosis	4.87(1.48–16.01)	0.009	3.81(1.04–14.02)	0.044
Malignancies	1.78(0.24–13.03)	0.572		
Coronary artery disease	3.43(0.47–25.11)	0.226		

HR, hazard ratio; CI, confidence interval; COPD, chronic obstructive pulmonary disease.
[a]All factors with $p<0.1$ in univariate analyses and age were included in the Cox multivariate analysis, and age, sex was enter in the Cox multivariate analysis.

Epidemiological studies have indicated that men and women are equally likely to develop bipolar disorder [24]. However, certain studies have revealed that sex steroid hormones play an essential role in immune response; specifically immune-stimulating effects caused by estrogen might trigger the inflammatory process. In other words, women are more vulnerable to immune dysfunction than men [25–27]. These findings might explain why women with RA had a higher risk of developing bipolar disorder than did women without RA.

When the patients were stratified according to follow-up duration, the incidence of bipolar disorder was significantly higher in the first year and more than 5 years after RA diagnosis. The first result might have been caused by detection bias; patients with symptoms of bipolar disorder might have been diagnosed shortly after RA diagnosis. The second result was compatible with our inflammation hypothesis regarding the association between RA and bipolar disorder. In contrast to acute inflammation, chronic inflammation persists for a prolonged period of time. We hypothesized that, in the long term, the chronic inflammatory process becomes a pathophysiology for the development of bipolar disorder [28].

Our analysis revealed that asthma, liver cirrhosis, and alcohol use disorder were independent risk factors associated with subsequent bipolar disorder in patients with RA. Evidence has indicated that chronic inflammatory processes in asthma and liver cirrhosis, like the pathophysiology of RA, involve cytokine interactions [29–31], and this combined and augmented chronic inflammatory effect might subsequently induce bipolar disorder. Moreover, cytokines that potentially cause depression and anxiety in liver cirrhosis [32] might also be associated with the development of bipolar disorder [33]. In addition, alcohol use disorder was associated with subsequent bipolar disorder in patients with RA. Several studies have indicated that alcohol consumption is associated with a lower incidence of disease and an improved quality of life among female patients with RA [34,35]. However, other studies have revealed that alcohol use disorders and bipolar disorder share certain genetic characteristics and are similar according to neuroimaging and biochemical findings [36,37]. Thus, alcohol use disorder might be an independent risk factor for the development of bipolar disorder among patients with RA.

Our study is the first retrospective study to examine RA as a risk factor for the development of bipolar disorder. A matched cohort study design comprising a population-based cohort of patients with RA and adequate controls for comorbidity constitute the strengths of our study. However, several limitations that are inherent to the use of claims databases should be considered. First, the diagnosis of RA in the NHIRD was based on the ICD-9-CM code and the issuance of a catastrophic illness certificate. Thus, the severity of RA as a risk factor for subsequent bipolar disorder was not explored. Second, the causal relationship was assessed mainly according to the chronological order in which the 2 conditions were diagnosed. However, both conditions might require long-term treatment, and the possibility that bipolar disorder causes RA cannot be excluded entirely. Third, information was unavailable on several demographic variables such as socioeconomic status, lifestyle, and family history, which might have provided useful information regarding factors that are potentially associated with RA and bipolar disorder [38,39]. Finally, this epidemiologic study was based on an observational design rather than an experimental design. Data on the relationship between the exacerbation of RA and the severity of bipolar disorder in patients with RA were unavailable. Therefore, the direction of causality in the association between the aforementioned possible risk factors and bipolar disorder development among patients with RA could not be determined.

In conclusion, this study revealed that RA increases the incidence of bipolar disorder development, suggesting that the RA-related inflammatory process is associated with increased expression of neuropsychiatric disturbances. Based on our data, we suggest that greater attention be focused on women, particularly those with asthma, liver cirrhosis, and alcohol use disorder. Additional prospective clinical studies on the relationship between RA and bipolar disorder are warranted.

Acknowledgments

We thank Huei-Sing Chang and Cheng-Fang Hong for their technical assistance. The study was based in part on data from the National Health Insurance Research Database provided by the Bureau of National Health Insurance, Department of Health, Taiwan and managed by the National Health Research Institutes. The interpretation and conclusion contained herein do not represent the views of the Bureau of National Health Insurance, the Department of Health, or the National Health Research Institutes.

Author Contributions

Conceived and designed the experiments: C-CH L-YH S-CC. Performed the experiments: C-JL C-CS Y-WH C-MY. Analyzed the data: C-CH L-YH C-JL TL. Contributed reagents/materials/analysis tools: C-JL P-MC T-JC. Contributed to the writing of the manuscript: S-CC C-CH L-YH.

References

1. Wasserman AM (2011) Diagnosis and management of rheumatoid arthritis. Am Fam Physician 84: 1245–1252.
2. Calabrese LH (1999) Rheumatoid arthritis and primary care: the case for early diagnosis and treatment. J Am Osteopath Assoc 99: 313–321.
3. Najjar S, Pearlman DM, Alper K, Najjar A, Devinsky O (2013) Neuroinflammation and psychiatric illness. J Neuroinflammation 10: 43.
4. Dickens C, McGowan L, Clark-Carter D, Creed F (2002) Depression in rheumatoid arthritis: a systematic review of the literature with meta-analysis. Psychosom Med 64: 52–60.
5. Torrey EF, Yolken RH (2001) The schizophrenia-rheumatoid arthritis connection: infectious, immune, or both? Brain Behav Immun 15: 401–410.
6. Nicassio PM (2010) Arthritis and psychiatric disorders: disentangling the relationship. J Psychosom Res 68: 183–185.
7. Abbott NJ, Ronnback L, Hansson E (2006) Astrocyte-endothelial interactions at the blood-brain barrier. Nat Rev Neurosci 7: 41–53.
8. Kivimaki M, Shipley MJ, Batty GD, Hamer M, Akbaraly TN, et al. (2013) Long-term inflammation increases risk of common mental disorder: a cohort study. Mol Psychiatry.
9. Stertz L, Magalhaes PV, Kapczinski F (2013) Is bipolar disorder an inflammatory condition? The relevance of microglial activation. Curr Opin Psychiatry 26: 19–26.
10. Wu CY, Chen YJ, Ho HJ, Hsu YC, Kuo KN, et al. (2012) Association between nucleoside analogues and risk of hepatitis B virus-related hepatocellular carcinoma recurrence following liver resection. JAMA 308: 1906–1914.
11. Lai NS, Tsai TY, Li CY, Koo M, Yu CL, et al. (2013) Increased frequency and costs of ambulatory medical care utilization prior to the diagnosis of rheumatoid arthritis: A national population-based study. Arthritis Care Res 27: 22146.
12. Lai CH, Lai MS, Lai KL, Chen HH, Chiu YM (2012) Nationwide population-based epidemiologic study of rheumatoid arthritis in Taiwan. Clin Exp Rheumatol 30: 358–363. Epub 2012 Jun 2026.
13. Khan NF, Perera R, Harper S, Rose PW (2010) Adaptation and validation of the Charlson Index for Read/OXMIS coded databases. BMC Fam Pract 11: 1.
14. Lampa J, Westman M, Kadetoff D, Agreus AN, Le Maitre E, et al. (2012) Peripheral inflammatory disease associated with centrally activated IL-1 system in humans and mice. Proc Natl Acad Sci U S A 109: 12728–12733.
15. Goldstein BI, Kemp DE, Soczynska JK, McIntyre RS (2009) Inflammation and the phenomenology, pathophysiology, comorbidity, and treatment of bipolar disorder: a systematic review of the literature. J Clin Psychiatry 70: 1078–1090.
16. Hamdani N, Tamouza R, Leboyer M (2012) Immuno- inflammatory markers of bipolar disorder: a review of evidence. Front Biosci (Elite Ed) 4: 2170–2182.
17. Drake C, Boutin H, Jones MS, Denes A, McColl BW, et al. (2011) Brain inflammation is induced by co-morbidities and risk factors for stroke. Brain Behav Immun 25: 1113–1122.
18. Ross R (1999) Atherosclerosis is an inflammatory disease. Am Heart J 138: S419–420.
19. Hu LY, Shen CC, Hu YW, Chen MH, Tsai CF, et al. (2013) Hyperthyroidism and risk for bipolar disorders: a nationwide population-based study. PLoS One 8: e73057.
20. Thomsen AF, Kessing LV (2005) Increased risk of hyperthyroidism among patients hospitalized with bipolar disorder. Bipolar Disord 7: 351–357.
21. Miller AH, Maletic V, Raison CL (2009) Inflammation and its discontents: the role of cytokines in the pathophysiology of major depression. Biol Psychiatry 65: 732–741.
22. Brietzke E, Stertz L, Fernandes BS, Kauer-Sant'anna M, Mascarenhas M, et al. (2009) Comparison of cytokine levels in depressed, manic and euthymic patients with bipolar disorder. J Affect Disord 116: 214–217.
23. Rege S, Hodgkinson SJ (2013) Immune dysregulation and autoimmunity in bipolar disorder: Synthesis of the evidence and its clinical application. Aust N Z J Psychiatry 47: 1136–1151.
24. Price AL, Marzani-Nissen GR (2012) Bipolar disorders: a review. Am Fam Physician 85: 483–493.
25. Cutolo M, Sulli A, Straub RH (2012) Estrogen metabolism and autoimmunity. Autoimmun Rev 11: A460–464.
26. Cutolo M, Villaggio B, Seriolo B, Montagna P, Capellino S, et al. (2004) Synovial fluid estrogens in rheumatoid arthritis. Autoimmun Rev 3: 193–198.
27. Cutolo M, Sulli A, Capellino S, Villaggio B, Montagna P, et al. (2004) Sex hormones influence on the immune system: basic and clinical aspects in autoimmunity. Lupus 13: 635–638.
28. Berk M, Williams LJ, Jacka FN, O'Neil A, Pasco JA, et al. (2013) So depression is an inflammatory disease, but where does the inflammation come from? BMC Med 11: 200.
29. Naik SR, Wala SM (2013) Inflammation, allergy and asthma, complex immune origin diseases: mechanisms and therapeutic agents. Recent Pat Inflamm Allergy Drug Discov 7: 62–95.
30. Shukla S, Shukla H, Kumar S, Aharwal RP, Gupta VK, et al. (2013) Allergy and inflammation: an immunological and therapeutic approach. Recent Pat Inflamm Allergy Drug Discov 7: 135–150.
31. Kocabayoglu P, Friedman SL (2013) Cellular basis of hepatic fibrosis and its role in inflammation and cancer. Front Biosci (Schol Ed) 5: 217–230.
32. Ko FY, Tsai SJ, Yang AC, Zhou Y, Xu LM (2013) Association of CD8 T cells with depression and anxiety in patients with liver cirrhosis. Int J Psychiatry Med 45: 15–29.
33. Liu HC, Yang YY, Chou YM, Chen KP, Shen WW, et al. (2004) Immunologic variables in acute mania of bipolar disorder. J Neuroimmunol 150: 116–122.
34. Bergman S, Symeonidou S, Andersson ML, Soderlin MK (2013) Alcohol consumption is associated with lower self-reported disease activity and better health-related quality of life in female rheumatoid arthritis patients in Sweden: data from BARFOT, a multicenter study on early RA. BMC Musculoskelet Disord 14: 218.
35. Lu B, Rho YH, Cui J, Iannaccone CK, Frits ML, et al. (2013) Associations of Smoking and Alcohol Consumption with Disease Activity and Functional Status in Rheumatoid Arthritis. J Rheumatol.
36. Farren CK, Hill KP, Weiss RD (2012) Bipolar disorder and alcohol use disorder: a review. Curr Psychiatry Rep 14: 659–666.
37. Pettinati HM, O'Brien CP, Dundon WD (2013) Current status of co-occurring mood and substance use disorders: a new therapeutic target. Am J Psychiatry 170: 23–30.
38. Waxmonsky JA, Thomas MR, Miklowitz DJ, Allen MH, Wisniewski SR, et al. (2005) Prevalence and correlates of tobacco use in bipolar disorder: data from the first 2000 participants in the Systematic Treatment Enhancement Program. Gen Hosp Psychiatry 27: 321–328.
39. Schoeyen HK, Birkenaes AB, Vaaler AE, Auestad BH, Malt UF, et al. (2011) Bipolar disorder patients have similar levels of education but lower socio-economic status than the general population. J Affect Disord 129: 68–74.

4

Risk of Developing Depressive Disorders following Rheumatoid Arthritis: A Nationwide Population-Based Study

Shu-Li Wang[2], **Cheng-Ho Chang**[1], **Li-Yu Hu**[1], **Shih-Jen Tsai**[3,4], **Albert C. Yang**[3,4,5], **Zi-Hong You**[6,7]*

1 Department of Psychiatry, Kaohsiung Veterans General Hospital, Kaohsiung, Taiwan, **2** Department of Dental Laboratory Technology, Central Taiwan University of Science and Technology, Taichung, Taiwan, **3** Department of Psychiatry, Taipei Veterans General Hospital, Taipei, Taiwan, **4** School of Medicine, National Yang-Ming University, Taipei, Taiwan, **5** Center for Dynamical Biomarkers and Translational Medicine, National Central University, Chungli, Taiwan, **6** Division of Nephrology, Department of Internal Medicine, Taichung Veterans General Hospital, Chia-Yi Branch, Chia-Yi, Taiwan, **7** Institute of Medicine, Chung Shan Medical University, Taichung, Taiwan

Abstract

Background & Aims: To evaluate the risk of depressive disorders among rheumatoid arthritis (RA) by using the Taiwan National Health Insurance Research Database (NHIRD).

Methods: We conducted a retrospective study of a matched cohort of 18 285 participants (3 657 RA patients and 14 628 control patients) who were selected from the NHIRD. Patients were observed for a maximum of 10 years to determine the rates of newly diagnosed depressive disorders, and Cox regression was used to identify the risk factors associated with depressive disorders in RA patients.

Results: During the 10-year follow-up period, 205 (11.2 per 1000 person-years) RA patients and 384 (5.1 per 1000 person-years) control patients were diagnosed with depressive disorders. In RA patients, most depressive disorders (n = 163, 80%) developed with five years of being diagnosed with RA. The incidence risk ratio of depressive disorders between RA patients and control patients was 2.20 (95% confidence interval [CI], 1.84–2.61, $P<.001$). After adjusting for age, sex, and comorbidities, RA patients were 2.06 times more likely to develop depressive disorders (95% CI, 1.73–2.44, $P<.001$) compared with the control patients. Hyperthyroidism (HR = 1.67) was an independent risk factor for depressive disorders in patients with RA.

Conclusions: The likelihood of developing depressive disorders is greater among RA patients than among patients without RA. Symptoms of depression should be sought in patients with RA.

Editor: Melvin G. McInnis, University of Michigan, United States of America

Funding: This study was supported by a grant from the Taipei Veterans General Hospital (V101D-001-2) and SJT received the funding. The funder had no role in study design, data collection and analysis, decision to publish, or preparation of the manuscript.

Competing Interests: The authors have declared that no competing interests exist.

* Email: zihongyou@gmail.com

These authors contributed equally to this work.

Introduction

Rheumatoid arthritis (RA) is a systemic chronic autoimmune disorder affecting primarily cartilage and bone. In addition, several organs such as lung, vessels, and kidney may be involved. In general, RA affects 0.5–1% of the population [1]. Despite of substantial advances in medical treatment, chronic pain, fatigue, and functional disability causes much psychosocial burden for these patients with RA [2,3].

Therefore, interest in the psychiatric aspects of rheumatoid arthritis has grown. Several studies have reported a high depression prevalence rate in patients with RA [4–12], and a significant correlation was observed among depression and increased pain levels in patients with RA [13]. Comorbid depression has been also shown to independently increase disability and a low quality of life in patients with RA [14–18]. In addition, depression has been demonstrated to be an independent risk factor for non-suicide mortality in patients with RA [19]. Hence, the depression symptoms should be examined in patients with RA because depression is a modifiable illness that is amenable to treatment.

However, in previous studies focusing on depression among patients with RA, depression was often evaluated by using rating scales, such as the Beck Depression Inventory or the Epidemiological Studies Depression Scale, rather than diagnosis by a psychiatrist [5–12]. The real prevalence rate of clinical depressive disorders in patients with RA remains unknown. In addition, the design of former studies prevented the temporal causal relationship between RA and depressive disorders from being clarified because the designs of these studies were almost cross-sectional studies [4–12]. Furthermore, whether there is an independent risk factor for newly diagnosed depressive disorders in patients with RA has never been studied.

We performed a population-based retrospective cohort study using data derived from the National Health Insurance (NHI) system in Taiwan. The purpose of our study was to determine whether RA was associated with an increased risk of clinical depressive disorders. Independent risk factors for newly diagnosed depressive disorders among the patients with RA were also identified.

Materials and Methods

Data Sources

Instituted in 1995, the NHI program is a mandatory health insurance program that offers comprehensive medical care coverage, including outpatient, inpatient, emergency, and traditional Chinese medicine, to all residents of Taiwan; the coverage rate is as high as 99% [20]. The NHI research database (NHIRD) contains comprehensive information regarding clinical visits, including prescription details and diagnostic codes based on the International Classification of Diseases, ninth revision, Clinical Modification (ICD-9-CM). The NHIRD is managed by the National Health Research Institutes (NHRI) and confidentiality is maintained according to the directives of the Bureau of the NHI. The data source for our study was the Longitudinal Health Insurance Database 2005 (LHID 2005), which is a dataset of NHIRD. Data for the LHID was collected by systematically and randomly sampling from the NHIRD; the database included the data of one million individuals. The NHRI of Taiwan reports that there were no significant differences in gender distribution, age distribution, or average insured payroll-related amount between the patients in the LHID and those in the original NHIRD [21]. Detailed information about the data source is provided on the NHRI website (http://nhird.nhri.org.tw). Comments, problems or requests about the data application could be sent to e-mail address at the NHRI (e-mail: nhird@nhri.org.tw).

Ethics Statement

The Institutional Review Board of the Taipei Veterans General Hospital approved this study (2013-03-035AC). Written consent from study patients was not obtained because the NHI dataset consists of de-identified secondary data for research purposes, and the Institutional Review Board of Taipei Veterans General Hospital issued a formal written waiver for the need for consent.

Study Population

Using data extracted from the LHID 2005, we conducted a retrospective cohort study of patients aged 20 years and older who were newly diagnosed with RA by a rheumatologist between January 1, 2000 and December 31, 2008. RA was defined as ICD-9-CM code: 714. We excluded patients who were diagnosed with depressive disorders (ICD-9-CM code: 296.2X-296.3X, 300.4, and 311.X) before enrollment. Insurance premiums, calculated according to the beneficiary's total income, were used to estimate monthly income. Monthly income was grouped into low income (monthly income <20,000 New Taiwan Dollar [NTD]), median income (20,000 NTD≤monthly income <40,000 NTD), and high income (monthly income ≥40,000 NTD). Urbanization was divided into three groups: urban, suburban, and rural. Urbanization and monthly income levels were used to represent socioeconomic status. For each cirrhotic patient included in the final cohort, 4 age-, sex-, and enrolment-date-matched control patients who were not diagnosed with rheumatoid arthritis or depressive disorder were randomly selected from the LHID 2005. All RA and control patients were observed until diagnosed with a depressive disorder by a psychiatrist, death, withdrawal from the NHI system, or December 31, 2009. The primary clinical outcome assessed was psychiatrist-diagnosed depressive disorder.

Statistical Analyses

The incidence of newly diagnosed depressive disorders in the RA and control patients, stratified by gender and age (equal or older than 60 years old or younger than 60 years old) was calculated. Independent *t*-tests and chi-squared tests were used to examine the differences in the demographic characteristics between the RA and control patients.

A Cox proportional-hazards regression model was used to identify variables that predicted depressive disorder in the RA and control patients, and in the RA patients only. Control variables, such as age; sex; common comorbidities, including hypertension, diabetes mellitus, dyslipidemia, coronary artery disease, congestive heart failure, cirrhosis, hyperthyroidism, hypothyroidism, cerebrovascular disease, and malignancy; urbanization; and monthly income were included as covariates in the univariate model. Factors that demonstrated a moderately significant statistical relationship in the univariate analysis ($P<.1$) were entered by forward selection in a multivariate Cox proportional-hazards regression model [22].

The Perl programming language (version 5.12.2) was used to extract and compute data. The Microsoft SQL Server 2005 (Microsoft Corp., Redmond, WA, USA) was used for data linkage, processing, and control sampling. IBM SPSS (version 19.0 for Windows; IBM Corp., New York, NY, USA) and SAS statistical software (version 9.2; SAS Institute Inc., Cary, NC, USA) were used to perform all statistical analyses. The comparisons resulting in a *P*-value of less than .05 were considered to indicate a statistically significant relationship.

Results

Participant Selection (Figure 1)

The sample comprised 3657 RA patients and 14 628 control patients without depression, among whom 72.8% were female. The median age at enrollment was 51 years (interquartile range [IQR], 41–61 years), and the median follow-up period was 4.72 years (IQR, 2.59–7.42 years) for RA patients and 4.92 years (IQR, 2.69.21–7.55 years) for control patients. The comorbidities, including hypertension, diabetes mellitus, dyslipidemia, congestive heart failure, hyperthyroidism, hypothyroidism, and cerebrovascular disease were more common in RA patients than control patients. The comparisons of the demographic and clinical variables between the RA and control patients are presented in Table 1.

Incidence Rate of Depressive Disorders

During the study period, 205 (11.2 per 1000 person-years) RA patients and 384 (5.1 per 1000 person-years) control patients were diagnosed with depressive disorders. The incidence risk ratio (IRR)

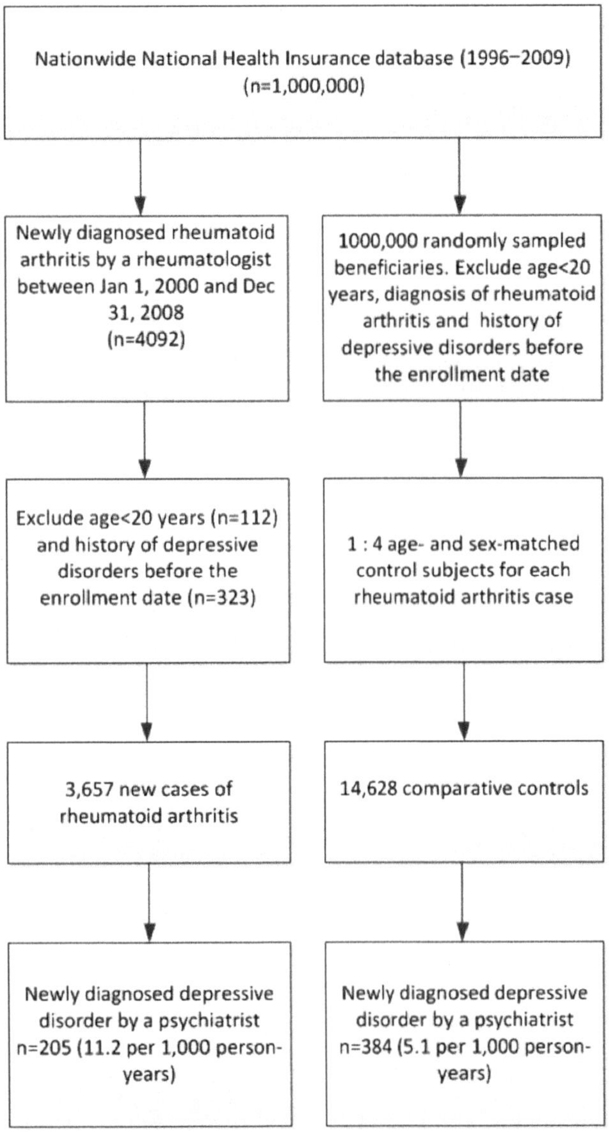

Figure 1. Flow chart of sample selection criteria.

of depressive disorders between RA patients and control patients was 2.20 (95% CI, 1.84–2.61, $P<.001$). When stratified by gender and age, the IRR of depressive disorders was still higher in the RA patients than in the control patients. The results are shown in Table 2. In RA patients, most depressive disorders (n = 163, 80%) developed with five years of being diagnosed with RA.

Rheumatoid arthritis on Risks of Clinical Depression

After adjusting for age, sex, comorbidities, urbanization, and monthly income, the hazard ratio (HR) for developing depressive disorders during the follow-up period was 2.06 times (95% CI, 1.73–2.44, $P<.001$) greater for the RA patients than for the control patients (Table 3 and figure 2).

Risks Factors for Depression in Rheumatoid arthritis Patients

In Table 4, we applied univariate analysis to predict the development of depressive disorders in the RA cohort, and the results demonstrated that the female sex (HR = 1.37, 95% CI, 0.98–1.90, $P = .063$), diabetes mellitus (HR = 1.39, 95% CI, 1.00–1.94, $P = .051$), hyperthyroidism (HR = 1.79, 95% CI, 1.09–2.94, $P = .022$), cerebrovascular disease (HR = 1.55, 95% CI, 0.99–2.41, $P = .054$) and high income (HR = 0.56, 95% CI, 0.34–0.94, $P = .028$) are significant prognostic factors. The multivariate analysis confirmed that hyperthyroidism (HR = 1.67, 95% CI, 1.01–2.76, $P = .045$) was an independent risk factor for depressive disorder in the patients with RA.

Discussion

The key findings of our study are that (1) the incidence rate of depressive disorders in patients with RA was 11.2 per 1000 person-year; (2) the risk of clinical depressive disorders was higher when patients with RA (HR = 2.06) and most depressive disorders (n = 163, 80%) developed within five years of being diagnosed with RA; (3) hyperthyroidism (HR = 1.67) might be an independent risk factor for depressive disorders among patients with RA.

The strengths of this study are the large sample size, the long follow-up period, and the diagnosis of clinical depressive disorders and rheumatoid arthritis by specialists. In addition, our study design involved an unbiased participant selection process. Because participation in the NHI is mandatory and all residents of Taiwan can access low-cost health care, referral bias is low and follow-up compliance is high.

Consistent with the results of previous studies [4–11], we found that the risk of depression in RA patients was higher than that in the non-RA control patients. Chronic inflammation is one of the possible causes. RA is a chronic inflammatory disease, and accumulating evidence implicates inflammation as a critical mediator in the pathophysiology of depressive disorders [23–26]. In the Cardiovascular Health Study of 4 268 patients, a significant association was noted between high levels of C-reactive protein and depression symptoms, even after adjusting for confounding factors [27]. Administration of cytokines including tumor necrosis factor-α in animal and human studies has been shown to induce depressive symptoms, including sleep disturbance, anorexia, loss of interest and mood disturbances [28]. Potential involved mechanisms include direct effects of pro-inflammatory cytokines on monoamine, dysregulation of the hypothalamic-pituitary-adrenal axis, impaired neuroplasticity and structural and functional brain changes [29].

The symptoms of RA such as pain and fatigue may be another possible cause for higher risk of depression in RA patients than that in the non-RA control patients. Symptoms of RA such as pain and fatigue may impair patients' function and quality of life and influence patients' perception of health status, and make the patients more prone to develop depressive symptoms [12,30]. RA patients often suffered pain and pain intensity was more clearly related to disability in RA patients [31]. Several studies have shown that chronic pain was an important risk factor for depression and suicidal behavior [32–34]. Previous study has shown that the degree of depression in RA patients varies in proportion to the level of pain [31].

Furthermore, physical comorbidities might be another possible cause for a higher prevalence of depressive disorder in RA patients. Our findings are consistent with the results of previous studies that found that a higher percentage of many physical comorbidities in RA patients, such as hypertension [35], diabetes mellitus [36], congestive heart failure [37], hypothyroidism [38], and cerebrovascular disease [39]. All of above diseases had been proposed to be related with increased the risk of depression [40–43].

Table 1. Baseline Characteristics of Patients with and without Rheumatoid Arthritis.

Demographic data	Patients with rheumatoid arthritis		Patients without rheumatoid arthritis		*P*-value
	n = 3,657		*n* = 14,628		
	n	%	*n*	%	
Age (years) (interquartile range)	51 (41–61)		51 (41–61)		
≥60	961	26.3	3,851	26.3	.966
<60	2,696	73.7	10,777	73.7	.
Sex					
Male	993	27.2	3972	27.2	.999
Female	2,664	72.8	10,656	72.8	.
Comorbidities					
Hypertension	1,186	32.4	4,032	27.6	<.001
Diabetes mellitus	687	18.8	2,305	15.8	<.001
Dyslipidemia	1,098	30.0	3,002	20.5	<.001
Coronary artery disease	45	1.2	168	1.1	.673
Congestive heart failure	172	4.7	533	3.6	.004
Cirrhosis	62	1.0	198	1.4	.117
Hyperthyroidism	219	6.0	477	3.3	<.001
Hypothyroidism	107	2.9	178	1.2	<.001
Cerebrovascular disease	316	8.6	929	6.4	<.001
Malignant neoplasms	96	2.6	338	2.3	.274
Degree of urbanization					
urban	2,238	61.2	8,787	60.1	.435
suburban	1,040	28.4	4,268	29.2	
rural	326	8.9	1,362	9.3	
Income group					
low income	1,731	47.3	7,151	48.9	.001
median income	1,430	39.1	5,820	39.8	
high income	496	13.6	1,657	11.3	
Follow-up years (median)	4.72 (2.59–7.42)		4.92 (2.69–7.55)		.004

Finally, long-term drug use in RA patients and inevitable side effects of various medications might also impaired quality of life in RA patients and increased the risk of depression in RA patients [44,45]. Previous study showed that disease-modifying drugs used for RA patients had been related to higher rates of depression, and suicidal ideation among RA patients, serving as an alert to the importance of considering also this factors in therapeutic decisions [46].

Table 2. Incidence of Depressive Disorders in Patients with and without Rheumatoid Arthritis.

	Patients with rheumatoid arthritis		Patients without rheumatoid arthritis		Risk ratio (95% CI)	*P* value
	No. of Depressive disorders	Per 1 000 person-years	No. of Depressive disorders	Per 1 000 person-years		
Total	205	11.2	384	5.1	2.20 (1.84–2.61)	<.001
Age						
≥60	49	2.8	109	1.4	1.85 (1.29–2.61)	<.001
<60	156	8.5	275	3.7	2.33 (1.91–2.85)	<.001
Sex						
Male	45	2.5	88	1.2	2.10 (1.44–3.05)	<.001
Female	160	8.7	296	3.9	2.22 (1.82–2.70)	<.001

CI indicates confidence interval.

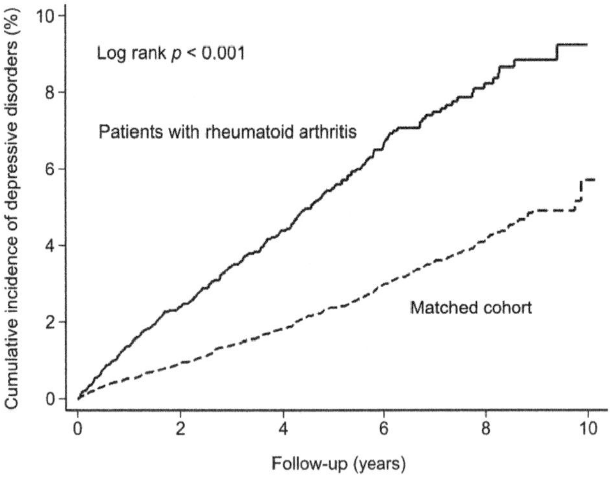

Figure 2. Cumulative incidence of depressive disorders in patients with rheumatoid arthritis (RA) and matched cohort.

According to previous studies, conservative estimates of the prevalence of depressive disorder among patients with RA ranged between 13 and 20% [13,45,47]. This prevalence rate was much higher than the rate calculated in this study. The possible reason for these two discrete findings might be partly due to difference in the methods of assessing depression [13]. In the most previous studies regarding RA and depression [5–12], rating scales, such as the Beck depression inventory, rather than diagnosis by a psychiatrist, were used for evaluation of depression in those studies. People who were recorded as depressed on rating scales may not meet the diagnostic criteria for clinical depressive disorders. However, depressive disorders in RA patients may be underdiagnosed in our study because symptoms of depressive disorders may mimic symptoms of RA, such as easily fatigue, sleep disturbance, and loss of interests with multiple somatic complaints. Physicians may have viewed RA patients' depressive symptoms as physical discomforts caused by RA and overlooked these symptoms, rather than viewing these symptoms as warning signs of depressive disorder.

There has been some discussion in the literature regarding the factors that influence the development of depression in patients with RA [48–50]. However, whether there is certain physical comorbidity as an independent risk factor for new-onset depressive disorders following a RA diagnosis has never been studied. In our study, we found that hyperthyroidism was an independent risk factor for depressive disorders in patients with RA. Studies have shown that mood disturbance, especially depressive disorders, often accompanies hyperthyroidism patients [51–54]. Alterations in components of the hypothalamic-pituitary-thyroid axis have been documented for the development of depressive disorder among patients with hyperthyroidism [53]. In addition, functional impairment caused by hyperthyroidism might play a vital role in causing psychological distresses including depressive disorders among patients with hyperthyroidism [55].

Table 3. Analyses of Risk Factors for Depressive Disorders in Patients with and without Rheumatoid Arthritis.

Predictive variables	Univariate analysis		Multivariate analysis	
	HR (95% CI)	*P* value	HR (95% CI)	*P* value
Rheumatoid arthritis	2.20 (1.86–2.60)	<.001	2.06 (1.73–2.44)	<.001
Age (<60 = 1, ≥60 = 0)	0.91 (0.76–1.10)	.327		
Sex (female = 1, male = 0)	1.34 (1.10–1.62)	.003	1.29 (1.06–1.57)	.011
Comorbidities				
Hypertension	1.39 (1.17–1.65)	<.001	1.00 (0.82–1.21)	.957
Diabetes mellitus	1.63 (1.34–1.99)	<.001	1.20 (0.96–1.50)	.116
Dyslipidemia	1.77 (1.48–2.12)	<.001	1.39 (1.14–1.71)	.001
Coronary artery disease	1.32 (0.62–2.77)	<.001	1.00 (0.47–2.13)	.995
Congestive heart failure	1.16 (0.75–1.79)	.505		
Cirrhosis	2.33 (1.39–3.89)	.001	1.91 (1.14–3.20)	.014
Hyperthyroidism	2.24 (1.61–3.12)	<.001	1.79 (1.27–2.52)	.001
Hypothyroidism	1.75 (1.01–1.76)	<.001	1.01 (0.57–1.78)	.973
Cerebrovascular disease	2.13 (1.65–2.76)	<.001	1.78 (1.36–2.33)	<.001
Malignant neoplasms	1.16 (0.65–2.05)	.622		
Degree of urbanization				
urban	Reference			
suburban	0.91 (0.76–1.10)	.319		
rural	0.85 (0.63–1.14)	.286		
Income group				
low income	Reference		Reference	
median income	0.94 (0.79–1.12)	.484	0.98 (0.83–1.17)	.847
high income	0.69 (0.51–0.92)	.013	0.75 (0.56–1.02)	.063

HR indicates hazard ratio; CI indicates confidence interval.

Table 4. Analyses of Risk factors for Depressive Disorders in Rheumatoid Arthritis Patients.

Predictive variables	Univariate analysis		Multivariate analysis	
	HR (95% CI)	*P* value	HR (95% CI)	*P* value
Age (<60 = 1, ≥60 = 0)	1.07 (0.77–1.47)	.701		
Sex (female = 1, male = 0)	1.37 (0.98–1.90)	.063	1.28 (0.92–1.79)	.146
Comorbidities				
Hypertension	1.13 (0.84–1.51)	.429		
Diabetes mellitus	1.39 (1.00–1.94)	.051	1.27 (0.90–1.78)	.171
Dyslipidemia	1.23 (0.91–1.66)	.174		
Coronary artery disease	0.97 (0.24–3.92)	.968		
Congestive heart failure	1.11 (0.57–2.16)	.766		
Cirrhosis	1.90 (0.85–4.29)	.120		
Hyperthyroidism	1.79 (1.09–2.94)	.022	1.67 (1.01–2.76)	.045
Hypothyroidism	1.34 (0.63–2.84)	.452		
Cerebrovascular disease	1.55 (0.99–2.41)	.054	1.46 (0.93–2.29)	.098
Malignant neoplasms	1.04 (0.43–2.54)	.925		
Degree of urbanization				
urban	Reference			
suburban	0.96 (0.71–1.31)	.793		
rural	0.78 (0.46–1.33)	.365		
Income group				
low income	reference		reference	
median income	1.04 (0.78–1.38)	.808	1.08 (0.81–1.44)	.603
high income	0.56 (0.34–0.94)	.028	0.62 (0.37–1.04)	.068

HR indicates hazard ratio; CI indicates confidence interval.

Our findings have certain limitations. Information regarding the family history of psychiatric disorders [56,57], lifestyle factors [58], self-perceived health, disability [59], and environmental factors (life stresses, such as recent major life event, domestic violence, childhood trauma, and social support) [60–63] are not included in the NHIRD, and all of which might be associated with the risk of development of depressive disorders. In addition, the severity of RA could not be ascertained. Whether the severity of RA influences the risk of developing depressive disorders warrants further study, despite previous studies indicating that disease activity of RA alone does not equate with depressive symptoms in RA patients reliably [47]. Furthermore, physicians may view RA patients' depressive symptoms as physical discomforts caused by RA and overlook these symptoms. Therefore, in our study, the incidence of clinical depressive disorders may be underestimated.

This population-based retrospective cohort study demonstrated that the risk of developing depressive disorders is higher among RA patients than those without RA, and that RA is an independent risk factor for depressive disorders. Hyperthyroidism is an independent risk factor for developing depressive disorders among patients with RA. Because depression was related to impairing the quality of life of RA patients, and depressive disorder is modifiable illness that is amenable to treatment, symptoms of depression should be sought in patients with RA. Future population-based prospective studies are needed to further investigate the association between RA and the risk of developing depressive disorders.

Acknowledgments

We thank Stephen Chow, Huei-Sing Chang, Cheng-Fang Hong, Chun-Hsin Hu, and Ai-Ling Hu for technical assistance. The study is based in part on data from the National Health Insurance Research Database, provided by the Bureau of National Health Insurance, Department of Health and managed by National Health Research Institutes. The interpretation and conclusions contained herein do not represent those of the Bureau of National Health Insurance, Department of Health or National Health Research Institutes.

Author Contributions

Conceived and designed the experiments: SLW LYH ZHY. Performed the experiments: SLW LYH SJT ACY. Analyzed the data: SLW LYH CHC. Contributed reagents/materials/analysis tools: SJT ACY. Contributed to the writing of the manuscript: SLW LYH ZHY.

References

1. Scott DL, Wolfe F, Huizinga TW (2010) Rheumatoid arthritis. Lancet 376: 1094–1108.
2. Rezvani A, Ayture L, Arslan M, Kurt E, Eroglu Demir S, et al. (2014) Affective temperaments in patients with rheumatoid arthritis. Int J Rheum Dis 17: 34–38.
3. Cross M, Smith E, Hoy D, Carmona L, Wolfe F, et al. (2014) The global burden of rheumatoid arthritis: estimates from the Global Burden of Disease 2010 study. Ann Rheum Dis.
4. Ahles TA, Khan SA, Yunus MB, Spiegel DA, Masi AT (1991) Psychiatric status of patients with primary fibromyalgia, patients with rheumatoid arthritis, and

subjects without pain: a blind comparison of DSM-III diagnoses. Am J Psychiatry 148: 1721–1726.
5. Callahan LF, Kaplan MR, Pincus T (1991) The Beck Depression Inventory, Center for Epidemiological Studies Depression Scale (CES-D), and General Well-Being Schedule depression subscale in rheumatoid arthritis. Criterion contamination of responses. Arthritis Care Res 4: 3–11.
6. Belza BL (1995) Comparison of self-reported fatigue in rheumatoid arthritis and controls. J Rheumatol 22: 639–643.
7. Serbo B, Jajic I (1991) Relationship of the functional status, duration of the disease and pain intensity and some psychological variables in patients with rheumatoid arthritis. Clin Rheumatol 10: 419–422.
8. Kasl SV, Cobb S (1969) The intrafamilial transmission of rheumatoid arthritis. V. Differences between rheumatoid arthritics and controls on selected personality variables. J Chronic Dis 22: 239–258.
9. Scheidt CE, Mueller-Becsangele J, Hiller K, Hartmann A, Goldacker S, et al. (2014) Self-reported symptoms of pain and depression in primary fibromyalgia syndrome and rheumatoid arthritis. Nord J Psychiatry 68: 88–92.
10. Allaire SH, Meenan RF, Anderson JJ (1991) The impact of rheumatoid arthritis on the household work performance of women. Arthritis Rheum 34: 669–678.
11. Lisitsyna TA, Zeltyn AE, Vel'tishchev D, Kovalevskaia OB, Seravina OF, et al. (2012) [Cognitive impairment and anxiety-depressive disorders in patients with rheumatoid arthritis]. Zh Nevrol Psikhiatr Im S S Korsakova 112: 96–103.
12. Coskun B, Coskun BN, Atis G, Ergenekon E, Dilek K (2014) Evaluation of sexual function in women with rheumatoid arthritis. Urol J 10: 1081–1087.
13. Dickens C, McGowan L, Clark-Carter D, Creed F (2002) Depression in rheumatoid arthritis: a systematic review of the literature with meta-analysis. Psychosom Med 64: 52–60.
14. Lowe B, Willand L, Eich W, Zipfel S, Ho AD, et al. (2004) Psychiatric comorbidity and work disability in patients with inflammatory rheumatic diseases. Psychosom Med 66: 395–402.
15. Lisitsyna TA, Veltishchev DY, Gerasimov AN, Seravina OF, Kovalevskaya OB, et al. (2013) [The magnitude of fatigue and its association with depression, pain, and inflammatory activity in rheumatoid arthritis]. Ter Arkh 85: 8–15.
16. van den Hoek J, Roorda LD, Boshuizen HC, van Hees J, Rupp I, et al. (2013) Long-term physical functioning and its association with somatic comorbidity and comorbid depression in patients with established rheumatoid arthritis: a longitudinal study. Arthritis Care Res (Hoboken) 65: 1157–1165.
17. Katz PP, Yelin EH (1994) Life activities of persons with rheumatoid arthritis with and without depressive symptoms. Arthritis Care Res 7: 69–77.
18. Wolfe F, Hawley DJ (1993) The relationship between clinical activity and depression in rheumatoid arthritis. J Rheumatol 20: 2032–2037.
19. Ang DC, Choi H, Kroenke K, Wolfe F (2005) Comorbid depression is an independent risk factor for mortality in patients with rheumatoid arthritis. J Rheumatol 32: 1013–1019.
20. Wu CY, Chen YJ, Ho HJ, Hsu YC, Kuo KN, et al. (2012) Association between nucleoside analogues and risk of hepatitis B virus-related hepatocellular carcinoma recurrence following liver resection. JAMA 308: 1906–1914.
21. Database. NHIR National Health Research Institutes.
22. Bednarek PH, Creinin MD, Reeves MF, Cwiak C, Espey E, et al. (2011) Immediate versus delayed IUD insertion after uterine aspiration. N Engl J Med 364: 2208–2217.
23. Lu Y, Feng L, Feng L, Nyunt MS, Yap KB, et al. (2013) Systemic inflammation, depression and obstructive pulmonary function: a population-based study. Respir Res 14: 53.
24. Pasco JA, Nicholson GC, Williams LJ, Jacka FN, Henry MJ, et al. (2010) Association of high-sensitivity C-reactive protein with de novo major depression. Br J Psychiatry 197: 372–377.
25. D'Mello C, Swain MG (2011) Liver-brain inflammation axis. Am J Physiol Gastrointest Liver Physiol 301: G749–761.
26. Madeeh Hashmi A, Awais Aftab M, Mazhar N, Umair M, Butt Z (2013) The fiery landscape of depression: A review of the inflammatory hypothesis. Pak J Med Sci 29: 877–884.
27. Kop WJ, Gottdiener JS, Tangen CM, Fried LP, McBurnie MA, et al. (2002) Inflammation and coagulation factors in persons >65 years of age with symptoms of depression but without evidence of myocardial ischemia. Am J Cardiol 89: 419–424.
28. Shimbo D, Chaplin W, Crossman D, Haas D, Davidson KW (2005) Role of depression and inflammation in incident coronary heart disease events. Am J Cardiol 96: 1016–1021.
29. Rosenblat JD, Cha DS, Mansur RB, McIntyre RS (2014) Inflamed moods: A review of the interactions between inflammation and mood disorders. Prog Neuropsychopharmacol Biol Psychiatry.
30. Katz PP, Yelin EH (2001) Activity loss and the onset of depressive symptoms: do some activities matter more than others? Arthritis Rheum 44: 1194–1202.
31. Peck JR, Smith TW, Ward JR, Milano R (1989) Disability and depression in rheumatoid arthritis. A multi-trait, multi-method investigation. Arthritis Rheum 32: 1100–1106.
32. Hassett AL, Aquino JK, Ilgen MA (2014) The risk of suicide mortality in chronic pain patients. Curr Pain Headache Rep 18: 436.
33. Hooley JM, Franklin JC, Nock MK (2014) Chronic pain and suicide: understanding the association. Curr Pain Headache Rep 18: 435.
34. Li JX (2014) Pain and depression comorbidity: A preclinical perspective. Behav Brain Res.
35. Manavathongchai S, Bian A, Rho YH, Oeser A, Solus JF, et al. (2013) Inflammation and hypertension in rheumatoid arthritis. J Rheumatol 40: 1806–1811.
36. Su CC, Chen Ie C, Young FN, Lian Ie B (2013) Risk of diabetes in patients with rheumatoid arthritis: a 12-year retrospective cohort study. J Rheumatol 40: 1513–1518.
37. Nicola PJ, Maradit-Kremers H, Roger VL, Jacobsen SJ, Crowson CS, et al. (2005) The risk of congestive heart failure in rheumatoid arthritis: a population-based study over 46 years. Arthritis Rheum 52: 412–420.
38. Raterman HG, van Halm VP, Voskuyl AE, Simsek S, Dijkmans BA, et al. (2008) Rheumatoid arthritis is associated with a high prevalence of hypothyroidism that amplifies its cardiovascular risk. Ann Rheum Dis 67: 229–232.
39. Wolfe F, Freundlich B, Straus WL (2003) Increase in cardiovascular and cerebrovascular disease prevalence in rheumatoid arthritis. J Rheumatol 30: 36–40.
40. Johansen A, Holmen J, Stewart R, Bjerkeset O (2012) Anxiety and depression symptoms in arterial hypertension: the influence of antihypertensive treatment. the HUNT study, Norway. Eur J Epidemiol 27: 63–72.
41. Freedland KE, Rich MW, Skala JA, Carney RM, Davila-Roman VG, et al. (2003) Prevalence of depression in hospitalized patients with congestive heart failure. Psychosom Med 65: 119–128.
42. Gothe F, Enache D, Wahlund LO, Winblad B, Crisby M, et al. (2012) Cerebrovascular diseases and depression: epidemiology, mechanisms and treatment. Panminerva Med 54: 161–170.
43. Guimaraes JM, de Souza Lopes C, Baima J, Sichieri R (2009) Depression symptoms and hypothyroidism in a population-based study of middle-aged Brazilian women. J Affect Disord 117: 120–123.
44. Pollard L, Choy EH, Scott DL (2005) The consequences of rheumatoid arthritis: quality of life measures in the individual patient. Clin Exp Rheumatol 23: S43–52.
45. Sheehy C, Murphy E, Barry M (2006) Depression in rheumatoid arthritis–underscoring the problem. Rheumatology (Oxford) 45: 1325–1327.
46. Pinho de Oliveira Ribeiro N, Rafael de Mello Schier A, Ornelas AC, Pinho de Oliveira CM, Nardi AE, et al. (2013) Anxiety, depression and suicidal ideation in patients with rheumatoid arthritis in use of methotrexate, hydroxychloroquine, leflunomide and biological drugs. Compr Psychiatry 54: 1185–1189.
47. Dickens C, Creed F (2001) The burden of depression in patients with rheumatoid arthritis. Rheumatology (Oxford) 40: 1327–1330.
48. Ramjeet J, Koutantji M, Barrett EM, Scott DG (2005) Coping and psychological adjustment in recent-onset inflammatory polyarthritis: the role of gender and age. Rheumatology (Oxford) 44: 1166–1168.
49. Covic T, Adamson B, Spencer D, Howe G (2003) A biopsychosocial model of pain and depression in rheumatoid arthritis: a 12-month longitudinal study. Rheumatology (Oxford) 42: 1287–1294.
50. Curtis R, Groarke A, Coughlan R, Gsel A (2005) Psychological stress as a predictor of psychological adjustment and health status in patients with rheumatoid arthritis. Patient Educ Couns 59: 192–198.
51. Placidi GP, Boldrini M, Patronelli A, Fiore E, Chiovato L, et al. (1998) Prevalence of psychiatric disorders in thyroid diseased patients. Neuropsychobiology 38: 222–225.
52. Kathol RG, Turner R, Delahunt J (1986) Depression and anxiety associated with hyperthyroidism: response to antithyroid therapy. Psychosomatics 27: 501–505.
53. Musselman DL, Nemeroff CB (1996) Depression and endocrine disorders: focus on the thyroid and adrenal system. Br J Psychiatry Suppl: 123–128.
54. Demet MM, Ozmen B, Deveci A, Boyvada S, Adiguzel H, et al. (2002) Depression and anxiety in hyperthyroidism. Arch Med Res 33: 552–556.
55. Lee H, Roh HS, Yoon JS, Lee SY (2010) Assessment of quality of life and depression in Korean patients with Graves' ophthalmopathy. Korean - J Ophthalmol 24: 65–72.
56. Kaur G, Tee GH, Ariaratnam S, Krishnapillai AS, China K (2013) Depression, anxiety and stress symptoms among diabetics in Malaysia: a cross sectional study in an urban primary care setting. BMC Fam Pract 14: 69.
57. Tenev VT, Robinson RG, Jorge RE (2009) Is family history of depression a risk factor for poststroke depression? Meta-analysis. Am J Geriatr Psychiatry 17: 276–280.
58. Psaltopoulou T, Sergentanis TN, Panagiotakos DB, Sergentanis IN, Kosti R, et al. (2013) Mediterranean diet and stroke, cognitive impairment, depression: A meta-analysis. Ann Neurol.
59. Becofsky K, Baruth M, Wilcox S (2013) Physical functioning, perceived disability, and depressive symptoms in adults with arthritis. Arthritis 2013: 525761.
60. Monroe SM, Slavich GM, Gotlib IH (2013) Life stress and family history for depression: The moderating role of past depressive episodes. J Psychiatr Res.
61. Chuang CH, Cattoi AL, McCall-Hosenfeld JS, Camacho F, Dyer AM, et al. (2012) Longitudinal association of intimate partner violence and depressive symptoms. Ment Health Fam Med 9: 107–114.
62. Heim C, Newport DJ, Mletzko T, Miller AH, Nemeroff CB (2008) The link between childhood trauma and depression: insights from HPA axis studies in humans. Psychoneuroendocrinology 33: 693–710.
63. Vilhjalmsson R (1993) Life stress, social support and clinical depression: a reanalysis of the literature. Soc Sci Med 37: 331–342.

5

5-Lipoxygenase Inhibitors Attenuate TNF-α-Induced Inflammation in Human Synovial Fibroblasts

Han-Ching Lin[1], Tzu-Hung Lin[1], Ming-Yueh Wu[1], Yung-Cheng Chiu[2], Chih-Hsin Tang[3], Mann-Jen Hour[4], Houng-Chi Liou[1], Huang-Ju Tu[1], Rong-Sen Yang[5]*, Wen-Mei Fu[1]*

1 Department of Pharmacology, College of Medicine, National Taiwan University and Hospital, Taipei, Taiwan, **2** Department of Orthopaedics, Taichung Veterans General Hospital, Taichung, Taiwan, **3** Department of Pharmacology, College of Medicine, China Medical University, Taichung, Taiwan, **4** School of Pharmacy, College of Medicine, China Medical University, Taichung, Taiwan, **5** Department of Orthopedics, College of Medicine, National Taiwan University and Hospital, Taipei, Taiwan

Abstract

The lipoxygenase isoform of 5-lipoxygenase (5-LOX) is reported to be overexpressed in human rheumatoid arthritis synovial tissue and involved in the progress of inflammatory arthritis. However, the detailed mechanism of how 5-lipoxygenase regulates the inflammatory response in arthritis synovial tissue is still unclear. The aim of this study was to investigate the involvement of lipoxygenase pathways in TNF-α-induced production of cytokines and chemokines. Human synovial fibroblasts from rheumatoid patients were used in this study. 5-LOX inhibitors and shRNA were used to examine the involvement of 5-LOX in TNF-α-induced cytokines and chemokines expression. The signaling pathways were examined by Western Blotting or immunofluorescence staining. The effect of 5-LOX inhibitor on TNF-α-induced chemokine expression and paw edema was also explored *in vivo* in C57BL/6 mice. Treatment with 5-LOX inhibitors significantly decreased TNF-α-induced pro-inflammatory mediators including interleukin-6 (IL-6) and monocyte chemo-attractant protein-1 (MCP-1) in human synovial fibroblasts. Knockdown of 5-LOX using shRNA exerted similar inhibitory effects. The abrogation of NF-κB activation was involved in the antagonizing effects of these inhibitors. Furthermore, 5-LOX inhibitor decreased TNF-α-induced up-regulation of serum MCP-1 level and paw edema in mouse model. Our results provide the evidence that the administration of 5-LOX inhibitors is able to ameliorate TNF-α-induced cytokine/chemokine release and paw edema, indicating that 5-LOX inhibitors may be developed for therapeutic treatment of inflammatory arthritis.

Editor: Chuen-Mao Yang, Chang Gung University, Taiwan

Funding: The work was supported by a grant from National Science Council (NSC 102-2314-B-002-045-MY3). RNAi reagents were obtained from the National RNAi Core Facility located at the Institute of Molecular Biology/Genomic Research Center, Academia Sinica. The funders had no role in study design, data collection and analysis, decision to publish, or preparation of the manuscript.

Competing Interests: The authors have declared that no competing interests exist.

* Email: rsyang@ntuh.gov.tw (R-SY); wenmei@ntu.edu.tw (W-MF)

Introduction

Rheumatoid arthritis (RA) is a chronic and systemic autoimmune syndrome, which is characterized by massive synovial proliferation and inflammation and leads to the destruction of joint cartilage and bone [1]. In addition, many kinds of cells infiltrate into the joint cavity during arthritis, including immune cells (such as macrophage, T cells and B cells) and erosive cells such as bone resorptive osteoclasts.

Arachidonic acid (AA) is a key inflammatory intermediate from the lipid composition. In response to a variety of stimuli, AA is released from membrane phospholipid by phospholipase. Pruzanski *et al.* [2] reported that the phospholipase A2 (PLA2) activity is increased in arthritis. Cytokines including TNF-α, IL-1 are reported to stimulate the activity of PLA2 [3,4]. Both cyclooxygenase (COX) and lipoxygenase (LOX) pathways are involved in the inflammatory actions related to AA [5].

The inflammatory synovial fluid in RA patients contains many kinds of cytokines including high levels of leukotrienes [6]. Leukotriene B4 (LTB4) is a downstream product of 5-lipoxygenase (5-LOX) and LTB4 is reported to be produced mainly by neutrophils, macrophages and mast cells [7]. LTB4 is considered as a powerful proinflammatory chemotactic agent and has been implicated as an important mediator of joint inflammation in RA. There are higher levels of LTB4 in the serum of RA patients than patients with inactive arthritis or normal subjects [8]. Ahmadzadeh *et al.* [9] demonstrate that the serum levels of LTB4 correlate with the disease severity. In addition, neutrophil-derived LTB4 is reported to contribute to arthritis induction and severity in a mouse inflammatory arthritis model [10].

The 5-LOX cascades and the role of LTB4 in RA are well documented. 5-LOX is required for the production of leukotrienes (LTC4, LTD4, and LTE4) which are reported to be potent broncho-constrictors and proinflammatory mediators [11]. These leukotrienes are known as the cysteinly leukotrienes (cys-LTs). 5-LOX enzyme is also involved in the production of LTB4. This lipid is primarily synthesized in neutrophils and macrophages, where the enzyme LTA4 hydrolase converts LTA4 to LTB4 [12]. In addition, 5-LOX enzyme is also involved in the production of bioactive metabolites of 5-hydroxyeicosatetraenoic acid (5-HETE) and 5-oxo-6,8,11,14-eicosatetraenoic acid (5-oxoETE) [13,14]. It

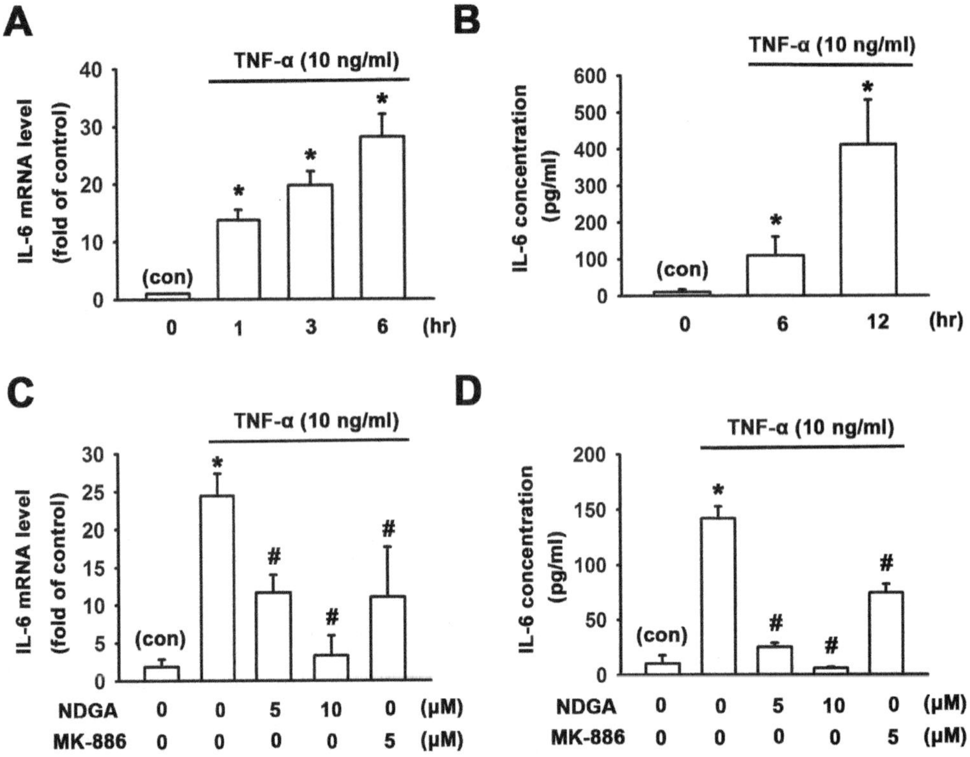

Figure 1. Inhibition of TNF-α-induced IL-6 expression by 5-LOX inhibitors in human synovial fibroblasts. Human synovial fibroblasts were incubated with TNF-α (10 ng/ml) for indicated time intervals. mRNA and released IL-6 were determined by QPCR and ELISA respectively. Treatment with TNF-α enhanced the IL-6 mRNA (A) expression and cytokine release (B) in a time-dependent manner. Pretreatment with two 5-LOX inhibitors, NDGA (5 or 10 μM) or MK-886 (5 μM) for 1 hr significantly inhibited the TNF-α-induced mRNA (C) or protein levels (D) of IL-6. Data are presented as mean ± SEM. *, $p<0.05$ compared with vehicle control (con). #, $p<0.05$ compared with TNF-α treatment alone.

has been reported that 5-LOX enzyme is present in the synovial lining of rheumatoid tissue [15]. Moreover, Gheroghe *et al.* [16] found that both 5-LOX and 15-LOX are present in RA and OA (osteoarthritis) synovium and 5-LOX is highly expressed in lining and sublining macrophages, neutrophils and mast cells.

PF-4191834, a novel selective 5-LOX inhibitor developed by Pfizer, is found to decrease arthritis-associated pain and inflammation in rat model [11]. However, the detailed mechanism of 5-LOX involved in inflammatory arthritis is still unclear. Here we found that blockade of 5-LOX by using commercial inhibitors or shRNA could decrease TNF-α-induced IL-6 and MCP-1 expression in human synovial fibroblasts. We then analyzed the signaling pathway and it was found that TNF-α-induced NF-κB activation was antagonized by 5-LOX inhibitors. In mouse model, it was also found that co-treatment of 5-LOX inhibitor could decrease TNF-α-induced MCP-1 serum level and paw edema. Our results demonstrate that 5-LOX is involved in TNF-α-induced inflammatory arthritis and may provide a new strategy for treating rheumatoid arthritis.

Methods

Ethics Statement

The study was approved by the Institutional Review Board of Taichung Veterans General Hospital (IRB TCVGH NO: C09248), and informed written consent was obtained from patients. All animal experiments were conducted in accordance with the Guidelines for Animals Research of Agriculture Council, ROC and approved by the Ethical Committee for Animal Research of the National Taiwan University (IACUC: 20120439).

Materials

Mouse monoclonal antibody for α-tubulin, C23, NF-κB p65 and rabbit polyclonal antibody for IgG, IKKα/β, IκBα, NF-κB p50, NF-κB p65 and goat anti-mouse or anti-rabbit secondary antibody conjugated with horseradish peroxidase were purchased from Santa Cruz Biotechnology (Santa Cruz, CA, USA). Mouse monoclonal antibody for phosphor-IκBα and rabbit monoclonal antibody for phosphor-IKKα/β were from Cell Signaling Technology (Danvers, MA, USA). Rabbit anti-5-LOX antibody was from Novus (Littleton, CO, USA). 5-LOX inhibitors, including MK-886, Nordihydroguaiaretic acid (NDGA); leukotriene B4 and leukotriene B4 receptor antagonist LY29311 were from Cayman Chemical Company (Ann Arbor, MI, USA). Collagenase and 4′,6-diamidino-2-phenylindole (DAPI) were from Sigma-Aldrich (St. Louis, MO, USA). Recombinant human TNF-α and enhanced chemiluminescent HRP substrate (ECL) were from Millipore (Bedford, MA, USA). We purchased RPMI-1640 medium, trypsin and anti-rabbit secondary antibody conjugated with Alexa Fluor 488 from Invitrogen (Carlsbad, CA, USA) and fetal bovine serum (FBS) from Biological Industries (Kibbutz Beit Haemek, Israel). Tri-zol was from MDBIO (Taipei, Taiwan). MMLV Reverse Transcriptase kit was from Promega (Madison, WI, USA). Taqman PCR Master Mix and qPCR probes were from Applied Biosystems/Invitrogen (Foster city, CA, USA).

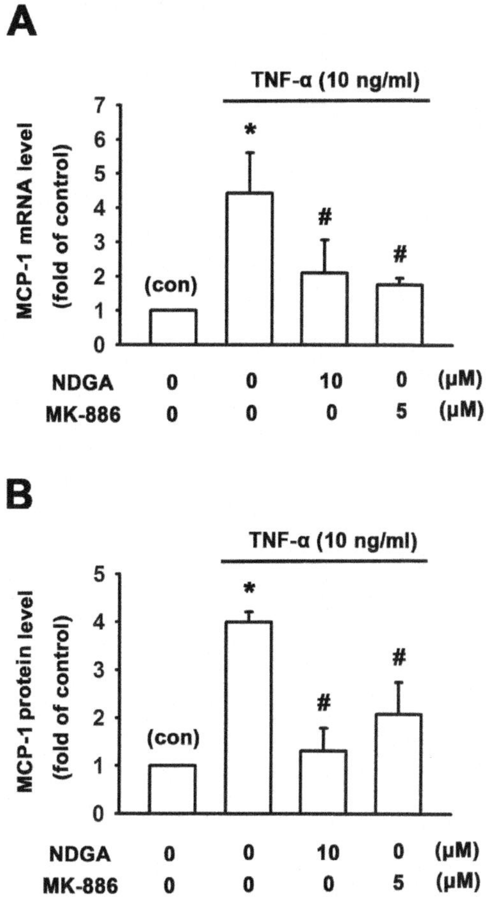

Figure 2. Attenuation of TNFα-induced MCP-1/CCL-2 expression by 5-LOX inhibitors in human synovial fibroblasts. Human synovial fibroblasts were pretreated with NDGA (10 μM) or MK-886 (5 μM) for 1 hr, and then treated with TNF-α for another 6 hr. Cell lysate was extracted for real-time PCR evaluation (A) and conditioned medium was collected for ELISA measurement of MCP-1 (B). Note that 5-LOX inhibitors NDGA and MK-886 antagonized TNF-α-induced mRNA and protein levels of MCP-1/CCL-2. Data are presented as mean ± SEM. *, $p<0.05$ compared with control (con). #, $p<0.05$ compared with TNF-α-treatment alone.

Cell cultures

Human synovial fibroblasts were isolated by collagenase treatment from synovial tissues obtained from patients with rheumatoid arthritis (RA) undergoing total knee replacement surgeries (Taichung Veterans General Hospital, Taichung, Taiwan) [17]. Patients with RA were fulfilled with diagnostic criteria of American College of Rheumatology (ACR). Fresh synovial tissues were minced and digested in a solution of collagenase, and DNase. Isolated synovial fibroblasts were filtered through 70 μm nylon filters. The cells were then grown on culture dishes in 95% air-5% CO_2 with RPMI-1640, which was supplemented with 10% heat-inactivated fetal calf serum, 100 U/ml penicillin, 100 μg/ml streptomycin, and 250 ng/ml fungizone (pH 7.6). Over 90% cultured cells were fibroblasts which were characterized by flow cytometry by using CD90 (Thy-1) antibody [18]. Synovial fibroblasts of passages four to nine were used in this study.

Quantitative real-time PCR

Total RNA were extracted from human synovial fibroblasts using a Tri-zol kit. The absorbance was measured in a spectrophotometer, Picodrop (Picodrop Ltd., Essex, UK) at 260 and 280 nm. RNA was used for RT-PCR by using two-step MMLV RT kit. Gene expression was detected by Real-Time PCR which was executed by using a SYBR Green PCR Master Mix (Applied Biosystems, Foster city, CA, USA) and an ABI StepOnePlus Real-time PCR system (Applied Biosystems). The cDNA was amplified with gene specific primers as shown below:

GAPDH: [19].
Forward primer: TGGGTGTGAACCATGAGAAG.
Reverse primer: GCTAAGCAGTTGGTGGTGC.
IL-6: [20].
Forward primer: TCACTGGTCTTTTGGAGTTTGA.
Reverse primer: AGAGCCCTCAGGCTGGACT.
MCP-1/CCL-2: [21].
Forward primer: ATGCAATCAATGCCCCAGTC.
Reverse primer: TGCAGATTCTTGGGTTGTGG.

Amplification was performed in the following cycling conditions: 50°C for 2 min and 95°C for 10 min and then 40 cycles at 95°C for 15 s followed by 60°C for 1 min. The optimal concentrations of primers and templates used in each reaction were established based on the standard curve created before reaction and corresponding to nearly 100% efficiency of the reaction. The reference household gene used to normalize the amount of mRNA was GAPDH. The fold change in gene expression relative to control was calculated by $2^{-\Delta\Delta CT}$.

Measurement of cytokines and chemokines

After treatment with TNF-α or test substances, the levels of IL-6 or MCP-1 in the culture medium of human synovial fibroblasts and serum from mice were determined by enzyme-linked immunosorbent assay (ELISA). The conditioned medium or serum from mice was obtained and IL-6 or MCP-1 was detected according to the manufacturer's protocol (R&D Systems, Minneapolis, MN, USA). All independent experiments were performed and the absorbance was determined using microplate reader (Bio-Tek, Winooski, VT, USA).

Transfection of RNA interference

The 5-LOX-shRNA conjugated on the vector of pLKO.1 with ampicillin-resistant region was purchased from National RNAi Core Facility (RNAi Core, Taipei, Taiwan). 3 μg 5-LOX-shRNA and 6 μl Lipofectamine 2000 (Invitrogen, Carlsbad, CA, USA) were premixed with OPTI-MEM separately for 5 min and then mixed with each other for 25 min and then applied to human synovial fibroblasts. The empty vector of shRNA was used as negative control. After 36 hr, the cells were harvested or the culture medium was replaced with serum-free medium and test substances.

Western Blot

After treatment with test substances, synovial fibroblasts were then washed with cold PBS and lysed for 30 min at 4°C with lysis buffer as described previously [18]. For the separation of cytoplasmic extracts (CE) and nuclear extracts, cells were cultured onto 10 cm dish. After reaching confluence, cells were treated with test substances, cytoplasmic extracts and nuclear extracts were separated by NE-PER (Thermo Scientific-Pierce, Rockford, IL, USA). Equal protein (30 μg) was applied per lane, and electrophoresis was performed under denaturing conditions on a 8% or 12% SDS gel and transferred to nitrocellulose membranes

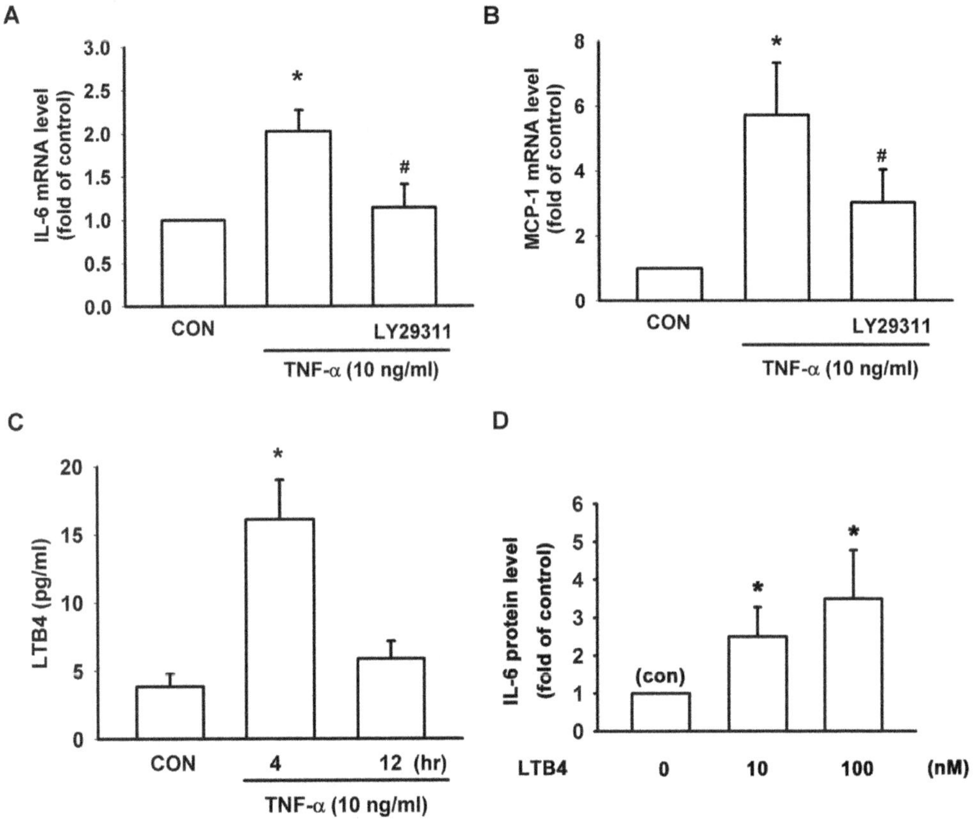

Figure 3. Involvement of leukotriene B4 in TNF-α-induced cytokine expression in human synovial fibroblasts. Human synovial fibroblasts were pretreated with LTB4 receptor antagonist LY29311 (1 μM) for 1 hr, and then treated with TNF-α for another 6 hr. TNF-α-induced up-regulation of IL-6 and MCP-1 were antagonized by LY29311 (A, B). RASFs were treated with TNF-α (10 ng/ml) for 4 and 12 hr, and the conditioned medium was collected for ELISA measurement of LTB4. Data show that LTB4 was increased at 4 hr (C). (D) Human synovial fibroblasts were treated with leukotriene B4 for 6 hrs at different concentrations, and conditioned medium was collected for ELISA assay. ELISA analysis showed that treatment with leukotriene B4 enhanced IL-6 release in a concentration-dependent manner. Data are presented as mean ± SEM. *, $p<0.05$ compared with control (con). #, $p<0.05$ compared with TNF-α-treatment alone.

(Invitrogen). The blots were blocked with 5% non-fat milk in TBS-T (0.5% Tween 20 in 20 mM Tris and 137 mM NaCl) for 1 h at room temperature and then probed with antibodies against 5-LOX, phosphor-IκBα, IκBα, phospho-IKKα/β, IKKα/β, NF-κB p50, NF-κB p65 (1:1000) at 4°C overnight. After 3 washes by TBS-T, the blots were subsequently incubated with goat anti-rabbit or anti-mouse peroxidase-conjugated secondary antibody (1:10000) for 1 h at room temperature. The blots were visualized by enhanced chemiluminescence using Amersham HyperfilmTM ECL (GE Healthcare, Pollards Wood, UK) or Biospectrum Imaging System (UVP, Upland, CA, USA). For normalization purposes, the same blot was also probed with mouse anti-α-tubulin antibody or mouse anti-C23 antibody (1:1000).

Immunofluorescent staining

For immunolabeling studies, synovial fibroblasts were seeded on glass overnight and then treated with test substances. After TNF-α (25 ng/ml) treatment for 30 min with or without inhibitors, 4% paraformaldehyde was used to fix the cells for 15 min. 0.1% triton was used to permeabilize the cells and 4% BSA was used for blocking non-specific binding for 1 hr. Synovial fibroblasts were stained with primary mouse monoclonal antibody against NFκB-p65 (1:200) (Santa Cruz sc-8008) (Lin *et al.*, 2011) overnight and then with Alexa Fluor 488-conjugated goat anti-mouse secondary antibody (Invitrogen, Carlsbad, California). The nucleus was counterstained by DAPI and the confocal images were obtained by using excitation wavelength 494 nm and emission wavelength 519 nm, respectively (for Alexa-488) (model SP5 TCS; Leica, Heidelberg, Germany) and the thickness of optical sections was set at 0.8 μm.

TNF-α-induced inflammation in animal models

8 weeks-old male C57BL/6 mice and 15-LOX knockout mice were purchased from the Laboratory Animal Center of National Taiwan University. All mice were kept under standard temperature, humidity, and timed lighting conditions and provided mouse chow and water ad libitum.

Recombinant mouse TNF-α (40 μg/kg) in the presence or absence of 5-LOX inhibitor NDGA (10 mg/kg) was injected intravenously from femoral vein of male C57BL/6 mice. Mice were sacrificed 6 hr later and serum was collected to perform ELISA analysis.

For the paw swelling experiment, TNF-α (200 ng dissolved in 10 μl PBS) in the presence or absence of NDGA (10 μM) or MK-886 (10 μM) was injected intraplantarly into the right hind paw and the PBS-injected left hind paw was used as control. Paw thickness was measured with digimatic caliper (Mitutoyo, Japan). The change of paw thickness was compared to the paw thickness at 0 hr.

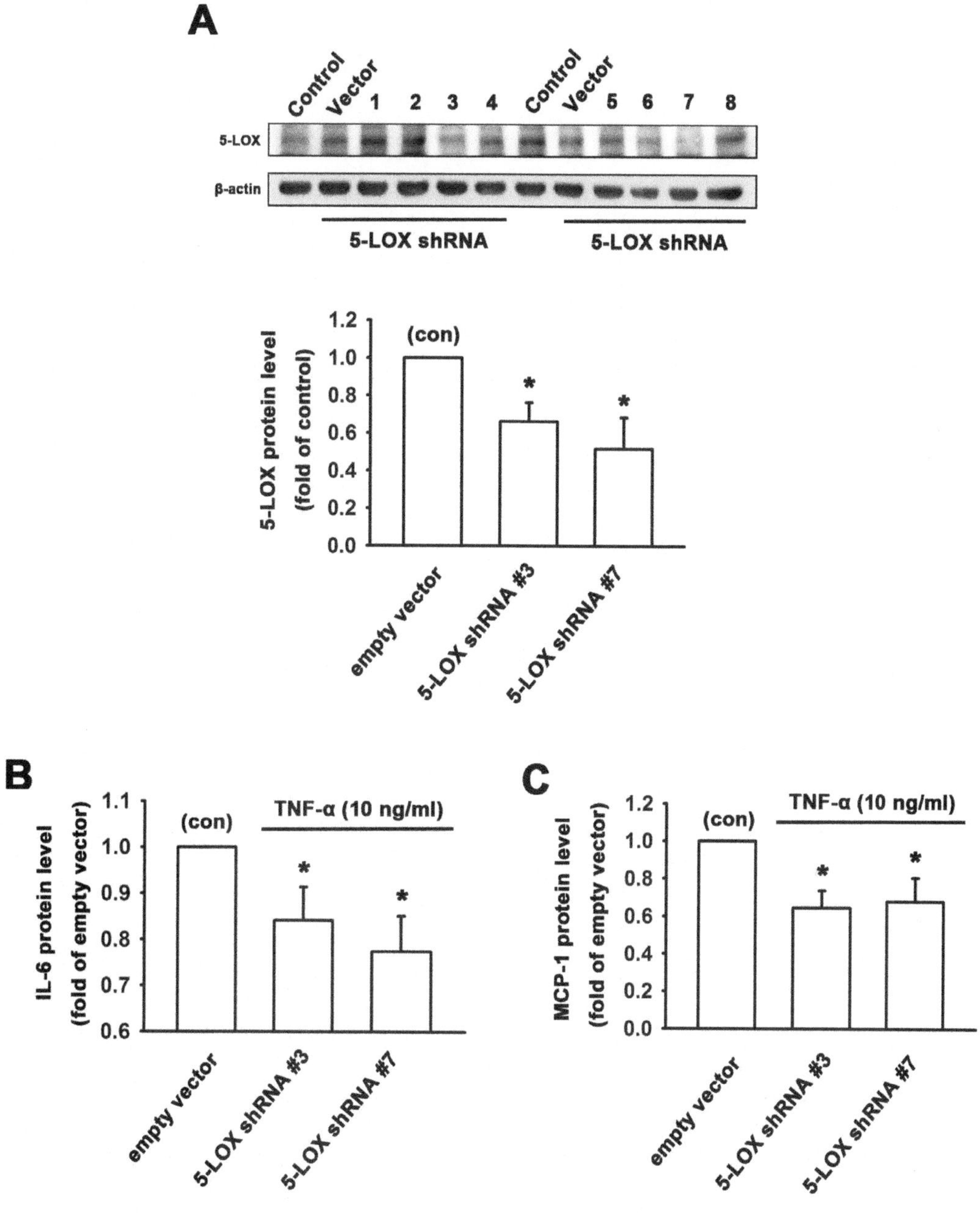

Figure 4. Knockdown of 5-LOX inhibits TNF-α-induced IL-6 and MCP-1 release in human synovial fibroblasts. Total protein extracts from RASFs transfected with empty vector or 5-LOX shRNA were used for Western blotting. (A) Immunoblotting showed that cells transfected with 5-LOX shRNA of clone No.3 and No.7 markedly decreased 5-LOX expression. Human synovial fibroblasts transfected with empty vector or 5-LOX shRNA were treated with TNF-α for 6 hr. IL-6 and MCP-1 protein release in the conditioned medium was evaluated by ELISA. Note that knockdown of 5-LOX decreased IL-6 (B) and MCP-1 (C) release following TNF-α treatment for 6 hr. Data are presented as mean ± SEM. *, $p<0.05$ compared with empty vector control (con).

Statistics

The data given were means ± S.E.M. The significance of difference between the experimental group and control was assessed by one-way analysis of variance (ANOVA) and 2-tailed Student's t-test. The difference is significant if the *p* value is less than 0.05.

Results

Effect of 5-LOX inhibitors on TNF-α-induced IL-6 expression in human synovial fibroblasts

In inflammatory arthritis, synovial fibroblasts contribute to synovium inflammation, angiogenesis, matrix degradation by its abilities to produce inflammatory cytokines, matrix degradation enzymes and angiogenic factor [22]. In addition, TNF-α is the potent inflammatory cytokine and is responsible for synovial fibroblasts-involved cartilage degradation. First of all, we examined whether TNF-α can enhance the production of pro-

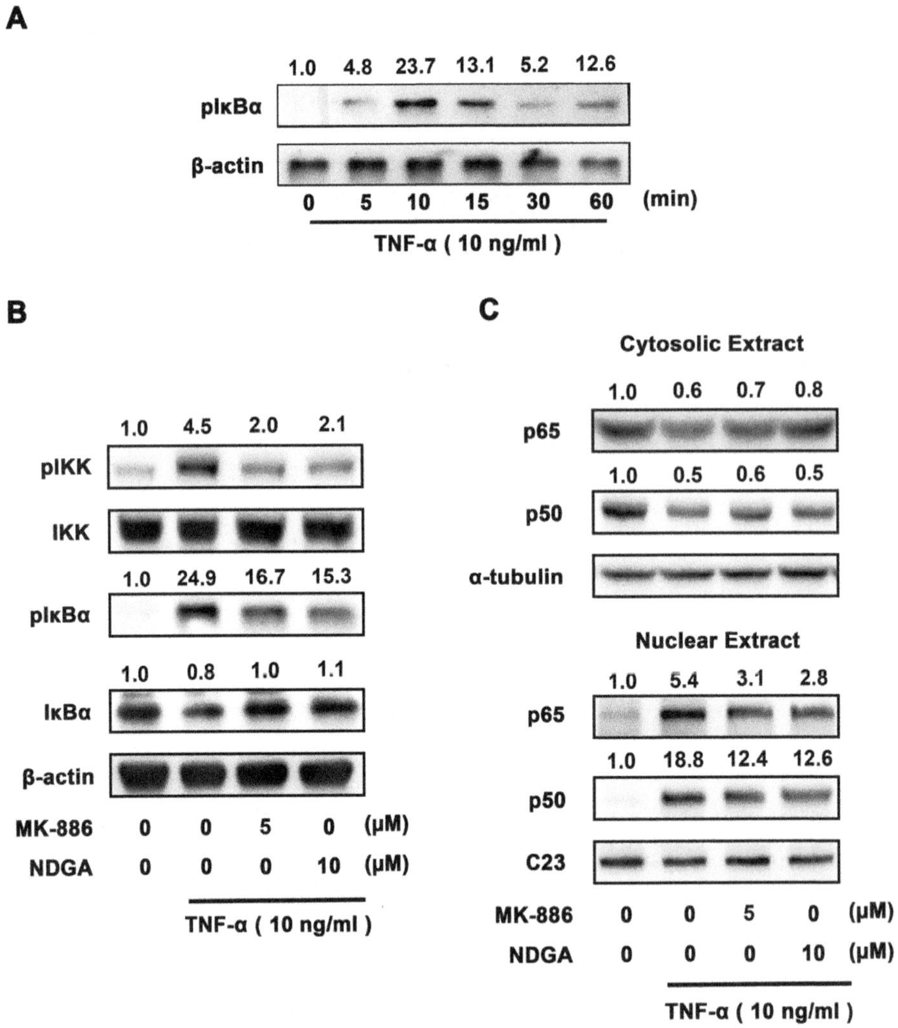

Figure 5. 5-LOX inhibitors antagonize TNF-α-induced IKKα/β activation, IκBα phosphorylation, IκBα degradation and NF-κB nuclear translocation in human synovial fibroblasts. (A) Immunoblotting showed that treatment of TNF-α (10 ng/ml) enhanced the phosphorylation of IκBα time-dependently in human synovial fibroblasts. (B) Human synovial fibroblasts were pre-incubated with 5-LOX inhibitors NDGA (10 μM) or MK-886 (5 μM) for 1 hr and then exposed to TNF-α for another 10 min. Note that pretreatment with NDGA or MK-886 could antagonize TNF-α-induced effects. (C) Human synovial fibroblasts were pretreated with NDGA (10 μM) or MK-886 (5 μM) for 1 hr. TNF-α (10 ng/ml) was then added for another 30 min. Cytosolic and nuclear extracts were separated by NE-PER kit. Note that NDGA or MK-886 significantly antagonized the nuclear translocation of NF-κB subunits of p65 and p50. C23 was used as nucleus marker.

inflammatory cytokine, IL-6. Human synovial fibroblasts were incubated with TNF-α (10 ng/ml) in serum-free medium for several time intervals. The mRNA and released protein level of IL-6 were evaluated by quantitative PCR and ELISA, respectively. Figures 1A and 1B showed that treatment with TNF-α enhanced the mRNA and protein levels of IL-6 in a time-dependent manner. Treatment of TNF-α for 6 hr increased mRNA expression of IL-6 to 28.2±3.9 fold of control (Figure 1A). In addition, treatment of TNF-α also increased IL-6 protein release to 9.9±2.3 fold and 40.0±7.0 fold of control at 6 or 12 hr, respectively (Figure 1B).

To investigate the role of 5-LOX in rheumatoid arthritis, human synovial fibroblasts were pretreated with 5-LOX inhibitors NDGA (5 and 10 μM) and MK-886 (5 μM) for 1 hr and then treated with TNF-α (10 ng/ml) for next 6 hr. mRNA extracted from cell lysates was evaluated by quantitative PCR and the conditioned medium collected was measured for IL-6 protein release by ELISA assay. Real-time PCR analysis showed that TNF-α significantly increased IL-6 mRNA levels and pretreatment with 5-LOX inhibitors NDGA (5 and 10 μM) and MK-886 (5 μM) could inhibit the upregulatory effect of TNF-α by 54.7±6.0%, 91.4±4.3% and 57.3±12.6%, respectively (Figure 1C). In addition, treatment with TNF-α increased the secreted IL-6 in the conditioned medium and pretreatment of 5-LOX inhibitors NDGA (5 and 10 μM) and MK-886 (5 μM) decreased the TNF-α-induced IL-6 protein levels by 83.0±1.1%, 96.3±0.4% and 48.1±2.8%, respectively (Figure 1D).

Effect of 5-LOX inhibitors on TNF-α-induced MCP-1/CCL-2 expression in human synovial fibroblasts

One of potential therapy in RA is targeting chemokines and a randomized clinical trial with an anti-CCL2/MCP-1 monoclonal antibody in RA patients has been reported previously [23]. MCP-1 plays a key role in leukocyte migration and recruitment of mononuclear phagocytes during inflammation in the joint and

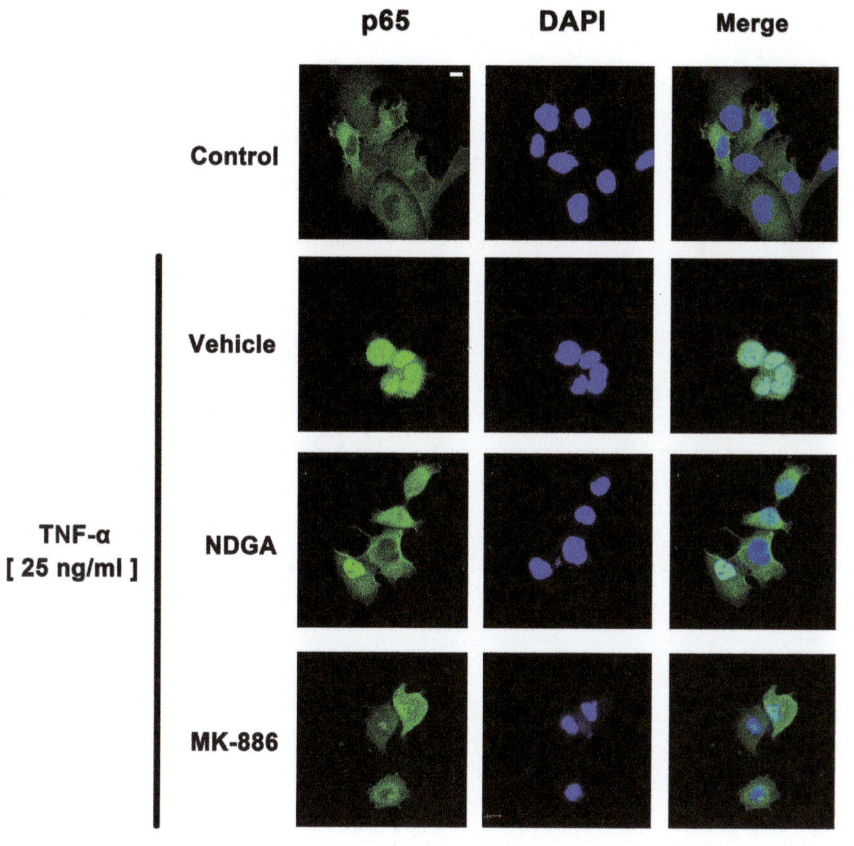

Figure 6. 5-LOX inhibitors antagonize TNF-α-induced nuclear translocation of p65. Immunofluorescent staining showed that p65 translocated into nucleus after treatment of TNF-α (25 ng/ml) for 30 min. Pretreatment of 5-LOX inhibitors NDGA (10 μM) or MK-886 (5 μM) antagonized the nuclear translocation of p65. DAPI staining was used to indicate the location of nucleus. Scale: 5 μm.

previous study indicated that there is overproduction of CCL-2/MCP-1 in RA patient's synovium [24]. To further elucidate the anti-inflammatory effects of 5-LOX inhibitors in the rheumatoid arthritis, human synovial fibroblasts were pretreated with 5-LOX inhibitors NDGA (10 μM) and MK-886 (5 μM) for 1 hr and then treated with TNF-α (10 ng/ml) for another 6 hr. mRNA levels extracted from cell lysates was evaluated by Real-time PCR and the supernatant was collected for measuring MCP-1 protein levels by ELISA assay. Real-time PCR analysis showed that TNF-α significantly increased MCP-1 mRNA expression to 4.5±0.5 fold of vehicle control (Figure 2A). Pretreatment of 5-LOX inhibitors NDGA (10 μM) and MK-886 (5 μM) decreased TNF-α-induced MCP-1 mRNA levels by 70.6±11.0%, and 77.9±3.2%, respectively (Figure 2A). The released MCP-1 was analysed by ELISA analysis and showed that treatment with TNF-α increased the secreted MCP-1 in the conditioned medium to 4.0±0.1 fold of vehicle control (Figure 2B). Pretreatment of 5-LOX inhibitors NDGA (10 μM) and MK-886 (5 μM) antagonized TNF-α-induced MCP-1 protein levels by 89.6±9.1%, and 63.8±12.7%, respectively (Figure 2B).

Involvement of leukotriene B4 in TNF-α-induced cytokine expression in human synovial fibroblasts

Leukotriene B4 (LTB4) is one of 5-Lipoxygenase downstream metabolites and plays an important role in pathogenesis of RA [25]. Recent study has suggested that LTB4 is an essential and non-redundant role in both acute and chronic inflammation of rheumatoid arthritis [10]. In addition, exogenous LTB4 could increase the expression of cytokines like TNF-α and IL-1β in human synovial fibroblasts [26]. We thus investigated whether LTB4 is involved incytokines release in human synovial fibroblasts. Human synovial fibroblasts were pretreated with LTB4 receptor antagonist LY29311 (1 μM) for 1 hr and then treated with TNF-α (10 ng/ml) for another 6 hr. mRNA were extracted for Real-time PCR analysis, and the results show that TNF-α-induced up-regulation of IL-6 and MCP-1 were reduced by LY29311 (Figure 3A, 3B). In addition, treatment of TNF-α for 4 hr increased the secretion of LTB4 from 3.9±0.9 to 16.1±2.9 (pg/ml) (Figure 3C). Treatmentwith LTB4 at different concentrations in serum-free RPMI medium for 6 hr and the quantity of IL-6 in conditioned medium was measured. It was found that treatment with LTB4 (10, 100 nM) increased secreted IL-6 protein levels to 2.5±0.5-fold and 3.5±0.3 fold of control, respectively (Figure 3D).

Knockdown of 5-LOX inhibits TNF-α-induced IL-6 and MCP-1 release in human synovial fibroblasts

To further examine the role of 5-LOX in TNF-α-induced IL-6 and MCP-1 expression, 5-LOX knockdown was performed by using 5-LOX shRNA and the protein release in the conditioned medium in response to TNF-α administration was measured. Total protein extracts from RASFs transfected with empty vector or 5-LOX shRNA were analyzed by immunoblotting. Figure 4A showed that cells transfected with 5-LOX shRNA No.3 and No.7 significantly decreased 5-LOX expression. Human synovial fibroblasts transfected with empty vector or 5-LOX shRNA clone No.3 and No.7 were then used to treat with TNF-α for 6 hr. IL-6

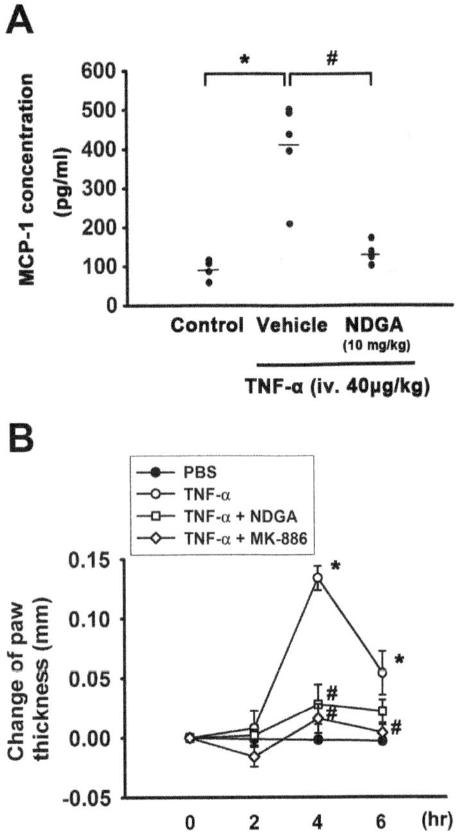

Figure 7. Antagonism by 5-LOX inhibitors on TNF-α-induced up-regulation of serum monocyte chemo-attractant protein-1 (MCP-1) level and paw edema in mice. (A) Male C57BL/6 mice (8 weeks-old) were injected with TNF-α (40 μg/kg in 0.2 ml saline) into femoral vein and 5-LOX inhibitor NDGA (10 mg/kg) was co-treated in another cohort. After 6 hr, mice were sacrificed and serum was collected for ELISA analysis. Note that mice injected with TNF-α markedly increased MCP-1 levels in serum, which was inhibited by co-treatment with 5-LOX inhibitor NDGA (10 mg/kg) (n = 4–5). (B) TNF-α was intraplantarly injected onto the paw of male C57BL/6 mice (8 weeks-old). 5-LOX inhibitors, NDGA (10 μM) or MK-886 (10 μM) was co-injected with TNF-α (10 μl). It was found that TNF-α induced acute paw edema and increased paw thickness during 4–6 hr. Note that co-administration of NDGA or MK-886 significantly attenuated TNF-α-induced paw edema (n = 5). Data are presented as mean ± SEM. *, $p < 0.05$ compared with vehicle control. #, $p < 0.05$ compared with TNF-α-treatment alone.

and MCP-1 protein release in the conditioned medium was evaluated by ELISA analysis. It was found that knockdown of 5-LOX with shRNA No.3 and No.7 decreased TNF-α-induced IL-6 protein release by 16.8±4.7% and 23.8±4.9%, respectively (Figure 4B). In addition, knockdown of 5-LOX with shRNA No.3 and No.7 reduced TNF-α-induced MCP-1 protein release by 36.6±5.2% and 32.6±7.9% following 6 hr treatment with TNF-α (Figure 4C).

Effect of 5-LOX inhibitors on TNF-α-induced IKKα/β activation, IκBα phosphorylation, IκBα degradation in human synovial fibroblasts

NF-κB is implicated in the transcriptional regulation of inflammatory response by TNF-α. Bondeson *et al.* [27] have demonstrated that the activation of NF-κB plays an important role

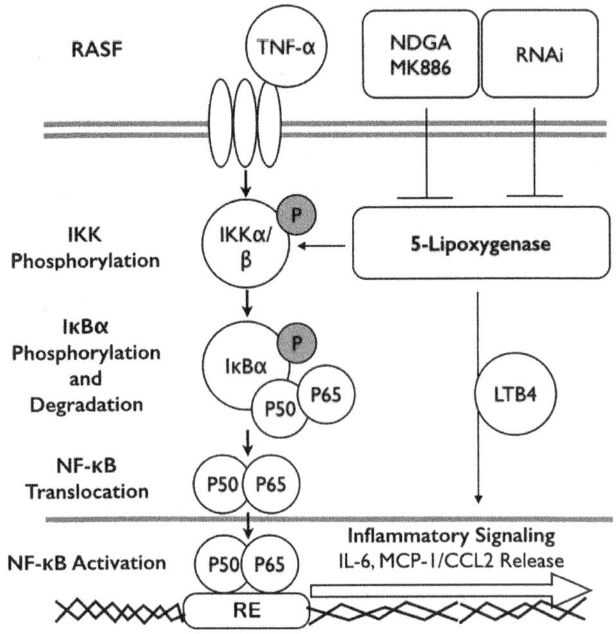

Figure 8. Schematic diagram of the involvement of 5-LOX in TNF-α-induced cytokine/chemokine release. TNF-α increased the release of IL-6 and MCP-1 via the activation of NF-κB signaling in RASFs. 5-LOX inhibitors, NDGA or MK886 inhibited TNF-α-induced activation of IKK and IκBα degradation. 5-LOX inhibitors also inhibited the translocation of NF-κB subunits of p50 and p65 into nucleus (response element) and then decreased TNF-α-induced IL-6 and MCP-1 release. Knockdown of 5-LOX by RNAi exerted similar inhibitory effects.

in the inflammatory action of TNF-α in synovial fibroblasts. To examine whether NF-κB pathway is involved in the antagonism of 5-LOX inhibitors on TNF-α-induced cytokine expression in human synovial fibroblasts, IKKα/β activation, IκBα phosphorylation, and IκBα degradation were evaluated by immunoblotting after stimulation by TNF-α. Since the canonical NF-κB pathway is induced by TNF-α and this activation leads to the recruitment and activation of an IKK complex comprising IKK alpha and/or IKK beta catalytic subunits. The IKK complex then phosphorylated IκBα at ser32 and ser36 to produce ubiquitination of IκBα at lysine residues and subsequent degradation by the 26 s proteasome. NF-κB complex (p50 and p65), which is associated with IκB to retain in the cytosol under resting state, is released and translocates to the nucleus [28]. Therefore, we first investigated the time-course of IκBα phosphorylation in human synovial fibroblasts. Cells were treated by TNF-α (10 ng/ml) for 5, 10, 15, 30, and 60 min and total proteins were extracted for Western blotting. The results showed that treatment with TNF-α (10 ng/ml) enhanced the phosphorylation of IκBα time-dependently in human synovial fibroblasts, and the phosphorylation of IκBα reached a peak at 10 min (Figure 5A). Human synovial fibroblasts were then pre-incubated with 5-LOX inhibitors NDGA (10 μM) or MK-886 (5 μM) for 1 hr and then exposed to TNF-α for another 10 min. It was found that pretreatment with NDGA or MK-886 could antagonize TNF-α-induced IKKα/β activation, IκBα phosphorylation and IκBα degradation (Figure 5B). Pretreatment of NDGA or MK-886 also inhibited the TNF-α-induced nuclear translocation of NF-κB subunits of p50 and p65 (Figure 5C). Immunofluorescence staining was also used to evaluate whether 5-LOX antagonized TNF-α-induced NF-κB nuclear translocation. Human synovial fibroblasts were treated with TNF-α (25 ng/ml) for 30 min and p65 translocated into nucleus (Figure 6). Pretreatment with 5-LOX inhibitors, including NDGA (10 μM) and MK-886 (5 μM) for 1 hr antagonized TNF-α-induced nuclear translocation of p65 (Figure 6). These results indicated that 5-LOX inhibitors decreased TNF-α-induced cytokine/chemokine expression via the abrogation of NF-κB signalling.

Effect of 5-LOX inhibitors on TNF-α-induced monocyte chemo-attractant protein-1 (MCP-1) release and paw edema in animal model

We have elucidated the role of 5-LOX in TNF-α-induced cytokines and chemokines production *in vitro*. We then examined the effect of 5-LOX inhibitor in animal model. Male C57BL/6 mice were injected with TNF-α (40 μg/kg, via femoral vein) with or without 5-LOX inhibitor NDGA (10 mg/kg). After 6 hr, mice were sacrificed and serum was collected to perform ELISA analysis. It was found that mice injected with TNF-α significantly increased MCP-1 levels in serum to 4.4±0.6 fold of vehicle-treated mice. However, co-treatment TNF-α with 5-LOX inhibitor NDGA (10 mg/kg) significantly reduced TNF-α-induced MCP-1 protein release in serum by 67.9±4.3% (Figure 7A). Moreover, we examined the effects of 5-LOX inhibitors on TNF-α-induced acute paw edema in mice model. As shown in figure 7B, intraplantar injection of TNF-α-increased the paw thickness and the thickness reached the peak at 4 hr. Co-administration with 5-LOX inhibitors, NDGA (10 μM) or MK-886 (10 μM) could markedly ameliorate TNF-α-induced paw edema. These results suggest that 5-LOX inhibitor can reduce TNF-α-induced chemokine production and paw edema *in vivo*.

Discussion

Synovial fibroblasts play a pivotal role in early events of rheumatoid arthritis [29]. Many factors contribute to synovial fibroblasts activation and enhance the bone destruction [22]. Various reports have indicated that cytokines such as TNF-α, IL-1β and IL-6 play key roles in driving the inflammation and synovial cell proliferation characterizing rheumatoid arthritis-associated joint destruction [30]. Moreover, synovial fibroblasts have capacities to produce and secrete a wide range of pro-inflammatory mediators, including cytokines like IL-1β, IL-6, TNF-α and chemokines like MCP-1, MIP-1a [31]. Inflammatory cytokines also can induce the release of additional inflammatory factors and enhance the activation of synovial fibroblasts [32]. Furthermore, cytokines themselves can further promote more inflammatory cytokines and chemokines in synovial fibroblasts, amplifying inflammatory events in the synovium [33]. Therefore, it is important to ameliorate the activation of synovial fibroblasts in the treatment of inflammatory arthritis.

Current therapies of biologic agents for rheumatoid arthritis have targeted these cytokines. Despite of the good efficacy of biologic agents such as TNF-α or IL-1β blocker for many patients with rheumatoid arthritis, augmented risk of some adverse side effects such as infection [34] and malignancy [35] still persist in concern. In addition, these biological therapies such as etanercept, abatacept, rituximab, and tocilizumab for rheumatoid arthritis directly target immune cells such as T and B cells and pro-inflammatory cytokines. It indicates that other therapies and new targets in the treatment of RA, especially ones targeting non-immune cells like synovial fibroblasts may be possible.

5-lipoxygenase is reported to be present in RA synovium and mostly expressed in macrophages, neutrophils and mast cells in the sublining layer [16]. Here we found that synovial fibroblasts isolated from rheumatoid arthritis patients express high protein levels of 5-LOX which is consistent with high levels of leukotriene B4, a 5-LOX downstream metabolite, found in synovial fluid in rheumatoid arthritis patients [6]. Leukotrienes are regarded as inflammatory mediators derived from the 5-LOX cascade of arachidonic acid [36] and implicated in the pathogenesis of several human acute and chronic inflammatory diseases such as atherosclerosis, dermatitis, cancer and rheumatoid arthritis [36]. Unlike diseases such as asthma, allergic rhinitis, and ischemia/stroke that associated with an overproduction of CysLTs, rheumatoid arthritis is more linked to an overproduction of LTB4, another branch downstream metabolite of 5-LOX [37]. LTB4 has long been considered to have deleterious effects in arthritis. In atherosclerosis, LTB4 can induce the overexpression of TNF-α, IL-6 and MCP-1 mRNA in cultured monocytes, causing an inflammatory environment [38]. In addition, we also found that exogenous LTB4 increased IL-6 protein release in a concentration-dependent manner in synovial fibroblasts, and the TNF-α-induced up-regulation of IL-6 and MCP-1 were antagonized by the pretreatment of leukotriene B4 receptor antagonist LY29311. TNF-α is reported to be involved in the arachidonic acid metabolism. TNF-α at 1 nM stimulates the lipoxygenase pathway, and 5-LOX metabolites including LTB4 and 5-HETE increase in human osteoblastic osteosarcoma cells [39]. Moreover, in immune inflammation, it is found that TNF-α is involved in ovalbumin-induced neutrophil migration through a LTB4-dependent mechanism so that MK-886, a 5-LOX inhibitor, inhibits the TNF-α-induced neutrophil migration. TNF-α can also stimulate the secretion of LTB4 from peritoneal cells [40]. LTB4 also promotes TNF-α-induced CCL27 expression via the NF-κB pathway in human keratinocytes [41]. Here we found that 5-LOX inhibitors, including MK-886 and NDGA significantly antagonized TNF-α-induced IL-6 and MCP-1 mRNA expression and protein release in a concentration-dependent manner in human synovial fibroblasts. In addition, it was also found that knockdown of 5-LOX by shRNA transient transfection reduced the protein release of IL-6 and MCP-1 in synovial fibroblasts, indicating that 5-LOX pathway or even its downstream metabolites play a crucial role in TNF-α-induced cytokine and chemokine upregulation in human synovial fibroblasts. These findings are also consistent with previous studies that mice lacking 5-LOX or treatment with 5-LOX inhibitor are protected from inflammatory arthritis [10].

NF-κB is activated during the early stage of joint inflammation in human synovial tissue [42]. LTB4, the downstream metabolite of 5-LOX, increases the mRNA expression of IL-6 and MCP-1 via BLT1 and BLT2, G protein-coupled receptors of leukotrienes, via a NF-κB-dependent mechanism in atherosclerosis [38]. Moreover, LTB4 may amplify the NF-κB activation through Stat1-dependent expression of MyD88 and reducing SOCS1 inhibition of MyD88 in mouse macrophages [43]. 5-LOX also plays a key role in LPS-induced monocyte adhesion to vascular endothelium by increasing expression of Mac-1 via NF-κB signaling pathways [44], indicating that 5-LOX enzyme activities or its downstream metabolites may be linked to NF-κB pathway. Here we found that 5-LOX inhibitors including MK-886 and NDGA antagonized TNF-α-induced IKKα/β activation, IκBα phosphorylation and IκBα degradation in human synovial fibroblasts. Furthermore, 5-LOX inhibitors also antagonized TNF-α-induced nuclear translocation of NF-κB subunits of p65 and p50 in Western blotting and immunofluorescent staining. Moreover, IκBα phosphorylation and TNF-α-induced nuclear translocation of NF-κB subunits of p65 were also antagonized by leukotriene B4 receptor antagonist LY29311 (figure S1). These results suggest that 5-LOX and its downstream products are involved in TNF-α-induced cytokines and chemokines expression via the inhibition of NF-κB signaling pathways in human synovial fibroblasts.

Here we found that mice treated with NDGA significantly reduced TNF-α-induced up-regulation of MCP-1 in the serum and TNF-α-induced paw edema, whereas 5-LOX inhibitor could not completely reverse TNF-α-induced expression of IL-6 and MCP-1, indicating that other signals are involved in this action. In addition to LOX, arachidonic acid could also be metabolized by COX-2 to produce the bioactive eicosanoids, which play another pivotal part in the inflammatory arthritis. Developing novel 5-LOX inhibitor or 5-LOX/COX-2 dual inhibitor is a therapeutic strategy to treat inflammatory diseases including arthritis [45]. Neuro-inflammation of brain damage induced by permanent cerebral ischemia and renal ischemia-reperfusion injury can be protected by treatment of zileuton, a 5-LOX inhibitor [46,47]. 5-LOX inhibitor, NDGA is reported to attenuate ovalbumin-induced lung inflammation in rats [48]. Oral administration with PF-4191834, which is developed by Pfizer, is able to ameliorate arthritis-associated pain and inflammation in rat model [11]. In addition, lecofelone, a COX/5-LOX inhibitor is reported to inhibit the progress of osteoarthritis [49]. It has also been demonstrated that PGE_2 and LTB4 were increased in collagen induced arthritis (CIA) paws, and combination of COX-2 and 5-LOX inhibitors is able to inhibit the development of CIA [50]. In RASF, TNF-α upregulates the secretion of PGE_2 and IL-6, and IL-6 can also be elevated by the addition of PGE_2 [51]. Furthermore, TNF-α-induced IL-6 expression was reduced by the treatment of selective COX-2 inhibitor NS-398. However, PGE_2 alone does not increase the expression of MCP-1 in RASF [52]. These results reveal that both 5-LOX and COX are involved in the TNF-α-induced up-regulation of cytokines. Other factors may also be related to MCP-1 expression [53,54].

In conclusion, 5-LOX exerts a crucial role in chronic systemic inflammation. We demonstrated that both 5-LOX inhibitors antagonized TNF-α-induced IL-6 and MCP-1 expression via inhibition of NF-κB activation in human RA synovial fibroblasts (Figure 8). Moreover, 5-LOX inhibitor can reduce the TNF-α-induced systemic inflammation and paw edema *in vivo*. Our results reveal a novel mechanism in TNF-α-induced inflammation and suggest new therapeutic strategies targeting 5-LOX for the treatment of rheumatoid arthritis.

Supporting Information

Figure S1 Leukotriene B4 receptor antagonist LY29311 reverses TNF-α-induced IκBα phosphorylation and NF-κB nuclear translocation in human synovial fibroblasts. Human synovial fibroblasts were pre-incubated with leukotriene B4 receptor antagonist LY29311 for 1 hr and then exposed to TNF-α (10 ng/ml) for another 30 min. The whole cell lysate results show that the phosphorylation of IκBα was decreased with the treatment of LY29311 in RASF. Cytosolic and nuclear extracts were separated by NE-PER kit. Note that LY29311 significantly antagonized the nuclear translocation of NF-κB subunits of p65. C23 was used as nucleus marker.

Author Contributions

Performed the experiments: H.C. Lin THL. Analyzed the data: H.C. Lin THL. Conceived the strategies and designed the experiments of this manuscript: RSY WMF. Prepared the manuscript: H.C. Lin THL. Supervised the project and edited the manuscript: RSY WMF. Performed the animal studies: MYW H.C. Liou HJT. Contributed to obtain the primary cell cultures: YCC CHT. Provided suggestions: MJH.

References

1. Brennan FM, McInnes IB (2008) Evidence that cytokines play a role in rheumatoid arthritis. The Journal of clinical investigation 118: 3537–3545.
2. Pruzanski W, Vadas P, Stefanski E, Urowitz MB (1985) Phospholipase A2 activity in sera and synovial fluids in rheumatoid arthritis and osteoarthritis. Its possible role as a proinflammatory enzyme. The Journal of rheumatology 12: 211–216.
3. Gilman SC, Chang J, Zeigler PR, Uhl J, Mochan E (1988) Interleukin-1 activates phospholipase A2 in human synovial cells. Arthritis and rheumatism 31: 126–130.
4. Bomalaski JS, Clark MA (1993) Phospholipase A2 and arthritis. Arthritis and rheumatism 36: 190–198.
5. Martel-Pelletier J, Lajeunesse D, Reboul P, Pelletier JP (2003) Therapeutic role of dual inhibitors of 5-LOX and COX, selective and non-selective non-steroidal anti-inflammatory drugs. Annals of the rheumatic diseases 62: 501–509.
6. Davidson EM, Rae SA, Smith MJ (1983) Leukotriene B4, a mediator of inflammation present in synovial fluid in rheumatoid arthritis. Annals of the rheumatic diseases 42: 677–679.
7. Lewis RA, Austen KF, Soberman RJ (1990) Leukotrienes and other products of the 5-lipoxygenase pathway. Biochemistry and relation to pathobiology in human diseases. The New England journal of medicine 323: 645–655.
8. Gursel T, Firat S, Ercan ZS (1997) Increased serum leukotriene B4 level in the active stage of rheumatoid arthritis in children. Prostaglandins, leukotrienes, and essential fatty acids 56: 205–207.
9. Ahmadzadeh N, Shingu M, Nobunaga M, Tawara T (1991) Relationship between leukotriene B4 and immunological parameters in rheumatoid synovial fluids. Inflammation 15: 497–503.
10. Chen M, Lam BK, Kanaoka Y, Nigrovic PA, Audoly LP, et al. (2006) Neutrophil-derived leukotriene B4 is required for inflammatory arthritis. The Journal of experimental medicine 203: 837–842.
11. Masferrer JL, Zweifel BS, Hardy M, Anderson GD, Dufield D, et al. (2010) Pharmacology of PF-4191834, a novel, selective non-redox 5-lipoxygenase inhibitor effective in inflammation and pain. The Journal of pharmacology and experimental therapeutics 334: 294–301.
12. Samuelsson B, Dahlen SE, Lindgren JA, Rouzer CA, Serhan CN (1987) Leukotrienes and lipoxins: structures, biosynthesis, and biological effects. Science 237: 1171–1176.
13. Miller TA, Ghosh J, Myers CE, Macdonald TL (2000) 5-HETE congeners as modulators of cell proliferation. Bioorganic & medicinal chemistry letters 10: 1913–1916.
14. Powell WS, Rokach J (2005) Biochemistry, biology and chemistry of the 5-lipoxygenase product 5-oxo-ETE. Progress in lipid research 44: 154–183.
15. Hashimoto A, Murakami Y, Kitasato H, Hayashi I, Endo H (2007) Glucocorticoids co-interact with lipoxin A4 via lipoxin A4 receptor (ALX) up-regulation. Biomedicine & pharmacotherapy = Biomedecine & pharmacotherapie 61: 81–85.
16. Gheorghe KR, Korotkova M, Catrina AI, Backman L, af Klint E, et al. (2009) Expression of 5-lipoxygenase and 15-lipoxygenase in rheumatoid arthritis synovium and effects of intraarticular glucocorticoids. Arthritis research & therapy 11: R83.
17. Tang CH, Chiu YC, Tan TW, Yang RS, Fu WM (2007) Adiponectin enhances IL-6 production in human synovial fibroblast via an AdipoR1 receptor, AMPK, p38, and NF-kappa B pathway. Journal of immunology 179: 5483–5492.
18. Lin TH, Tang CH, Wu K, Fong YC, Yang RS, et al. (2011) 15-deoxy-Delta(12,14) -prostaglandin-J2 and ciglitazone inhibit TNF-alpha-induced matrix metalloproteinase 13 production via the antagonism of NF-kappaB activation in human synovial fibroblasts. Journal of cellular physiology 226: 3242–3250.
19. Folco EJ, Sheikine Y, Rocha VZ, Christen T, Shvartz E, et al. (2011) Hypoxia but not inflammation augments glucose uptake in human macrophages: Implications for imaging atherosclerosis with 18fluorine-labeled 2-deoxy-D-glucose positron emission tomography. Journal of the American College of Cardiology 58: 603–614.
20. Philippe L, Alsaleh G, Suffert G, Meyer A, Georgel P, et al. (2012) TLR2 expression is regulated by microRNA miR-19 in rheumatoid fibroblast-like synoviocytes. Journal of immunology 188: 454–461.
21. Cakmak H, Basar M, Seval-Celik Y, Osteen KG, Duleba AJ, et al. (2012) Statins inhibit monocyte chemotactic protein 1 expression in endometriosis. Reproductive sciences 19: 572–579.
22. Neumann E, Lefevre S, Zimmermann B, Gay S, Muller-Ladner U (2010) Rheumatoid arthritis progression mediated by activated synovial fibroblasts. Trends in molecular medicine 16: 458–468.
23. Haringman JJ, Smeets TJ, Reinders-Blankert P, Tak PP (2006) Chemokine and chemokine receptor expression in paired peripheral blood mononuclear cells and synovial tissue of patients with rheumatoid arthritis, osteoarthritis, and reactive arthritis. Annals of the rheumatic diseases 65: 294–300.
24. Koch AE, Kunkel SL, Harlow LA, Johnson B, Evanoff HL, et al. (1992) Enhanced production of monocyte chemoattractant protein-1 in rheumatoid arthritis. The Journal of clinical investigation 90: 772–779.

25. Mathis S, Jala VR, Haribabu B (2007) Role of leukotriene B4 receptors in rheumatoid arthritis. Autoimmunity reviews 7: 12–17.
26. Xu S, Lu H, Lin J, Chen Z, Jiang D (2010) Regulation of TNFalpha and IL1beta in rheumatoid arthritis synovial fibroblasts by leukotriene B4. Rheumatology international 30: 1183–1189.
27. Bondeson J, Lauder S, Wainwright S, Amos N, Evans A, et al. (2007) Adenoviral gene transfer of the endogenous inhibitor IkappaBalpha into human osteoarthritis synovial fibroblasts demonstrates that several matrix metalloproteinases and aggrecanases are nuclear factor-kappaB-dependent. The Journal of rheumatology 34: 523–533.
28. Perkins ND (2007) Integrating cell-signalling pathways with NF-kappaB and IKK function. Nature reviews Molecular cell biology 8: 49–62.
29. Muller-Ladner U, Ospelt C, Gay S, Distler O, Pap T (2007) Cells of the synovium in rheumatoid arthritis. Synovial fibroblasts. Arthritis research & therapy 9: 223.
30. Park JY, Pillinger MH (2007) Interleukin-6 in the pathogenesis of rheumatoid arthritis. Bulletin of the NYU hospital for joint diseases 65 Suppl 1: S4–10.
31. Abeles AM, Pillinger MH (2006) Statins as antiinflammatory and immunomodulatory agents: a future in rheumatologic therapy? Arthritis and rheumatism 54: 393–407.
32. Noss EH, Brenner MB (2008) The role and therapeutic implications of fibroblast-like synoviocytes in inflammation and cartilage erosion in rheumatoid arthritis. Immunological reviews 223: 252–270.
33. Bartok B, Firestein GS (2010) Fibroblast-like synoviocytes: key effector cells in rheumatoid arthritis. Immunological reviews 233: 233–255.
34. Dixon WG, Hyrich KL, Watson KD, Lunt M, Galloway J, et al. (2010) Drug-specific risk of tuberculosis in patients with rheumatoid arthritis treated with anti-TNF therapy: results from the British Society for Rheumatology Biologics Register (BSRBR). Annals of the rheumatic diseases 69: 522–528.
35. Strangfeld A, Hierse F, Rau R, Burmester GR, Krummel-Lorenz B, et al. (2010) Risk of incident or recurrent malignancies among patients with rheumatoid arthritis exposed to biologic therapy in the German biologics register RABBIT. Arthritis research & therapy 12: R5.
36. Peters-Golden M, Henderson WR, Jr. (2007) Leukotrienes. The New England journal of medicine 357: 1841–1854.
37. Di Gennaro A, Haeggstrom JZ (2012) The leukotrienes: immune-modulating lipid mediators of disease. Advances in immunology 116: 51–92.
38. Sanchez-Galan E, Gomez-Hernandez A, Vidal C, Martin-Ventura JL, Blanco-Colio LM, et al. (2009) Leukotriene B4 enhances the activity of nuclear factor-kappaB pathway through BLT1 and BLT2 receptors in atherosclerosis. Cardiovascular research 81: 216–225.
39. Zhang W, Dziak R (1996) Tumor necrosis factor alpha stimulates arachidonic acid metabolism in human osteoblastic osteosarcomal cells. Prostaglandins, leukotrienes, and essential fatty acids 54: 427–431.
40. Canetti C, Silva JS, Ferreira SH, Cunha FQ (2001) Tumour necrosis factor-alpha and leukotriene B(4) mediate the neutrophil migration in immune inflammation. British journal of pharmacology 134: 1619–1628.
41. Kanda N, Watanabe S (2007) Leukotriene B(4) enhances tumour necrosis factor-alpha-induced CCL27 production in human keratinocytes. Clinical and experimental allergy: journal of the British Society for Allergy and Clinical Immunology 37: 1074–1082.
42. Gilston V, Jones HW, Soo CC, Coumbe A, Blades S, et al. (1997) NF-kappa B activation in human knee-joint synovial tissue during the early stage of joint inflammation. Biochemical Society transactions 25: 518S.
43. Serezani CH, Lewis C, Jancar S, Peters-Golden M (2011) Leukotriene B4 amplifies NF-kappaB activation in mouse macrophages by reducing SOCS1 inhibition of MyD88 expression. The Journal of clinical investigation 121: 671–682.
44. Lee SJ, Choi EK, Seo KW, Bae JU, Kim YH, et al. (2013) 5-Lipoxygenase plays a pivotal role in endothelial adhesion of monocytes via an increased expression of Mac-1. Cardiovascular research 99: 724–733.
45. Leone S, Ottani A, Bertolini A (2007) Dual acting anti-inflammatory drugs. Current topics in medicinal chemistry 7: 265–275.
46. Patel NS, Cuzzocrea S, Chatterjee PK, Di Paola R, Sautebin L, et al. (2004) Reduction of renal ischemia-reperfusion injury in 5-lipoxygenase knockout mice and by the 5-lipoxygenase inhibitor zileuton. Molecular pharmacology 66: 220–227.
47. Tu XK, Yang WZ, Wang CH, Shi SS, Zhang YL, et al. (2010) Zileuton reduces inflammatory reaction and brain damage following permanent cerebral ischemia in rats. Inflammation 33: 344–352.
48. Kim SY, Kim TB, Moon KA, Kim TJ, Shin D, et al. (2008) Regulation of pro-inflammatory responses by lipoxygenases via intracellular reactive oxygen species in vitro and in vivo. Experimental & molecular medicine 40: 461–476.
49. Brune K (2004) Safety of anti-inflammatory treatment–new ways of thinking. Rheumatology 43 Suppl 1: i16–20.
50. Anderson GD, Keys KL, De Ciechi PA, Masferrer JL (2009) Combination therapies that inhibit cyclooxygenase-2 and leukotriene synthesis prevent disease in murine collagen induced arthritis. Inflammation research: official journal of the European Histamine Research Society [et al] 58: 109–117.
51. Kunisch E, Jansen A, Kojima F, Loffler I, Kapoor M, et al. (2009) Prostaglandin E2 differentially modulates proinflammatory/prodestructive effects of TNF-alpha on synovial fibroblasts via specific E prostanoid receptors/cAMP. Journal of immunology 183: 1328–1336.
52. Largo R, Diez-Ortego I, Sanchez-Pernaute O, Lopez-Armada MJ, Alvarez-Soria MA, et al. (2004) EP2/EP4 signalling inhibits monocyte chemoattractant protein-1 production induced by interleukin 1beta in synovial fibroblasts. Annals of the rheumatic diseases 63: 1197–1204.
53. Kunisch E, Chakilam S, Gandesiri M, Kinne RW (2012) IL-33 regulates TNF-alpha dependent effects in synovial fibroblasts. International journal of molecular medicine 29: 530–540.
54. Villiger PM, Terkeltaub R, Lotz M (1992) Production of monocyte chemoattractant protein-1 by inflamed synovial tissue and cultured synoviocytes. Journal of immunology 149: 722–727.

6

Influence of Adult Height on Rheumatoid Arthritis: Association with Disease Activity, Impairment of Joint Function and Overall Disability

Ying Chen[1,2], Zanzhe Yu[2], Jonathan C. Packham[1], Derek L. Mattey[1,2]*

1 Haywood Rheumatology Centre, Haywood Hospital, High Lane, Burslem, Stoke-on-Trent, Staffordshire, United Kingdom, **2** Institute of Science and Technology in Medicine, Keele University, Staffordshire, United Kingdom

Abstract

Objectives: To investigate whether normal variation of adult height is associated with clinical characteristics in rheumatoid arthritis (RA), including disease activity (DAS28), impairment of joint function (mechanical joint score, MJS) and overall disability (health assessment questionnaire, HAQ).

Methods: A cohort (134 males, 287 females) of consecutively recruited RA patients of Northern European origin was studied. Height, weight and demographic information were obtained. A core set of disease measurements, including DAS28, MJS and HAQ, were recorded at baseline, 12 and 24 months. Other clinical variables (e.g. disease duration, IgM rheumatoid factor, antibodies to cyclic citrullinated peptide, C-reactive protein, erythrocyte sedimentation rate) were recorded at baseline. Socioeconomic status, smoking status, comorbid condition, other autoimmune conditions and drug therapy were also recorded. Associations were analyzed using univariate statistics and multivariate linear regression models. Mediation tests were also carried out for evaluating the relationship between gender, height and disease measures.

Results: In males, height was inversely associated with DAS28, MJS and HAQ (at baseline and over 24 months) independent of other factors (e.g. weight, body mass index, age, disease duration, osteoporosis, autoantibodies, erosive disease, joint replacement, steroid use, smoking status, socioeconomic status and comorbid disease). In females, a similar trend was seen but the relationships were non significant. In the whole population, the association of female gender with more active disease and poor function disappeared after adjustment for height. Mediation analysis indicated that height served as a full mediator in the relationship of gender with disease activity and overall disability. Confirmation of these findings was demonstrated in a second RA population (n = 288).

Conclusion: Adult height is inversely associated with disease activity, impairment of joint function and overall disability in RA, particularly in males. The association of female sex with more severe disease activity and disability appears to be mediated by smaller stature.

Editor: Massimo Pietropaolo, University of Michigan Medical School, United States of America

Funding: Funding was provided by the Medical Research Council and the Haywood Rheumatism Research and Development Foundation (Charity number 507273). The funders had no role in study design, data collection and analysis, decision to publish, or preparation of the manuscript.

Competing Interests: The authors have declared that no competing interests exist.

* E-mail: d.l.mattey@keele.ac.uk

Introduction

Body height is among the most visible of human characteristics, and is highly heritable ($h^2 = 0.8$) [1]. It has been associated with numerous genomic loci (n>100), with each contributing a small amount of effect [2]. It is a complex trait also influenced by a variety of environmental factors, including diet and the prenatal environment [3].

Normal variation of height in adulthood is associated with several disease conditions, including various cancers (short stature/ decreased risk) [4,5], cardiovascular diseases (CVD) (short stature/ increased risk) [6], type 2 diabetes (short stature/increased risk) [7], periodontitis (short stature/increased risk) [8], and chronic obstructive pulmonary disease (short stature/increased risk) [9]. Previous studies have found no relationship between height and the risk of developing rheumatoid arthritis (RA) [10,11], but as far as we are aware there have been no studies on whether there is a relationship between height and disease activity or severity in rheumatoid arthritis (RA).

It has been suggested that the association of short stature with CVD and other diseases may be related to an increased inflammatory burden in such individuals due to early-life infections which have impact on eventual adult height [12]. We hypothesized that there may be an association between adult height and disease activity and/or severity in patients with RA. In the present study we investigated whether there was a relationship between height and a number of major disease characteristics in RA, including disease activity, impairment of mechanical joint function and global degree of disability. Our results suggest that, in men particularly, height is inversely associated with increased disease activity, and overall severity in RA. The well described association of female sex with more severe disease activity and poor functional outcome appears to be mediated by smaller stature.

Methods

Patients

This study was based on a cohort (n = 430) of consecutively recruited RA patients of Northern European origin, resident in North Staffordshire and attending the Clinical Rheumatology Unit at the Haywood Hospital. All patients had a diagnosis of RA, and met the 1987 American College of Rheumatology criteria [13]. Nine (2.1%) samples were excluded from the current report, on the basis that information on height, sex or any key outcome variable was incomplete. Inclusion or exclusion of these samples made no difference to the associations found.

Body height (standing height) and weight were measured on each patient at baseline. Height (in cm to the nearest 0.1 cm) was measured with a stadiometer with a measuring slide and a heel plate. Position of the head was standardized by asking the sampled subject to stand straight, without shoes and with the heels together. Weight (in kg to the nearest 0.1 kg) was measured with a reliable weighing scale while the participant was wearing light clothing and no shoes. Body mass index (BMI) was obtained by weight (in kg)/ $height^2$ (in m). Five of the 421 patients were wheelchair users, but with support it was possible for them to stand straight enough for height measurements. All of these patients were women. Other demographic data (e.g. age, gender, post code of residence, occupation) was also recorded at recruitment. Socioeconomic status was estimated by the Carstairs index of deprivation based on postcode address [14]. A history of current or past cigarette smoking was obtained from a questionnaire completed by each patient at baseline, as described previously [15].

Clinical variables, including disease duration, disease activity, IgM rheumatoid factor (RF), anti-cyclic citrullinated peptide antibody (anti-CCP), levels of C-reactive protein (CRP) and erythrocyte sedimentation rate (ESR), presence of extra-articular disease (e.g. nodules, vasculitis, interstitial lung disease), and presence of erosive disease were obtained at baseline. RA disease activity was measured by the Disease Activity Score 28 (DAS28). Evaluation of DAS28 includes the number of swollen and tender joints (based on 28 joints), the global visual analogue scale, and ESR [16]. The Mechanical Joint Score (MJS) and the Health Assessment Questionnaire (HAQ) score were used to assess the total amount of joint impairment of mechanical function and the overall degree of disability, respectively [17,18]. These three outcome variables were obtained at baseline, 12 and 24 months follow-up. Complete data at all time points over 24 months was available on 305/430 (72.4%) patients.

Patients were also categorized into those with or without osteoporosis at the time of study entry. Patients were classified has having osteoporosis if their T scores obtained by bone densitometry were less than −2.5, and/or if they were being treated with anti-osteoporotic drugs. Previous/current medication and any major comorbid conditions (e.g. ischaemic heart disease (IHD), diabetes, chronic pulmonary disease, renal disease, neoplasia) on each patient were recorded at recruitment, as described previously [15]. Other variables recorded included evidence of other autoimmune conditions (e.g. Sjogren's syndrome, autoimmune thyroid disease, inflammatory bowel disease), any hypothyroidism, and any history of knee or hip joint replacement.

A second study population of patients (n = 288, median age 62.0, median disease duration 8.0 years, female n = 175) was used in a replication study of the association of height with clinical characteristics. DAS28 scores were obtained on the majority of patients (n = 285), although HAQ scores were only available for 94 patients. MJS data were not collected. This group was on standard disease modifying anti-rheumatic drug (DMARD) therapy and had been recruited as a control group for patients on biologic therapy in previous studies.

Ethics statement

Written informed consent was provided by each patient according to the Declaration of Helsinki. The research was approved by the North Staffordshire Local Research Ethics Committee.

Statistical analysis

The relationship between binary variables was assessed using contingency tables. The relationship between binary variables and quantitative variable was assessed using two-sample T-test (Student's, Aspin-Welch or Mann-Whitney U Test, according to the distribution and the variance). Correlation testing (Pearson's or Spearman's Correlation, according to the distribution) was used to assess the relationship between quantitative variables. Multivariate linear modelling (multivariate multiple regression) was used to assess the influence of independent variable (e.g. body height, sex) on dependent variable (e.g. disease activity) with or without adjustment for other covariates. The selection of other covariates in each model was based on an all possible regressions procedure to determine which candidate variables should be included in the final model. This algorithm seeks a subset that provides a maximum value of R-squared. Multiple regression analyses were then run to determine the regression coefficients and p values for each of the independent variables chosen in the final model. Each regression analysis was examined for multicollinearity by looking at the variance inflation factors, tolerances and condition number test. The mediation effect was assessed by using the Preacher and Hayes' method for assessing and comparing indirect effects in mediator models [19]. The macro for this method, called INDIRECT, can be accessed at http://www.afhayes.com/spss-sas-and-mplus-macros-and-code.html. This macro estimates the path coefficients and generates bootstrap confidence intervals for indirect effects through mediator variables, and allows for adjustment for other covariates. Analyses were all carried out using the Number Cruncher Statistical System for Windows (version NCSS 2007), except for the mediation tests (SPSS version 20 with the INDIRECT macro). The significance level was set at a p value of 0.05, and all p values were based on 2-tailed tests. MJS did not fit a normal distribution and was square root transformed in multiple regression models to fit normality.

Results

Characteristics of patients

The cohort consisted of 134 (31.8%) male and 287 female patients with RA. Table 1 shows the demographic and clinical variables at baseline. In this particular population, female patients were younger, and a significantly higher percentage of female patients were currently receiving methotrexate. As expected, females were shorter with lower body weight. There was no difference in BMI between genders. Ever-smoking was less frequent in females than males. Female patients with RA were associated with earlier onset, higher DAS28 (non-significant), higher HAQ score, and a greater frequency of osteoporosis and hypothyroidism. Males were more likely to be associated with common co-morbid conditions (e.g. hypertension, IHD, diabetes).

Table 1. Demographic and clinical characteristics compared between female and male patients.

Parameter	All patients, n = 421	Male, n = 134	Female, n = 287	p value¶
Demographic variable				
Age, yrs	62.0 (54.0–69.0)	64.5 (57.8–72.0)	60.0 (54.0–67.0)	0.0002
Body weight, kg	76.2±15.3	84.2±13.6	72.4±14.6	<0.0001
Height, cm	165.3±9.0	174.2±6.5	161.1±6.6	<0.0001
BMI, kg/m^2	27.8±5.1	27.8±4.4	27.9±5.5	>0.10
Ever-smoking	275/418 (65.8)	109/133 (82.0)	166/285 (58.2)	<0.0001
Carstairs score	1.10 (−1.63–3.0)	1.30 (−2.55–3.25)	1.10 (−1.50–3.0)	>0.10
RA clinical variable				
Age at onset, yrs	49.6±13.1	51.8±12.6	48.5±13.2	0.016
Duration, yrs	9.0 (3.0–17.3)	8.5 (4.0–18.3)	9.0 (2.7–17.0)	>0.10
RF status	238/419 (56.8)	75/133 (56.4)	163/286 (57.0)	>0.10
Anti-CCP status	308/408 (75.5)	96/130 (73.8)	212/278 (76.3)	>0.10
CRP, mg/l	11.0 (4.5–20.0)	11.8 (5.0–22.9)	10.3 (4.0–19.0)	>0.10
ESR, mm/hrs†	20.0 (10.0–35.8)	16.0 (7.5–37.0)	22.0 (11.0–35.0)	0.067
PGA†	43.0 (21.0–57.0)	46.0 (22.0–62.5)	39.5 (20.8–54.0)	>0.10
TJC†	4 (1–9)	3 (1–8)	4 (1–9)	>0.10
SJC†	3 (1–6)	2 (0–5)	3 (1–7)	>0.10
DAS28	4.20±1.38	4.05±1.48	4.27±1.33	>0.10
MJS	7.0 (3.0–15.0)	7.0 (3.0–14.0)	7.0 (3.0–16.0)	>0.10
HAQ score	1.625 (1.0–2.0)	1.50 (0.875–2.0)	1.625 (1.125–2.125)	0.046
Osteoporosis	59/421 (14.0)	12/134 (9.0)	47/287 (16.4)	0.041
Joint replacement*	66/419 (15.8)	24/133 (18.0)	42/286 (14.7)	>0.10
Drug treatment for RA				
DMARD use	392/421 (93.1)	122/134 (91.0)	270/287 (94.1)	>0.10
Methotrexate use	255/421 (60.6)	71/134 (53.0)	184/287 (64.1)	0.030
Steroid use	41/420 (9.8)	15/134 (11.2)	26/286 (9.1)	>0.10
Biologic agent use	60/421 (14.3)	19/134 (14.2)	41/287 (14.3)	>0.10
Co-morbid condition				
Hypertension	166/418 (39.7)	66/134 (49.3)	100/284 (35.2)	0.0062
IHD	84/420 (20.0)	43/133 (32.3)	41/287 (14.3)	<0.0001
Diabetes‡	32/420 (7.6)	17/133 (12.8)	15/287 (5.2)	0.0066
Hypothyroidism	27/420 (6.4)	1/133 (0.75)	26/287 (9.05)	0.001
Asthma	44/419 (10.5)	13/133 (9.8)	31/286 (10.8)	>0.10

Values are n (%), mean ± standard deviation (SD) or median (interquartile range (IQR)).
¶Comparison between male and female patients, un-adjusted;
*hip or knee replacement;
†components of DAS28;
‡types I and II combined.

These remained significantly associated after adjustment for age and disease duration.

Body height and RA in sex-separated analysis

Body height in males ranged between 157 and 197 cm, and in females between 146 and 180.5 cm. Table 2 shows the selected characteristics compared between patients below (<), and equal or above (≥) median height for male (173.3 cm) and female patients (160.5 cm) separately.

It was a prerequisite of the present study to avoid the confounding effect of age on body height and on other parameters e.g. the younger generation tends to be taller, and increasing age may be associated with reduction in height. The correlations between height (continuous variable) and age in males and females were ($r = -0.22$, $p = 0.010$) and ($r = -0.15$, $p = 0.014$), respectively. All analyses were therefore adjusted for age.

Association with disease activity and outcome indices

In males, patients <median height were associated with higher DAS28, MJS (borderline association) and HAQ score, compared to those ≥median height (Table 2). The correlations of height (continuous variable) with DAS28, MJS and HAQ score were ($r = -0.25$, $p = 0.0039$), ($r = -0.22$, $p = 0.0095$) and ($r = -0.23$, $p = 0.0066$), respectively. In females, the association of <median height with worse RA outcome (DAS28, MJS and HAQ score) was not significant, but showed a similar trend to that in males

Table 2. Demographic and clinical characteristics compared between patients with below (<) and equal or above (≥) median height in sex-separated setting.

Parameter	Male patients, n = 134			Female patients, n = 287		
	<median, n = 67	≥median, n = 67	p value¶	<median, n = 143	≥median, n = 144	p value¶
Age, yrs	65.0 (59.0–72.0)	64.0 (52.0–72.0)	>0.10	62.0 (54.0–69.0)	59.0 (53.3–66.0)	>0.10
Body weight, kg	80.8±12.7	87.6±13.7	0.0034	68.8±13.5	75.9±14.8	<0.0001
BMI, kg/m^2	28.3±4.6	27.3±4.2	>0.10	28.3±5.5	27.4±5.4	>0.10
Ever smoke	53/67 (79.1)	56/66 (84.8)	>0.10	85/142 (59.9)	81/143 (56.6)	>0.10
Carstairs score	1.30 (−1.40–3.40)	1.15 (−2.73–2.88)	>0.10	1.20 (−1.60–3.10)	1.10 (−1.40–3.0)	>0.10
Duration, yrs	7.0 (4.0–14.0)	11.0 (5.0–21.0)	0.019	11.0 (3.0–18.0)	9.0 (2.50–17.0)	>0.10
RF status	36/66 (54.5)	39/67 (58.2)	>0.10	85/143 (59.4)	78/143 (54.5)	>0.10
Anti-CCP status	48/65 (73.8)	48/75 (73.8)	>0.10	112/138 (81.2)	100/140 (71.4)	0.057
CRP, mg/l	12.3 (5.0–31.2)	11.0 (4.8–20.0)	>0.10	10.0 (4.3–19.0)	11.0 (4.0–19.0)	>0.10
ESR, mm/hrs†	16.0 (9.0–44.3)	15.0 (6.0–28.0)	0.071	22.0 (12.0–38.0)	19.5 (11.0–34.0)	>0.10
PGA†	46.0 (33.0–60.0)	46.0 (16.8–65.5)	>0.10	43.0 (23.0–54.0)	36.0 (19.0–54.0)	>0.10
TJC†	3 (2–8)	3 (0–7)	>0.10	5 (1–10)	4 (1–8)	>0.10
SJC†	2 (1–6)	2 (0–5)	>0.10	3 (1–6)	3 (1–7)	>0.10
DAS28	4.34±1.31	3.75±1.59	0.023	4.34±1.37	4.20±1.29	>0.10
MJS	9.0 (3.0–17.0)	6.0 (2.8–12.0)	0.076	8.0 (3.0–17.0)	6.0 (3.0–15.0)	>0.10
HAQ score	1.75 (1.25–2.125)	1.25 (0.625–1.875)	0.0046	1.75 (1.25–2.125)	1.625 (1.0–2.0)	>0.10
Osteoporosis	10/67 (14.9)	2/67 (3.0)	0.016	28/143 (19.6)	19/143 (13.2)	>0.10
Joint replacement*	13/67 (19.4)	11/66 (16.7)	>0.10	20/142 (14.1)	22/142 (15.3)	>0.10
DMARD use	60/67 (89.6)	62/67 (92.5)	>0.10	136/143 (95.1)	134/144 (93.1)	>0.10
Methotrexate use	38/67 (56.7)	33/67 (49.3)	>0.10	86/143 (60.1)	98/144 (68.1)	>0.10
Steroid use	6/67 (9.0)	9/67 (13.4)	>0.10	14/143 (9.8)	12/143 (8.4)	>0.10
Biologic agent use	12/67 (17.9)	7/67 (10.4)	>0.10	20/143 (14.0)	21/144 (14.6)	>0.10
Hypertension	34/67 (50.7)	32/67 (47.8)	>0.10	57/141 (40.4)	43/143 (30.1)	0.068
IHD	20/67 (29.9)	23/66 (34.8)	>0.10	25/143 (17.5)	16/144 (11.1)	>0.10
Diabetes‡	7/67 (10.4)	10/66 (15.2)	>0.10	10/143 (7.0)	5/144 (3.5)	>0.10
Hypothyroidism	1/67 (1.5)	0/66 (0.0)	>0.10	13/143 (9.1)	13/144 (9.0)	>0.10
Asthma	7/67 (10.4)	6/66 (9.1)	>0.10	21/142 (14.8)	10/144 (6.9)	0.033

Values are n (%), mean ± SD or median (IQR).
¶Comparison within gender, un-adjusted;
*hip or knee replacement;
†components of DAS28;
‡types I and II combined.

(Table 2). Correlation analysis indicated that height (continuous variable) was significantly correlated with HAQ score ($r = -0.14$, $p = 0.017$) but not with DAS28 or MJS.

To determine whether demographic, clinical and other variables were likely to be potential confounders or effect modifiers of the associations with height we carried out univariate linear regression analyses to determine which variables were most significantly associated with disease activity/severity measures. Variables with a p value of 0.2 or less were chosen for inclusion in further multivariate analyses. An all possible regressions procedure was run for each disease measure to determine which subset of candidate variables should be run in the final multiple regression models. Introduction of weight, BMI or other variables into these multivariate models made little or no difference to the association with height in men, although a number of other variables were also significant in these models. Notably, the presence of any co-morbid disease was significantly associated with DAS28 and HAQ, while the use of steroids was independently associated with HAQ and MJS. The presence of RF was associated only with DAS28, CRP was associated only with MJS, and the Carstairs index was associated only with the HAQ. (Table 3).

In females, height was not significantly associated with any of the disease activity/severity parameters in multivariate models which included other significant variables (Table 4). Other anthropometric measurements (weight or BMI) were not significantly associated. As in men, co-morbid disease and presence of RF was associated with DAS28, although steroid use was also associated in women. The strongest associations with MJS were disease duration, presence of RF and osteoporosis, while the HAQ was associated with disease duration, ESR, Carstairs index, steroid use and hip replacement.

The relationships between height and the mean-time-averaged DAS28, MJS and HAQ score over 24 months (MTA-DAS28, MJS, and HAQ score at baseline, 12 and 24 months) were also analyzed on 103 (76.9%) male and 202 (70.4%) female patients using similar regression models. Height showed very significant

Table 3. Multivariate multiple regression analyses showing variables most strongly associated with DAS28, MJS and HAQ score in male patients with RA.

Model 1, dependent variable: DAS28			Model 2, dependent variable: MJS*			Model 3, dependent variable: HAQ		
Independent variable	Regression coefficient (SE)	p value	Independent variable	Regression coefficient (SE)	p value	Independent variable	Regression coefficient (SE)	p value
Height, cm	−0.050 (0.018)	0.005	Height, cm	−0.058 (0.016)	0.0008	Height, cm	−0.026 (0.009)	0.006
Comorbid disease†	1.682 (0.412)	<0.0001	Duration, yrs	0.074 (0.010)	<0.0001	Duration, yrs	0.018 (0.0060)	0.0027
RF (+/−)	0.572 (0.239)	0.018	CRP mg/l	0.009 (0.004)	0.015	Comorbid disease†	0.771 (0.207)	0.0003
			Steroid use	0.870 (0.346)	0.013	Carstairs index	0.064 (0.021)	0.003
						Steroid use	0.454 (0.190)	0.018

Variables were baseline values.
*MJS was square root transformed to fit normality.
†Presence of any comorbid disease (e.g ischaemic heart disease, diabetes, chronic pulmonary disease, renal disease, neoplasia).
RF, rheumatoid factor; CRP, C-reactive protein.
R-squared values: Model 1 = 0.2320, Model 2 = 0.3967, Model 3 = 0.2760.

Table 4. Multivariate multiple regression analyses showing variables most strongly associated with DAS28, MJS and HAQ score in female patients with RA.

Model 1, dependent variable: DAS28			Model 2, dependent variable: MJS*			Model 3, dependent variable: HAQ		
Independent variable	Regression coefficient (SE)	p value	Independent variable	Regression coefficient (SE)	p value	Independent variable	Regression coefficient (SE)	p value
RF (+/−)	0.607 (0.153)	<0.0001	Duration, yrs	0.098 (0.0089)	<0.0001	Duration, yrs	0.025 (0.0044)	<0.0001
Comorbid disease†	0.594 (0.211)	0.005	RF (+/−)	0.618 (0.150)	<0.0001	ESR, mm/h	0.014 (0.002)	<0.0001
Steroid use	0.534 (0.262)	0.042	Osteoporosis	0.879 (0.202)	<0.0001	Carstairs index	0.049 (0.016)	0.003
						Steroid use	0.329 (0.137)	0.017
						Hip replacement	0.296 (0.140)	0.035

Variables were baseline values.
*MJS was square root transformed to fit normality.
†Presence of any comorbid disease (e.g ischaemic heart disease, diabetes, chronic pulmonary disease, renal disease, neoplasia).
RF, rheumatoid factor; ESR, erythrocyte sedimentation rate.
R-squared values: Model 1 = 0.1023, Model 2 = 0.4189, Model 3 = 0.2721.

associations with MTA-DAS28, MTA-MJS and MTA-HAQ score in males after adjusting for other significant independent variables (Table 5). In females there were no associations between height and mean time-averaged disease measures in models containing the most significant baseline variables associated with each measure (Table 6). BMI was significantly associated with the MTA-DAS28 in a model which also included RF and comorbid disease.

Gender vs. height in association with disease activity and outcome indices

Comparison between genders showed that female patients tended to have higher scores for the DAS28 and HAQ score, although the DAS28 association was not significant in univariate analysis (Table 1). We hypothesized that the association of females with more severe RA may be related to females having a generally shorter stature than males.

In multivariate multiple regression models of the whole population, female sex was associated with higher DAS28 and HAQ scores after adjusting for other variables, but excluding height (Table S1). However, after inclusion of height (continuous variable) as a covariate in these models, the association of female sex with higher DAS28 and HAQ score totally disappeared (Table 7). The association of height with disease activity/severity measures was significant in all models with or without adjustment for gender, although the significance levels for the DAS28 and HAQ associations were attenuated after adjusting for gender (Table 7). Height also showed significant associations with MTA-DAS28, MTA-MJS and MTA-HAQ score over 24 months after adjusting for other confounding factors (Table S2).

We postulated that height may be acting as a mediator in the relationship of gender, with disease activity and outcome indices (Figure 1). To formally investigate this, we applied Preacher and Hayes' method for assessing and comparing indirect effects in mediator models using the INDIRECT macro. The results demonstrated that although the total effect of gender on DAS28 and HAQ was significant (c path, models 1 and 3 respectively, Table 8), the direct effect contributed little or nothing to this (c' path, models 1 and 3 respectively, Table 8). The indirect effect through the mediator (i.e. height) played the major role, based on the significance of both a and b paths, and the quantified a×b effect (a, b, a×b paths, models 1 and 3 respectively, Table 8). Gender did not have a significantly effect on MJS (c path, model 2, Table 8). However, the effect of height on MJS was significant (b path, model 2, Table 8). The analyses were adjusted for age and disease duration, and further adjustment made no significant difference to the results (data not shown). Similar results were also obtained on index records over 24 months (Table S3).

To investigate whether sex influenced disease measurements in patients with equal height, we examined a subgroup of 54 females with height between 161.4 and 180.5 cm and a randomly selected group of 54 height matched males with height between 161.4 and 180.5 cm. This was the maximum number of patients that could be examined in order to achieve two groups with an equal median height and interquartile range (median 170 cm, IQR 167–173). Patients with osteoporosis were excluded from the analysis in order to prevent a disproportionate number of shorter men suffering from osteoporosis being matched for height with women. Multivariate, multiple regression analysis showed that gender was not associated with any disease measurement in any of the models tested (Table 9). In contrast, in subgroups of men (n = 50) and women (n = 50) with disparate height, containing males between 176 and 197 cm (median 180 cm), and females between 146 and 156.8 cm (median 153 cm), female sex was associated

Table 5. Multivariate multiple regression analyses showing baseline variables most strongly associated with DAS28, MJS and HAQ score over time (24 months) in male patients with RA.

Model 1, dependent variable: MTA-DAS28			Model 2, dependent variable: MTA-MJS*			Model 3, dependent variable: MTA-HAQ		
Independent variable	Regression coefficient (SE)	p value	Independent variable	Regression coefficient (SE)	p value	Independent variable	Regression coefficient (SE)	p value
Height, cm	−0.063 (0.018)	0.0005	Height, cm	−0.055 (0.017)	0.0018	Height, cm	−0.031 (0.009)	0.0016
Comorbid disease†	1.470 (0.434)	0.001	Duration, yrs	0.069 (0.011)	<0.0001	Comorbid disease†	0.717 (0.234)	0.003
			Steroid use	1.090 (0.323)	0.0011	Duration, yrs	0.017 (0.0068)	0.005
						Carstairs index	0.056 (0.022)	0.011
						Steroid use	0.414 (0.201)	0.042

MTA: mean-time-averaged values over 24 months, scored at baseline, 12 and 24 months. Based on 103 (76.9%) male patients who had been followed up for 24 months with measurements at each time point available. Independent variables were baseline values.
*MTA-MJS was square root transformed to fit normality. ,
†Presence of any comorbid disease (e.g ischaemic heart disease, diabetes, chronic pulmonary disease, renal disease, neoplasia).
R-squared values: Model 1 = 0.2327, Model 2 = 0.3967, Model 3 = 0.3058.

Table 6. Multivariate multiple regression analyses showing baseline variables most strongly associated with DAS28, MJS and HAQ score over time (24 months) in female patients with RA.

Model 1, dependent variable: MTA-DAS28			Model 2, dependent variable: MTA-MJS*			Model 3, dependent variable: MTA-HAQ		
Independent variable	Regression coefficient (SE)	p value	Independent variable	Regression coefficient (SE)	p value	Independent variable	Regression coefficient (SE)	p value
RF (+/−)	0.018 (0.007)	0.0036	Duration, yrs	0.093 (0.0086)	<0.0001	Duration, yrs	0.025 (0.0047)	<0.0001
BMI	0.038 (0.014)	0.0088	RF (+/−)	0.435 (0.160)	0.007	ESR, mm/h	0.009 (0.002)	0.0002
Age, yrs	0.018 (0.0076)	0.020				Carstairs index	0.045 (0.018)	0.012
Comorbid disease†	0.437 (0.215)	0.044				Hip replacement	0.350 (0.159)	0.033

MTA: mean-time-averaged values over 24 months, scored at baseline, 12 and 24 months. Based on 202 (70.4%) female patients who had been followed up for 24 months with measurements at each time point available.
Independent variables were baseline values.
*MTA-MJS was square root transformed to fit normality.
†Presence of any comorbid disease (e.g ischaemic heart disease, diabetes, chronic pulmonary disease, renal disease, neoplasia).
RF, rheumatoid factor; BMI, body mass index; ESR, erythrocyte sedimentation rate.
R-squared values: Model 1 = 0.1464, Model 2 = 0.4056, Model 3 = 0.2358.

Table 7. Multivariate multiple regression analyses showing variables most strongly associated with DAS28, MJS and HAQ score in all patients with RA (adjusted for gender).

Model 1, dependent variable: DAS28			Model 2, dependent variable: MJS*			Model 3, dependent variable: HAQ		
Independent variable	Regression coefficient (SE)	p value	Independent variable	Regression coefficient (SE)	p value	Independent variable	Regression coefficient (SE)	p value
Height, cm	−0.0222 (0.009)	0.023	Height, cm	−0.0142 (0.007)	0.029	Height, cm	−0.0122 (0.003)	0.019
RF (+/−)	0.605 (0.130)	<0.0001	Duration, yrs	0.085 (0.006)	<0.0001	Duration, yrs	0.021 (0.003)	<0.0001
Comorbid disease†	0.841 (0.190)	<0.0001	Osteoporosis	0.769 (0.183)	<0.0001	ESR, mm/h	0.008 (0.002)	<0.0001
Steroid use	0.500 (0.216)	0.021	CRP, mg/l	0.0084 (0.0026)	0.002	Carstairs index	0.059 (0.013)	<0.0001
Female	−0.0145 (0.189)	0.93	RF (+/−)	0.295 (0.126)	0.020	Comorbid disease†	0.318 (0.098)	0.001
			Female	−0.190 (0.182)	0.30	Steroid use	0.308 (0.114)	0.007
						Hip replacement	0.234 (0.117)	0.048
						Female	0.048 (0.098)	0.62

Variables were baseline values.
*MJS was square root transformed to fit normality,
†Presence of any comorbid disease (e.g ischaemic heart disease, diabetes, chronic pulmonary disease, renal disease, neoplasia).
RF, rheumatoid factor; CRP, C-reactive protein; ESR, erythrocyte sedimentation rate. Models shown adjusted for gender. In models unadjusted for gender the associations with height remained significant (DAS28, p = 0.002; MJS, p = 0.043, HAQ, p = 0.0002).
R-squared values: Model 1 = 0.1359, Model 2 = 0.3833, Model 3 = 0.2792.

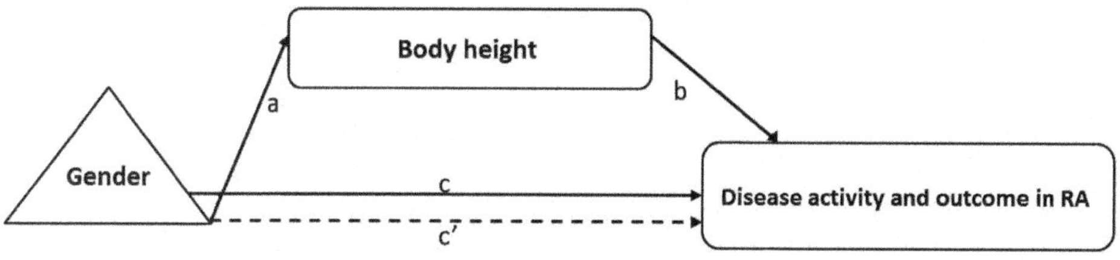

Figure 1. Mediation model for height as a mediator in the relationship between gender and disease measures in RA. Gender, independent variable; body height, mediator variable; disease activity and outcome in RA, dependent variable. Path of effect: a, effect of independent variable on mediator variable; b, effect of mediator variable on dependent variable; c, total effect of independent variable on dependent variable; a×b, indirect effect of independent variable on dependent variable; c', direct effect of independent variable on dependent variable; c = c'+a×b.

with a higher DAS28 and HAQ score in models adjusted for other significant variables. No association was seen with MJS (Table S4).

Replication study

Replication of these analyses in a second population of RA patients provided confirmation of the influence of height on disease activity and function. In all patients there was a significant inverse correlation of height with DAS28 (−0.174, p = 0.0030) and HAQ (−0.346, p = 0.0006). The DAS28 and HAQ were again significantly higher in females than males (5.0 v 4.59, p = 0.016 and 1.65 v 1.19, p = 0.0050), but these associations were lost after adjusting for height in multiple regression models (data not shown). The mediation effect also reached significance in this smaller dataset for HAQ (a×b effect: 0.261 (0.074–0.506)).

We also examined subgroups of male and female patients who were either height matched (median 168 cm), or were disparate in height (female median 153 cm, male median 178 cm). Multiple regression analysis on height matched patients showed that gender was not associated with DAS28 (p = 0.20) or HAQ (p = 0.70) in models containing age, disease duration and body weight (or BMI) as independent variables. However, in the subgroup with disparate height, female sex was associated with a higher DAS28 (p = 0.030) and HAQ score (p = 0.0004) in models adjusted for age, disease duration and body weight (or BMI).

Discussion

This study has demonstrated for the first time that the normal variation of adult height is strongly associated with major disease characteristics in RA. Furthermore, the association of female sex with more active RA and worse function is lost after adjustment for height, suggesting that this relationship may be due to the smaller stature of females. Analysis of the mediation effect showed that height may serve as a full mediator in the relationship of gender with disease activity and overall disability in RA. In gender specific analysis, short stature in male patients was significantly associated with worse disease activity, impairment of mechanical joint function and disability, whilst in females, the relationship was weaker with a significant correlation being found only with disability. However the latter association disappeared when adjusted for other variables associated with the HAQ score.

Different gender specific associations are common in RA, with females often reported as having higher levels of disease activity and worse functional outcome [20–25], while males have greater autoantibody production [26]. Higher DAS/DAS28 scores in women have been reported in early disease (<12 months) in some [21,25], but not all studies [20,24], but consistently higher female DAS28 scores have been observed in early RA patients followed up prospectively for 5 years [25], and in cross sectional studies of longstanding RA [21,22]. Higher HAQ scores in women have invariably been found patients with early and established disease [20–25]. It has been suggested that higher DAS28 and HAQ in women is possibly due to higher pain perception and less muscular strength. However we did not find a significant difference in pain scores between men and women in this group (unpublished observations). Also, it does not explain why height matched men and women had similar HAQ scores, since we would still have expected the men to have greater muscular strength than the women. Another suggestion is that the menopausal state is responsible for a major part of the differences in outcome between men and women, with postmenopausal women having worse disability and damage [20]. However, we have found that although postmenopausal women have significantly higher DAS28 and HAQ scores than men and premenopausal women, these associations disappear when adjusted for height (unpublished observations).

Further evidence for the influence of height was provided by sub-group analysis which showed no differences in gender for disease activity or functional outcome after matching for height. Differences in height are associated with differences in bone geometry, limb proportions, joint angles, etc. Although height is largely affected by gender, these differences, rather than other sex-related factors (e.g. sex hormones), may be more influential in affecting joint damage.

Body height is likely to be marker for some other environmental or biological process rather than be a causal factor itself. Potential factors influencing height include socio-economic status, smoking, in utero maternal health, nutritional status in childhood and early-life infections. In this study adjustment for the Carstairs deprivation index and smoking history made no difference to the associations with height, but no information was available on childhood infections or nutrition in this cohort. Increased burden of infection, immunity and inflammation in children/teenagers have an adverse impact on linear growth and pubertal development, and hence adult height [8,12]. Early-onset chronic autoimmune/inflammatory diseases, such as type I diabetes, celiac disease and paediatric inflammatory bowel disease (particularly Crohn's disease), are associated with growth impairment in children/teenagers, although other factors contribute, including nutritional deficit and/or abnormality of the growth hormone/insulin-like growth factor 1 (GH/IGF-1) axis [27–29].

Growth hormone (GH) is fundamental to linear growth, and primarily acts as a promoter of skeletal long bone growth/development and chondrocyte maturation [30]. GH stimulates insulin-like growth factor 1 (IGF-1) synthesis, and the latter is responsible for stimulating cartilage and bone extracellular matrix protein synthesis [30]. Deficiency in these proteins thus results in growth retardation, short adult stature, low bone mineral density

Table 8. Mediation models demonstrating the mediator effect of height on the relationship between gender and measures of disease activity and outcome in all patients with RA.

Model 1, dependent variable: DAS28				Model 2, dependent variable: MJS				Model 3, dependent variable: HAQ			
Path of effect	Regression coefficient (SE)	p value	*Bootstrap results: regression coefficient (95% CI)	Path of effect	Regression coefficient (SE)	p value	*Bootstrap results: regression coefficient (95% CI)	Path of effect	Regression coefficient (SE)	p value	*Bootstrap results: regression coefficient (95% CI)
a	−13.491 (0.690)	<0.0001	-	a	−13.491 (0.690)	<0.0001	-	a	−13.501 (0.688)	<0.0001	-
b	−0.0226 (0.010)	0.031	-	b	−0.0285 (0.098)	0.0037	-	b	−0.0177 (0.005)	0.0009	-
a×b	0.305 (-)	-	0.301 (0.019–0.579)	a×b	0.384 (-)	-	0.383 (0.113–0.671)	a×b	0.239 (-)	-	0.239 (0.093–0.380)
c	0.298 (0.146)	0.043	-	c	0.156 (0.138)	0.26	-	c	0.232 (0.075)	0.0021	-
c′	−0.0070 (0.203)	0.97	-	c′	−0.229 (0.190)	0.23	-	c′	−0.0074 (0.103)	0.94	-

Gender as the independent variable; height as the proposed mediator; disease activity and outcome index (i.e. DAS28, MJS or HAQ) at baseline as dependent variable. MJS was square root transformed to fit normality. Models shown adjusted for age and disease duration as standard; adjustment for further confounding factors made no significant difference to the results. Path of effect: a, effect of gender on height; b, effect of height on disease indices; a×b, indirect effect through mediation; c, total effect; c′, direct effect; c can be expressed as the sum of the direct and indirect effects (i.e. c=c′+a×b).
*Bootstrap results for indirect effect through proposed mediation: number of bootstrap resamples, n=5,000.

Table 9. Multivariate multiple regression analyses showing variables most strongly associated with DAS28, MJS and HAQ score in height-matched male and female patients with RA.

Model 1, dependent variable: DAS28			Model 2, dependent variable: MJS*			Model 3, dependent variable: HAQ		
Independent variable	Regression coefficient (SE)	p value	Independent variable	Regression coefficient (SE)	p value	Independent variable	Regression coefficient (SE)	p value
Comorbid disease†	1.141 (0.395)	0.005	Duration, yrs	0.095 (0.012)	<0.0001	Duration, yrs	0.035 (0.0063)	<0.0001
			CRP, mg/l	0.015 (0.004)	0.001	Carstairs index	0.072 (0.022)	0.002
						ESR, mm/h	0.007 (0.003)	0.006

Variables were baseline values. Based on 54 males with height between 161.4 and 180.5 cm, and 54 females with height between 161.4 and 180.5 cm.
†Presence of any comorbid disease (e.g ischaemic heart disease, diabetes, chronic pulmonary disease, renal disease, neoplasia). Patients with osteoporosis were excluded.
*MJS was square root transformed to fit normality. Gender was not significantly associated in any model.
R-squared values: Model 1=0.0741, Model 2=0.3347, Model 3=0.4066.

and bone mass. This would be likely to increase the risk of more severe erosive damage in patients with RA. Recently, a possible association of GH deficiency with autoimmunity and inflammation was suggested [31,32]. Furthermore, low levels of IGF-1 in RA synovial fluid were found to be associated with systemic inflammation [33]. It is noteworthy that in genome wide association studies (GWAS) a genetic variant in the IFG1 gene was found to be associated with adult height in eastern Asian populations (but not in Caucasians) [34,35].

It has been proposed that early-life infections may impose a life-long inflammatory burden which may lead to the development of atherosclerotic and thrombotic conditions in late-life [12]. This model also links maternal infections and inflammation with fetal and infant inflammation and reduced growth. In line with this argument, short stature has been associated with increased risk for CVD, type II diabetes and periodontitis [6–8]. Interestingly, RA shows numerous characteristics and pathogenetic processes that have similarities to periodontitis [36]. We speculate that this pathophysiological model may provide some explanation for our observation that short stature is associated with more severe RA.

Another important consideration is the effect of the large number of genetic variants which underlie growth/development, and hence adult height. Based on recent large-scale genome-wide association studies (GWAS), a single-nucleotide polymorphism (SNP) in the CDK6 gene, a key controller of cell cycle progression, was found to be associated with both adult height and the susceptibility to RA [37,38]. GWAS also identified a SNP in the GDF5 gene which is strongly associated both with low adult height and susceptibility to osteoarthritis (OA) [39–41]. GDF5 is a member of the TGF-beta superfamily, and is involved in bone growth and differentiation and joint development, both in adult and embryonic tissues [42–45]. Rare mutations in the GDF5 gene have been associated with several disorders of skeletal development [39]. The allele, associated with decrease in stature/ susceptibility to OA, has been shown to be associated with decreased GDF5 transcriptional activity in chondrogenic cells and with *in vivo* reduced expression of GDF5 in articular cartilage [39,40]. GDF5 may play a role in repair of damaged joint tissues (e.g. cartilage), and decrease in GDF5 expression may lead to less regeneration.

Other possible genetic candidates include the ESR1 gene which is associated with both adult height and age at onset of RA [2,46], and several genes implicated in both the extracellular matrix pathway and adult height, including MMP24, ECM2, EFEMP1, ADAMTS13 and ACAN [2,36,47]. Further work on the relationship between genetic variants, height and disease severity in RA may provide novel insights into the understanding of the aetiology/pathology of the disease.

There are some limitations to this study due to its cross-sectional nature. Analysis of the relationship between height and disease measures is complicated by secular trends in adult height over recent generations in which there is increased height in younger generations [48]. Furthermore the height in older generations may be reduced due to age related reduction in intervertebral disc height or a loss of vertebral height from osteoporotic vertebral collapse. Adult height also decreases with general ill health and immobility, so the possibility of established, severe RA leading to a greater reduction in height (reverse causation) is a major consideration. However, we found that the inverse association of height with greater disease activity/severity in men remained significant in models adjusted for age, disease duration, osteoporosis, comorbid disease or the presence of other autoimmune conditions. Moreover, other possible confounders such as steroid use, erosive disease, joint replacement, extra-articular disease, presence of autoantibodies and socio-economic status had no significant effect on the relationship between height and disease activity/severity. However, it is clear from the R-squared values in our models that a large amount of the variance in the dependent variables is unexplained by the variables in each of the models. Other unknown/untested factors are therefore important. We were unable to investigate some associations, such as the reported relationship between low serum 25-hydroxyvitamin D (25(OH)D) levels and decreased height [49]. A possible relationship of 25(OH)D deficiency with more severe disease activity in RA [50] suggests that this variable should be considered in future studies on body height and severity of disease.

Further prospective studies of recent onset RA and studies in larger cohorts are needed to confirm our findings. Future studies should also include measurement of leg length since the effects of age and disease severity are likely to have less effect on this component of adult height.

Supporting Information

Table S1 Multivariate multiple regression analyses showing variables most strongly associated with DAS28, MJS and HAQ score in all patients with RA, excluding adjustment for height.

Table S2 Multivariate multiple regression analyses showing baseline variables most strongly associated with DAS28, MJS and HAQ score over 24 months in all patients with RA.

Table S3 Mediation models demonstrating the mediator effect of height on the relationship between gender and measures of disease activity and outcome over 24 months in all patients with RA.

Table S4 Multivariate multiple regression analysis showing variables most strongly associated with DAS28, MJS and HAQ score in male and female RA patients of disparate height.

Acknowledgments

We wish to thank Mrs Michelle Kirwan, Mrs Ann Barcroft (research nurses), Mrs Janet Turner and Ms Chantel-lea Birchall (research assistants) for their help with data collection and entry.

Author Contributions

Conceived and designed the experiments: YC JCP DLM. Performed the experiments: YC DLM. Analyzed the data: YC ZY DLM. Contributed reagents/materials/analysis tools: YC ZY JCP. Wrote the paper: YC JCP DLM.

References

1. Lettre G (2011) Recent progress in the study of the genetics of height. Hum Genet 129:465–72.
2. Allen HL, Estrada K, Lettre G, Berndt SI, Weedon MN, et al. (2010) Hundreds of variants clustered in genomic loci and biological pathways affect human height. Nature 467:832–8.
3. Silventoinen K, Sammalisto S, Perola M, Boomsma DJ, Cornes BK, et al. (2003) Heritability of adult body height: a comparative study of twin cohort in eight countries. Twin Res 6:399–408.
4. Gunnell D, Okasha M, Smith GD, Oliver SE, Sandhu J, et al. (2001) Height, leg length, and cancer risk: A systematic review. Epidemiol Rev 23:313–42.

5. Green J, Cairns BJ, Casabonne D, Wright FL, Reeves G, et al. (2011) Height and cancer incidence in the Million Women Study: prospective cohort, and meta-analysis of prospective studies of height and total cancer risk. Lancet Oncol 12:785–94.
6. Paajanen TA, Oksala NKJ, Kuukasjärvi P, Karhunen PJ (2010) Short stature is associated with coronary heart disease: a systematic review of the literature and a meta-analysis. Eur Heart J 31:1802–9.
7. Lawlor DA, Ebrahim S, Davey Smith G (2002) The association between components of adult height and Type II diabetes and insulin resistance: British Women's Heart and Health Study. Diabetologia 45:1097–106.
8. Meisel P, Kohlmann T, Kocher T (2007) Association of height with inflammation and periodontitis: the Study of Health in Pomerania (SHIP). J Clin Periodontol 34:390–6.
9. Ward K, Hubbard R (2011) Is adult height related to the risk of having Chronic Obstructive Pulmonary Disease? Epidemiol Community Health 65:226–9.
10. Vessey MP, Villard-Mackintosh L, Yeates D (1987) Oral contraceptives, cigarette smoking and other factors in relation to arthritis. Contraception 35:457–64.
11. Cerhan JR, Saag KG, Criswell LA, Merlino LA, Mikuls TR (2002) Blood transfusion, alcohol use, and anthropometric risk factors for rheumatoid arthritis in older women. J Rheumatol 29:246–54.
12. Crimmins EM, Finch CE (2006) Infection, inflammation, height, and longevity. PNAS 103:598–503.
13. Arnett FC, Edworthy SM, Bloch DA, McShane DJ, Fries JF, et al. (1988) The American Rheumatism Association 1987 revised criteria for the classification of rheumatoid arthritis. Arthritis Rheum 31:315–24.
14. Carstairs V (1995) Deprivation indices: their interpretation and use in relation to health. J Epidemiol Community Health (suppl 2):s3–8
15. Chen Y, Dawes PT, Packham JC, Mattey DL (2011) Interaction between smoking and polymorphism in the promoter region of the VEGFA gene is associated with ischemic heart disease and myocardial infarction in rheumatoid arthritis. J Rheumatol 38:802–9.
16. Prevoo ML, van't Hof MA, Kuper HH, van Leeuwen MA, van de Putte LB, et al. (1995) Modified disease activity scores that include twenty-eight-joints counts: development and validation in a prospective longitudinal study of patients with rheumatoid arthritis. Arthritis Rheum 38:44–8.
17. Johnson AH, Hassell AB, Jones PW, Mattey DL, Saklatvala J, et al. (2002) The mechanical joint score: a new clinical index of joint damage in rheumatoid arthritis. Rheumatology (Oxford) 41:189–95.
18. Fries J, Spitz P, Young D (1982) Dimensions of health outcomes: the health assessment questionnaire, disability and pain scales. J Rheumatol 9:789–93.
19. Preacher KJ, Hayes AF (2008) Asymptotic and resampling strategies for assessing and comparing indirect effects in multiple mediator models. Behav Res Methods 40:879–891.
20. Kuiper S, van Gestel AM, Swinkels HL, de BOO TM, da Silva JA, et al. (2001) Influence of sex, age, and menopausal state on the course of early rheumatoid arthritis. J Rheumatol 28:1809–16.
21. Tengstrand B, Ahlmen M, Hafstrom I, for the BARFOT Study Group (2004) The influence of sex on RA: A prospective study of onset and outcome after 2 years. J Rheumatol 31:207–13.
22. Sokka T, Toloza S, Cutolo M, Kautiainen H, Makinen H, et al. (2009) Women, men, and rheumatoid arthritis: analyses of disease activity, disease characteristics, and treatments in the QUEST-RA Study. Arthritis Res Ther 11:R7.
23. Jawaheer D, Olsen J, Lahiff M, Forsberg S, Lähteenmäki J, et al. (2010) Gender, body mass index and rheumatoid arthritis disease activity: results from the QUEST-RA Study. Clin Exp Rheumatol 28:454–61.
24. Jawaheer D, Maranian P, Park G, Lahiff M, Amjadi SS, et al. (2010) Disease progression and treatment responses in a prospective DMARD-naïve seropositive early rheumatoid arthritis cohort: does gender matter? J Rheumatol 37:2475–85.
25. Ahlmen M, Svensson B, Albertsson K, Forslind K, Hafstrom I, for the BARFOT Study Group (2010) Influence of gender on assessments of disease activity and function in early rheumatoid arthritis in relation to radiographic joint damage. Ann Rheum Dis 69:230–33.
26. Jawaheer D, Lum RF, Gregersen PK, Criswell LA (2006) Influence of male sex on disease phenotype in familial rheumatoid arthritis. Arthritis Rheum 54:3087–94.
27. Chiarelli F, Giannini C, Mohn A (2004) Growth, growth factors and diabetes. Eur J Endocrinol 151 Suppl 3:U109–17.
28. Nemet D, Raz A, Zifman E, Morag H, Eliakim A (2009) Short stature, celiac disease and growth hormone deficiency. J Pediatr Endocrinol Metab 22:979–83.
29. Griffiths AM (2009) Growth retardation in early-onset inflammatory bowel disease: should we monitor and treat these patients differently? Dig Dis 27:404–11.
30. Malemud CJ (2007) Growth hormone, VEGF and FGF: Involvement in rheumatoid arthritis. Clin Clim Acta 375:10–9.
31. De Bellis A, Colao A, Tirelli G, Ruocco G, Di Somma C, et al. (2008) Autoimmunity as a possible cause of growth hormone deficiency. J Endocrinol Invest 31:1132–4.
32. Pass C, MacRae VE, Ahmed SF, Farquharson C (2009) Inflammatory cytokines and the GH/IGF-I axis: novel actions on bone growth. Cell Biochem Funct 27:119–27.
33. Boström EA, Svensson M, Andersson S, Jonsson IM, Ekwall AK, et al. (2011) Resistin and insulin/insulin-like growth factor signalling in rheumatoid arthritis. Arthritis Rheum 63:2894–904.
34. Okada Y, Kamatani Y, Takahashi A, Matsuda K, Hosono N, et al. (2010) A genome-wide association study in 19633 Japanese subjects identified LHX3-QSOX2 and IGF1 as adult height loci. Hum Mol Genet 19:2303–12.
35. Kim JJ, Lee HI, Park T, Kim K, Lee JE, et al. (2010) Identification of 15 loci influencing height in a Korean population. J Hum Genet 55:27–31.
36. Detert J, Pischon N, Burmester GR, Buttgereit F (2010) The association between rheumatoid arthritis and periodontal disease. Arthritis Res Ther 12:218.
37. Raychaudhuri S, Remmers EF, Lee AT, Hackett R, Guiducci C, et al. (2008) Common variants at CD40 and other loci confer risk of rheumatoid arthritis. Nat Genet 40:1216–23.
38. Weedon MN, Lango H, Lindgren CM, Wallace C, Evans DM, et al. (2008) Genome-wide association analysis identifies 20 loci that influence adult height. Nat Genet 40:575–83.
39. Miyamoto Y, Mabuchi A, Shi D, Kubo T, Takatori Y, et al. (2007) A functional polymorphism in the 5′-UTR of GDF5 is associated with susceptibility to osteoarthritis. Nat Genet 39:529–33.
40. Southam L, Rodriguez-Lopez J, Wilkins JM, Pombo-Suarez M, Snelling S, et al. (2007) An SNP in the 5′-UTR of GDF5 is associated with osteoarthritis susceptibility in Europeans and with in vivo differences in allelic expression in articular cartilage. Hum Mol Genet 16:2226–32.
41. Sanna S, Jackson AU, Nagaraja R, Willer CJ, Chen WM, et al. (2008) Common variants in the GDF5-BFZB region are associated with variation in human height. Nat Genet 40:198–203.
42. Francis-West P, Abdelfattah A, Chen P, Allen C, Parish J, et al. (1999) Mechanisms of GDF-5 action during skeletal development. Development 126:1305–15.
43. Francis-West P, Parish J, Lee K, Archer C (1999) BMP/GDF-signalling interactions during synovial joint development. Cell Tissue Res 296:111–9.
44. Chang SC, Hoang B, Thomas JT, Vukicevic S, Luyten FP, et al. (1994) Cartilage-derived morphogenetic proteins. New members of the transforming growth factor-beta superfamily predominantly expressed in long bones during human embryonic development. J Biol Chem 269:28227–34.
45. Chujo T, An HS, Akeda K, Miyamoto K, Muehleman C, et al. (2006) Effects of growth differentiation factor-5 on the intervertebral disc–in vitro bovine study and in vivo rabbit disc degeneration model study. Spine 31:2909–17.
46. Ushiyama T, Mori K, Inoue K, Huang J, Nishioka J, et al. (1999) Association of oestrogen receptor gene polymorphisms with age at onset of rheumatoid arthritis. Ann Rheum Dis 58:7–10.
47. Lanktree MB, Guo Y, Murtaza M, Glessner JT, Bailey SD, et al. (2011) Meta-analysis of dense genecentric association studies reveals common and uncommon variants associated with height. Am J Hum Genet 88:6–18.
48. Cole TJ (2003) The secular trend in human physical growth: a biological view. Econ Hum Biol 1:161–8.
49. Kremer R, Campbell PP, Reinhardt T, Gilsanz V (2009) Vitamin D status and its relationship to body fat, final height, and peak bone mass in young women. J Clin Endocrinol 94:67–73.
50. Song GG, Bae SC, Lee YH (2012) Association between vitamin D intake and the risk of rheumatoid arthritis. Clin Rheumatol Sep 2 [Epub ahead of print]

7

Functional Phenotype of Synovial Monocytes Modulating Inflammatory T-Cell Responses in Rheumatoid Arthritis (RA)

Bo Ruem Yoon[1], Su-Jin Yoo[2], Yeon ho Choi[1,4], Yeon-Ho Chung[1], Jinhyun Kim[2], In Seol Yoo[2], Seong Wook Kang[2*], Won-Woo Lee[1,3,4,5*]

1 Department of Microbiology and Immunology, Seoul National University College of Medicine, Seoul, Korea, 2 Department of Internal Medicine, Chungnam National University School of Medicine, Daejon, Korea, 3 Department of Biomedical Sciences, Seoul National University College of Medicine, Seoul, Korea, 4 Cancer Research Institute, Seoul National University, Seoul, Korea, 5 Ischemic/Hypoxic Disease Institute, and Institute of Infectious Diseases, Seoul National University College of Medicine, Seoul, Korea

Abstract

Monocytes function as crucial innate effectors in the pathogenesis of chronic inflammatory diseases, including autoimmunity, as well as in the inflammatory response against infectious pathogens. Human monocytes are heterogeneous and can be classified into three distinct subsets based on CD14 and CD16 expression. Although accumulating evidence suggests distinct functions of monocyte subsets in inflammatory conditions, their pathogenic roles in autoimmune diseases remain unclear. Thus, we investigated the phenotypic and functional characteristics of monocytes derived from synovial fluid and peripheral blood in RA patients in order to explore the pathogenic roles of these cells. In RA patients, $CD14^{+}CD16^{+}$, but not $CD14^{dim}CD16^{+}$, monocytes are predominantly expanded in synovial fluid and, to a lesser degree, in peripheral blood. Expression of co-signaling molecules of the B7 family, specifically CD80 and CD276, was markedly elevated on synovial monocytes, while peripheral monocytes of RA and healthy controls did not express these molecules without stimulation. To explore how synovial monocytes might gain these unique properties in the inflammatory milieu of the synovial fluid, peripheral monocytes were exposed to various stimuli. CD16 expression on $CD14^{+}$ monocytes was clearly induced by TGF-β, although co-treatment with IL-1β, TNF-α, or IL-6 did not result in any additive effects. In contrast, TLR stimulation with LPS or zymosan significantly downregulated CD16 expression such that the $CD14^{+}CD16^{+}$ monocyte subset could not be identified. Furthermore, treatment of monocytes with IFN-γ resulted in the induction of CD80 and HLA-DR expression even in the presence of TGF-β. An *in vitro* assay clearly showed that synovial monocytes possess the unique capability to promote Th1 as well as Th17 responses of autologous peripheral CD4 memory T cells. Our findings suggest that the cytokine milieu of the synovial fluid shapes the unique features of synovial monocytes as well as their cardinal role in shaping inflammatory T-cell responses in RA.

Editor: Eui-Cheol Shin, KAIST, Graduate School of Medical Science & Engineering, Republic of Korea

Funding: This work was supported by a grant of the Korea Healthcare Technology R&D Project, Ministry for Health & Welfare Affairs, Republic of Korea [Grant No. HI11C1705(A111752)]. The funder had no role in study design, data collection and analysis, decision to publish, or preparation of the manuscript.

Competing Interests: The authors have declared that no competing interests exist.

* Email: wonwoolee@snu.ac.kr (WWL); kangsw@cnuh.co.kr (SWK)

These authors contributed equally to this work.

Introduction

Monocytes are circulating mononuclear phagocytes that have been generally regarded as systemic precursors for tissue macrophages and inflammatory dendritic cells (DCs) [1–3]. Besides their primary role as a precursor, monocytes function as important innate effectors against pathogens through phagocytosis, production of reactive oxygen species (ROS), and secretion of proinflammatory cytokines [4]. It is clear that monocytes are also involved in the pathogenesis of many chronic inflammatory diseases such as RA, Crohn's diseases, and atherosclerosis [5].

Circulating monocytes are highly plastic and heterogeneous [6–9]. In humans, differential expression of CD14 (LPS co-receptor) and CD16 (FcγIII receptor) allows monocytes to be divided into at least two major subsets that have distinct functional activities. The $CD14^{+}CD16^{-}$ monocytes, which are referred to as *'classical'* monocytes, are the most prevalent subset representing 80–90% of blood monocytes in a healthy individual. In contrast, $CD16^{+}$ monocytes comprise a relatively smaller subset in circulating human monocytes but are markedly expanded during infection and inflammatory conditions. Thus, they are generally referred to as *'proinflammatory'* or *'nonclassical'* monocytes. Recent studies demonstrated that $CD16^{+}$ monocytes could be further divided into $CD14^{+}CD16^{+}$ and $CD14^{dim}CD16^{+}$ subsets. Of note, these two subsets differ in their gene signatures and capacity to secrete inflammatory cytokines in response to external stimuli [8]. $CD14^{+}CD16^{+}$ monocytes share many features of $CD14^{+}CD16^{-}$ monocytes including a high capacity for phagocytosis and proinflammatory cytokine production in response to TLR ligands. In comparison, CD14^{dim}CD16$^+$ monocytes exhibit a reduced capacity for phagocytosis and produce less ROS, but have the unique ability to patrol the blood vessel endothelium for signs of damage and infection. Since perturbation of monocyte subsets, especially significant expansion of CD16$^+$ monocytes, is seen in many chronic inflammatory conditions, it has been suggested that CD16$^+$ monocytes play a pivotal role in the pathophysiology of many autoimmune diseases.

RA is a systemic and chronic autoimmune disease that primarily targets synovial membranes [10]. Despite extensive studies, the cause of RA is still unknown although a complex interplay among genetic factors and environmental triggers are thought to be involved [11]. The presence of autoantibodies generated via T-cell-dependent processes in RA patients and mouse models underscore the importance of adaptive immunity as the central contributor to early pathogenesis [11]; however, a growing body of evidence has revealed that a variety innate effector cells, such as monocytes/macrophage, are also closely involved in the development of synovial inflammation in RA [10]. In particular, massive infiltration of activated monocytes/macrophages are frequently observed in synovial membranes of RA patients where they are a major source of many cytokines including TNF-α, IL-1β, IL-8, and GM-CSF in the inflamed joints. Of note, accumulating monocytes in synovial tissue of RA patients express significantly increased CD16 on their surface and produce enormous amounts of TNF-α in response to TLR stimulation [12,13].

Given the presence of monocytes at the sites of both T-cell priming and antigen entry, their possible roles in the regulation of T-cell responses have been suggested [7]. Indeed, it has become clear from recent studies that inflammatory monocytes influence T cell polarization and expansion and shape T-cell responses [7,14]. Recently, *in vivo* activated-monocytes derived from the inflamed joint fluid of active RA patients have been shown to specifically promote pathogenic T-cell responses, mainly in a cell contact-dependent manner [15]. In this context, monocytes are not just producers of inflammatory cytokines, but are closely linked to the modulation of adaptive immune responses, especially T-cell responses, in autoimmune diseases [7,15,16].

In the present study, we sought to investigate the phenotypic and functional characteristics of monocytes derived from synovial fluid and peripheral blood of RA patients in order to further explore their pathogenic roles. Here we found that CD14$^+$CD16$^+$, but not CD14^{dim}CD16$^+$, monocytes were predominantly expanded in synovial fluid and to a lesser degree in peripheral blood of RA patients. Further, the synovial monocytes differentially expressed co-signaling molecules such as CD80 and CD276, suggesting distinct regulatory roles for T-cell responses. Our findings also suggest the possibility that the cytokine milieu of the synovial fluid confers unique phenotypic features to synovial monocytes and hence, shapes their roles in directing the inflammatory T-cell response during RA.

Materials and Methods

Cell preparation

The study protocols were reviewed and approved by the institutional review board of Chungnam National University Hospital (IRB No. 2012-01-024) and the institutional review board of Seoul National University Hospital (IRB No.1109-055-378). All RA patients and healthy volunteers provided their written informed consent to participate in this study. Peripheral blood and synovial fluid of RA patients were collected after obtaining the written informed consent at Department of Internal Medicine, Chungnam National University Hospital. Peripheral blood of healthy volunteers was drawn after obtaining the written informed consent at Seoul National University College of Medicine. Mononuclear cells were isolated from peripheral blood and synovial fluid by density gradient centrifugation (Bicoll separating solution; BIOCHROM Inc, Cambridge, UK). Monocytes were positively separated from peripheral blood mononuclear cells (PBMC) and synovial fluid mononuclear cells (SFMC) with anti-CD14 microbeads (Miltenyi Biotec Inc, Auburn, CA). In some experiments, CD14$^+$CD16$^-$ monocytes were positively purified using anti-CD14$^+$ microbeads from PBMC in which CD16$^+$ monocyte were depleted by CD16 monocyte isolation kit (Miltenyi Biotec Inc). CD4 memory T cells were negatively isolated from PBMC with human memory CD4$^+$ T cell enrichment kit (EasySep negative selection; STEMCELL technologies Inc, Vancouver, Canada).

Flow cytometric analysis

PBMC and SFMC were stained for 30 min at 4 degree with the following antibodies: APC-CD3, PE-Cy5-CD4, APC-Cy7-CD14, PE-Cy5-CD16, APC-CD19, APC-CD56, PE-CD80, PE-CD86, APC-CD276, FITC-HLA-DR (all from BD Bioscience, San Jose, CA), PE-CX$_3$CR1 (eBioscience, San Diego, CA), and PE-CCR2 (R&D systems, Minneapolis, MN). Stained cells were acquired by a BD LSRII (BD bioscience) and analyzed by using Flowjo software (Tree star, Ashland, OR).

Cell culture

Purified monocytes and CD4 memory T cells were cultured in RPMI 1640 medium supplemented with 10% fetal bovine serum (FBS), 1% penicillin/streptomycin (penicillin 100units/ml and streptomycin 100 ug/ml) and 1% L-glutamine (2 mM). For T cell-monocyte coculture, purified monocytes were seeded at 5×10^3 into each well of U-bottomed 96-well plate and incubated with soluble anti-CD3 and anti-CD28 antibodies (1 μg/ml of each; BD bioscience) in the presence of 100ng/ml LPS (Sigma-Aldrich Inc, St. Louis, MO). After incubation for 1 hour, 2.5×10^4 CD4$^+$ memory T cells were added into each well and co-cultured with LPS-activated monocytes for 7 days. In some experiments, purified monocytes were treated for 18 hours with TGF-β (10 ng/ml; R&D systems) in the presence or absence of the indicated recombinant human cytokines such as IL-1β, IL-6 (25 ng/ml of each; both from R&D system), TNF-α (25 ng/ml; ProSpec, East Brunswick, NJ) and IFN-γ (25 ng/ml; eBioscience) and SB431542 (TGF-β signaling inhibitor; Calbiochem, La Jolla, CA), After 18 hour-treatment, the monocytes were stained with the following antibodies: APC-Cy7-CD14, PE-CD16, PE-CD80, and FITC-HLA-DR. The stained cells were acquired by a BD LSRII (BD bioscience).

Intracellular cytokine staining (ICS) and enzyme-linked immunosorbent assay (ELISA)

For intracellular cytokine staining, CD4 T cells co-cultured with monocytes for 7 days were re-stimulated 6 hours with 50ng/ml PMA (Sigma-Aldrich Corp. St. Louis, MO) and 1 ug/ml ionomycin (Sigma-Aldrich) in the presence with Golgiplug (BD Bioscience) for last 4 hours. The cells were fixed and permeablized with BD Cytofix/Cytoperm kit and stained with the following antibodies: PE-IL-17A (eBioscience), PE-Cy7-IFN-γ, and PE-Cy5-CD4 (both from BD Biosciences), followed by analysis using a BD LSRII. In some experiments, intracellular cytokine staining was performed with freshly isolated PBMC and SFMC from RA patients. The amount of IL-17A and IFN-γ in coculture supernatant was quantified by commercial ELISA kits (eBioscience for IL-17A ELISA kit and BioLegend for IFN-γ ELISA kit). The measurement of OD (Optical density) was performed using DTX 880/multimode detector (Beckman coulter, Brea, CA).

Quantitative RT-PCR

Total RNA was extracted from freshly isolated or cocultured cells using TRIzol reagents (life technologies, Grand Island, NY) and cDNA was synthesized by GoScript reverse transcription system (Promega, Madison, WI). Real-time quantitative RT-PCR was performed in triplicates on a 7500 PCR system (Applied Biosystems, Grand Island, NY) using following primers: *CD16*:5′-GCTCCGGATATCTTTGGTGA-3′ and 5′-CTCCCTGGC-ACTTCAGAGTC-3′; *CD68*:5′-ACTGAACCCCAACAAAAC-CA-3′ and 5′-TTGTACTCCACCGCCATGTA3′; *CD80*:5′-GGGAAAGTGTACGCCCTGTA-3′ and 5′-GCTACTTCT-GTGCCCACCAT-3′; *CD86*:5′-TGGAACCAACACAATGGA-GA-3′and 5′-GGTTGCCCAGGAACTTACAA-3′; *CX_3CR1*:5′-GCAAGAAGCCCAAGAGTGTC-3′ and 5′-ATGCTGATGA-CGGTGATGAA-3′; *CD276*:5′-ACCATCACACCCCAGAGA-AG-3′ and 5′-GCCAGATGAGGTTGAGCTGT-3′; *CCR2*:5′-CTGTCCACATCTCGTTCTCGGTTTA-3′ and 5′-CTGAA-CTTCTCCCCAACGAA-3′; *CCR5*; 5′-CTGAGACATCCGT-TCCCCTA-3′ and 5′-TTGCCCACAAAACCAAAGAT-3′; *TLR2*:5′-ATTGTGCCCATTGCTCTTTC-3′and 5′-CTGCC-CTTGCAGATACCATT-3′; *TLR4*:5′-TCTTCAACCAGACC-TCTACATTCCA-3′ and 5′-GGAACATCCAGA GTGACAT-CACAG-3′; *TLR7*:5′-TCACTCCATGCCATCAAGAA-3′ and 5′-ACCATCTAGCCCCAAGGAGT-3′; *TLR8*:5′-TTTTCTT-CATTGGGCCAAAC-3′ and 5′-GAATGGCTGAAA ATTCA-GTTCC-3′; *β-actin*: 5′-GGACTTCGAGCAAGAGATGG-3′and 5′-AGCACTGTGTTGGCGTACAG-3′. The levels of gene expression were normalized to the expression of *β-actin*. The comparative C_T method ($\Delta\Delta C_T$) was used for the quantification of gene expression.

Statistical analysis

Two-tailed paired *t*-test or unpaired *t*-test was done to analyze data using Prism 5 software (GraphPad Software Inc, La Jolla, CA) as indicated in the figure legends. *P* values of less than 0.05 were considered statistically significant.

Results

$CD14^+CD16^+$, but not $CD14^{dim}CD16^+$, monocytes are predominantly expanded in RA patients

Perturbation in the proportions of circulating monocyte subsets has been observed in many inflammatory conditions [9,13]. We first examined whether the frequency of different monocyte subsets was changed in RA patients compared to healthy controls. Based on the phenotypic definition of human monocytes in previous reports [4,9], CD14 and CD16 expression on peripheral blood monocytes (PBMO) from healthy controls and RA patients were analyzed. For this study, monocytes were defined as cells expressing the pan-monocyte marker, HLA-DR, but not bearing any B, T, or NK cell lineage markers in order to avoid contamination with HLA-DR or CD16 expressing B or NK cells, respectively. In agreement with previous reports [4,9], $CD16^+$ monocytes were further divided into two subsets, "intermediate" $CD14^+CD16^+$ and "nonclassical" or "patrolling" $CD14^{dim}CD16^+$ monocytes, by their CD14 expression level (Fig. 1A). As shown in the Figure 1B, the frequency of $CD14^+CD16^+$ monocytes was significantly enhanced in the peripheral blood of RA patients compared with age-matched healthy controls (Mean ± S.E.M., 16.96±3.05% vs. 7.02±1.50%, $p = 0.0207$). However, the frequency of peripheral $CD14^{dim}CD16^+$ monocytes did not significantly differ between RA patients and healthy controls, (2.92±0.54% vs. 1.81±0.33%). Although both monocyte subsets express CD16, these subsets are considered phenotypically and functionally distinct [4,9]. Consequently, the ratio of $CD14^+CD16^+$ to $CD14^{dim}CD16^+$ monocytes in RA patients was six times higher than that in healthy controls (21.83±5.49 fold vs. 3.54±0.94 fold), indicating the selective expansion of $CD14^+CD16^+$ monocytes in the peripheral blood of RA patients. However, the frequency of monocytes, defined as $HLA\text{-}DR^+CD14^+$, among PBMCs did not differ between RA patients and healthy controls (Fig. 1C). To examine clinical relevance of $CD14^+CD16^+$ monocyte, we analyzed the association between the frequency of $CD14^+CD16^+$ monocyte and clinical parameters in the patient. As seen in Figure 1D, the frequency of peripheral $CD14^+CD16^+$ monocytes was significantly correlated with disease activity measured by serum C-reactive protein levels among the RA patients (Fig. 1D).

We next investigated whether the $CD14^+CD16^+$ monocyte population was more expanded in synovial fluid, which is the site of inflammation in RA patients (Fig. 2). To this end, monocyte subsets were compared between the periphery and synovial fluids, which were prepared simultaneously from the same RA patients. In synovial fluid, the percentage of classical $CD14^+CD16^-$ monocytes was significantly reduced compared to that of the peripheral blood of the same patients (Fig. 2B, 59.76±4.95% vs. 83.06±2.48%; $p<0.0005$). Conversely, there was a significant increase of $CD14^-CD16^-HLA\text{-}DR^+$ cells as well as $CD14^+CD16^+$ monocytes in synovial fluid, while $CD14^{dim}CD16^+$ monocytes were only minimally changed. In 15 out of 18 patients tested, $CD14^+CD16^+$ monocytes were increased more than two fold in synovial fluid when compared with peripheral blood (21.33±3.18% vs. 11.97±2.25%; $p<0.05$). We also revealed that the frequency of $HLA\text{-}DR^+CD14^+$ monocytes, which includes $CD14^+CD16^+$ monocytes, is significantly increased in synovial fluid ($p<0.05$), suggesting that the absolute number of $CD14^+CD16^+$ monocytes is also likely increased in synovial fluid (Fig. 2C). Enhanced CD16 expression in synovial monocyte was also confirmed at the level of gene expression and found to be significantly higher in $CD14^+$ monocytes purified from synovial fluids than those purified from peripheral blood of the same RA patient (Fig. 2D).

Co-signaling molecules are differentially expressed in synovial and peripheral monocytes in RA patients

In vivo activated monocytes derived from the synovial fluid of RA patients play a critical role in inducing pathogenic CD4 T-cell responses in a cell contact-dependent manner [15]. Thus, the differential expression of surface molecules by synovial monocytes may be responsible for this finding. To explore a pathogenic role of synovial monocytes in RA patients, we evaluated the expression of major co-signaling molecules on monocytes freshly prepared from paired peripheral blood and synovial fluid samples in RA.

Among the molecules tested, the most prominent differences were observed in the expression of CD80 (B7.1) and CD276 (B7–H3), which are members of B7 co-signaling family [17], between synovial and peripheral monocytes in RA patients (Fig. 3). Expression of CD80 and CD276 mRNAs in purified synovial monocytes were drastically upregulated (Mean ± S.E.M., 12.52±1.91 folds and 66.67±16.68 folds, respectively) when compared with peripheral monocytes from the same RA patient. In contrast, expression of CD86, another B7 co-stimulatory molecule, and CD68, a marker of tissue macrophages, were not

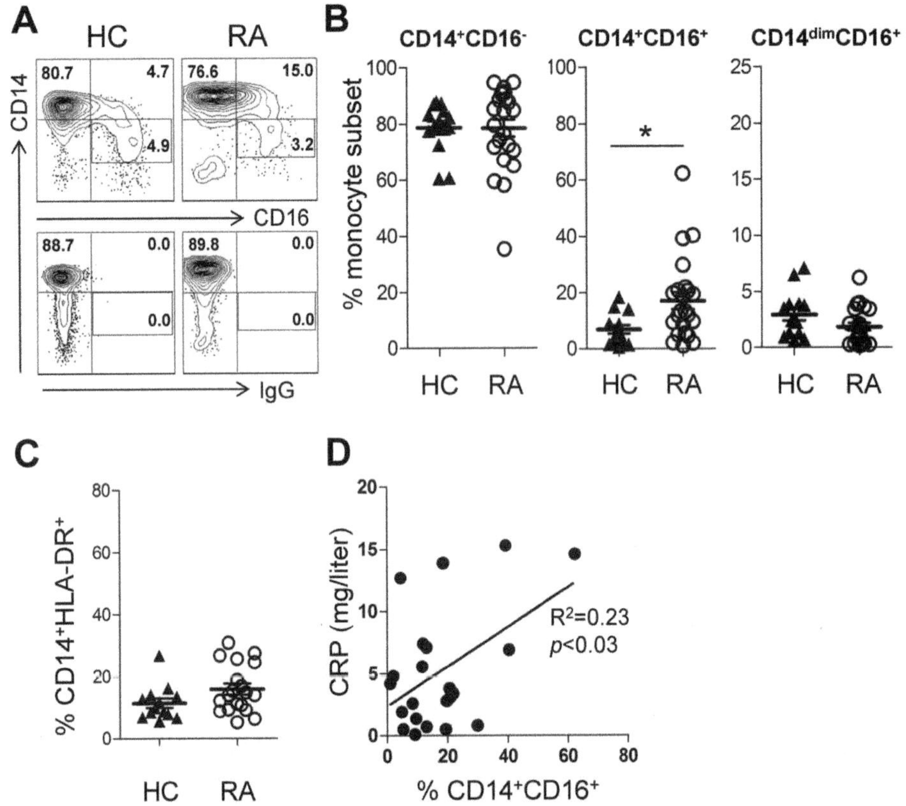

Figure 1. Frequency of $CD14^+CD16^+$, but not $CD14^{dim}CD16^+$, monocytes is increased in peripheral blood of rheumatoid arthritis (RA) patients compared with healthy controls (HC). (**A**) Representative contour plot of peripheral monocytes from HC (left) and RA patients (right). Monocytes were defined as cells expressing HLA-DR but not expressing any lineage markers, such as CD3 (T cells), CD19 (B cells), or CD56 (NK cells). Gated cells were subdivided into three monocyte subsets by their expression of CD14 and CD16. Number in rectangular gate indicates the frequency of $CD14^{dim}CD16^+$ monocytes. (**B**) Frequencies (%) of three monocyte subsets in peripheral blood from HC (n = 14) and RA patients (n = 23) (**C**) Frequencies (%) of monocytes expressing CD14 and HLA-DR among peripheral blood mononuclear cells (PBMC) between HC and RA patients. (**D**) The frequency of peripheral $CD14^+CD16^+$ monocyte was plotted against serum C-reactive protein levels (CRP) among RA patients (n = 22). Each data point represents an individual subject; horizontal bars and error bars show the mean ± SEM. * = $P<0.05$ by unpaired *t*-test (B). *P* value in (D) was obtained using the Pearson correlation analysis.

changed in synovial monocytes (1.50±0.32 and 1.33±0.21 fold, respectively. Not significant) (Fig. 3A). Furthermore, peripheral monocytes from both healthy controls (data not shown) and RA patients constitutively express CD86 at high levels, but do not express CD80 or CD276 (Fig. 3B). Thus, elevated CD80 and CD276 expression appeared to be a feature unique to synovial monocyte in RA patients, a finding that was confirmed by examining the surface expression of these molecules by flow cytometric analysis ($p<0.05$ and $p<0.05$, respectively; Fig. 3C). HLA-DR is a human MHC class II molecule that complexes with cognate antigen and gives the first signal to the T cell receptor (TCR) on CD4 T cells [18]. In humans, monocytes constitutively expressed HLA-DR at high levels, but HLA-DR expression on synovial monocytes was found to be significantly higher than that of peripheral monocytes (MFI; 4,907±1,132 vs. 17,817±2,917, $p<0.0001$, Fig. 3C). Upregulated expression of CD80, CD276, and HLA-DR by synovial monocytes suggests that these cells differentially regulate T cell responses. When the expressions of CD80 and CD86 were compared among three different monocyte subsets in RA patients, CD80 expression was significantly higher in $CD14^+CD16^+$ monocytes in synovial fluid (Fig. 3D, $p<0.01$), whereas CD86 expression was markedly lower in synovial $CD14^{dim}CD16^+$ (Fig. 3E, $p<0.05$).

Differential expression of chemokine receptors and TLRs in synovial and peripheral monocytes of RA patients

Chemokines and their receptors are critical for mediating monocyte recruitment into sites of inflammation [6,19]. Since perturbation of monocyte subsets derived from synovial fluid were clearly seen in RA patients (Fig. 2), we next examined whether the expression of chemokine receptors differ between synovial and peripheral monocytes in the same RA patients. Consistent with previous findings [19,20], CCR5 gene expression in synovial monocytes was markedly upregulated, by 30.41 fold (±9.19), compared with peripheral monocytes ($p<0.05$). In contrast to CCR5, mRNA expression of CX_3CR1 was significantly reduced by 50% in synovial monocyte (Fig. 4A). $CD16^+$ monocytes are known to express high levels of CX_3CR1 and low levels of CCR2. In addition, the CX_3CR1-CX_3CL1 interaction is critical for efficient trans-endothelial migration of $CD16^+$ monocyte [6]. In spite of prominent expansion of $CD14^+CD16^+$ monocyte in RA patients (Fig. 1B and 2B), the expression of CX_3CR1 was decreased moderately on peripheral $CD16^+$ monocytes and more strikingly on synovial $CD16^+$ monocytes from RA patients (Fig. 4B and 4C). Of note, CX_3CR1 expression was almost comparable among the three monocyte subsets in RA synovial monocytes (Fig. 4D). The expression of CCR2, another monocyte subset-

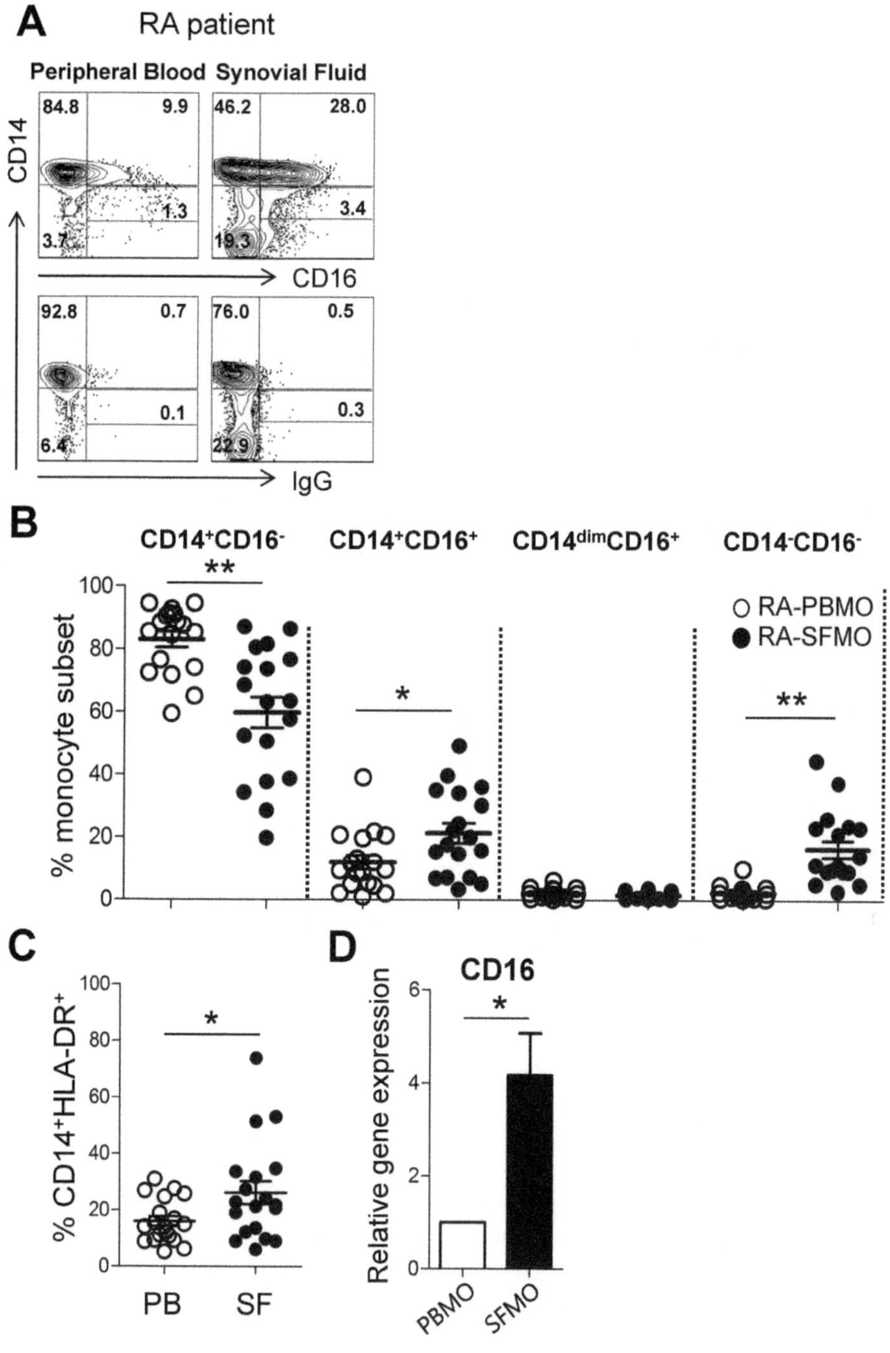

Figure 2. CD14^{+}CD16^{+} monocytes are more expanded in synovial fluid (SF), which is the site of inflammation in RA patients. (A) Representative contour plot of CD14 and CD16 expression on paired peripheral (left) and synovial monocytes (right) from RA patients. Number in rectangular gate indicates the frequency of CD14^{dim}CD16^{+} monocytes. **(B)** Frequencies (%) of different monocyte subsets which were subdivided by differential expression of CD14 and CD16, in paired peripheral blood and synovial fluid RA patient samples (n = 18) **(C)** Frequencies (%) of CD14^{+}HLA-DR^{+} monocytes in peripheral blood and synovial fluid derived from the same RA patients (n = 18) **(D)** Relative gene expression of CD16 in monocytes purified from peripheral blood and synovial fluid of the same RA patients (n = 5). Each data point represents an individual subject; horizontal bars and error bars show the mean ± SEM. * = $P<0.05$; ** = $P<0.01$ by paired *t*-test in **(B and C)**. Bars show the mean ± SEM. * = $P<0.05$ by paired *t*-test in **(D)**. PBMO (peripheral blood monocytes) and SFMO (synovial fluid monocytes).

specific chemokine receptor, did not differ significantly between healthy controls and RA patients (Fig. 4A).

Several studies have recently demonstrated that TLR-stimulated monocytes are required for optimal induction of Th17 cells, which are involved in the pathogenesis of various autoimmune diseases [15,16]. Thus, we analyzed TLR expression in monocytes from blood and synovial fluid of RA patients or healthy controls. In peripheral monocytes, quantitative PCR analysis revealed that TLR8 gene expression was markedly elevated in RA patients, whereas TLR2, TLR4, and TLR7 (Fig. 5A) were comparably expressed between RA patients and healthy controls. In monocytes from the same RA patients, the levels of TLR4 gene

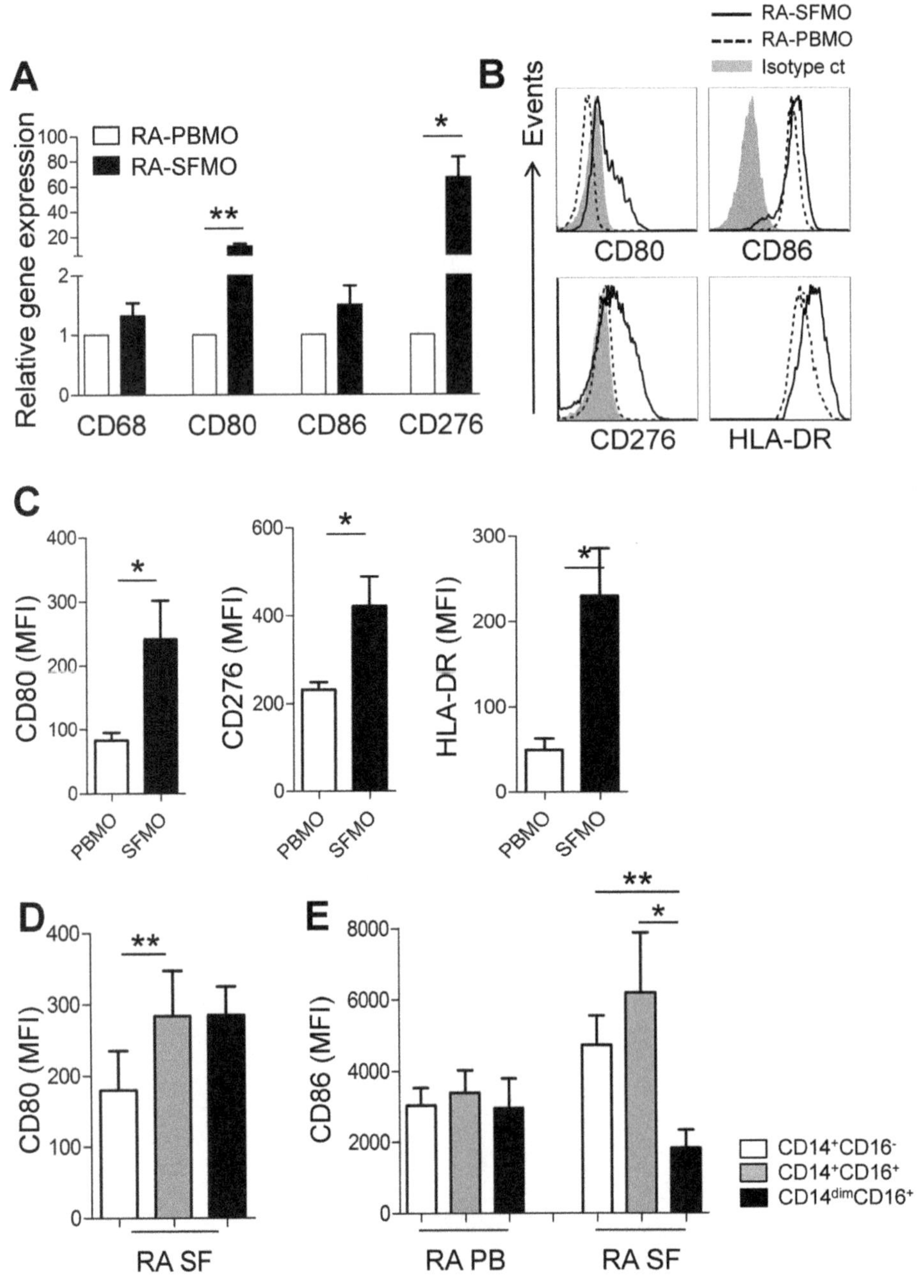

Figure 3. RA patient-derived synovial monocytes predominantly express B7 family member co-signaling molecules, CD80 and CD276. (**A**) Quantitative RT-PCR analysis of CD68, CD80, CD86, and CD276 gene expression in paired peripheral and synovial monocytes from RA patients (n = 4 or 5). (**B**) Representative flow cytometric analysis of CD80, CD86, CD276, and HLA-DR expression on paired peripheral and synovial monocytes from RA patients (solid line: synovial monocytes; dashed line: peripheral monocytes; gray shaded: isotype control). (**C**) Surface expression of CD80, CD276, and HLA-DR on peripheral and synovial monocytes from RA patients (n = 7 or 12). (**D**) Expression of CD80 on three different monocyte subsets of synovial monocytes from RA patients (n = 8). (**E**) Expression of CD86 on three different monocyte subsets of synovial and peripheral monocytes from RA patients (n = 8). Bars show the mean ± SEM. * = $P<0.05$; ** = $P<0.01$ by paired *t*-test in (**A, D, and E**) and unpaired *t*-test (**C**). MFI means mean fluorescent intensity. PBMO (peripheral blood monocytes) and SFMO (synovial fluid monocytes).

expression in those derived from synovial fluid was approximately 10 fold greater than in the peripheral monocytes (Fig. 5B).

Cytokines shape the unique functional phenotype of synovial monocytes

The expansion of circulating $CD16^+$ monocytes has been associated with various acute or chronic inflammatory diseases [21]. We, and others, have shown that $CD14^+CD16^+$, but not $CD14^{dim}CD16^+$, monocytes are markedly enhanced at sites of inflammation in chronic autoimmune disorders such as RA and Crohn's diseases (Fig. 2B) [14]. One possible mechanism for this is the *de novo* expression of CD16 on monocytes caused by exposure to the inflammatory milieu of synovial fluid. To test this possibility, purified $CD14^+$ monocytes from healthy donor were stimulated with TLR ligands or various cytokines and CD16 expression

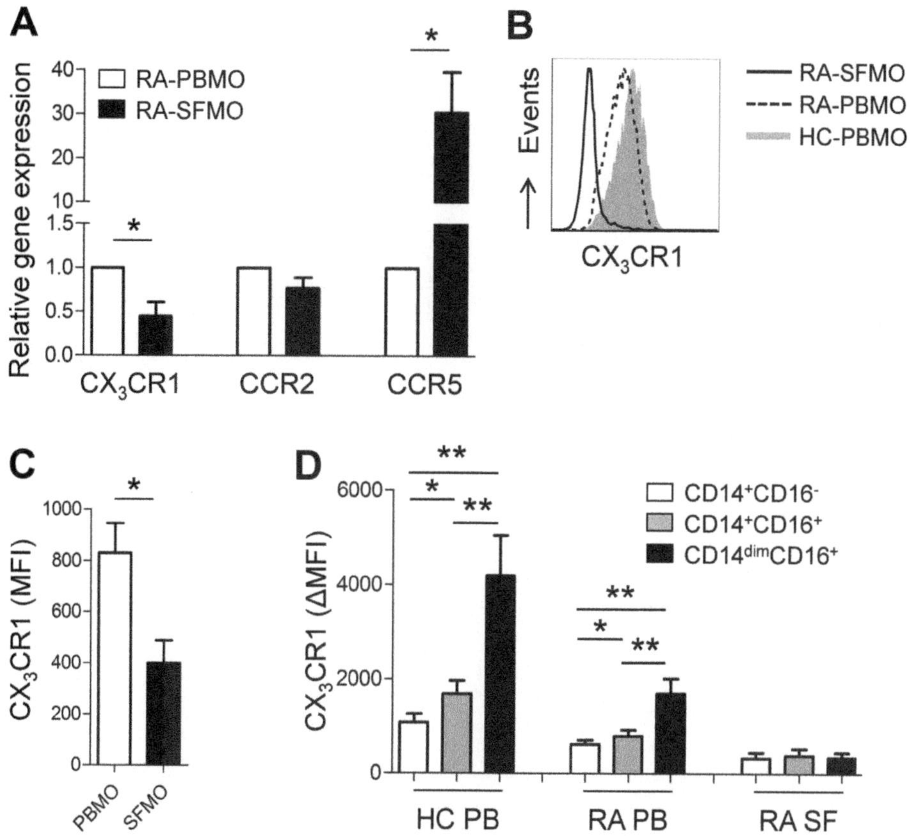

Figure 4. Expression of monocyte subset-specific chemokine receptors differs between peripheral and synovial monocytes from RA patients. (**A**) Quantitative RT-PCR analysis of CX_3CR1, CCR2, and CCR5 gene expression in paired peripheral and synovial monocytes from RA patients (n = 4 or 5). (**B**) Representative flow cytometric analysis of CX_3CR1 expression on peripheral monocytes from HC and paired peripheral and synovial monocytes from RA patients (solid line: RA synovial monocytes; dashed line: RA peripheral monocytes; gray shaded: HC peripheral monocytes). (**C**) Flow cytometric analysis of CX_3CR1 expression on paired peripheral and synovial monocytes from RA patients (n = 8). (**D**) Expression of CX_3CR1 on three different monocyte subsets of peripheral monocytes from HC (n = 8) and peripheral and synovial monocytes from RA patients (n = 8). Bars show the mean ± SEM. * = $P<0.05$; ** = $P<0.01$ by paired *t*-test (**A, C, and D**). MFI = mean fluorescent intensity.

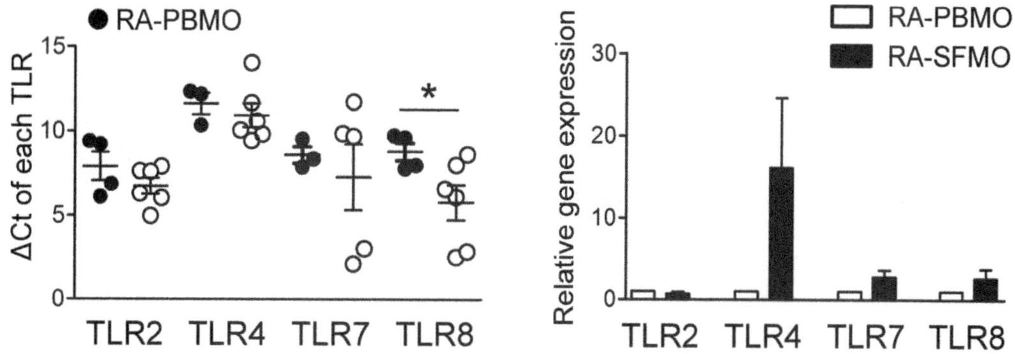

Figure 5. Expression of toll-like receptors differs between peripheral and synovial monocytes derived from RA patients. (**A**) Quantitative RT-PCR analysis of TLR2, 4, 7, and 8 gene expression in peripheral monocytes between HC and RA patients. Expression was normalized to β-actin and ΔCt was calculated by subtracting the Ct of β-actin from the Ct of each TLR gene. Each data point represents an individual subject. (**B**) Comparison of TLR2, 4, 7, and 8 gene expression in paired peripheral and synovial monocytes from RA patients (n = 6); Horizontal bars and error bars show the mean ± SEM. * = $P<0.05$ by unpaired *t*-test with Welch's correction in (**A**).

assessed by flow cytometric analysis. As seen in Figure 6A, the $CD14^+CD16^+$ monocyte subset almost completely disappeared following stimulation with LPS (ligand for TLR4) or zymosan (ligand for TLR2) for 18 hours ($p<0.01$ and $p<0.05$, respectively). In the noninfectious setting of chronic inflammatory diseases such as RA, it is likely that cytokines in synovial fluid contribute to monocyte activation. To this end, we found that TGF-β clearly induced elevated CD16 expression on $CD14^+$ monocytes from healthy controls (Fig. 6B). Approximately 20% of monocytes induced CD16 expression on their cell surface following TGF-β treatment and this induction was successfully inhibited by treatment with a selective blocker of TGF-β signaling, SB431542, confirming this effect was due to TGF-β (Fig. 6C). No additive effects of co-treatment with pro-inflammatory cytokine such as IL-1β, TNF-α, or IL-6 were observed in the present experiments, whereas co-treatment with IL-1β induced a weak inhibitory effect on CD16 induction ($p<0.05$) (Fig. 6D). We next explored the cytokine environment in which expression of CD80 and HLA-DR are induced by monocytes. Since TGF-β is a key inducer of CD16 on monocytes, purified monocytes were incubated with various cytokines in the presence of TGF-β. The results clearly revealed that IFN-γ is a potent inducer of CD80 and HLA-DR expression on monocytes (Fig. 7A–D). Furthermore, TGF-β treatment exhibited no significant effect on the expression of CD80 or HLA-DR (Fig. 7A–D). Likewise, CD80 mRNA expression with IFN-γ alone or TGF-β plus IFN-γ treatment was markedly enhanced, by 18.09 fold (±10.36) and 14.53 fold (±7.04), respectively (Fig. 7B). Of note, TGF-β plus IFN-γ treatment significantly induced CD16 expression, although not as much TGF-β treatment alone (Fig. 7D). We finally examined whether RA synovial fluid could up-regulate CD16 expression on monocytes. As seen in Figure 7E, synovial fluid enhanced the expression of CD16 on $CD14^+$ monocyte from healthy donor with dose-dependent manner. This up-regulation was greatly inhibited by SB431542, a specific blocker of TGF-β signaling. These findings suggest that the distinct functional phenotype of synovial monocytes seen in RA patients may be induced by the cytokine milieu specific to their synovial fluid.

Synovial monocytes have a unique capability to promote proinflammatory Th17 and Th1 responses in RA patients

The $CD14^+CD16^+$ monocyte subset is known to be responsible for pathogenesis of chronic inflammatory diseases and therefore, these cells are referred as to as inflammatory monocytes [14]. To examine whether synovial monocytes in RA patients have a unique capability to modulate T-cell responses, we conducted crisscross cocultures using CD4 memory T cells and monocytes from the synovial fluid and peripheral blood of the same RA patients for 7 days in the presence of soluble anti-CD3, anti-CD28 antibodies and LPS (Fig. 8A). On day 7, cytokine production of co-cultured CD4 T cells was analyzed using intracellular cytokine staining and ELISA. As shown in Figure 8A, proportions of $IL\text{-}17A^+$ and/or IFN^+ $CD4^+$ T cells were significantly higher in peripheral CD4 memory T cells when cultured with synovial monocytes than with peripheral monocytes from the same RA patients. In contrast, induction of $IL\text{-}17A^+$ and/or $IFN\text{-}\gamma^+$ cells from synovial CD4 memory T cells was not affected regardless of monocyte origin in RA patients (Fig. 8A). Consistent with data from the flow cytometric analysis, the amount of IL-17A and IFN-γ in the culture supernatant was significantly increased when peripheral CD4 memory T cells were co-cultured with synovial monocytes (Fig. 8B). Taken together, activated monocytes derived from synovial fluid possess a unique capability to promote production of proinflammatory IL-17 and IFN-γ from peripheral CD4 memory T cells.

Discussion

In the present study, we demonstrate that proinflammatory $CD14^+CD16^+$, but not $CD14^{dim}CD16^{+,}$ monocytes are moderately expanded in peripheral blood and prominently in synovial fluid of RA patients compared to healthy controls. Synovial monocytes have a unique B7 family co-signaling molecule and chemokine receptor expression profile and these distinct functional phenotypes could be induced under the specific cytokine milieu within the synovial fluid. Moreover, RA patient synovial monocytes, but not peripheral monocytes, possess the capability to promote pathogenic Th17 and Th1 responses from autologous peripheral CD4 memory T cells *in vitro*.

One pathologic hallmark of RA is the massive infiltration of activated monocytes/macrophages into inflamed joints where these cells are the primary producers of TNF-α, the major pro-inflammatory cytokine in RA pathogenesis [22]. In addition, activated monocytes from synovial fluid of RA patients function as antigen presenting cells to promote pathogenic CD4 T cell responses at sites of inflammation [7,15,16]. Therefore, monocytes/macrophages have become a major target in the treatment of RA. Given that peripheral $CD16^+$ monocytes are markedly expanded in active RA patients, and their levels correlate with disease severity and responsiveness to therapy, these cells have been implicated in the pathophysiology of RA [19].

Our data clearly reveal that the expansion of peripheral and synovial $CD16^+$ monocytes in RA patients was restricted to the $CD14^+CD16^+$ (and not $CD14^{dim}CD16^+$) monocyte subset (Fig. 1B and 2B). The level of $CD14^{dim}CD16^+$ was not significantly changed in RA patients, indicating that $CD14^{dim}CD16^+$ cells were not responsible for the expansion of $CD16^+$ monocytes in RA (Fig. 1B and 2B). The $CD14^{dim}CD16^+$ monocyte subset was reported to be a functional homolog of the *patrolling* murine $LY6C^{low}$ ($Gr1^-$) monocyte subset. These cells have an important role in innate local surveillance of tissues and in antiviral immunity through sensing of viral DNA. The $CD14^{dim}CD16^+$ monocyte subset produces a greater amount of both the IL-1 receptor antagonist (IL-1Ra), which prevents IL-1-mediated signaling responses by competing with IL-1, and the IL-10 receptor [4]. Thus, in this context, $CD14^{dim}CD16^+$ monocytes appear to have an anti-inflammatory role, if any, and are not likely involved in the pathogenesis of RA. In contrast, $CD14^+CD16^+$ monocytes are the most potent producers of TNF-α, IL-1β, and IL-6 in response to various stimuli. Thus, expanded $CD14^+CD16^+$ monocytes in RA patients play a central role contributing to the pathogenic environment of inflamed joints.

Co-signaling molecule networks among immune cells are critical for controlling the immune response [17]. Among these, the B7 superfamily is major co-signaling molecules acting as a checkpoint in the modulation of T-cell responses [23]. Given that *in vivo* activated-monocytes derived from synovial fluid of active RA patients promote pathogenic Th17 responses through cell contact, it was suggested that differential expression of co-signaling molecules might be responsible. Here we show the upregulation of CD80 (B7-1) and CD276 (B7–H3), which are members of B7 superfamily, on synovial monocytes and not on peripheral monocytes in RA patients (Fig. 3). Both CD80 and CD276 are known to be inducibly expressed on monocytes under stimulation conditions, whereas CD86 (B7-2) is constitutively expressed on resting monocytes. As CD80 and CD276 were found to be induced on monocytes by TLR or cytokine stimulation, our data

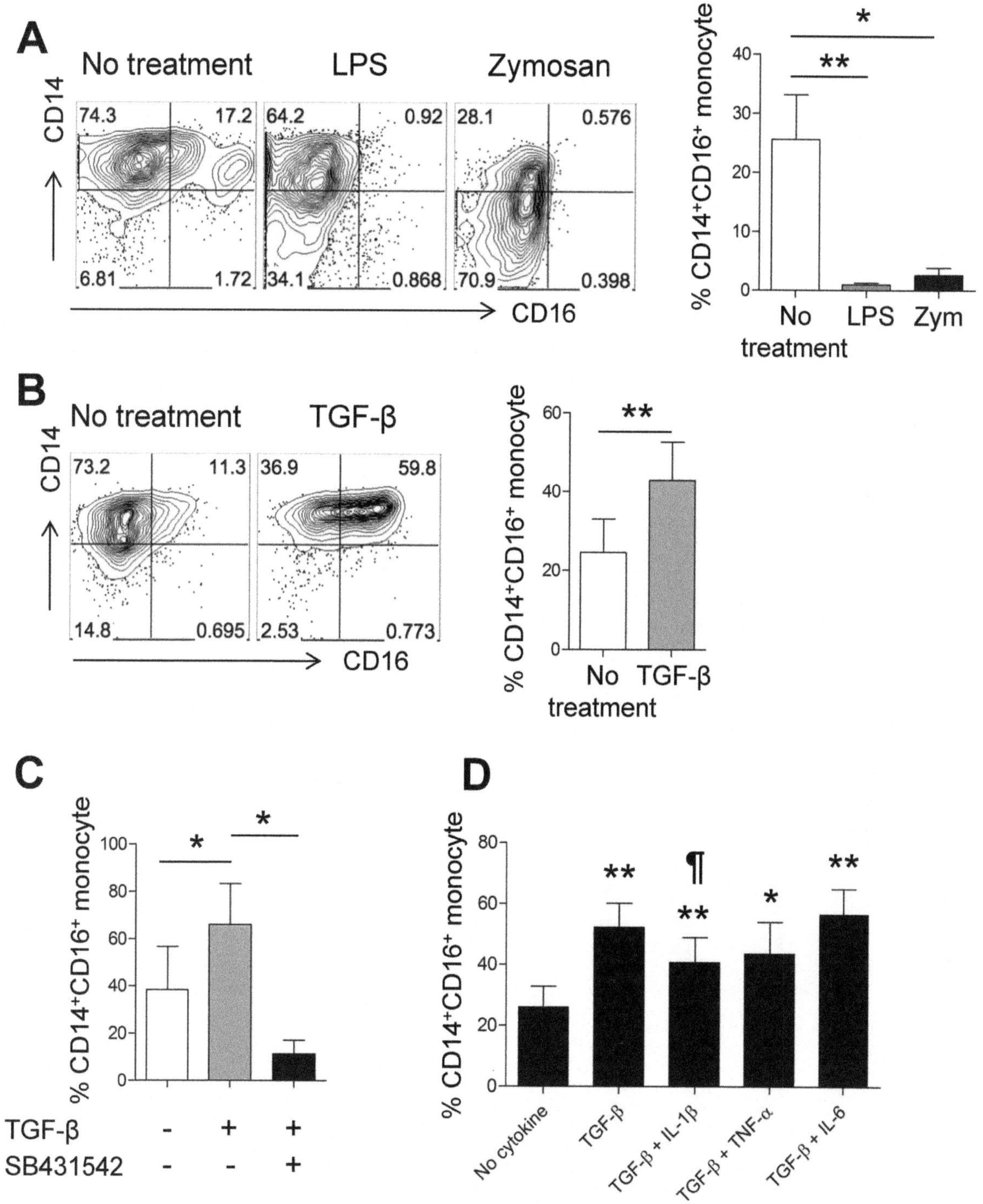

Figure 6. Cytokines shape the unique functional phenotype of synovial monocytes. PBMC or purified monocytes derived from HC were stimulated for 18 hours with the indicated TLR agonists or cytokines and expression of CD14 and CD16 were analyzed by flow cytometry. (**A**) Representative flow cytometric analysis of change in CD16 expression on monocytes (left) and bar graph showing the decreased frequency of the $CD14^{+}CD16^{+}$ monocytes after stimulation with LPS (10 ng/ml) or zymosan (Zym; 10 ug/ml) (right; n = 5). (**B**) Representative flow cytometric analysis of change in CD16 expression on monocytes (left) and bar graph showing the increased frequency of $CD14^{+}CD16^{+}$ monocytes (right; n = 10) after treatment with recombinant human TGF-β (10 ng/ml). (**C**) Purified $CD14^{+}CD16^{-}$ monocytes were treated with TGF-β in the absence or presence of TGF-β signaling blocker, SB431542. TGF-β-induced CD16 expression on monocytes is significantly inhibited by SB431542 (n = 3). (**D**) Frequency of the $CD14^{+}CD16^{+}$ monocytes treated with the indicated proinflammatory cytokines [IL-1β (25 ng/ml), IL-6 (25 ng/ml), and TNF-α (25 ng/ml)] in the presence of TGF-β (n = 9). Bars show the mean ± SEM. * = $P<0.05$; ** = $P<0.01$ by Mann Whitney test in (**A**) and paired *t*-test in (**B and C**). * = $P<0.05$; ** = $P<0.01$ versus no cytokine group in (**D**) and ¶ = $P<0.05$ versus TGF-β group by paired *t*-test in (**D**).

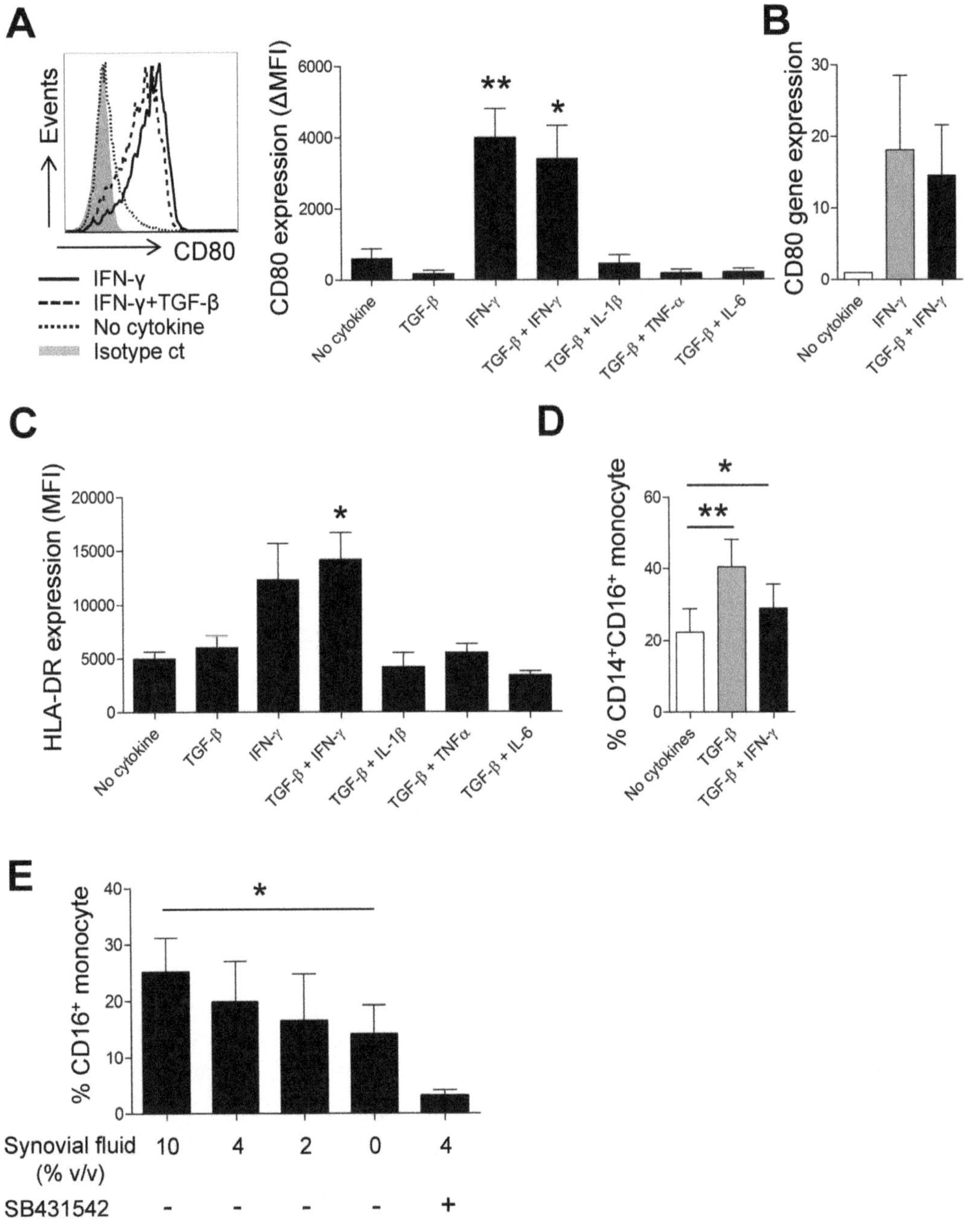

Figure 7. Cytokines are contributing factors for the unique functional phenotypes of RA synovial monocytes. PBMC or purified monocytes derived from HC were stimulated for 18 hours with the indicated cytokines or synovial fluid and expression of indicated molecules were analyzed by flow cytometry (**A**). Representative flow cytometric analysis of CD80 expression on monocytes treated with the indicated cytokines [left; solid line: IFN-γ (25 ng/ml), dashed line: IFN-γ plus TGF-β, dotted line: no cytokine, gray shaded: isotype control]. The change in CD80 expression on monocytes treated with various combinations of cytokines (right; n = 6). MFI, mean fluorescent intensity. (**B**). Quantitative RT-PCR analysis of CD80 gene expression on monocytes after treatment with IFN-γ alone or IFN-γ plus TGF-β (n = 3). (**C**) The change in HLA-DR expression on monocytes treated with various combinations of cytokines (n = 5). (**D**) Frequency of the $CD14^{+}CD16^{+}$ monocytes treated with TGF-β alone or IFN-γ plus TGF-β (n = 13). (**E**) Induced CD16 on $CD14^{+}$ monocytes treated for 18 hours with various concentration of synovial fluid derived from RA patients with or without SB431542 (n = 5). Bars show the mean ± SEM. * = $P<0.05$; ** = $P<0.01$ versus no cytokine group in (**A, C, and D**). * = $P<0.05$; versus no treatment group in (**E**).

suggest that synovial monocytes, but not peripheral monocytes, from RA patients are in an activated state, presumably due to the surrounding cytokine milieu [24,25]. Although induction of CD276 is closely linked to activation and differentiation of monocytes, its exact functional role is still controversial [26]. Whether CD276-mediated signaling in T cells plays a pathogenic role in RA remains to be elucidated.

Trafficking of $CD16^{+}$ monocytes is directly dependent on the CX_3CR1- CX_3CL1 interaction under both steady-state and inflammatory conditions [6,27,28]. Therefore, it is reasonable to assume that CX_3CR1 would be more highly expressed on synovial

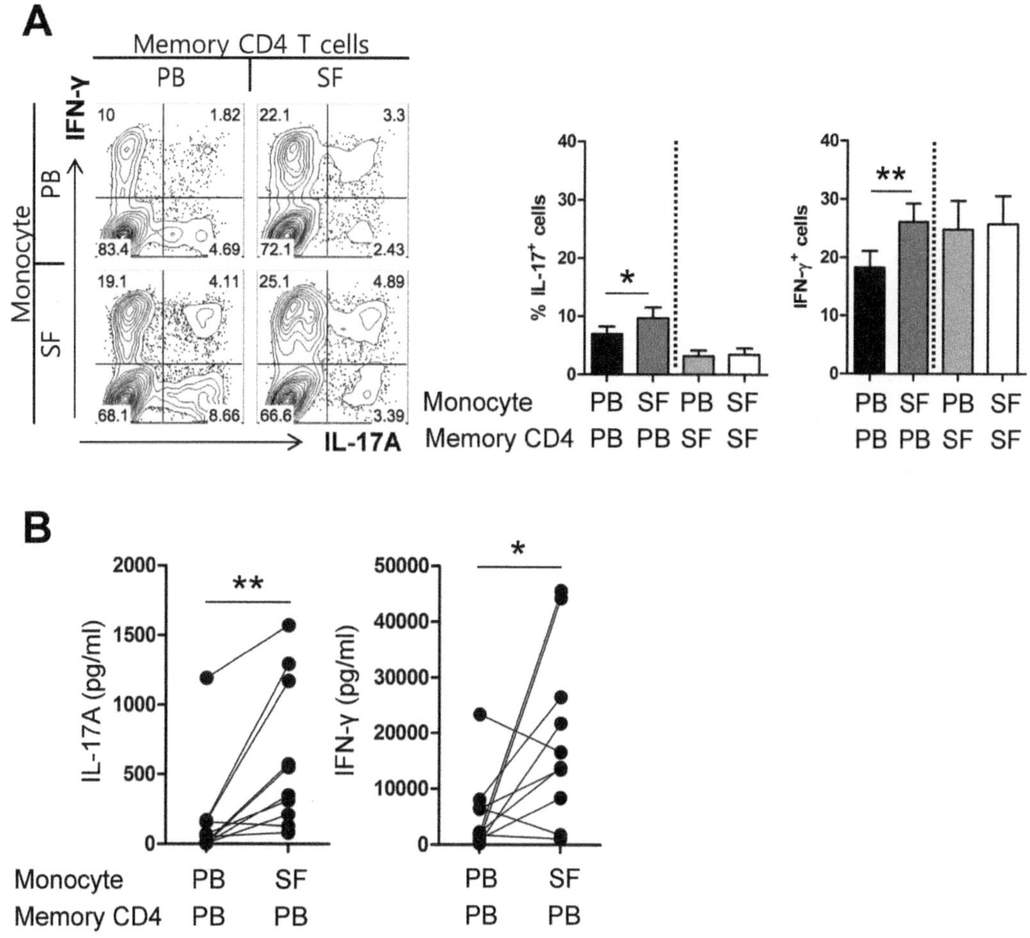

Figure 8. RA patient-derived synovial monocytes have a unique capacity to promote inflammatory Th17 and Th1 responses. Monocytes and $CD4^+$ memory T cells were isolated from peripheral blood and synovial fluid of RA patients and were cocultured in a crisscross pattern for 7 days in the presence of soluble anti-CD3 and anti-CD28 antibodies (1 μg/ml of each) and LPS (100 ng/ml) as described in Material and Methods. (**A**) Representative contour plot of ICS (left) and frequency (%) of IL-17A- and IFN-γ-producing CD4 T cells in the cirsscross colculture (right; n = 14). (**B**) The amounts of IL-17A (left) and IFN-γ (right) in the culture supernatant were quantified using conventional ELISA kits (n = 10). Each pair of symbols represents one experiment. Bars show the mean ± SEM. * = $P<0.05$; ** = $P<0.01$ by paired *t*-test in in (**A and B**).

monocytes than on peripheral monocytes, if the increase in synovial $CD14^+CD16^+$ monocytes observed here is due to selective migration from the periphery; however, the expression of CX_3CR1 mRNA was found to be decreased considerably in synovial monocytes of RA patients (Fig. 4A). More interestingly, CX_3CR1 expression on synovial monocytes was very similar among the three monocyte subsets (Fig. 4D). This implies that $CD14^+CD16^-$ monocytes may be recruited into inflamed joints and gain expression of the CD16 molecule under inflammatory conditions present within synovial fluid. To this point, it should be noted that the majority of $CD14^+CD16^+$ monocytes in the mucosa of intestinal bowel disease (IBD) patients are derived from $CD14^+CD16^-$ cells, and these cells undergo a phenotypic switch to CD16 expression under inflammatory conditions [14].

Thus, the key question is how synovial monocytes gain this unique phenotypic feature in inflamed joints of RA. Since $CD14^+CD16^+$ monocytes are markedly expanded in cancer patients repeatedly treated with LPS and in sepsis patients, it has been suggested that the increase in cytokines caused by LPS or septicemia contribute to the induction of CD16 on monocytes [29,30]. Indeed, CD16 expression can be induced by certain cytokines found in inflammatory conditions such as TGF-β, IL-10, and M-CSF [31]. In this study, we showed that CD16 expression on monocytes was significantly elevated following treatment of cells with TGF-β, an effect that was successfully inhibited by a specific blocker of TGF-β signaling, SB431542 (Fig. 6C). However, major pro-inflammatory cytokines such as TNF-α, IL-1β, and IL-6, which are abundant in inflamed joints, did not positively influence CD16 induction on monocytes (Fig. 6D). In spite of the role of TGF-β for CD16 induction, our ELISA showed that the average amount of TGF-β in the plasma of healthy controls was comparable to that in RA patients (data not shown). TGF-β mainly exists in a latent form and the amount of active TGF-β in most of biological samples is below the detection limit using conventional ELISA. Since TGF-β activation locally occurs at the cell surface, local concentration of bioactive TGF-β is presumably more important for their biological functions than total amount of latent TGF-β. In this context, it should be noted that purified $CD14^+CD16^-$ monocyte aggregated with activated platelet, one of major source of bioactive TGF-β, markedly induced CD16 with TGF-β signaling dependent manner [32]. The interplay between TGF-β and monocytes is responsible for amplification of monocyte-mediated inflammatory responses in an autocrine fashion. TGF-β is produced by monocytes at sites of inflammation and TGF-β-stimulated monocytes release an inactive, latent form of TGF-β that in turn, is activated by monocytes [33,34]. In the present study, the expression of CD80 and HLA-DR on synovial monocytes (Fig. 3) was also predominantly enhanced by IFN-γ, which is abundant in inflamed joints and probably released by Th1 cells [35]. Given that HLA-DR and CD80 play a critical role for delivering 'signal 1' and 'signal 2' to T cells, respectively, synovial monocytes could have immunostimulatory effects on T cell responses at the site of inflammation.

Activated monocytes exert fundamental effects on the polarization and expansion of T cells and can contribute to shaping primary and secondary T-cell responses [7]. Thus, synovial monocytes with distinct functional phenotypes can modulate T-cell responses in RA. Recently, it was reported that Th17 responses are selectively promoted by *in vivo*-activated synovial monocytes derived from active RA patients. In addition, Rossol et al. showed that LPS-treated $CD14^{+}CD16^{+}$ monocytes preferentially promote the expansion of the Th17, but not Th1, subset and none of the monocyte subsets influence Th1 expansion in healthy donors [36]. However, our findings clearly show that synovial monocytes, and not peripheral monocytes, derived from RA patients markedly facilitate production of IFN-γ as well as IL-17 from autologous, peripheral $CD4^{+}$ memory T cells (Fig. 8). It is unclear why not only Th17, but also Th1 subsets are significantly expanded in our experimental system. Perhaps differences in culture systems utilized by us and others are responsible for this disparate result. Another possible cause is our use of RA patient-derived CD4 memory T cells and not total CD4 T cells. In the clinical setting, CD4 T cells, which have a chance to associate with activated monocytes in the inflamed joints, are likely to be memory T cells due to the inability of naive T cells to be recruited into the site of inflammation. Indeed, a majority of synovial T cells belong to the memory subset (data not shown). Although Th17 cells undeniably play a critical role in RA pathogenesis, it should be noted that in RA patients a large proportion of synovial $CD4^{+}$ T cells are also IFN-γ-producing Th1 cells [35]. It is therefore possible that synovial monocytes provide the recruited CD4 memory T cells with a favorable environment for the enhancement of IFN-γ and IL-17 production in the inflamed joints.

In summary, our study reveals the phenotypic and functional characteristics of monocytes in the synovial fluid and peripheral blood of RA patients, which may be affected by the synovial fluid environment and thus, critically affect the pathogenesis of RA. Thus, this suggests that the synovial fluid cytokine milieu imparts unique features upon synovial monocytes and thus, affects their critical roles in inflammatory T-cell responses during RA.

Author Contributions

Conceived and designed the experiments: BRY SWK WWL. Performed the experiments: BRY SJY Yeon ho Choi Yeon-Ho Chung. Analyzed the data: BRY SJY Yeon ho Choi Yeon-Ho Chung SWK WWL. Contributed reagents/materials/analysis tools: SJY JK ISY SWK. Contributed to the writing of the manuscript: BRY SWK WWL.

References

1. Randolph GJ, Inaba K, Robbiani DF, Steinman RM, Muller WA (1999) Differentiation of phagocytic monocytes into lymph node dendritic cells in vivo. Immunity 11: 753–761.
2. Geissmann F, Jung S, Littman DR (2003) Blood monocytes consist of two principal subsets with distinct migratory properties. Immunity 19: 71–82.
3. Varol C, Landsman L, Fogg DK, Greenshtein L, Gildor B, et al. (2007) Monocytes give rise to mucosal, but not splenic, conventional dendritic cells. J Exp Med 204: 171–180.
4. Cros J, Cagnard N, Woollard K, Patey N, Zhang SY, et al. (2010) Human CD14dim monocytes patrol and sense nucleic acids and viruses via TLR7 and TLR8 receptors. Immunity 33: 375–386.
5. Woollard KJ, Chin-Dusting J (2010) P-selectin antagonism in inflammatory disease. Curr Pharm Des 16: 4113–4118.
6. Shi C, Pamer EG (2011) Monocyte recruitment during infection and inflammation. Nat Rev Immunol 11: 762–774.
7. Geissmann F, Auffray C, Palframan R, Wirrig C, Ciocca A, et al. (2008) Blood monocytes: distinct subsets, how they relate to dendritic cells, and their possible roles in the regulation of T-cell responses. Immunol Cell Biol 86: 398–408.
8. Ingersoll MA, Platt AM, Potteaux S, Randolph GJ (2011) Monocyte trafficking in acute and chronic inflammation. Trends Immunol 32: 470–477.
9. Wong KL, Yeap WH, Tai JJ, Ong SM, Dang TM, et al. (2012) The three human monocyte subsets: implications for health and disease. Immunol Res 53: 41–57.
10. McInnes IB, O'Dell JR (2010) State-of-the-art: rheumatoid arthritis. Ann Rheum Dis 69: 1898–1906.
11. McInnes IB, Schett G (2011) The pathogenesis of rheumatoid arthritis. N Engl J Med 365: 2205–2219.
12. Iwahashi M, Yamamura M, Aita T, Okamoto A, Ueno A, et al. (2004) Expression of Toll-like receptor 2 on CD16+ blood monocytes and synovial tissue macrophages in rheumatoid arthritis. Arthritis Rheum 50: 1457–1467.
13. Ziegler-Heitbrock L (2007) The CD14+ CD16+ blood monocytes: their role in infection and inflammation. J Leukoc Biol 81: 584–592.
14. Koch S, Kucharzik T, Heidemann J, Nusrat A, Luegering A (2010) Investigating the role of proinflammatory CD16+ monocytes in the pathogenesis of inflammatory bowel disease. Clin Exp Immunol 161: 332–341.
15. Evans HG, Gullick NJ, Kelly S, Pitzalis C, Lord GM, et al. (2009) In vivo activated monocytes from the site of inflammation in humans specifically promote Th17 responses. Proc Natl Acad Sci U S A 106: 6232–6237.
16. Evans HG, Suddason T, Jackson I, Taams LS, Lord GM (2007) Optimal induction of T helper 17 cells in humans requires T cell receptor ligation in the context of Toll-like receptor-activated monocytes. Proc Natl Acad Sci U S A 104: 17034–17039.
17. Yi KH, Chen L (2009) Fine tuning the immune response through B7–H3 and B7–H4. Immunol Rev 229: 145–151.
18. Gay D, Maddon P, Sekaly R, Talle MA, Godfrey M, et al. (1987) Functional interaction between human T-cell protein CD4 and the major histocompatibility complex HLA-DR antigen. Nature 328: 626–629.
19. Kawanaka N, Yamamura M, Aita T, Morita Y, Okamoto A, et al. (2002) CD14+, CD16+ blood monocytes and joint inflammation in rheumatoid arthritis. Arthritis Rheum 46: 2578–2586.
20. Katschke KJ Jr, Rottman JB, Ruth JH, Qin S, Wu L, et al. (2001) Differential expression of chemokine receptors on peripheral blood, synovial fluid, and synovial tissue monocytes/macrophages in rheumatoid arthritis. Arthritis Rheum 44: 1022–1032.
21. Sanchez-Torres C, Garcia-Romo GS, Cornejo-Cortes MA, Rivas-Carvalho A, Sanchez-Schmitz G (2001) CD16+ and CD16- human blood monocyte subsets differentiate in vitro to dendritic cells with different abilities to stimulate CD4+ T cells. Int Immunol 13: 1571–1581.
22. Davignon JL, Hayder M, Baron M, Boyer JF, Constantin A, et al. (2013) Targeting monocytes/macrophages in the treatment of rheumatoid arthritis. Rheumatology (Oxford) 52: 590–598.
23. Greenwald RJ, Freeman GJ, Sharpe AH (2005) The B7 family revisited. Annu Rev Immunol 23: 515–548.
24. Linsley PS, Greene JL, Brady W, Bajorath J, Ledbetter JA, et al. (1994) Human B7-1 (CD80) and B7-2 (CD86) bind with similar avidities but distinct kinetics to CD28 and CTLA-4 receptors. Immunity 1: 793–801.
25. Hathcock KS, Laszlo G, Pucillo C, Linsley P, Hodes RJ (1994) Comparative analysis of B7-1 and B7-2 costimulatory ligands: expression and function. J Exp Med 180: 631–640.
26. Hofmeyer KA, Ray A, Zang X (2008) The contrasting role of B7–H3. Proc Natl Acad Sci U S A 105: 10277–10278.
27. Ancuta P, Rao R, Moses A, Mehle A, Shaw SK, et al. (2003) Fractalkine preferentially mediates arrest and migration of CD16+ monocytes. J Exp Med 197: 1701–1707.
28. Auffray C, Fogg DK, Narni-Mancinelli E, Senechal B, Trouillet C, et al. (2009) CX3CR1+ CD115+ CD135+ common macrophage/DC precursors and the role of CX3CR1 in their response to inflammation. J Exp Med 206: 595–606.
29. Blumenstein M, Boekstegers P, Fraunberger P, Andreesen R, Ziegler-Heitbrock HW, et al. (1997) Cytokine production precedes the expansion of CD14+CD16+ monocytes in human sepsis: a case report of a patient with self-induced septicemia. Shock 8: 73–75.
30. Mackensen A, Galanos C, Wehr U, Engelhardt R (1992) Endotoxin tolerance: regulation of cytokine production and cellular changes in response to endotoxin application in cancer patients. Eur Cytokine Netw 3: 571–579.
31. Welch GR, Wong HL, Wahl SM (1990) Selective induction of Fc gamma RIII on human monocytes by transforming growth factor-beta. J Immunol 144: 3444–3448.
32. Mazzieri R, Munger JS, Rifkin DB (2000) Measurement of active TGF-beta generated by cultured cells. Methods Mol Biol 142: 13–27.

33. Wahl SM, McCartney-Francis N, Allen JB, Dougherty EB, Dougherty SF (1990) Macrophage production of TGF-beta and regulation by TGF-beta. Ann N Y Acad Sci 593: 188–196.
34. McCartney-Francis N, Mizel D, Wong H, Wahl L, Wahl S (1990) TGF-beta regulates production of growth factors and TGF-beta by human peripheral blood monocytes. Growth Factors 4: 27–35.
35. Yamada H, Nakashima Y, Okazaki K, Mawatari T, Fukushi JI, et al. (2008) Th1 but not Th17 cells predominate in the joints of patients with rheumatoid arthritis. Ann Rheum Dis 67: 1299–1304.
36. Rossol M, Kraus S, Pierer M, Baerwald C, Wagner U (2012) The CD14(bright) CD16+ monocyte subset is expanded in rheumatoid arthritis and promotes expansion of the Th17 cell population. Arthritis Rheum 64: 671–677.

IL-6 Amplifies TLR Mediated Cytokine and Chemokine Production: Implications for the Pathogenesis of Rheumatic Inflammatory Diseases

Ivan Caiello[1], Gaetana Minnone[1], Dirk Holzinger[2,3], Thomas Vogl[2], Giusi Prencipe[1], Antonio Manzo[4], Fabrizio De Benedetti[1]*, Raffaele Strippoli[1,5]*

1 Division of Rheumatology, Bambino Gesù Children's Hospital, Rome, Italy, **2** Department of Paediatric Rheumatology and Immunology, University Children's Hospital Muenster, Muenster, Germany, **3** Institute of Immunology, University Hospital Muenster, Muenster, Germany, **4** Rheumatology and Translational Immunology Research Laboratories (LaRIT), Division of Rheumatology, IRCCS Policlinico S. Matteo Foundation/University of Pavia, Pavia, Italy, **5** Department of Cellular Biotechnologies and Haematology, Sapienza University of Rome, Rome, Italy

Abstract

The role of Interleukin(IL)-6 in the pathogenesis of joint and systemic inflammation in rheumatoid arthritis (RA) and systemic juvenile idiopathic arthritis (s-JIA) has been clearly demonstrated. However, the mechanisms by which IL-6 contributes to the pathogenesis are not completely understood. This study investigates whether IL-6 affects, alone or upon toll like receptor (TLR) ligand stimulation, the production of inflammatory cytokines and chemokines in human peripheral blood mononuclear cells (PBMCs), synovial fluid mononuclear cells from JIA patients (SFMCs) and fibroblast-like synoviocytes from rheumatoid arthritis patients (RA synoviocytes) and signalling pathways involved. PBMCs were pre-treated with IL-6 and soluble IL-6 Receptor (sIL-6R). SFMCs and RA synoviocytes were pre-treated with IL-6/sIL-6R or sIL-6R, alone or in combination with Tocilizumab (TCZ). Cells were stimulated with LPS, S100A8-9, poly(I-C), CpG, Pam2CSK4, MDP, IL-1β. Treatment of PBMCs with IL-6 induced production of TNF-α, CXCL8, and CCL2, but not IL-1β. Addition of IL-6 to the same cells after stimulation with poly(I-C), CpG, Pam2CSK4, and MDP induced a significant increase in IL-1β and CXCL8, but not TNF-α production compared with TLR ligands alone. This enhanced production of IL-1β and CXCL8 paralleled increased p65 NF-κB activation. In contrast, addition of IL-6 to PBMCs stimulated with LPS or S100A8-9 (TLR-4 ligands) led to reduction of IL-1β, TNF-α and CXCL8 with reduced p65 NF-κB activation. IL-6/IL-1β co-stimulation increased CXCL8, CCL2 and IL-6 production. Addition of IL-6 to SFMCs stimulated with LPS or S100A8 increased CXCL8, CCL2 and IL-1β production. Treatment of RA synoviocytes with sIL-6R increased IL-6, CXCL8 and CCL2 production, with increased STAT3 and p65 NF-κB phosphorylation. Our results suggest that IL-6 amplifies TLR-induced inflammatory response. This effect may be relevant in the presence of high IL-6 and sIL-6R levels, such as in arthritic joints in the context of stimulation by endogenous TLR ligands.

Editor: Wenyu Lin, Harvard Medical School, United States of America

Funding: This study was supported by research funding from the IRCCS Bambino Gesú Children's Hospital "Ricerca Corrente" to FDB. IRCCS Bambino Gesú Hospital "Ricerca Corrente" had no role in study design, data collection and analysis, decision to publish, or preparation of the manuscript.

Competing Interests: Dr De Benedetti's Institution received unrestricted research grants from Pfizer, Abbvie, Novartis, Novimmune, Roche, SOBI and travel support from Roche. The other authors declare that they have no competing interests.

* Email: fabrizio.debenedetti@opbg.net (FDB); rafstrippoli@libero.it (RS)

Introduction

Interleukin-6 (IL-6) is a pleiotropic cytokine with multiple functions in different pathophysiologic systems [1,2]. Data from animal models have shown that IL-6 plays a non-redundant role in several pathophysiological events, such as fever, liver acute-phase response, and in the transition from acute to chronic inflammation [3]. The recent introduction of tocilizumab (TCZ), an IL-6 receptor blocker, in the treatment of rheumatoid arthritis (RA) and systemic juvenile idiopathic arthritis (s-JIA), clearly demonstrated a major role of this cytokine in the pathogenesis of joint and systemic inflammation [4,5]. However, the cellular and molecular mechanisms by which high levels of IL-6, which are present in blood and synovial fluids contribute to the pathogenesis are not completely understood.

In recent years, many efforts in understanding the pathogenic role of IL-6 in arthritis have been focused on the effect of IL-6 on adaptive immunity. Indeed, IL-6 has a role in the differentiation of B lymphocyte into auto-antibody producing plasma cells, which participate in the pathogenesis of arthritis through the formation of immune complexes (IC) [6]. Moreover, high levels of IL-6 may cause a Th17/Treg cell imbalance during RA, which is corrected upon treatment with TCZ [7,8]. Accordingly, IL-6 mediated B and T lymphocyte dysregulation may lead to abnormal production of inflammatory cytokines, chemokines and metalloproteases by both leukocytes and cells of the synovial stroma, leading to synovial tissue degradation and bone erosions.

However, little is known about possible direct effects of IL-6 on innate immune mechanisms. Toll like receptors (TLRs) are a family of trans-membrane glycoproteins with conserved extracellular domains and a cytoplasmic signaling domain homologous to that of IL-1R, called the Toll/IL-1R domain. They bind a wide array of bacterial and viral peptides [9]. Signals from the various TLR ligands generally converge to activate the mitogen-activated protein kinases (MAPKs), p65 nuclear-factor kappa B (p65 NF-κB), and interferon regulatory factor 3 (IRF-3)/IRF-7 pathways, which mediate inflammatory cytokine and type I interferon secretion, thus controlling the response to pathogens [9]. TLR response may be relevant for the pathogenesis of rheumatic diseases also in the absence of infections. Indeed, a number of endogenous TLR ligands, especially for TLR2 and TLR4, has recently emerged as potential players in chronic inflammation [10]. For example, TLR4 ligands belonging to the S100 family may play a role in pathogenesis of s-JIA, and immunocomplexes (IC) including citrullinated proteins have been involved in the pathogenesis of RA [11–13].

We have previously shown that IL-6 directly enhances TRL ligand-induced response [14] both in vitro and ex vivo. IL-6 transgenic (IL-6TG) mice undergo an exaggerated inflammatory response when treated with TLR ligands and peritoneal macrophages from these mice produce increased levels of IL-6 and IL-1β when stimulated *ex vivo* with TLR ligands [14].

The aim of this study was to evaluate whether IL-6 directly affected inflammatory cytokine and chemokine production upon TLR stimulation with various TLR ligands in human mononuclear cells and RA synoviocytes.

Methods

Antibodies and chemicals

Polyclonal antibodies against phospho-STAT3 (Tyr705) phospho-NFκB (Ser536) were from Cell Signaling (Cell Signaling Technology, Danvers, MA); monoclonal antibodies against tubulin were from Sigma (Saint Louis, MO). Recombinant human IL-6 ad soluble IL-6 receptor (sIL-6R) were from R&D Systems (Minneapolis, MN). LPS was from Sigma Aldrich, (St Louis, MO) CpG-DNA, Pam3CSK4, Muramyl dipeptide (MDP) and Poly(IC) were from Invivogen (San Diego, CA); S100A8 and S100A9 were from Vogl lab. TCZ (RoActemra) was from Roche, Milan, Italy.

Isolation and culture of peripheral blood mononuclear cells (PBMCs) synovial fluid mononuclear cells (SFMCs) and synovial fibroblasts form RA patients

Peripheral blood mononuclear cells (PBMCs) were derived from healthy donors by centrifugation on a LSF-Lymphocyte Separation Ficoll (LiStarFish). For ELISA studies, cells were put at 1×10^6/well in 24 wells plate in DMEM supplemented with 10% fetal calf serum (FCS) (HyClone). For western blot assays, cells were starved in DMEM supplemented with 0.5% FCSfor 2 hours before stimulation. In some experiments, cells were left to adhere on plastic for 3 hours in DMEM supplemented with 10% FCS.

Synovial fluid mononuclear cells from 10 oligoarticular JIA patients (SFMCs) were isolated by Ficoll density centrifugation. 1×10^6 cells/well were put in 24 wells plate and were left to adhere on plastic for 3 hours in DMEM supplemented with 10% FCS. Cells were then washed and treated with different stimuli. Due to limited amount of supernatants obtained by culture of SFMCs, it was not possible to measure all cytokines in the supernatants of the SFMCs obtained by each patient.

Synoviocytes were obtained from 5 RA patients undergoing ultrasound-guided synovial biopsy. [15]. Cells isolated from synovial tissue by enzymatic digestion with collagenase and were cultured in DMEM supplemented with 10% FCS. For ELISA assays, cells were grown to confluence in a p24 plate (approximately 50.000 cells per well). For western blot assays, cells were starved at 0.5% FCS for two hours before stimulation.

The part of the study involving JIA patients (SFMCs) was approved by the Ethical Committee of the Bambino Gesù Children's Hospital Rome, Italy, and written consent was obtained from the parents of each child. The part of the study involving RA patients (synoviocytes) was approved by the Ethical Committee of the IRCCS Policlinico San Matteo Foundation, Pavia, Italy, and written consent was obtained from all patients.

Reverse transcription–polymerase chain reaction (PCR)

Total RNA was extracted using TRIzol (Invitrogen), and cDNA was obtained using the Superscript Vilo kit (Invitrogen). The following gene expression assay was used in the real-time PCR assays: human TLR4 (Hs00152939_ml). Gene expression data

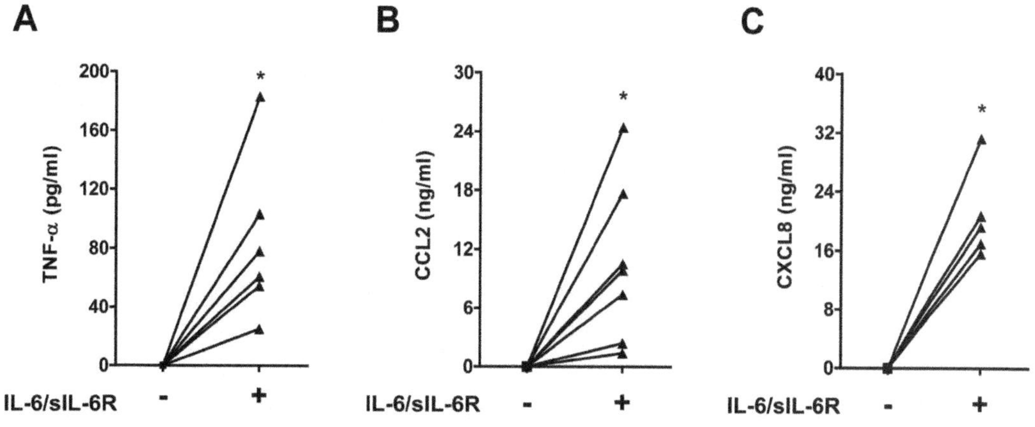

Figure 1. TNF-α, CCL2 and CXCL8 production in human PBMCs exposed to IL-6. Human PBMCs were exposed to IL-6 (10 ng/ml) in combination with sIL-6R (125 ng/ml) (IL-6/sIL-6R) for 18 hours. TNF-α, CCL2 and CXCL8 levels were measured by ELISA. *$p<0.05$ for values from IL-6/sIL-6R stimulated compared with not treated (NT) cells.

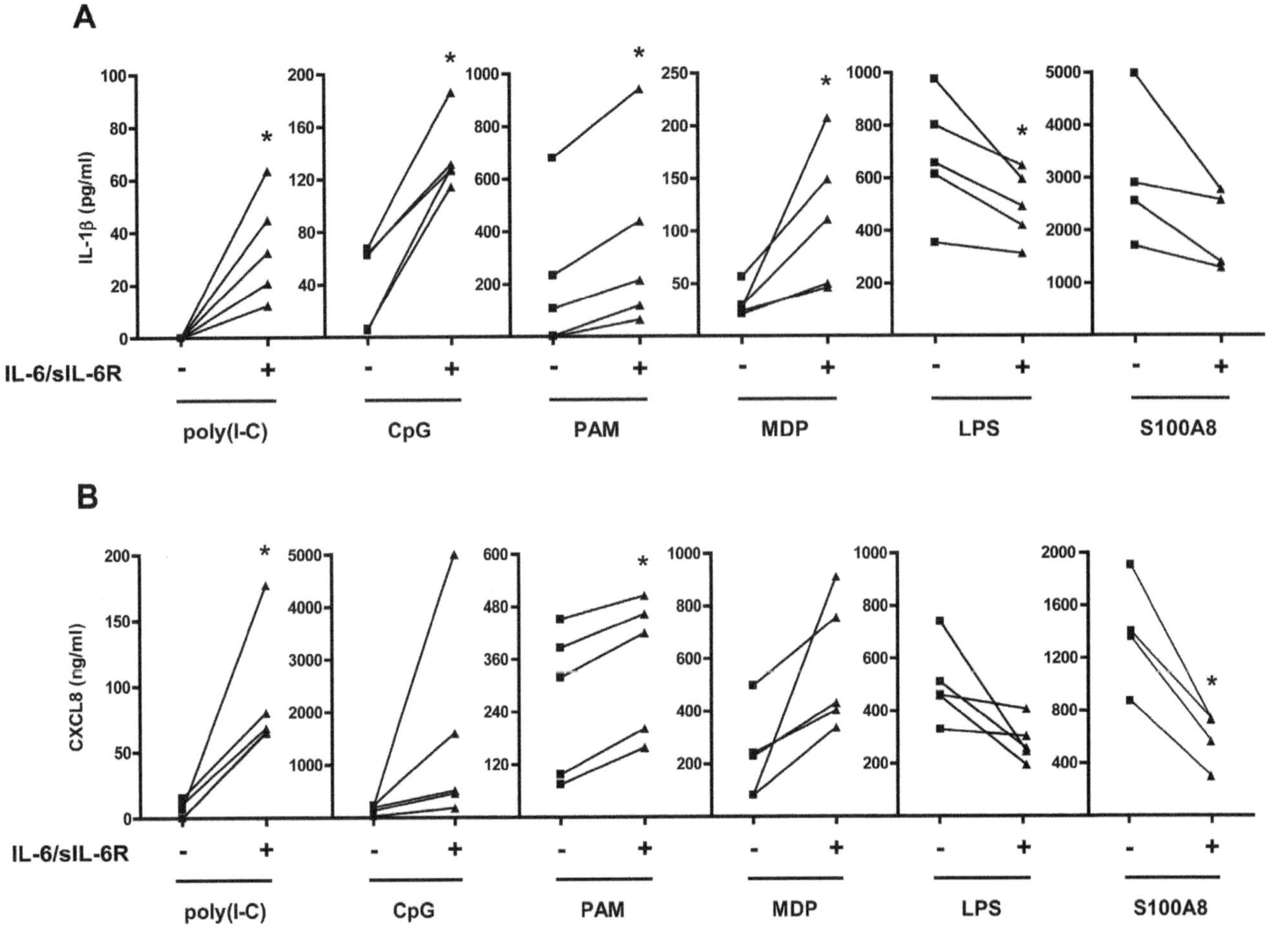

Figure 2. Exposure to IL-6 affects the production of inflammatory cytokines and chemokines in human PBMCs in response to TLR ligands. Human PBMCs were pre-exposed to IL-6/sIL-6R for 1 hour. Cells were then stimulated with poly(I-C) (20 μg/ml), CpG (5 μg/ml), PAM (200 ng/ml), MDP (10 μg/ml), LPS (10 ng/ml), S100A8 (5 μg/ml) for 18 hours. IL-1β (**A**) and CXCL8 (**B**) levels were measured by ELISA. *p<0.05 for values from IL-6/sIL-6R-stimulated compared with NT cells.

were normalized using GAPDH (Hs99999905_m1) as an endogenous control and analyzed using the $2^{\Delta\Delta ct}$ method.

Western blotting

Cells were lysed and Western blots were performed as in [14].

Cytokine measurement

Human IL-6, IL-1β, TNF-α, CXCL8, CCL2 ELISA kits were from R&D Systems, Minneapolis, MN. All cytokines were quantified according to the manufacturers' instructions.

Statistical analysis

Data are expressed as the mean ± SEM. Statistical analysis was performed by one-way analysis of variance, followed by Student's unpaired *t*-test or the Mann-Whitney U test. *P* values less than 0.05 were considered significant.

Results

IL-6 induces production of inflammatory chemokines by peripheral blood mononuclear cells

We first analyzed the effect of IL-6 on inflammatory cytokine and chemokine production by peripheral blood mononuclear cells (PBMCs). In all experiments, we used IL-6 in combination with the sIL-6R (IL-6/sIL-6R) in order to obtain a response also in cells expressing gp130, but not membrane IL-6 receptor (IL-6R) [2]. We used IL-6/sIL-6R at concentrations comparable con that observed in biological fluids (blood, synovial fluid) in physiopathological conditions [16].

Stimulation with IL-6/sIL-6R for 18 hours induced production of TNF-α, CCL2 and CXCL8 (Figure 1). In contrast, no detectable levels of IL-1β protein were found (data not shown).

IL-6 induces increased production of inflammatory cytokines and chemokines following TLR stimulation of mononuclear cells

We then analysed the production of inflammatory cytokines and chemokines in response to TLR ligands in PBMCs in the presence or in the absence of pre-treatment with IL-6/sIL-6R. When IL-6/sIL-6R were added together with poly(I-C) (TLR-3 ligand), CpG (TLR-9 ligand), Pam2CSK4 (PAM) (TLR-2 ligand), or the NOD2 specific agonist MDP, we observed a marked increase in IL-1β production. IL-6 enhanced IL-1β production to a different extent when using different TLR ligands (Figure 2A). IL-6 induced ex novo IL-1β production upon poly(I-C) stimulation, a 6 fold increase upon MDP stimulation and a 1.7 fold increase when

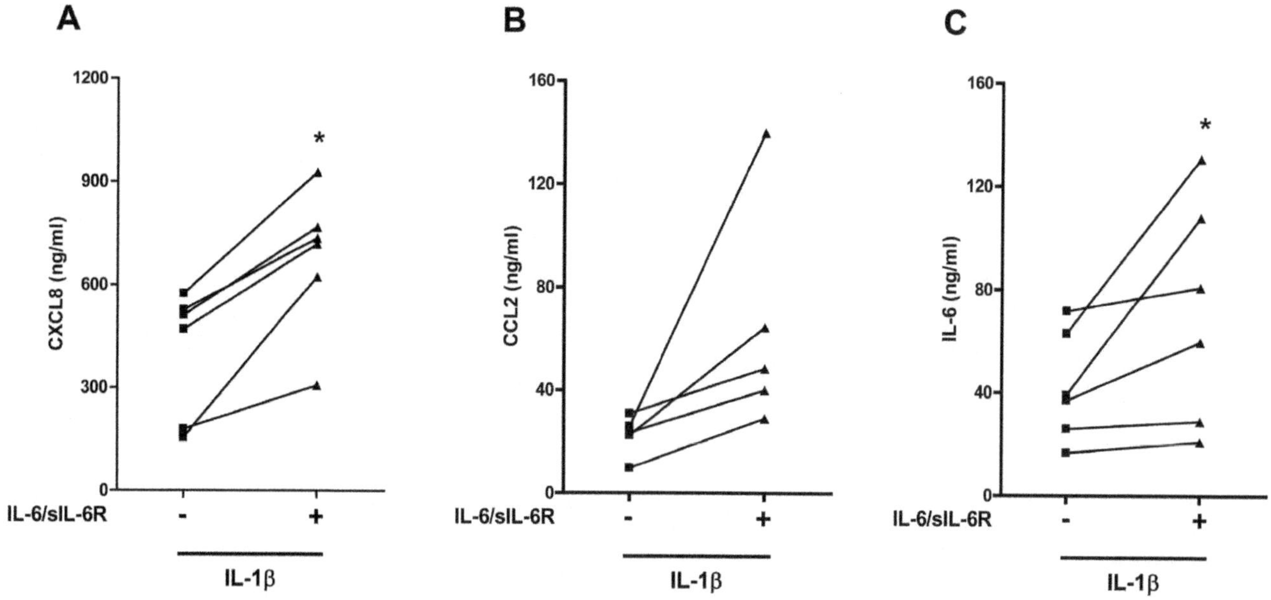

Figure 3. Exposure to IL-6 affects the production of inflammatory cytokines and chemokines in human PBMCs in response to IL-1β. Human PBMCs were pre-exposed to IL-6/sIL-6R for 1 hour. Cells were then stimulated with IL-1β (1 ng/ml) for 18 hours. CXCL8 (**A**), CCL2 (**B**), and IL-6 (**C**) levels were measured by ELISA. In (**C**), the levels of exogenous IL-6 were subtracted after the ELISA measurement. *p<0.05 for values from IL-6/sIL-6R-stimulated compared with NT cells.

stimulating cells with PAM. In contrast, and similarly to what has been previously reported by others [17], when IL-6/sIL-6R were added together with LPS, a TLR4 ligand, we found a decrease in IL-1β production. The same result was obtained using S100A8, as well as S100A9, endogenous ligands of TLR4 (Figure 2A and Figure S1A). Also, CXCL8 production was increased following stimulation with poly(I-C), CpG, PAM, and MDP in the presence of IL-6/sIL-6R. In contrast, CXCL8 production induced by LPS, S100A8 and S100A9 was inhibited by the addition of IL-6/sIL-6R (Figure 2B and Figure S1B). In order to enrich for monocytes, we performed adherence on plastic before stimulation. Similarly to unseparated PBMCs, IL-1β and CXCL8 production was increased in the presence of IL-6/sIL-6R following stimulation with all TLR ligands analyzed, except LPS (Figure S2A–B).

In accordance with previously published results, TNF-α production induced by LPS was significantly reduced by the presence of IL-6/sIL-6R, whereas production by CpG, PAM, and MDP was not significantly affected (Figure S3).

IL-6 potentiates IL-1β-induced inflammatory chemokine production

Since the IL-1 receptor shares structural and functional similarities with TLRs, we analyzed the effect of IL-6 on IL-1β-induced inflammatory cytokine and chemokine production in PBMCs. IL- 6/sIL-6R enhanced IL-1β-induced production of CXCL8 (Figure 3A), CCL2 production (Figure 3B), and IL-6 (Figure 3C). On the other hand, IL-6/sIL-6R treatment did not significantly affect IL-1β-induced TNF-α production (Figure S4).

IL-6 affects TLR signalling in PBMCs

We hypothesized that TLR and the IL-6 receptor cooperate in the induction of an increased pro inflammatory signalling in

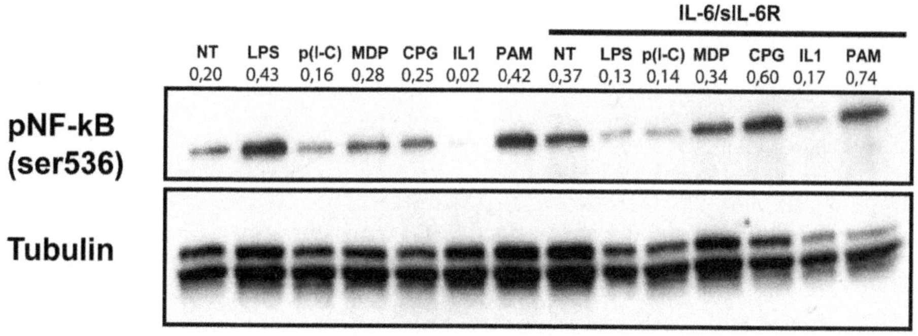

Figure 4. Increased p65 NF-κB activation in response to inflammatory stimuli in human PBMCs pre-exposed to IL-6/IL-6R. Western blots showing the expression of phospho–p65 NF-kB (Ser^{536}) in total lysates from human PBMCs pre-exposed to IL-6 (10 ng/ml) in combination with sIL-6R (125 ng/ml) for 1 hour and stimulated with LPS, poly(I-C), MDP, CpG, IL-1β, PAM (used at the same concentrations as in Figure 2) for 90 minutes. Expression of α-tubulin was used as a loading control. Results of densitometric analysis are shown above each blot. Data are representative of 3 independent experiments.

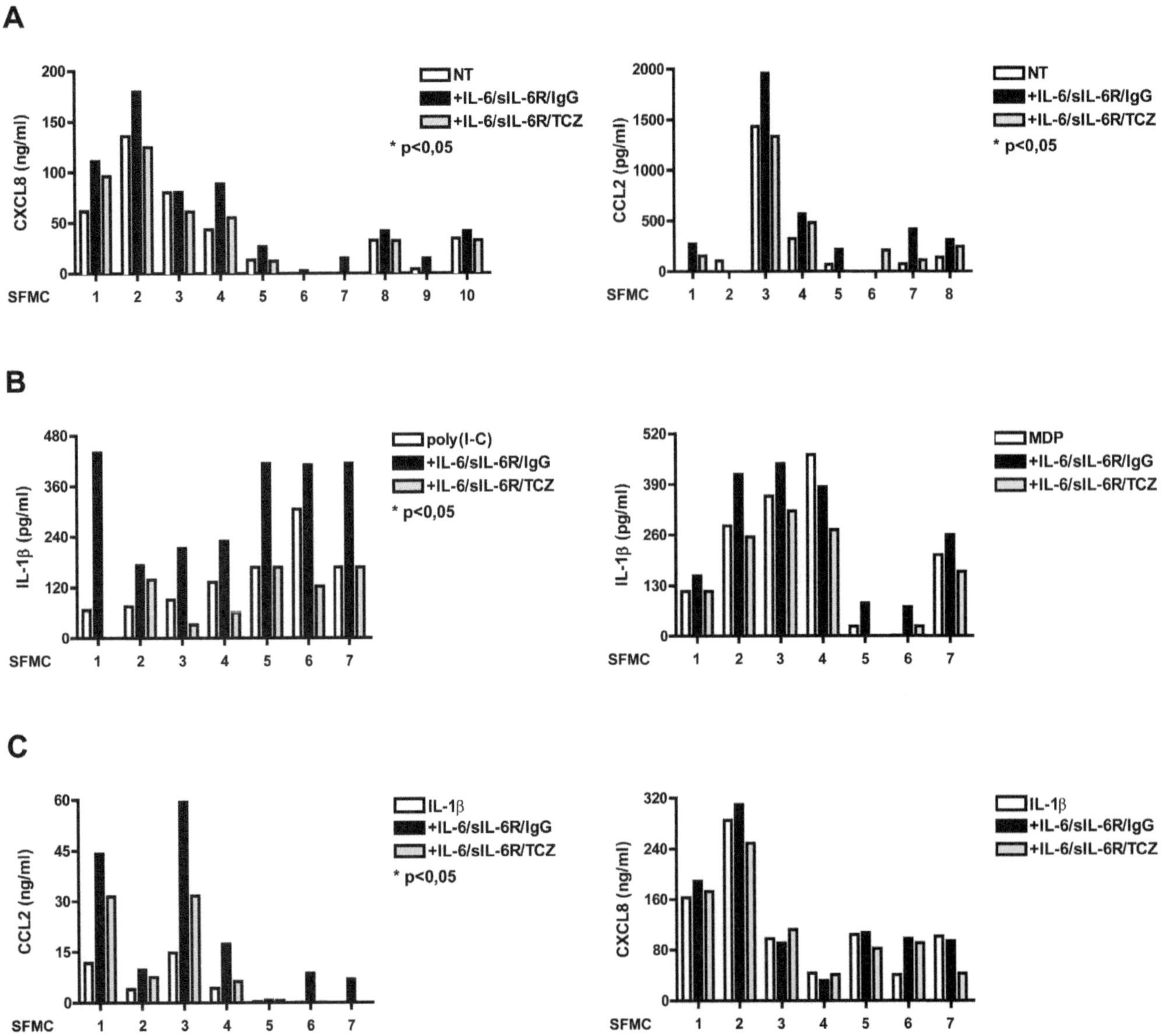

Figure 5. Exposure to IL-6 enhances cytokine and chemokine production in SFMC. SFMC were left to adhere on plastic for 3 hours in DMEM supplemented with 10% fetal calf serum (FCS). SFMC were pre-exposed to IL-6/sIL-6R in combination with IgG1 or with TCZ (50 μg/ml) for 1 hour. Cells were then left untreated (**A**) or stimulated with poly(I-C) and MDP (**B**), IL-1β (1ng/ml) (**C**). CXCL8, CCL2 and IL-1β levels were measured by ELISA. *$p<0.05$ for values from IL-6/sIL-6R-stimulated compared with NT cells.

PBMCs. We focused on p65 NF-κB, where signals elicited by TLR and IL-6 may converge, as previously suggested by us and others [9,14]. p65 NF-κB plays a major role in inflammatory cytokine and chemokine production upon TLR ligand stimulation and is involved in arthritis pathogenesis [9,18]. We analyzed by western blot analysis Ser536 phosphorylation, which is linked to p65 NF-κB activity [19]. Differently from IκBα phosphorylation, Ser536 phosphorylation is not followed by p65 NF-κB ubiquitination and degradation and may better allow an analysis of the persistence of p65 NF-κB activation [20]. p65 NF-κB-DNA binding activity is often evaluated after cell stimulation for 1–2 h [20,21]. Densitometry values were ratio-ed to that of tubulin. Treatment with IL-6/sIL-6R alone led to an increase in p65NF-κB phosphorylation induced by CpG, MDP, PAM and IL-1β (Figure 4). No changes were found in p65 NF-κB phosphorylation upon stimulation with poly(I-C). In contrast, IL-6/sIL-6R pretreatment led to a decrease in p65 NF-κB phosphorylation induced by LPS stimulation, consistently with the effect on cytokine production. Since different response to LPS upon exposure to IL-6 may be due to changes in receptor expression, we analyzed TLR4 expression by RT-PCR analysis, and we did not find clear changes (Figure S5). Thus, our results suggest that IL-6 may modify TLR mediated cytokine production through an effect on p65 NF-κB activation. Moreover, the reduced TLR4-mediated signaling upon exposure to IL-6 is not related to changes in TLR4 expression.

IL-6 enhances inflammatory cytokine and chemokine production in SFMCs stimulated with TLR ligands

In order to investigate the direct patho-physiological relevance of our finding, we analyzed whether IL-6 has a pro-inflammatory activity in mononuclear cells from synovial fluid (SFMCs) of JIA patients. IL-6 levels in synovial fluids of patients with JIA are

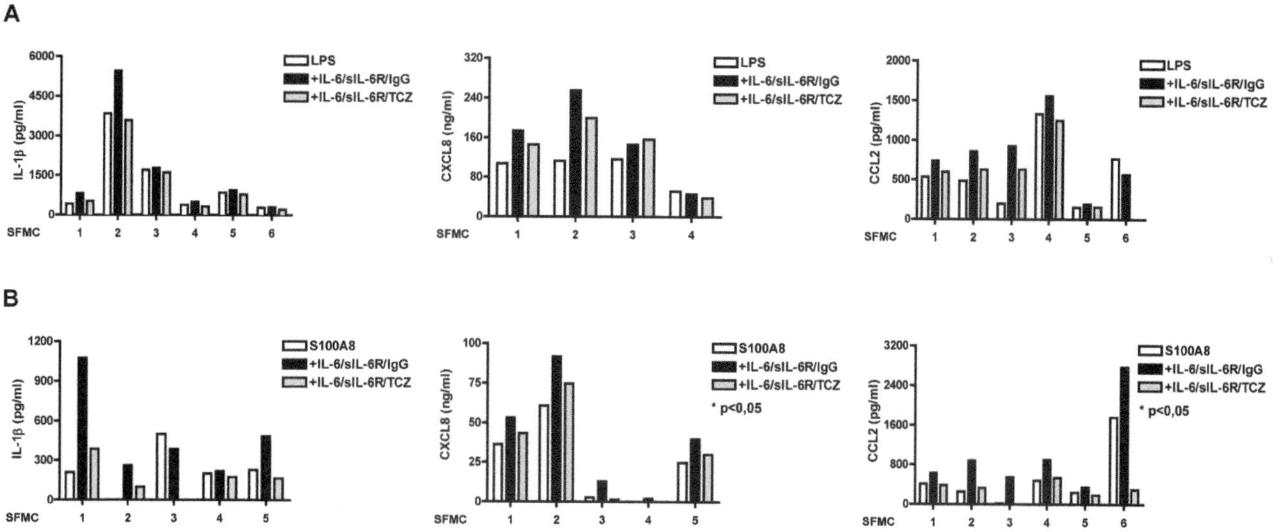

Figure 6. Exposure to IL-6 enhances cytokine and chemokine production in SFMC. SFMC were left to adhere on plastic for 3 hours in DMEM supplemented with 10% fetal calf serum (FCS). SFMC were pre-exposed to IL-6/sIL-6R in combination with IgG1 or with TCZ for 1 hour. Cells were then stimulated for 18 hours with LPS (10 ng/ml) (**A**), and S100A8 (5 μg/ml) (**B**). IL-1β, CXCL8 and CCL2 levels were measured by ELISA. *$p<0.05$ for values from IL-6/sIL-6R -stimulated compared with NT cells.

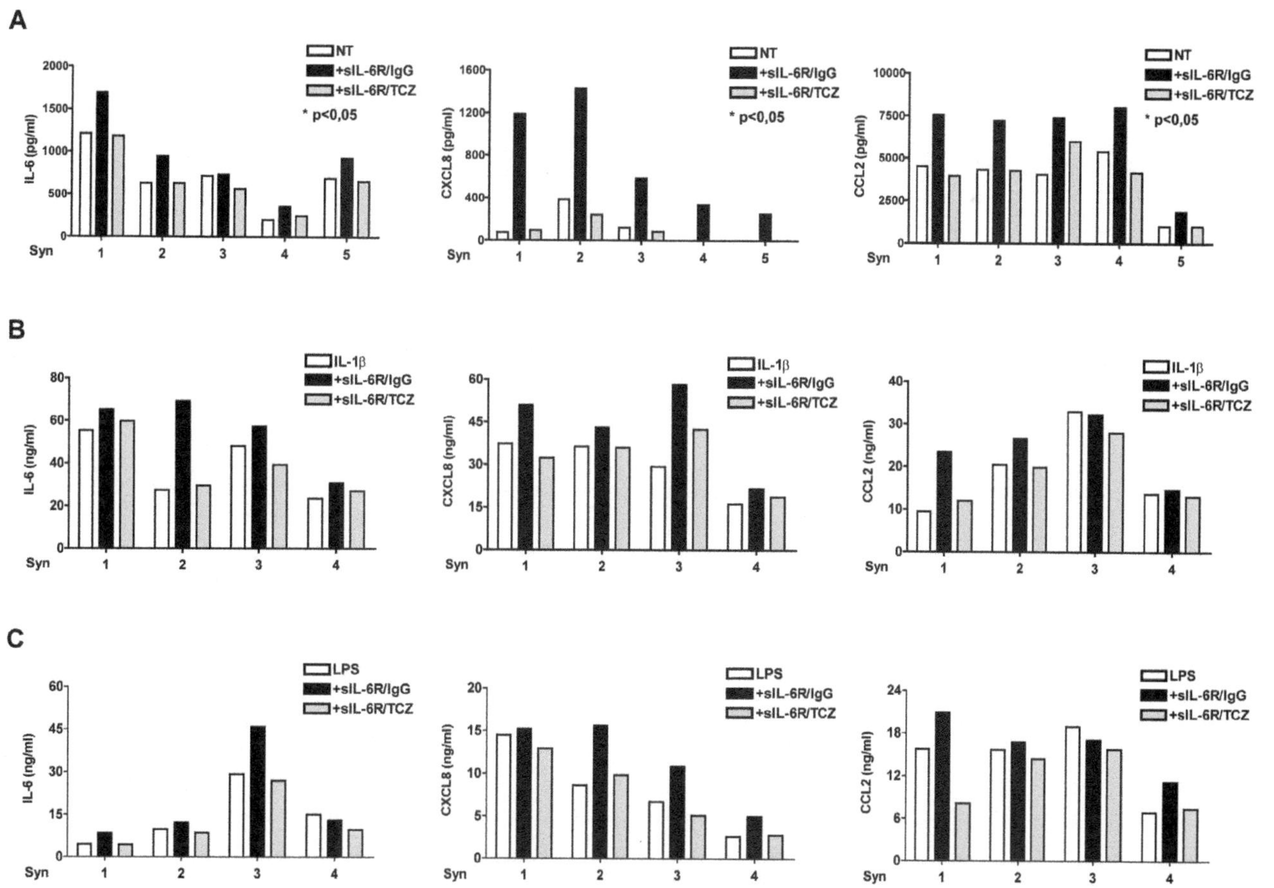

Figure 7. Exposure to sIL-6R enhances cytokine and chemokine production in RA synoviocytes. (**A**) Cells were treated with control IgG1, with sIL-6R in combination with IgG1 (sIL-6/IgG1) or with TCZ (sIL-6R/TCZ) for 18 hours. IL-6, CXCL8 and CCL2 levels were measured by ELISA. (**B–C**) RA synoviocytes were treated with control IgG1, with sIL-6/IgG1 or with sIL-6R/TCZ for 1 hour. Cells were then left untreated or stimulated with IL-1β (1 ng/ml) (**B**) or LPS (10 ng/ml) (**C**). CXCL8 and CCL2 levels were measured by ELISA. *$p<0.05$ for values from IL-6/sIL-6R -stimulated compared with NT cells.

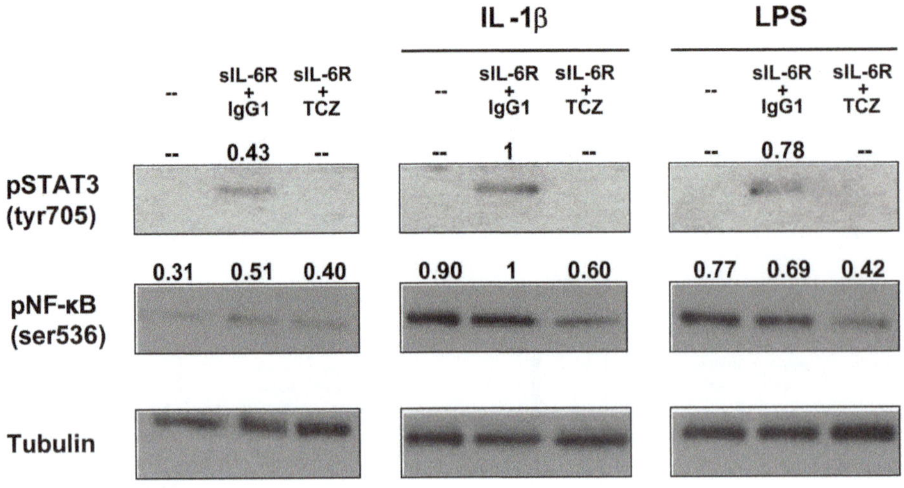

Figure 8. Western blots showing the expression of phospho-STAT3 (Tyr^{705}), phospho-NF-kB (Ser^{536}) in total lysates of RA synoviocytes pretreated as in Figure 7B for 1 hour and then stimulated with IL-1β (1 ng/ml) or LPS (10 ng/ml) for 90 minutes. Expression of α-tubulin was used as a loading control. Results of densitometric analysis are shown above each blot. Data are representative of 3 independent experiments.

markedly elevated [16]. We separated adherent cells in order to enrich for macrophages. In unstimulated conditions, these cells showed undetectable IL-1β production (data not shown), but produced high amounts of CXCL8 and CCL2 (Figure 5A). In these cells, IL-6/sIL-6R treatment increased CXCL8 and CCL2 production, which were reduced upon treatment with TCZ (Figure 5A). Similarly to PBMCs from human donors, IL-1β production in these cells was increased upon stimulation with poly(I-C) and MDP in the presence of IL-6/sIL-6R (Figure 5B). Accordingly, when stimulating these cells with IL-1β, treatment with IL-6/sIL-6R led to a further increase of CCL2, but not of CXCL8 production (Figure 5C).

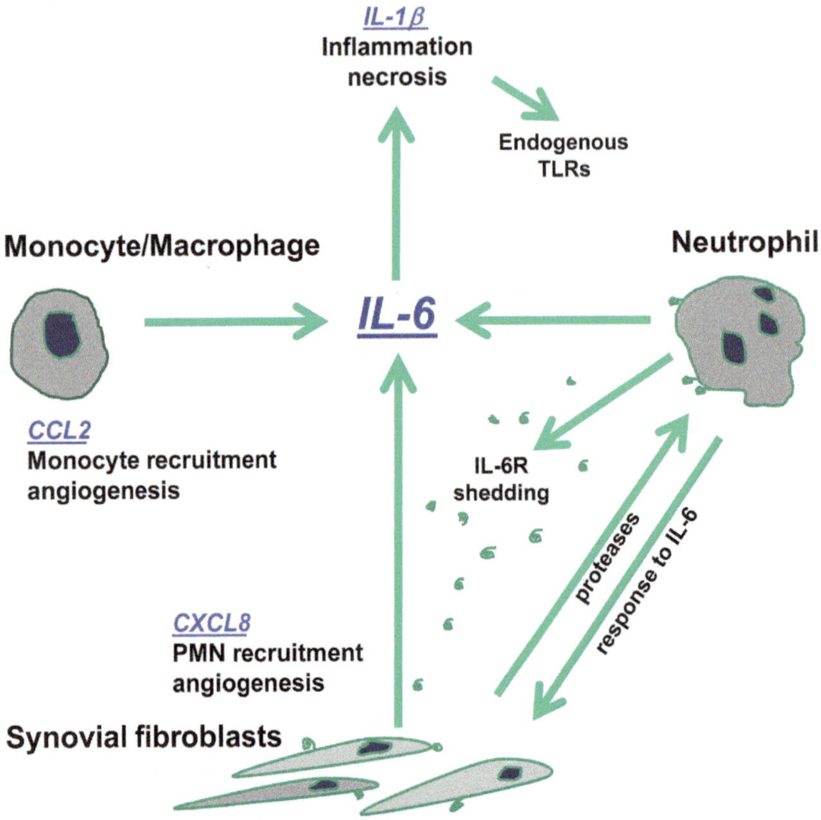

Figure 9. IL-6 amplifies the inflammatory response through a direct effect on stromal and innate immunity cells.

Interestingly, and differently from what observed with PBMCs when stimulating these cells with LPS or S100A8, as TLR4 ligands, pre-treatment with IL-6/sIL-6R led to increased CXCL8, CCL2, and IL-1β production (Figure 6A–B).

IL-6 enhances inflammatory cytokine and chemokine production in RA synoviocytes

We analyzed whether IL-6 exhibits its pro-inflammatory effect also in RA synoviocytes. Since these cells do not express the membrane IL-6R, they respond to IL-6 only in the presence of sIL-6R [22]. RA synoviocytes constitutively produced IL-6, which was increased by treatment with sIL-6R and inhibited by the addition of TCZ (Figure 7A). Treatment with sIL-6R alone led also to increased production of CXCL8 and CCL2 (Figure 7A). Moreover, addition of sIL-6R led to increased production of IL-6, CXCL8 and CCL2 following stimulation with IL-1β (Figure 7B) or LPS (Figure 7C). Analysis of lysates from RA synoviocytes showed that tyrosine phosphorylation of STAT3 was increased, confirming the activation of the IL-6 signalling pathway following addition of sIL-6R (Figure 8). Serine536-NF-κB phosphorylation was increased in the presence of sIL-6R alone and was markedly reduced by TCZ both in untreated cells and in cells stimulated with IL-1β and LPS. Overall, these results demonstrate that high levels of IL-6/sIL-6R, as those present in joints of patients with arthritis, may contribute to the amplification of the inflammatory response enhancing the production of IL-1β, CXCL8 and CCL2 by SFMCs and by RA synoviocytes.

Discussion

Since its discovery, IL-6 has been described as a cytokine able to exert pro- as well as anti-inflammatory activities [17,23–26]. Early studies unequivocally demonstrated that IL-6 inhibits the LPS-induced release of IL-1 and TNF-α in peripheral blood mononuclear cells [17,27]. Our findings confirm and extend these results, obtained using LPS, showing that addition of IL-6 to PBMCs led to the inhibition of IL-1β and CXCL8 production not only when induced by LPS, but also when induced by S100A8-9, as an endogenous TLR4. In contrast, we found that, when PBMCs were stimulated with other stimuli such as poly(I-C), CpG and MDP, IL-6 cooperates with pro-inflammatory signals increasing IL-1β and CXCL8 production. To the best of our knowledge this has not been reported before. Overall, for all TLR ligands analysed, with the exception of TLR4-specific ligands, IL-6 enhanced IL-1β and CXCL8 production by PMBCs.

The inhibition observed with TLR4 ligands versus the stimulatory effect observed with other TLRs has no clear explanation in terms of different signaling pathways involved [9]. LPS-induced response is intense and has often been considered as a paradigm of TLR mediated response. However, it may not reflect the complexity of the activity of multiple TLR ligands. Indeed, TLR4 engagement leads to the induction of Myd88 dependent, as well as MyD88-independent pathways, involving the recruitment of TRIF adaptor protein upon activation. Dose response experiments with S100A8/9 and LPS ruled out that the inhibitory effect was related to the intensity of the response (data not shown). Also, expression of TLR4 was not affected by exposure to IL-6. Notably, we found that the addition of IL-6 led to reduced NF-κB activity upon LPS, but not other TLR ligand stimulation, suggesting profound, and yet to be clarified differences in the interactions between multiple signaling pathways.

We also focused on the IL-1β/IL-6 mutual regulation. IL-1β/IL-6 co-stimulation led to an increased production of CXCL8, CCL2 and IL-6. This potentiation between IL-1 and IL-6 may have a translational relevance. In patients with systemic JIA, recent results in clinical trials underscore a role for both IL-6 and IL-1β overproduction [4,28]. It is well known that IL-1 induces IL-6 [17]; our data show synergy in the induction of pro-inflammatory chemokines. All together these data show multiple levels of interactions between IL-1β and IL-6 in vitro and led us to hypothesize an IL-6/IL-1β axis, rather than an IL-6/TNF-α axis, occurring during inflammation in the presence of TLR ligands. Clarifying IL-1/IL-6 mutual regulations and interactions in vivo, in patients with sJIA, may lead to a better understanding of disease pathogenesis and, possibly, of a way to predict response to treatments. A functional link between IL-1β and IL-6 is also suggested by the observation that patients with familial Mediterranean fever (FMF), an auto-inflammatory disease, were successfully treated with TCZ [29,30].

In order to investigate whether the results observed with PBMCs were also reproduced in cells originating from inflammatory site, i.e. inflamed joints, we used adherent MCs obtained from synovial fluids of patients with JIA and synovial fibroblasts obtained from synovial tissue of patients with RA. Differently from PBMCs, SFMCs produce in steady state high levels of cytokines and chemokines. Treatment with IL-6 increased basal CXCL8 and CCL2 production and IL-1β production following poly(I-C) and MDP stimulation. More importantly, in contrast with PBMCs, we did not observe any inhibitory effect of IL-6 on CXCL8 and CCL2 production following TLR4 stimulation with both LPS and S100A8-9. Rather, a stimulatory effect was observed. In RA synoviocytes treatment with sIL-6R led to a *de novo* production of CXCL8 and to an increased production of IL-6 and CCL2. Noteworthy, addition of sIL-6R to IL-1β or LPS stimulated RA synoviocytes did not inhibit the production of IL-6, CXCL8 and CCL2. Similarly to what observed with SFMCs, a stimulatory effect was observed.

These data, with SFMCs and with RA synoviocytes suggest that the inhibitory effect of IL-6 on LPS induced cytokine production is cell and cell context specific. It is conceivable to speculate that cells who have been exposed to an inflammatory environment, such as SFMCs and RA synoviocytes, have abnormal regulation of their responses to *pro*-inflammatory stimuli. Our results point to a differential regulation of the p65 NF-κB pathway activation under these circumstances.

IL-6 has been demonstrated to enhance p65 NF-κB activation in intestinal epithelia, but no information to date has been provided about its activity in synoviocytes [31]. Our results led us to hypothesize that IL-6 and TLR induced intracellular signals may converge at the level of p65 NF-κB phosphorylation or upstream. Additional connections between the two pathways cannot be excluded. For instance, STAT-3 and p65 NF-κB have been shown to physically interact, enhancing CXCL8 transcription activity [32].

Our results in the context of the pathophysiological events occurring in inflamed joints suggest that the high levels of IL-6 may have a relevant role in amplifying inflammation. The interactions between stromal and innate immunity cells orchestrated by IL-6 are summarized in in Figure 9. IL-6 in the presence of its soluble receptor induces CXCL8 production by RA synoviocytes. CXCL8 induces polymorphonuclear neutrophil leukocyte (PMN) chemotaxis and activation. IL-6 is known to prolong the survival of these cells [33]. Proteases present in the synovial fluid will enhance the shedding of sIL-6R from the plasma membrane of PMNs, increasing IL-6 activity on RA synoviocytes [24]. IL-6 also plays a direct role in monocyte chemotaxis and in the differentiation of monocytes towards macrophages [33,34]. Moreover, CXCL8 may contribute to neo-angiogenesis, which is a characteristic of inflamed synovia [35]. CCL2 also may enhance angiogenesis and contribute to chemotaxis of mononuclear cells [35]. Furthermore, our data point to endogenous TLR ligands released from necrotic synovial fluid cells cooperating with IL-6 in amplifying local inflammation [36].

Overall, our study shed light on the role of IL-6 in the pathogenesis of inflammatory arthritides. We demonstrated a direct effect of IL-6 in enhancing TLR ligand induced inflammatory cytokine and chemokine production. These IL-6 mediated effects support the presence of a positive loop between components of the innate immunity, such as monocyte/macrophages and neutrophils, and cells from the synovial stroma, such as RA synoviocytes.

Supporting Information

Figure S1 Effects of exposure to IL-6 on the production of IL1-β in human PBMCs in response to S110A9. Human PBMCs were pre-exposed to IL-6/sIL-6R for 1 hour. Cells were then stimulated with S100A9 (5 μg/ml) for 18 hours. IL1-β (**A**) and CXCL8 levels (**B**) were measured by ELISA. $*p<0.05$ for values from IL-6/sIL-6R-stimulated compared with NT cells.

Figure S2 Exposure to IL-6 affects the production of IL1-β and CXCL8 in adherent human PBMCs in response to TLR ligands. Human PBMCs cells were left to adhere on plastic for 3 hours in DMEM supplemented with 10% fetal calf serum (FCS). Cells were pre-exposed to IL-6/sIL-6R for 1 hour. Cells were then stimulated with poly(I-C) (20 μg/ml), CpG (5 μg/ml), PAM (200 ng/ml), MDP (10 μg/ml), LPS (10 ng/ml) for 18 hours. IL-1β (**A**) and CXCL8 (**B**) levels were measured by ELISA. $*p<0.05$ for values from IL-6/sIL-6R-stimulated compared with NT cells.

Figure S3 Effects of exposure to IL-6 on the production of TNF-α in human PBMCs in response to TLR ligands. Human PBMCs were pre-exposed to IL-6/sIL-6R for 1 hour. Cells were then stimulated with CpG (5 μg/ml), PAM (200 ng/ml), poly(I-C) (20 μg/ml), MDP (10 μg/ml), LPS (10 ng/ml) for 18 hours. TNF-α levels were measured by ELISA. $*p<0.05$ for values from IL-6/sIL-6R-stimulated compared with NT cells.

Figure S4 Effects of exposure to IL-6 on the production of TNF-α in human PBMCs in response to IL-1β. Human PBMCs were pre-exposed to IL-6/sIL-6R for 1 hour. Cells were then stimulated with IL-1β (1 ng/ml) for 18 hours. CXCL8. TNF-α levels were measured by ELISA.

Figure S5 Effects of exposure to IL-6 on the expression of TLR4 in human PBMCs in response to LPS. Human PBMCs were pre-exposed to IL-6/sIL-6R for 1 hour. Cells were then stimulated with LPS (10 ng/ml) for 6 hours. Quantitative reverse transcription–polymerase chain reaction was performed on total RNA, with TLR4 mRNA normalized to GAPDH mRNA expression.

Author Contributions

Conceived and designed the experiments: IC GP FD RS. Performed the experiments: IC DH GM RS. Analyzed the data: IC DH GP TV FDB RS. Contributed reagents/materials/analysis tools: DH TV AM FDB. Contributed to the writing of the manuscript: DH GP FDB RS.

References

1. Nishimoto N, Kishimoto T (2006) Interleukin 6: from bench to bedside. Nat Clin Pract Rheumatol 2: 619–626.
2. Heinrich PC, Behrmann I, Haan S, Hermanns HM, Muller-Newen G, et al. (2003) Principles of interleukin (IL)-6-type cytokine signalling and its regulation. Biochem J 374: 1–20.
3. Naugler WE, Karin M (2008) The wolf in sheep's clothing: the role of interleukin-6 in immunity, inflammation and cancer. Trends Mol Med 14: 109–119.
4. De Benedetti F, Brunner HI, Ruperto N, Kenwright A, Wright S, et al. (2012) Randomized trial of tocilizumab in systemic juvenile idiopathic arthritis. N Engl J Med 367: 2385–2395.
5. Smolen JS, Beaulieu A, Rubbert-Roth A, Ramos-Remus C, Rovensky J, et al. (2008) Effect of interleukin-6 receptor inhibition with tocilizumab in patients with rheumatoid arthritis (OPTION study): a double-blind, placebo-controlled, randomised trial. Lancet 371: 987–997.
6. Choy E (2012) Understanding the dynamics: pathways involved in the pathogenesis of rheumatoid arthritis. Rheumatology (Oxford) 51 Suppl 5: v3–11.
7. Ogura H, Murakami M, Okuyama Y, Tsuruoka M, Kitabayashi C, et al. (2008) Interleukin-17 promotes autoimmunity by triggering a positive-feedback loop via interleukin-6 induction. Immunity 29: 628–636.
8. Samson M, Audia S, Janikashvili N, Ciudad M, Trad M, et al. (2012) Brief report: inhibition of interleukin-6 function corrects Th17/Treg cell imbalance in patients with rheumatoid arthritis. Arthritis Rheum 64: 2499–2503.
9. Takeuchi O, Akira S (2010) Pattern recognition receptors and inflammation. Cell 140: 805–820.
10. Erridge C (2010) Endogenous ligands of TLR2 and TLR4: agonists or assistants? J Leukoc Biol 87: 989–999.
11. Gerss J, Roth J, Holzinger D, Ruperto N, Wittkowski H, et al. (2012) Phagocyte-specific S100 proteins and high-sensitivity C reactive protein as biomarkers for a risk-adapted treatment to maintain remission in juvenile idiopathic arthritis: a comparative study. Ann Rheum Dis 71: 1991–1997.
12. Holzinger D, Frosch M, Kastrup A, Prince FH, Otten MH, et al. (2012) The Toll-like receptor 4 agonist MRP8/14 protein complex is a sensitive indicator for disease activity and predicts relapses in systemic-onset juvenile idiopathic arthritis. Ann Rheum Dis 71: 974–980.
13. Sokolove J, Zhao X, Chandra PE, Robinson WH (2011) Immune complexes containing citrullinated fibrinogen costimulate macrophages via Toll-like receptor 4 and Fcgamma receptor. Arthritis Rheum 63: 53–62.
14. Strippoli R, Carvello F, Scianaro R, De Pasquale L, Vivarelli M, et al. (2012) Amplification of the response to Toll-like receptor ligands by prolonged exposure to interleukin-6 in mice: implication for the pathogenesis of macrophage activation syndrome. Arthritis Rheum 64: 1680–1688.
15. Scire CA, Epis O, Codullo V, Humby F, Morbini P, et al. (2007) Immunohistological assessment of the synovial tissue in small joints in rheumatoid arthritis: validation of a minimally invasive ultrasound-guided synovial biopsy procedure. Arthritis Res Ther 9: R101.
16. De Benedetti F, Pignatti P, Gerloni V, Massa M, Sartirana P, et al. (1997) Differences in synovial fluid cytokine levels between juvenile and adult rheumatoid arthritis. J Rheumatol 24: 1403–1409.
17. Schindler R, Mancilla J, Endres S, Ghorbani R, Clark SC, et al. (1990) Correlations and interactions in the production of interleukin-6 (IL-6), IL-1, and tumor necrosis factor (TNF) in human blood mononuclear cells: IL-6 suppresses IL-1 and TNF. Blood 75: 40–47.
18. Brown KD, Claudio E, Siebenlist U (2008) The roles of the classical and alternative nuclear factor-kappaB pathways: potential implications for autoimmunity and rheumatoid arthritis. Arthritis Res Ther 10: 212.
19. Buss H, Dorrie A, Schmitz ML, Hoffmann E, Resch K, et al. (2004) Constitutive and interleukin-1-inducible phosphorylation of p65 NF-{kappa}B at serine 536 is mediated by multiple protein kinases including I{kappa}B kinase (IKK)-{alpha}, IKK{beta}, IKK{epsilon}, TRAF family member-associated (TANK)-binding kinase 1 (TBK1), and an unknown kinase and couples p65 to TATA-binding protein-associated factor II31-mediated interleukin-8 transcription. J Biol Chem 279: 55633–55643.
20. Strippoli R, Benedicto I, Foronda M, Perez-Lozano ML, Sanchez-Perales S, et al. (2010) p38 maintains E-cadherin expression by modulating TAK1-NF-kappa B during epithelial-to-mesenchymal transition. J Cell Sci 123: 4321–4331.
21. Prencipe G, Minnone G, Strippoli R, De Pasquale L, Petrini S, et al. (2014) Nerve Growth Factor Downregulates Inflammatory Response in Human Monocytes through TrkA. J Immunol 192: 3345–3354.
22. Nishimoto N, Ito A, Ono M, Tagoh H, Matsumoto T, et al. (2000) IL-6 inhibits the proliferation of fibroblastic synovial cells from rheumatoid arthritis patients in the presence of soluble IL-6 receptor. Int Immunol 12: 187–193.

23. Xing Z, Gauldie J, Cox G, Baumann H, Jordana M, et al. (1998) IL-6 is an antiinflammatory cytokine required for controlling local or systemic acute inflammatory responses. J Clin Invest 101: 311–320.
24. Scheller J, Chalaris A, Schmidt-Arras D, Rose-John S (2011) The pro- and anti-inflammatory properties of the cytokine interleukin-6. Biochim Biophys Acta 1813: 878–888.
25. Alonzi T, Fattori E, Lazzaro D, Costa P, Probert L, et al. (1998) Interleukin 6 is required for the development of collagen-induced arthritis. J Exp Med 187: 461–468.
26. Fattori E, Cappelletti M, Costa P, Sellitto C, Cantoni L, et al. (1994) Defective inflammatory response in interleukin 6-deficient mice. J Exp Med 180: 1243–1250.
27. Aderka D, Le JM, Vilcek J (1989) IL-6 inhibits lipopolysaccharide-induced tumor necrosis factor production in cultured human monocytes, U937 cells, and in mice. J Immunol 143: 3517–3523.
28. Ruperto N, Brunner HI, Quartier P, Constantin T, Wulffraat N, et al. (2012) Two randomized trials of canakinumab in systemic juvenile idiopathic arthritis. N Engl J Med 367: 2396–2406.
29. Dinarello CA (2010) IL-1: discoveries, controversies and future directions. Eur J Immunol 40: 599–606.
30. Stein N, Witt M, Baeuerle M, Proft F, Schulze-Koops H, et al. (2012) Familial Mediterranean Fever: Inhibition of IL-6 Signalling As a New Therapeutic Option in a Frequent Autoinflammatory Syndrome. ACR abstract 747.
31. Wang L, Walia B, Evans J, Gewirtz AT, Merlin D, et al. (2003) IL-6 induces NF-kappa B activation in the intestinal epithelia. J Immunol 171: 3194–3201.
32. Yoshida Y, Kumar A, Koyama Y, Peng H, Arman A, et al. (2004) Interleukin 1 activates STAT3/nuclear factor-kappaB cross-talk via a unique TRAF6- and p65-dependent mechanism. J Biol Chem 279: 1768–1776.
33. Asensi V, Valle E, Meana A, Fierer J, Celada A, et al. (2004) In vivo interleukin-6 protects neutrophils from apoptosis in osteomyelitis. Infect Immun 72: 3823–3828.
34. Chomarat P, Banchereau J, Davoust J, Palucka AK (2000) IL-6 switches the differentiation of monocytes from dendritic cells to macrophages. Nat Immunol 1: 510–514.
35. Zlotnik A, Yoshie O (2012) The chemokine superfamily revisited. Immunity 36: 705–716.
36. Brentano F, Schorr O, Gay RE, Gay S, Kyburz D (2005) RNA released from necrotic synovial fluid cells activates rheumatoid arthritis synovial fibroblasts via Toll-like receptor 3. Arthritis Rheum 52: 2656–2665.

9

Poor Survival in Rheumatoid Arthritis Associated with Bronchiectasis: A Family-Based Cohort Study

Xavier Puéchal[1,2*], Emmanuelle Génin[3], Thierry Bienvenu[4], Claire Le Jeunne[1], Daniel J. Dusser[5]

1 National Referral Center for Rare Systemic Autoimmune Diseases, Department of Internal Medicine, Hôpital Cochin, Assistance Publique-Hôpitaux de Paris, Université Paris Descartes, Paris, France, **2** INSERM U1016, CNRS UMR 8104, Institut Cochin, Paris, France, **3** INSERM UMR-1078, Centre Hospitalier Universitaire, Brest, France, **4** Biochemistry and Molecular Biology Laboratory, Hôpital Cochin, Assistance Publique-Hôpitaux de Paris, Université Paris Descartes, Paris, France, **5** Department of Respiratory Diseases, Hôpital Cochin, Assistance Publique-Hôpitaux de Paris, Université Paris Descartes, Paris, France

Abstract

Background: Diffuse bronchiectasis (DB) may occur in rheumatoid arthritis (RA). *CFTR* (cystic fibrosis transmembrane conductance regulator) mutations predispose RA patients to DB, but the prognosis of RA-associated DB (RA-DB) is unclear.

Methods: We report long-term mortality data from a nationwide family-based association study of patients with RA only, DB only or RA-DB. We assessed mortality as a function of clinical characteristics and CF/*CFTR*-RD (*CFTR*-related disorders) mutations in 137 subjects from 24 kindreds. Potential risk factors were investigated by Cox proportional-hazard analysis with shared Gaussian random effects to account for within-family correlations.

Results: During a median follow-up of 11 years after inclusion, 18 patients died, mostly from cardiorespiratory causes. Survival was significantly lower for RA-DB patients than for unaffected relatives and for patients with RA or DB only. RA patients with DB had also a poorer prognosis in terms of survival after RA diagnosis (HR, 8.6; 95% CI, 1.5–48.2; $P = 0.014$) and from birth (HR, 9.6; 95% CI, 1.1–81.7; $P = 0.039$). Early onset of DB (HR, 15.4; 95% CI, 2.1–113.2; $P = 0.007$) and CF/*CFTR*-RD mutation (HR, 7.2; 95% CI, 1.4–37.1; $P = 0.018$) were associated with poorer survival in patients with RA-DB. Thus, CF/*CFTR*-RD mutations in RA patients with early-onset DB defined a subgroup of high-risk patients with higher mortality rates (log-rank test $P = 1.28 \times 10^{-5}$).

Conclusion: DB is associated with poorer survival in patients with RA. Early-onset DB and *CFTR* mutations are two markers that identify RA patients at a high risk of death, for whom future therapeutic interventions should be designed and evaluated.

Editor: Dominique Heymann, Faculté de médecine de Nantes, France

Funding: This work was supported by grants from the Assistance Publique-Hôpitaux de Paris (Contrat de Recherche et d'Innovation Clinique CRC98046) (to XP) and the Société Française de Rhumatologie (to XP). The funders had no role in study design, data collection and analysis, decision to publish, or preparation of the manuscript.

Competing Interests: The authors have declared that no competing interests exist.

* Email: xavier.puechal@cch.aphp.fr

Introduction

Rheumatoid arthritis (RA) is a systemic autoimmune disease, of unknown origin, that affects 0.5–1.0% of the adult population worldwide [1]. It primarily involves the joints, but extra-articular manifestations, such as lung involvement, have been observed and may increase the burden of this frequently disabling disease. Most studies in RA patients have reported higher mortality rates than for the general population and have shown that extra-articular manifestations contribute to premature death [2,3].

There is a well-established association between RA and diffuse bronchiectasis (DB). In prospective blind studies based on high-resolution computed tomography (HRCT) in patients with RA, the prevalence of diffuse bronchiectasis has been reported to range from 5.6% to 30% [4–9]. Conversely, RA is found in 2.7% to 5.2% of patients with DB referred to respiratory medicine departments for investigation [10,11]. In cases of symptomatic DB in RA patients, respiratory symptoms precede the onset of RA in more than 90% of cases, with a mean interval of more than 30 years between the onset of the two diseases (early-onset, mostly childhood DB) [10,12–16]. In less than 10% of patients, respiratory symptoms of DB occur concomitantly with the onset of arthritis (late-onset and adulthood DB) [17]. The prognosis of these two subtypes of DB in RA patients remains unclear. Recent data have suggested that the lung may be an early site of autoimmune-related injury in RA patients and a potential site involved in RA-related autoimmunity [18,19]. Further analyses of the link between RA and DB are, therefore, required.

Cystic fibrosis transmembrane conductance regulator (*CFTR*) gene mutations have been identified as the cause of cystic fibrosis (CF) [20], a disease associated with DB and impaired survival due to respiratory insufficiency in most cases [21]. Beside CF, some DB may be classified as *CFTR*-related diseases (*CFTR*-RD), defined as a clinical entity associated with CFTR dysfunction not fulfilling the diagnostic criteria for CF [22].

We previously reported a higher prevalence of CF/*CFTR*-RD mutations in patients suffering from RA-associated DB (RA-DB) than in the general population [16]. We found a strong association and linkage between mutations in the CF/*CFTR*-RD gene and RA-DB phenotypes in a French nationwide family-based association study [23]. CF/*CFTR*-RD mutations were five times more frequent in RA-DB patients than in patients with RA only (no DB) and cosegregated with RA-DB in the families. Furthermore, RA-DB patients carrying at least one abnormal *CFTR* allele but not fulfilling the diagnostic criteria for CF more frequently had chronic sinusitis, a trend toward more severe pulmonary involvement, and CFTR protein dysfunction, as demonstrated by the lower nasal potential difference of these patients than of patients with both RA and DB but without CF/*CFTR*-RD mutations [16]. These data suggest that CF/*CFTR*-RD mutations may predispose patients with RA to DB, but the vital prognosis of the RA-DB association has not been investigated in detail, and the influence of the clinical onset of DB and the presence of CF/*CFTR*-RD mutations on survival has not been studied.

We therefore investigated long-term mortality and variables predictive of the risk of death in a well characterized, prospectively followed family-based cohort of patients with a diagnosis of RA only, DB only, or RA-DB.

Methods

The study protocol was reviewed and approved by the institutional review board for clinical research of *Assistance Publique-Hôpitaux de Paris* and the ethics committee of the Medical Faculty of Paris Descartes University. Written informed consent was obtained from all participants.

Study population

The study was performed in a prospectively followed family-based cohort recruited between September 1999 and February 2002, which has been described elsewhere [23]. Briefly, for inclusion in the study, each family had to include at least one proband with both RA and symptomatic DB and one affected first-degree relative with RA and/or DB. Once a family was deemed eligible for inclusion, all affected subjects and unaffected relatives were interviewed and blood samples were taken for *CFTR* genotyping.

Interview and clinical assessment at inclusion

At inclusion, pedigree analysis was carried out and each family member underwent face-to-face semi-structured interviews and clinical assessment. Given the known association of RA and DB and the possibility of asymptomatic or paucisymptomatic DB, all RA patients underwent HRCT of the lungs. An HRCT scan of the lungs was also conducted for other participants presenting respiratory symptoms. All cases of DB were confirmed by two independent observers finding evidence of diffuse (more than one lobe) bronchiectasis on HRCT scan, without knowledge of the *CFTR* mutational status of the individual concerned. In patients with both RA and DB, DB was defined as early-onset DB if respiratory symptoms preceded RA by more than 10 years (mostly childhood DB) and as late-onset DB for patients whose respiratory symptoms occurred at the same time or less than 10 years before RA onset (adulthood DB). Participants were classified into four categories: RA-DB, RA without DB (RA only), DB only and unaffected.

CFTR genotyping

We checked the entire coding region and exon/intron junctions of *CFTR* for CF/*CFTR*-RD mutations, which were subsequently confirmed by direct DNA sequencing, as previously described [23]. Nucleotide substitutions were classified according to their known or predicted functional consequences [23] and groups of mutations were considered collectively in the analyses.

Survival

The primary outcome measure was survival between November 2011 and December 2012. Data were censored on December 31st, 2012. Vital status was recorded in this family-based cohort, with a new questionnaire that was sent to each participant and a follow-up interview carried out for all families. Information about the cause of death was collected retrospectively from a family questionnaire and medical reports. Survival from inclusion was determined for all participants and survival from birth and from RA diagnosis was also analyzed.

Statistical analysis

The characteristics of the patients (sex ratio, age at inclusion, age at diagnosis, median follow-up) were compared between the groups in chi-squared tests, Fisher's exact tests or Kruskal-Wallis tests, as appropriate.

Survival analysis was performed with the R package "survival" [24]. Kaplan-Meier survival curves were plotted with the "plot.survfit" function and the log-rank test, implemented in the "survdiff" function, was used to compare survival between groups.

We adjusted for the effect of covariates and estimated hazard ratios (HR) while accounting for family correlations, by fitting Cox models with Gaussian random effects models to the data with the R package "coxme" [25]. Each individual was assumed to have a random genetic risk, but risks were correlated between individuals according to the strength of their pedigree relationship, as assessed by their kinship coefficient. We report HR and 95% confidence intervals (95% CI) and the *P*-value of the *z* test.

We compared survival from inclusion, adjusted for age at inclusion, between the individuals included in the study, as a function of their disease status. We then focused on RA patients and compared their survival from birth and from RA diagnosis as a function of whether or not they had DB (comparison of RA-DB with RA only). Finally, we focused on patients with both RA and DB and investigated the factors potentially influencing their survival from birth or from RA diagnosis.

All analyses were conducted with R version 2.15.1 [26].

Results

Patients' characteristics

The family-based cohort comprised 137 subjects from 24 kindreds, including 30 patients with RA-DB, 25 patients with RA only and eight patients with DB only; the remaining participants constituted the unaffected relatives.

The main demographic features of the participants enrolled in the family-based cohort are shown in Table 1. The median follow-up time after inclusion was 10, 11, 11, and 12 years for patients with RA-DB, RA only, DB only, and unaffected relatives, respectively.

Survival in different groups of individuals

At the time of analysis, vital status was known for all subjects. Eighteen patients and 11 unaffected relatives from the study cohort had died (Table 1). In patients with RA-DB, the reported cause of death was identified in 12 of the 14 patients who died, and

Table 1. Characteristics and outcome of the 137 participants in the family-based cohort study.

Characteristics	RA-DB	RA only	DB only	Unaffected relatives	P value
	(N=30)	(N=25)	(N=8)	(N=74)	
Sex ratio (F/M)	25/5	17/8	5/3	37/37	0.011[a]
Median (mean) age at RA onset – yr	45 (45.1)	39 (42.0)	-	-	0.35[b]
Median (mean) age at inclusion – yr	64.0 (60.1)	51.0 (51.1)	45.5 (50.1)	52.0 (54.7)	0.08[b]
Symptoms at inclusion					
Dyspnea – no. (%)	24 (80%)		7 (86%)		1[a]
Cough and sputum – no. (%)	24 (80%)		7 (86%)		1[a]
>1 respiratory infection/year – no. (%)	19 (63%)		6 (71%)		0.69[a]
Sinus involvement – no. (%)	14 (47%)		5 (63)%		0.69[a]
Hemoptysis – no. (%)	7 (23%)		3 (38%)		0.41[a]
Subjects with at least one *CFTR* mutation – no. (%)	18 (60%)	5 (20%)	6 (75%)	16 (22%)	5.5×10^{-5} [a]
Age when last seen – yr					0.15[b]
Median	70.5	62	56	65.5	
Mean±SD	69.57±9.74	62.80±12.70	61.00±17.74	67.07±14.45	
Median (mean) follow-up time – yr	10 (9.5)	11 (11.7)	11 (10.9)	12 (12.4)	0.06[b]
Deaths – no. (%)	14 (46.7%)	2 (8.0%)	2 (25.0%)	11 (14.9%)	0.0015[a]
Cause of death - no.					
cardiorespiratory	8	1		1	
others	4*	1[†]	1[‡]	5[¥]	
unknown	2		1	5	

RA: rheumatoid arthritis; DB: diffuse bronchiectasis. *CFTR*: cystic fibrosis transmembrane conductance regulator gene.
Plus-minus values are means±SD.
[a] *P*-values of Fisher exact tests.
[b] *P*-values of Kruskal-Wallis tests.
* Causes of death included CVA, Hodgkin lymphoma, cancer, and refractory RA, in one patient each.
[†] Cause of death was CVA.
[‡] Cause of death was cancer.
[¥] Causes of death included cancer in 4 patients and degenerative neurological disease in one patient.
doi:10.1371/journal.pone.0110066.t001

cardiorespiratory disease was the principal cause of death reported for eight of these patients.

There were more deaths after inclusion among the patients with RA-DB than among the other groups (RA only, DB only, unaffected relatives) (Table 1), even after adjustment for age at inclusion (Fig. 1A). RA-DB patients tended to be older at inclusion than patients with RA only or DB only (Table 1). We therefore also compared survival from birth between the different groups (Fig. S1A). For patients with RA or DB only, survival after inclusion or since birth was not significantly different from the survival of unaffected relatives (log-rank test $P=0.71$ and $P=0.21$, respectively). By contrast, survival was a mean of 8.6 years shorter for RA-DB patients than for unaffected relatives (log-rank test $P=6.2\times10^{-5}$) (Fig. 1A and Fig. S1A). In mixed effect Cox models, with unaffected relatives as the reference group, the HR for death was significant only for patients with RA-DB, whether we took inclusion in the study (HR, 7.61; 95% CI, 2.68–21.59; *z*-test $P=0.00014$) (Fig. 1B) or birth as the starting points (Fig. S1B).

Survival in rheumatoid arthritis patients with and without bronchiectasis

The survival of RA-DB patients after RA diagnosis was significantly lower than that of patients with RA only, even after adjusting for age of diagnosis (Fig. 2). Kaplan-Meier estimates of the probability of survival 15 years after RA diagnosis were 82.8% (95% CI, 70.2% to 97.8%) for RA-DB patients and 95.2% (95% CI, 86.6% to 100%) for patients with RA only ($P=0.022$). In the mixed effect Cox model adjusted for age at RA diagnosis, the HR for death associated with the presence of DB was 8.6 (95% CI, 1.5 to 48.2; *z*-test $P=0.014$) (Fig. 2B). We obtained similar results if we considered survival from birth, with a HR for death associated with the presence of DB of 9.6 (95% CI, 1.1 to 81.7; *z*-test $P=0.039$).

Factors influencing survival in patients with both rheumatoid arthritis and bronchiectasis

We found that 18 of the 30 patients with RA-DB (60%) had early-onset DB, whereas the other 12 patients with RA-DB (40%) had late-onset DB. Individuals with early-onset DB tended to be diagnosed with RA at younger ages than those with late-onset DB. We therefore studied survival from birth in RA-DB patients.

In univariate analyses of survival from birth, early-onset DB, CF/*CFTR*-RD mutations and being male were associated with poorer survival (Table 2).

Multivariate analysis of survival from birth showed that, in patients with RA-DB, an early onset of DB (HR, 15.4; 95% CI, 2.1 to 113.2; $P=0.0072$) and CF/*CFTR*-RD mutations (HR, 7.2; 95% CI, 1.4 to 37.1; $P=0.018$) were the two major determinants associated with poorer survival (Table 2). Eight of the 14 RA-DB

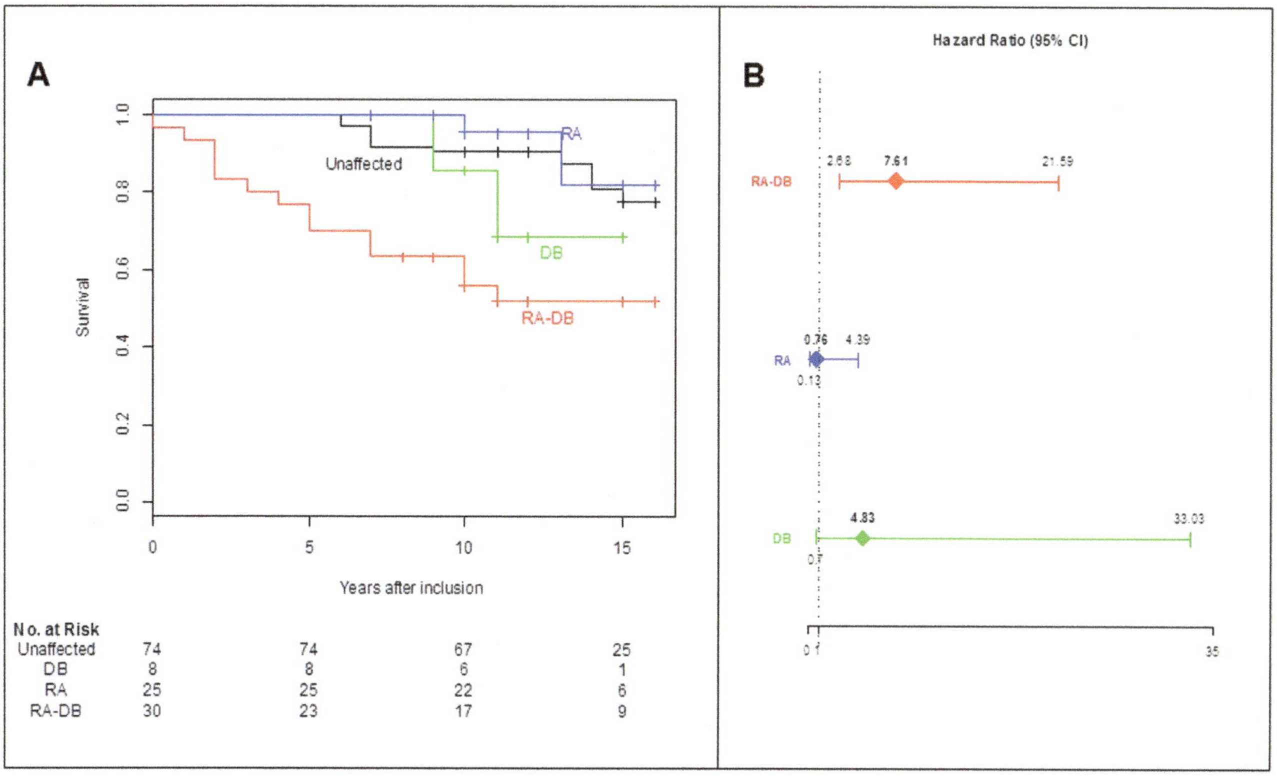

Panel A. Kaplan-Meier survival curves from inclusion in the study for the various groups of individuals.
Panel B. Hazard ratios (95% CI) of death after inclusion for the various disease groups, compared with unaffected relatives as the reference group.
A mixed effect Cox model was fitted, taking inclusion as the starting point and adjusting for age at inclusion. Individual random effects were assumed to be correlated as a function of the corresponding kinship coefficients. The variance of the random effect was 1.48.
RA: rheumatoid arthritis; DB: diffuse bronchiectasis.

Figure 1. Kaplan-Meier probability of survival from inclusion of the various participants in the study cohort, according to their phenotype. Panel A. Kaplan-Meier survival curves from inclusion in the study for the various groups of individuals. **Panel B.** Hazard ratios (95% CI) of death after inclusion for the various disease groups, compared with unaffected relatives as the reference group. A mixed effect Cox model was fitted, taking inclusion as the starting point and adjusting for age at inclusion. Individual random effects were assumed to be correlated as a function of the corresponding kinship coefficients. The variance of the random effect was 1.48. RA: rheumatoid arthritis; DB: diffuse bronchiectasis.

patients who died (57.1%) carried CF/*CFTR*-RD mutations and 10 (71.4%) had early-onset DB. The corresponding figures were six of 16 (37.5%) and 8 of 16 (50%) for the surviving RA-DB patients. The analysis classified RA patients with DB into categories of low or high risk of death. CF/*CFTR*-RD mutations in RA patients with early-onset DB defined a subgroup of high-risk patients with higher mortality rates (log-rank test $P = 1.28 \times 10^{-5}$). Only RA patients with both an early onset of DB and CF/*CFTR*-RD mutations were found to have significantly poorer survival and these patients tended to develop RA at a younger age than the other RA-DB patients. Survival from birth did not differ significantly between patients with late-onset DB and no mutation, patients with late-onset DB and CF/*CFTR*-RD mutations and patients with early-onset DB and no mutation (log-rank test = 2.8; 2 df; $P = 0.251$). Survival in RA-DB patients is shown according to risk of death categories in Figure 3.

Discussion

In this prospective cohort study, DB was associated with poorer survival in RA patients. This analysis further identified early-onset DB and CF/*CFTR*-RD mutation as factors associated with a poorer survival in RA-DB patients.

This study provides the first evidence of long-term poor survival in patients with DB-associated RA, who were found to have an eight times higher probability of death after RA diagnosis than family members with RA only. Cardiorespiratory causes were the most frequently reported causes of death in this population. These results are similar to those of a previous controlled study, in which the five-year probability of mortality in patients with RA-DB was found to be five times that of a matched control group of patients with RA alone and 2.4 times that of a group of patients with DB alone [14]. Most of the deaths of patients with RA-DB (60%) in this previous study were attributed to respiratory infection, whereas the severity of RA, as assessed by HAQ, grip strength, nodules and steroid treatment, was not significantly associated with poorer survival [14].

In patients with RA, childhood-onset DB is much more prevalent than late-onset DB [10,12-16]. Most (60%) of the 30 patients from our cohort with both RA and DB had early-onset DB, beginning more than 10 years before the onset of RA. These data are consistent with the hypothesis that the lung may be an early target of systemic RA autoimmunity or a site at which RA-related autoimmunity is initiated, with an initial autoimmune response in the lung [18,19]. We found that RA-DB patients with early-onset DB had a poorer prognosis than those with late-onset

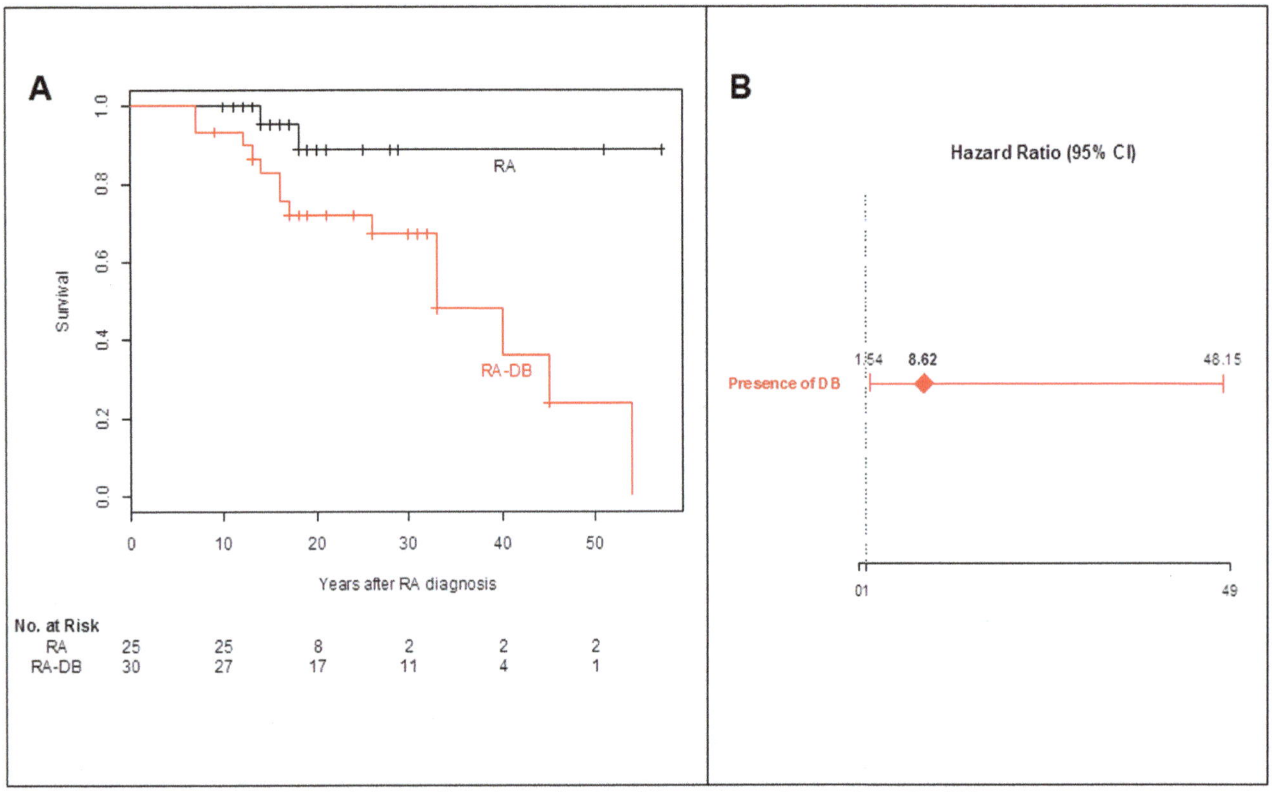

Panel A. Kaplan-Meier curves of survival after RA diagnosis, as a function of the presence or absence of associated DB.
Panel B. Hazard ratios (95% CI) for death after RA diagnosis associated with the presence of DB.
A mixed effect Cox model was fitted, taking RA diagnosis as the starting point. Individual random effects were assumed to be correlated as a function of the corresponding kinship coefficients. The variance of the random effect was 4 10^{-4}.
RA: rheumatoid arthritis; DB: diffuse bronchiectasis.

Figure 2. Kaplan-Meier probability of survival after RA diagnosis in patients, as a function of the presence or absence of associated DB. Panel A. Kaplan-Meier curves of survival after RA diagnosis, as a function of the presence or absence of associated DB. **Panel B.** Hazard ratios (95% CI) for death after RA diagnosis associated with the presence of DB. A mixed effect Cox model was fitted, taking RA diagnosis as the starting point. Individual random effects were assumed to be correlated as a function of the corresponding kinship coefficients. The variance of the random effect was 4 10^{-4}. RA: rheumatoid arthritis; DB: diffuse bronchiectasis.

DB, and early-onset DB was identified as a major determinant of survival in RA patients in multivariate analysis. The role of CF/*CFTR*-RD mutation in the association between RA and DB has been described before [23] and such mutations were found in 50% of the RA-DB patients with early-onset DB and 42% of those with late-onset DB. Not only do CF/*CFTR*-RD mutations predispose RA patients to DB, they are also associated with poorer survival. The prognostic implications of *CFTR* gene mutations have been considered to date only for in patients with CF. Our results demonstrate that RA patients with both early-onset DB and CF/*CFTR*-RD mutations should be considered at high risk of death and should receive more aggressive treatment, including smoking cessation and physiotherapy. Most of our patients were enrolled before the widespread use of biological agents likely to modify

Table 2. Analysis of survival from birth of 30 patients with both RA and DB.

	Univariate analysis	Multivariate analysis	
	***P* value**	**Hazard ratio [95% CI]**	***P* value**
Early-onset DB	0.009	15.4 [2.1; 113.2]	0.0072
***CFTR* mutations**	0.073	7.2 [1.4; 37.1]	0.018
Male versus female	0.06	1.1 [0.2; 5.6]	0.92

RA: rheumatoid arthritis; DB: diffuse bronchiectasis.
Early-onset DB: respiratory symptoms preceding RA by >10 years (mostly childhood DB).
CFTR: cystic fibrosis transmembrane conductance regulator gene.
A mixed effect Cox model was used, with shared random effects, depending on the kinship coefficient of individuals.
The variance of the random effect was 4×10^{-4}.

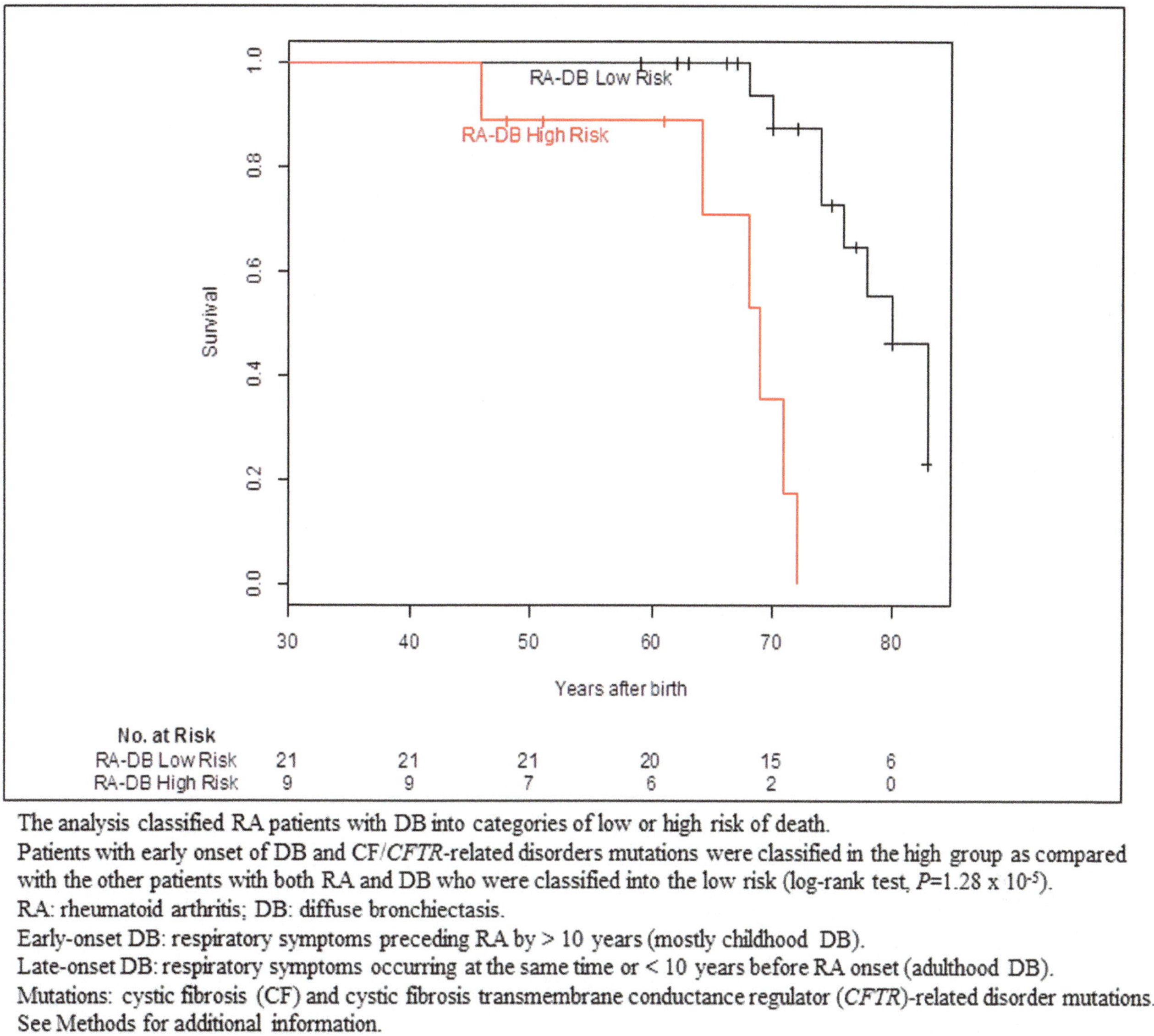

Figure 3. Kaplan-Meier probability of survival from birth of patients with both RA and DB according to risk of death categories. The analysis classified RA patients with DB into categories of low or high risk of death. Patients with early onset of DB and CF/*CFTR*-related disorders mutations were classified in the high group as compared with the other patients with both RA and DB who were classified into the low risk. RA: rheumatoid arthritis; DB: diffuse bronchiectasis. Early-onset DB: respiratory symptoms preceding RA by >10 years (mostly childhood DB). Late-onset DB: respiratory symptoms occurring at the same time or <10 years before RA onset (adulthood DB). Mutations: cystic fibrosis (CF) and cystic fibrosis transmembrane conductance regulator (*CFTR*)-related disorder mutations. See Patients and Methods for additional information.

mortality [27], but frequent pulmonary superinfections may constitute a contraindication for such treatments in these patients [15]. These high-risk patients should be eligible in priority in protocols evaluating new treatment interventions such as long-term macrolide therapy which may be beneficial in patients with non-CF bronchiectasis [28–33] and significantly improve the signs and symptoms of RA [34,35]. It remains unclear which patients should receive antibiotic treatment [36], but we suggest that RA patients with early-onset DB carrying CF/*CFTR*-RD mutations should be among those treated and evaluated for long-term azithromycin therapy.

Our study has several strengths. It is a family-based study, which made it possible to gather long-term data for all the individuals included. Such a family-based design limits research bias, by providing appropriate controls and follow-up. Furthermore, phenotypic characterization was carried out and mutational *CFTR* status was determined for all individuals. We systematically checked for DB on HRCT scans for all RA patients and for all individuals with respiratory symptoms. These scans were assessed by two investigators blind to the results of genetic tests.

Several limitations of this study merit further comment. The predictors of mortality in RA include severe extra-articular manifestations [2,37–41]. One of the limitations of this nationwide study is the lack of information regarding other risk factors for mortality in RA patients. These confounding factors may influence the outcome, but the strongest predictor of mortality has been shown to be extra-articular manifestations of the disease [2,40] and the leading cause of death of our RA-DB patients was cardiorespiratory complications. Sample size is another potential limitation of this study. The limited number of patients in each subgroup restricts the power of this study to detect differences. However, this series of patients with RA-DB is one of the largest ever studied, and differences in age at onset of DB and genetic background appear to have a significant, independent, and strong effect on mortality. In addition, our patients were selected from families with a history of RA or DB. It therefore remains unclear to what extent these results can be extrapolated to patients with no such family history. Another limitation of this study is the possible overestimation of the survival of patients with RA and late-onset DB with respect to that of patients with RA and early-onset DB. Indeed, for recruitment in the study, a family had to include at least one patient with RA and DB. Thus, if this patient had late-onset DB, there is the possibility of a survival advantage because he or she must have lived long enough after the onset of RA to develop DB meeting the late-onset criterion. However, this should not have biased the results concerning the deleterious effects of CF/*CFTR*-RD mutations on survival in patients with early-onset DB, in whom the presence of a mutation was found to lead to a mean decrease in survival of 7.1 years on average (log rank test = 6.3; 1 df; $P = 0.012$).

Conclusions

In this prospective family cohort, DB in RA patients was associated with lower overall survival. CF/*CFTR*-RD mutations predispose RA patients with early-onset DB to more severe disease, associated with a shorter lifespan. The identification of early-onset DB and the genotyping of such patients may make it possible to define high-risk patients for whom new treatments should be developed and evaluated specifically.

Supporting Information

Figure S1 Kaplan-Meier probability of survival from birth of the various participants in the study cohort as a function of their phenotype. Panel A. Kaplan-Meier survival curves from birth for the various groups of individuals. **Panel B.** Hazard ratios (95% CI) for death since birth for the various disease groups, compared with unaffected relatives as the reference group. A mixed effect Cox model was fitted, taking birth as the starting point and age as the scale. Individual random effects were assumed to be correlated as a function of the corresponding kinship coefficient. The variance of the random effect was 1.35. RA: rheumatoid arthritis; DB: diffuse bronchiectasis.

Acknowledgments

We thank the patients and their families for their participation. We thank Paul Legmann for HRCT scan analysis. We thank Eglantine Rouanet for assistance with data management, and the French Society of Rheumatology and the French National Society of Internal Medicine. We thank Philippe Saint Pierre for his helpful comments and advice on the analysis of correlated survival data.

Author Contributions

Conceived and designed the experiments: XP EG TB DD. Performed the experiments: EG TB. Analyzed the data: XP EG TB CLJ DD. Contributed reagents/materials/analysis tools: EG TB. Wrote the paper: XP EG TB CLJ DD.

References

1. Firestein GS (2003) Evolving concepts of rheumatoid arthritis. Nature 423: 356–361.
2. Turesson C, O'Fallon WM, Crowson CS, Gabriel SE, Matteson EL (2002) Occurrence of extraarticular disease manifestations is associated with excess mortality in a community based cohort of patients with rheumatoid arthritis. J Rheumatol 29: 62–67.
3. Aviña-Zubieta JA, Choi HK, Sadatsafavi M, Etminan M, Esdaile JM, et al. (2008) Risk of cardiovascular mortality in patients with rheumatoid arthritis: a meta-analysis of observational studies. Arthritis Rheum 59: 1690–1697.
4. Fewins HE, McGowan I, Whitehouse GH, Williams J, Mallya R (1991) High definition computed tomography in rheumatoid arthritis associated pulmonary disease. Br J Rheumatol 30: 214–216.
5. McDonagh J, Greaves M, Wright AR, Heycock C, Owen JP, et al. (1994) High resolution computed tomography of the lungs in patients with rheumatoid arthritis and interstitial lung disease. Br J Rheumatol 33: 118–122.
6. Hassan WU, Keaney NP, Holland CD, Kelly CA (1995) High resolution computed tomography of the lung in lifelong non-smoking patients with rheumatoid arthritis. Ann Rheum Dis 54: 308–310.
7. Vergnenègre A, Pugnere N, Antonini MT, Arnaud M, Melloni B, et al. (1997) Airway obstruction and rheumatoid arthritis. Eur Respir J 10: 1072–1078.
8. Perez T, Remy-Jardin M, Cortet B (1998) Airways involvement in rheumatoid arthritis: clinical, functional, and HRCT findings. Am J Respir Crit Care Med 157: 1658–1665.
9. Zrour SH, Touzi M, Bejia I, Golli M, Rouatbi N, et al. (2005) Correlations between high-resolution computed tomography of the chest and clinical function in patients with rheumatoid arthritis: prospective study in 75 patients. Joint Bone Spine 72: 41–47.
10. Solanki T, Neville E (1992) Bronchiectasis and rheumatoid disease: is there an association? Br J Rheumatol 31: 691–693.
11. Pasteur MC, Helliwell SM, Houghton SJ, Webb SC, Foweraker JE, et al. (2000) An investigation into causative factors in patients with bronchiectasis. Am J Respir Crit Care Med 162: 1277–1284.
12. Mathieu JP, Stack BH, Dick WC, Buchanan WW (1978) Pulmonary infection and rheumatoid arthritis. Br J Dis Chest 72: 57–61.
13. McMahon MJ, Swinson DR, Shettar S, Wolstenholme R, Chattopadhyay C, et al. (1993) Bronchiectasis and rheumatoid arthritis: a clinical study. Ann Rheum Dis 52: 776–779.
14. Swinson DR, Symmons D, Suresh U, Jones M, Booth J (1997) Decreased survival in patients with co-existent rheumatoid arthritis and bronchiectasis. Br J Rheumatol 36: 689–691.
15. Puéchal X (1998) Bronchiectasis in rheumatoid arthritis. Rev Rhum Engl Ed 65: 447–450.
16. Puéchal X, Fajac I, Bienvenu T, Desmazes-Dufeu N, Hubert D, et al. (1999) Increased frequency of cystic fibrosis deltaF508 mutation in bronchiectasis associated with rheumatoid arthritis. Eur Respir J 13: 1281–1287.
17. Shadick NA, Fanta CH, Weinblatt ME, O'Donnell W, Coblyn JS (1994) Bronchiectasis. A late feature of severe rheumatoid arthritis. Medicine (Baltimore) 73: 161–170.
18. Demoruelle MK, Weisman MH, Simonian PL, Lynch DA, Sachs PB, et al. (2012) Airways abnormalities and rheumatoid arthritis-related autoantibodies in subjects without arthritis: early injury or initiating site of autoimmunity? Arthritis Rheum 64: 1756–1761.
19. Reynisdottir G, Karimi R, Joshua V, Olsen H, Hensvold AH, et al. (2014) Structural changes and antibody enrichment in the lungs are early features of anti-citrullinated protein antibody-positive rheumatoid arthritis. Arthritis Rheumatol 66: 31–39.
20. Knowles MR, Durie PR (2002) What is cystic fibrosis? N Engl J Med 347: 439–442.
21. McKone EF, Emerson SS, Edwards KL, Aitken ML (2003) Effect of genotype on phenotype and mortality in cystic fibrosis: a retrospective cohort study. Lancet 361: 1671–1676.
22. Bombieri C, Claustres M, De Boeck K, Derichs N, Dodge J, et al. (2011) Recommendations for the classification of diseases as CFTR-related disorders. J Cyst Fibros 10 Suppl 2: S86–S102.
23. Puéchal X, Bienvenu T, Génin E, Berthelot JM, Sibilia J, et al. (2011) Mutations of the cystic fibrosis gene in patients with bronchiectasis associated with rheumatoid arthritis. Ann Rheum Dis 70: 653–659.
24. Therneau T (2013) A package for survival analysis in S. R package version 2.37–4. Available: http://CRAN.R-project.org/package=survival. Accessed 2014 Sep 19.
25. Therneau T (2012) Coxme: Mixed Effects Cox Models. R package version 2.2–3. Available: http://CRAN.R-project.org/package=coxme. Accessed 2014 Sep 19.
26. R Core Team (2012) R: A language and environment for statistical computing. R Foundation for Statistical Computing, Vienna, Austria. ISBN 3-900051-07-0. Available: http://www.R-project.org/. Accessed 2014 Sep 19.
27. Jacobsson LT, Turesson C, Nilsson JA, Petersson IF, Lindqvist E, et al. (2007) Treatment with TNF blockers and mortality risk in patients with rheumatoid arthritis. Ann Rheum Dis 66: 670–675.
28. Koh YY, Lee MH, Sun YH, Sung KW, Chae JH (1997) Effect of roxithromycin on airway responsiveness in children with bronchiectasis: a double-blind, placebo-controlled study. Eur Respir J 10: 994-999.
29. Tsang KW, Ho PI, Chan KN, Ip MS, Lam WK, et al. (1999) A pilot study of low-dose erythromycin in bronchiectasis. Eur Respir J 13: 361–364.

30. Wong C, Jayaram L, Karalus N, Eaton T, Tong C, et al. (2012) Azithromycin for prevention of exacerbations in non-cystic fibrosis bronchiectasis (EMBRACE): a randomised, double-blind, placebo-controlled trial. Lancet 380: 660–667.
31. Altenburg J, de Graaff CS, Stienstra Y, Sloos JH, van Haren EH, et al. (2013) Effect of azithromycin maintenance treatment on infectious exacerbations among patients with non-cystic fibrosis bronchiectasis: the BAT randomized controlled trial. JAMA 309: 1251–1259.
32. Serisier DJ, Martin ML, McGuckin MA (2013) Effect of long-term, low-dose erythromycin on pulmonary exacerbations among patients with non-cystic fibrosis bronchiectasis: the BLESS randomized controlled trial. JAMA 309: 1260–1267.
33. Elborn JS, Tunney MM (2013) Macrolides and bronchiectasis: clinical benefit with a resistance price. JAMA 309: 1295–1296.
34. Ogrendik M, Karagoz N (2011) Treatment of rheumatoid arthritis with roxithromycin: a randomized trial. Postgrad Med 123: 220–227.
35. Ogrendik M (2007) Effects of clarithromycin in patients with active rheumatoid arthritis. Curr Med Res Opin 23: 515–522.
36. Wilson R, Wells AU (2012) Azithromycin in bronchiectasis: when should it be used? Lancet 380: 627–629.
37. Foster CS, Forstot SL, Wilson LA (1984) Mortality rate in rheumatoid arthritis patients developing necrotizing scleritis or peripheral ulcerative keratitis. Effects of systemic immunosuppression. Ophthalmology 91: 1253–1263.
38. Erhardt CC, Mumford PA, Venables PJ, Maini RN (1989) Factors predicting a poor life prognosis in rheumatoid arthritis: an eight year prospective study. Ann Rheum Dis 48: 7–13.
39. Turesson C, Jacobsson L, Bergström U (1999) Extra-articular rheumatoid arthritis: prevalence and mortality. Rheumatology (Oxford) 38: 668–674.
40. Gabriel SE, Crowson CS, Kremers HM, Doran MF, Turesson C, et al (2003) Survival in rheumatoid arthritis: a population-based analysis of trends over 40 years. Arthritis Rheum 48: 54–58.
41. Turesson C, McClelland RL, Christianson TJ, Matteson EL (2007) Severe extra-articular disease manifestations are associated with an increased risk of first ever cardiovascular events in patients with rheumatoid arthritis. Ann Rheum Dis 66: 70–75.

Expression of the Inherently Autoreactive Idiotope 9G4 on Autoantibodies to Citrullinated Peptides and on Rheumatoid Factors in Patients with Early and Established Rheumatoid Arthritis

Geraldine Cambridge[1]*, Rita A. Moura[1,2], Tania Santos[2], Akif A. Khawaja[1,3], Joaquim Polido-Pereira[2,4], Helena Canhão[2,4], Maria J. Leandro[1], João E. Fonseca[2,4]

1 Centre for Rheumatology, University College London, London, United Kingdom, 2 Rheumatology Research Unit, Instituto de Medicina Molecular, Faculdade de Medicina da Universidade de Lisboa, Lisbon, Portugal, 3 Centre for Inflammation and Tissue Repair, University College London, London, United Kingdom, 4 Rheumatology Department, Centro Hospitalar de Lisboa Norte, EPE, Hospital de Santa Maria, Lisbon, Portugal

Abstract

Background: The pre-symptomatic stage of Rheumatoid arthritis (RA) is associated with pro-inflammatory cytokines and autoantibodies. High levels and epitope spread by Rheumatoid factors (RhF) and autoantibodies to citrullinated proteins signify progression towards disease expression. In established RA, the persistence of high autoantibody levels reflects production by both long-lived plasma cells and short-lived plasmablasts. Neither the relative contributions to pathogenesis by autoantibodies from either source, nor the factors responsible for deciding the fate of autoantigen specific 'parent' B-cells, is understood. Phenotypic markers identifying subsets of autoreactive B-cells are therefore of interest in understanding the origin and perpetuation of the autoimmune response in RA. One such phenotypic marker is the rat monoclonal antibody, 9G4, which recognises an idiotope on immunoglobuins derived from the inherently autoreactive VH-gene, VH4-34. We therefore investigated whether the 9G4 idiotope was expressed on autoantibodies in patients with RA.

Methodology/Principal Findings: Sera from 19 patients with established RA and those with <1year history of untreated polyarthritis either resolving into RA (n = 42) or non-RA diagnosis (n = 31) were included. Autoantibodies to cyclic citrullinated peptides (CCP), RhF and co-expression of the 9G4 idiotope were measured by ELISA. 9G4 recognised a population of anti-CCP antibodies in the majority of sera from patients with established disease and also in samples from patients with early disaese. 9G4+RhF levels were generally lower and not associated with positivity for, or levels of 9G4+CCP.

Conclusions/Significance: The persistence of 9G4+ immunoglobulins, of any isotype, in serum is rare. We describe here the novel finding of 9G4 expression on anti-CCP antibodies in patients from the earliest symptoms of RA through to established disease. Our results suggest that 9G4 expression on anti-CCP autoantibodies was not due to polyclonal expansion of VH4-34-encoded immunoglobulins. These studies may therefore provide a new focus for investigation into the evolution of the autoimmune response in RA patients.

Editor: Peter Szodoray, Institute of Immunology, Rikshospitalet, Norway

Funding: RAM was supported with a fellowship from Fundação para a Ciência e a Tecnologia (FCT, SFRH/BPD/81936/2011). TS was supported with a grant from Erasmus Programme. The funders had no role in study design, data collection and analysis, decision to publish, or preparation of the manuscript.

Competing Interests: The authors have declared that no competing interests exist.

* Email: g.cambridge@ucl.ac.uk

Introduction

The serology of patients with Rheumatoid arthritis (RA) is characterised by persistently raised levels of autoantibodies of two main specificities, being those against Fc of IgG (Rheumatoid factors, RhF) and to peptide sequences on a number of different proteins which have undergone citrullination (anti-citrullinated protein/peptide antibodies - ACPA) [1–3]. Multiple isotypes of both RhF and ACPA and epitope spread of ACPA can precede the development of clinical disease by many months or years [4–8]. Detection of ACPA in the clinical setting however is usually through binding to commercially prepared combinations of cyclic citrullinated peptides (CCP), which detect antibodies of most but not all specificities [9]. The RhF response can also be both exaggerated and show evidence of somatic hypermutation [10,11]. Although unaffected relatives and relatives with undifferentiated arthritis can also have ACPA and RhF, albeit at much lower titres, the number of isotypes is more limited and sera from patients with undifferentiated arthritis also recognise fewer citrullinated epitopes [12].

The usage of some genes encoding particular variable heavy chains of immunoglobulins (IGVH) has been associated with the development of autoantibodies [11,13,14], with those encoded by VH4-34 being the prototype [15]. Identification of B-cells and antibodies using this VH gene is possible using the rat monoclonal antibody, 9G4, which recognises a unique comformational epitope largely confined within framework 1 of VH4-34-derived immunoglobulins (Igs) [16]. This epitope is inherently autoreactive as it recognises N-acetyllactosamine (NAL) on a number of microbial glycolipids, self glycoproteins and on cells undergoing apoptosis [17–19]. 9G4+ B-cells can constitute up to 10% of peripheral B-cells although VH4-34-derived serum Igs constitute less than 1% of total Igs [20]. The level of VH4-34-derived Igs can however transiently increase in response to infections [19,21–23]. The ability to recognise a number of self-antigens via the NAL-epitope may thus be advantageous in clearing damaged, apoptotic or neoplastic cells, but may also increase the risk of autoimmunity, particularly if the conventional binding site on the same molecule undergoes mutation to an autoreactive specificity. VH4-34 gene usage has been shown to be obligatory for the production of most pathogenic IgM cold-agglutinins and has been for demonstrated in IgM-RhF, IgG anti-dsDNA antibodies in systemic lupus erythematosus (SLE), and IgM anti-myeloperoxidase antibodies in systemic vasculitis [24–27]. The consequence of allowing the inherently autoreactive VH4-34-derived B cell populations to persist within the B-cell repertoire, across all ethic groups, implies that differentiation to antibody secretion, except in the context of infection, must be under strict physiological control. Censoring of 9G4+ B-cells may be due to anergy associated with high-dose antigen exposure, as the apparent block to maturation into Ig secretion can be overcome by culturing isolated 9G4+ cells *in vitro* with cytokines and CD70 stimulation [22].

Preliminary studies in our laboratory showed that sera from some patients with established RA contained 9G4+ antibodies to CCP [28]. In the present cross-sectional study, we have extended analysis of 9G4 expression to include sera from patients with the earliest symptoms of RA (<6 weeks polyarthritis) and disease controls, and in patients with established disease, using samples from a well-described cohort [29]. We have also measured serum autoantibody levels and class and included anti-microbial antibodies in the analysis.

Patients and Methods

Patients

Patients were attending the Rheumatology Department in the Hospital de Santa Maria, Lisbon Academic Medical Centre and Hospital da Luz, Lisbon, Portugal. Serum samples were collected from 40 consecutive patients with untreated polyarthritis of less than 6 weeks duration of symptoms and from 33 untreated early polyarthritis patients with >6 weeks and <1 year of disease history. Serum samples were also collected from 19 patients with established seropositive RA from Lisbon Academic Medical Centre (Est-RA) Samples from Lisbon centers were stored at Biobanco-IMM, Lisbon Academic Medical Centre. All patients with established disease had received a variety of therapies but patients currently or previously treated with rituximab were excluded. Serum samples from 21 healthy controls (HC) were also collected. The local ethics committees (Comissão de Ética do Hospital de Santa Maria, Lisbon, Portugal and University College London Ethics Committee, London, United Kingdom) approved the study and all patients signed an informed consent prior to any protocol-specific procedure.

Measurement of IgM and IgA Rheumatoid factor (RhF)

RhF were detected using affinity purified rabbit IgG (Sigma Aldrich, St Louis, USA) as substrate. Binding of sera (diluted 1/200) on coated and uncoated wells was measured using goat-anti-human IgA- or IgM-horeradish peroxidase (HRP) conjugate (The Binding Site, Birmingham, UK). In all ELISAs, color development was with tetramethylbenzidine (TMB-Sigma-Aldrich, Gillingham, UK). After subtracting background binding (to uncoated wells), arbitrary units (AU) of binding were calculated by reference to control sera and a standard curve constructed from high positive control sera for each isotype. Cuts-off were 10 AU/ml and 23 AU/ml for IgM and IgA-RhF respectively. IgG-RhF was detected following pepsin digestion of sera with detection of IgG-Fab_2 fragments using HRP-conjugated goat anti-IgG-Fab_2, as previously described [30]. Reagents were supplied by TheraTest (Chicago, USA).

Anti-cyclic citrullinated peptide antibodies

Antibodies to citrullinated peptides were measured using commercial ELISA plates coated with second generation citrullinated peptides (CCP2) (FCCP600; Axis Sheild Diagnostics, Dundee, UK). Sera was added to plates at a dilution of 1/200. HRP-conjugated sheep anti-human IgG, −IgM or −IgA (The Binding Site, UK) were used to detect classes of anti-CCP2, and the assay was developed as above for RhF. Levels of IgG-CCP2 were calculated as per manufacturers instructions and IgM- and IgA-CCP2 calculated following in-house protocol. Cut-off values were defined according to the manufacturer's instructions for IgG-CCP2 (5 U/ml) or defined as mean ± 3SD from healthy controls for IgM-CCP2 and IgA-CCP2 (26 AU/mL and 10 AU/mL, respectively).

Expression of 9G4 on RhF and on antibodies to CCP2

For detection of 9G4 expression on either RhF or CCP2, sera (diluted 1/50 in RD6Q diluent, R & D Systems, Abingdon, UK) were added to respective antigen coated wells of ELISA plates. Following initial incubation, the 9G4 reagent (IGM Bioscience, Palo Alto, USA) was added at a concentration of 2 μg/ml to one side of the plate, the duplicate serum-incubated wells receiving diluent buffer instead of 9G4. 9G4 binding to RhF was detected using biotinylated goat anti-rat IgG (Abcam, Cambridge, UK), and a streptavidin–HRP visualization system. An affinity purified HRP-conjugated sheep anti-rat-IgG reagent (Amersham, UK) was used to detect 9G4 recognition of CCP2-binding antibodies. Results were calculated and presented as optical densities (OD at 450 nm) following the subtraction of any background binding in the absence of the 9G4 reagent. Results exceeding mean ± 3 SD of 5 HC sera were regarded as positive.

Separation of sera using Protein G columns

Sera from 4 patients with established RA which had both IgM- and IgG-class autoantibodies to CCP2, which also bound the 9G4 reagent, were separated on Protein G columns using conventional techniques [31]. Eluted fractions (using low-pH) and flow-through fractions were then tested for IgM-, IgG- and 9G4-CCP2 activity, as described above.

Statistical analysis

Statistical differences were determined using GraphPad Prism (GraphPad, San Diego, USA). For populations not following a normal distribution, non-parametric statistics were used (Mann-Whitney U test) to compare independent groups. Linear regression (Spearman's rank correlation) was used to determine relationships between variables. Differences were considered statistically significant for $p<0.05$.

Results

Characteristics of patient cohorts

Clinical details of patients with established RA, untreated polyarthritis, together with HC, are shown in Table 1. In patients with a history of polyathritis of <6 weeks (n = 40), after a minimum follow-up of 3 months, 14/40 patients fulfilled the 2010 American College of Rheumatology (ACR)/European League Against Rheumatism (EULAR) criteria for RA [32] and were classified as Very Early Rheumatoid Arthritis (VERA) patients. The remaining early polyarthritis patients (n = 26), who did not evolve into RA, were classified as Very Early Non-RA (VENRA). Patients in the VENRA group were resolved into diagnostic categories of spondyloarthritis (6), SLE (5), polymyalgia rheumatica (4), microcrystalline arthritis (2), Sjögren syndrome (1), undifferentiated diffuse connective tissue disease (1), viral polyarthritis (1), arthritis associated with malignancy (1) and 5 patients entered spontaneously into remission (self-limiting polyarthritis). In the second group of untreated polyarthritis patients (n = 33), who had more than 6 weeks history but less than one year of disease duration, those who after a minimum follow-up of 2 years fulfilled the 2010 ACR/EULAR criteria for RA (n = 28) were classified as Early RA (ERA) [32]. The remaining 5 untreated early polyarthritis patients who did not evolve into RA were classified as Early Non-RA (ENRA) (all with undifferentiated arthritis). Comparing VERA with VENRA and ERA with ENRA, there were no significant differences with respect to age, number of tender joints, ESR or DAS28, although patients in the ERA cohort had significantly more swollen joints than ENRA (Table 1).

9G4+autoantibodies in early and established RA

Although the numbers of patients in each early RA cohort were low, relative levels of 9G4 binding to each autoantigen specificity in patients and HC showed that overall, 9G4 binding to the citrullinated substrate appeared greater than that by RhF (Figure 1A and B). 9G4 expression on autoantibodies in VERA patients was largely restricted to those targeting citrullinated peptides (6/14 compared with 1/14 for RhF). 9G4 expression was borderline positive on CCP2-binding antibodies in 2 samples in the VENRA control group. In the ERA cohort, 9G4 expression was similar for both autoantibody specificities but in Est-RA, virtually all sera contained 9G4+CCP2 activity (18/19) compared with 6/19 positive for 9G4+RhF. In Figure 2A and B, IgG-CCP2 and IgM-RhF were the main specificities present in patients with the earliest disease (VERA cohort). IgM class autoantibodies of both specificities, but not IgA- or IgG- autoantibodies, were also present in a proportion of VENRA patients (4/26 with IgM-CCP2 and 2/26 with IgM-RhF), but not in patients in the ENRA cohort (0/5). 9G4+ expression was borderline positive on CCP2-binding antibodies in 2 samples in the VENRA control group, both of which contained IgM-CCP2 only (Figure 2A). The percentage of samples positive for 9G4+CCP2 in the ERA cohort was the same as that for 9G4+RhF (39%). The percentage of samples positive for 9G4 binding in the established RA cohort however was nearly 100% whereas the percentage containing 9G4+RhF remained around 30%. Levels of binding also appeared considerably lower for 9G4+RhF than for 9G4+CCP2 (Figure 2B; Figure 1).

Comparison of isotypes and 9G4 expression in individual patients

Figures 3–5 show autoantibody isotypes (anti-CCP2 and RhF) and corresponding 9G4 expression in sera from individual patients in the VERA, ERA and Est-RA cohorts respectively. Serum autoantibody results were ranked on the basis of the relative levels of IgG-CCP2 antibodies in order to compare positivity for individual specificities in each patient. In the VERA cohort (Figure 3), 9G4 expression on CCP2-binding antibodies was evident in all samples which also had significant IgG-CCP2, although 2 had very low/borderline expression. IgM- and IgA-CCP2 were present in only 2 of these samples. IgM-RhF was present in 8 samples, 2 of which were also positive for IgA-RhF,

Table 1. Demographic data of healthy controls, patients with untreated polyarthritis and patients with established RA.

Clinical features	Healthy Controls	VERA	VENRA	ERA	ENRA	Est-RA
Median and range						
unless otherwise indicated	**(n = 21)**	**(n = 14)**	**(n = 26)**	**(n = 28)**	**(n = 5)**	**(n = 19)**
Age (years)	52 (22–66)	50 (26–94)	41 (24–83)	48 (17–79)	45 (41–66)	54 (21–77)
Sex (% female)	67	93	73	82	80	68
Disease duration	NA	<6	<6	8 (2–12)	3 (3–11)	5 (1–20)
(time)		weeks	weeks	months	months	years
Swollen joints	NA	16 (0–28)	2 (0–22)	6 (0–26)*	1 (0–7)*	3 (1–22)
Tender joints	NA	12 (1–28)	7 (0–25)	6 (0–26)	3 (1u7–7)	4 (1–22)
ESR (mm/1st hour)	ND	39 (3–95)	27 (4–120)	21 (2–120)	9 (6–33)	25 (5–95)
DAS28 (mean ± SD)	NA	6.1±1.7	4.9±1.9	5.1±1.4	3.8±1.3	4.7±1.4

NA[a]: not applicable, ND[b]: not determined, *p<0.05 (Mann Whiney Rank sum).
Results for healthy controls (HC) and patients with untreated polyarthritis of either ≤6 weeks duration (Very Early-VE) and subsequently diagnosed as RA (VERA) or Non-RA (VENRA) and patients with >6 weeks and ≤1 year history of polyarthritis (Early-E) subsquently diagnosed with RA (ERA) or a different clinical diagnosis Non-RA (ENRA). Est-RA: Established RA.

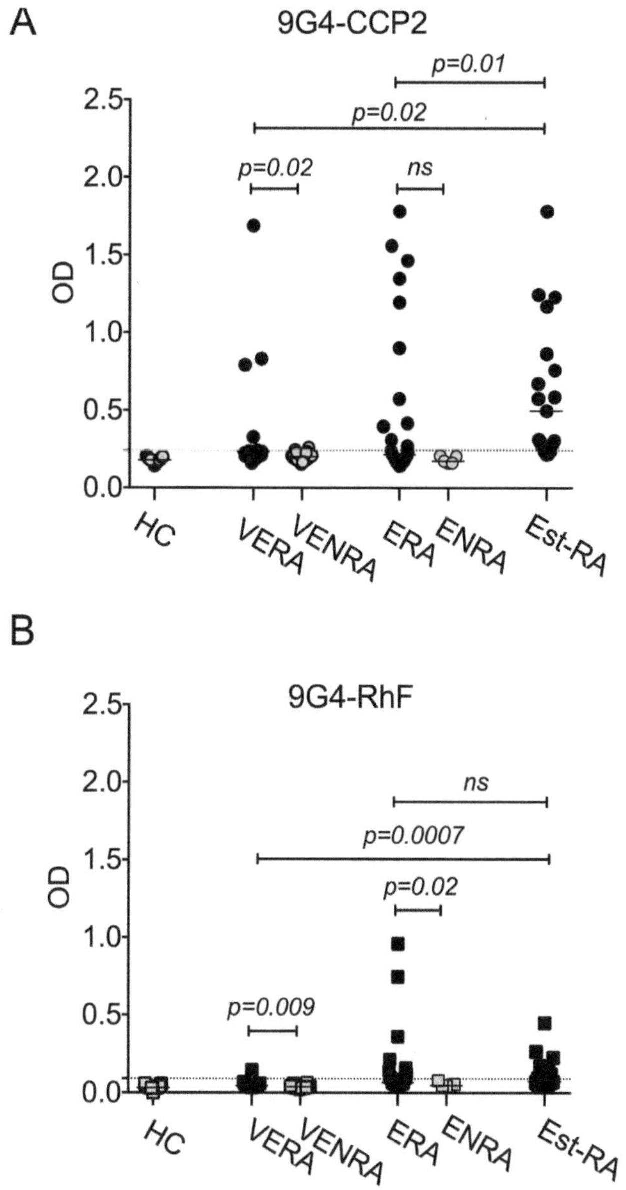

Figure 1. 9G4 expresssion on antibodies to CCP2 and on RhF in early and established RA. 9G4 expression on CCP2 (A) and RhF (B) in sera from healthy controls (HC), patients with very early RA (VERA), very early non-RA (VENRA), early RA (ERA), early non-RA (ENRA) and a cohort of seropositive established RA (Est-RA). Comparisons were with Mann Whitney U test at 5% level.

with only 1 sample being 9G4+RhF. Figure 4 similarly shows results for patients within the ERA group. IgG-CCP2 positivity was usually accompanied in the same sample by IgM-CCP2, IgA-CCP2 and 9G4+CCP2. The presence and level of the RhF response and 9G4+RhF expression did not correlate with presence or levels of anti-CCP2 antibodies in the same patient. In the Est-RA cohort (Figure 5), samples with the highest levels of IgG-CCP2 also contained IgM- and IgA-CCP2 and most were also positive for IgM-RhF. The pattern of 9G4+CCP2 positivity corresponded most closely with that of samples containing IgM- and IgA-CCP2 as well as IgG-CCP2.

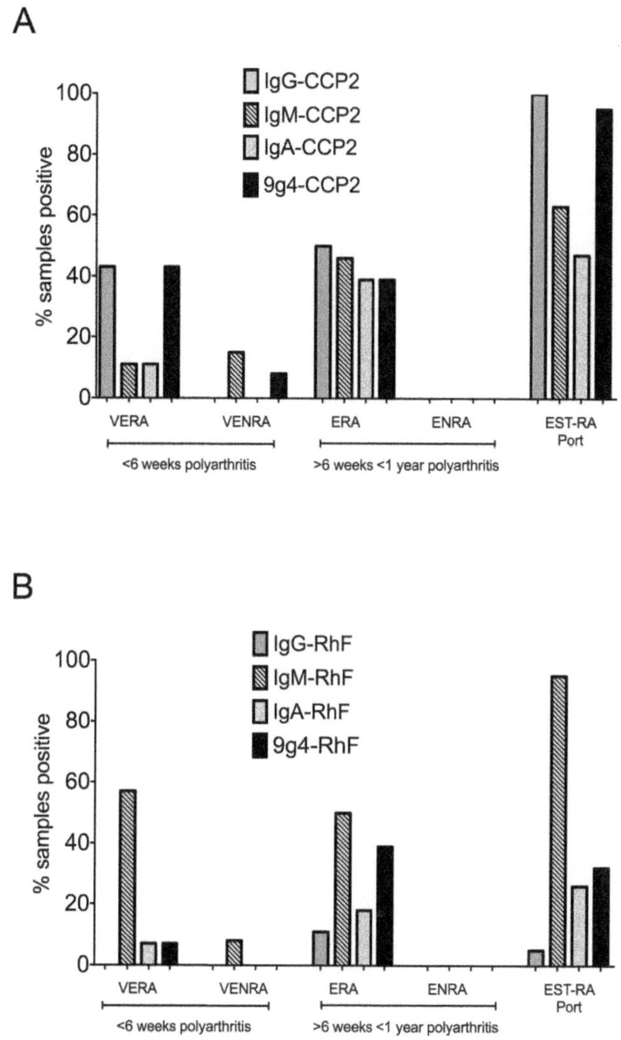

Figure 2. Percentages of samples positive for IgG-, IgA- and IgM- anti-CCP2 antibodies and RhF and for 9G4 expression. Isotypes of anti-CCP2 antibodies and 9G4 expression on CCP2 binding antibodies are shown in (A) and isotypes of RhF and 9G4 expression of antibodies binding to rabbit-IgG are shown in (B).

Is 9G4 expression on IgM or IgG-anti-CCP2 antibodies?

Protein G columns were used to separate sera from 4 patients with established RA (Figure S1). Following separation, results suggested most 9G4 activity associated with the eluted fraction. However, the eluted fractions contained both IgM- and IgG-CCP2 activity, probably due to interference by Rheumatoid factors. In the flow-through fractions only 1 serum was positive for 9G4-CCP2 binding. This fraction also had CCP2 binding activity in both IgM- and -IgG-CCP2 assays, which may also be due to the presence of high levels of Rheumatoid factors blocking Fcγ binding to Protein G. Results were therefore equivocal but suggested that at least a proportion of 9G4+CCP2 were within the IgG fraction.

Discussion

The ability to bind the rat monoclonal anti-idiotope antibody, 9G4, was used as a surrogate measure of the utilisation of the VH4-34 heavy chain by the 2 main autoantibody specificities present in sera from patients with RA. Our results showed that in

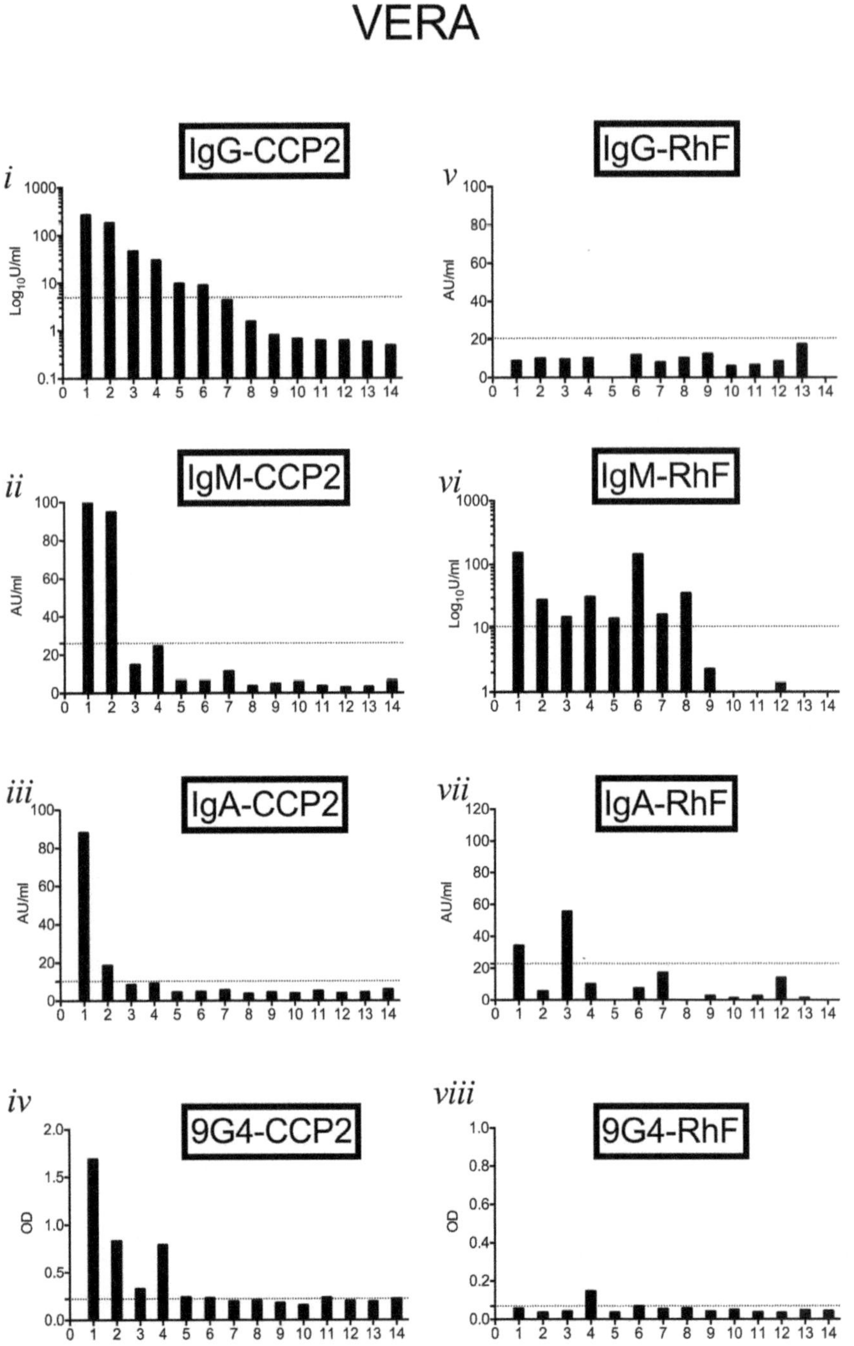

Figure 3. 9G4 expression and relative levels of autoantibodies in individual patients in the ERA cohort. Results for all autoantibody isotypes and for 9G4 expression were ranked in order of the relative levels of IgG-CCP2 in order to follow results for individual patients (as numbered on x-axis). Horizontal dotted lines show upper limit of normal ranges determined for each parameter as described in the text.

patients with early RA and with established disease, there was a remarkably consistent recognition of anti-CCP2 antibodies by the 9G4 reagent. Positivity for binding of 9G4 to RhF was also found but less frequently. Further, levels of binding to each autoantibody specificity did not correlate in individual patients. This report is the first, to our knowledge, to describe the apparent usage of the inherently autoreactive VH4-34 gene by anti-CCP2 antibodies in patients with RA from the very earliest signs of disease.

Unaffected relatives of RA patients, as well those with an undifferentiated arthritis, can test positive for ACPA (and RhF) [33]. In the present study, we found that although IgM-CCP2 and IgM-RhF could both be present in sera from VENRA and ENRA patients, where synovitis failed to develop into RA, 9G4 expression on anti-CCP2 antibodies was present in only 2 samples, and at very low levels. Both samples were from VENRA patients, and contained only IgM-class anti-CCP2.

In normal individuals, VH4-34 usage by total serum immunoglobulins (both IgM and IgG) is disproportionately low (~0.7% of serum IgM; no IgG) given that 5–10% of peripheral B-cells express the 9G4 idiotope [20,34]. Consistent with a lack of class-

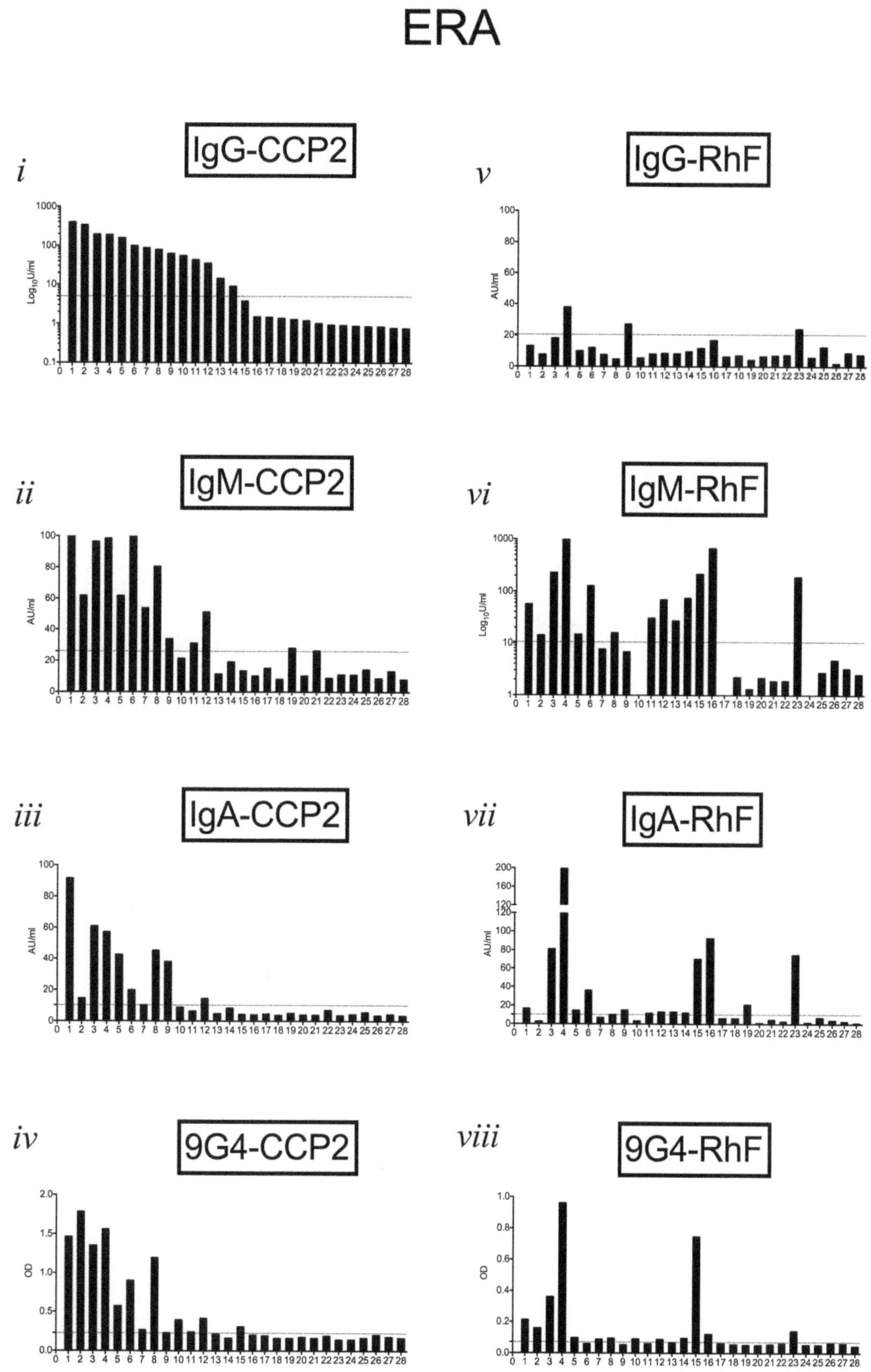

Figure 4. 9G4 expression and relative levels of autoantibodies in individual patients in the ERA cohort. Results for all autoantibody isotypes and for 9G4 expression were ranked in order of the relative levels of IgG-CCP2 in order to follow results for individual patients (as numbered on x-axis). Horizontal dotted lines show upper limit of normal ranges determined for each parameter as described in the text.

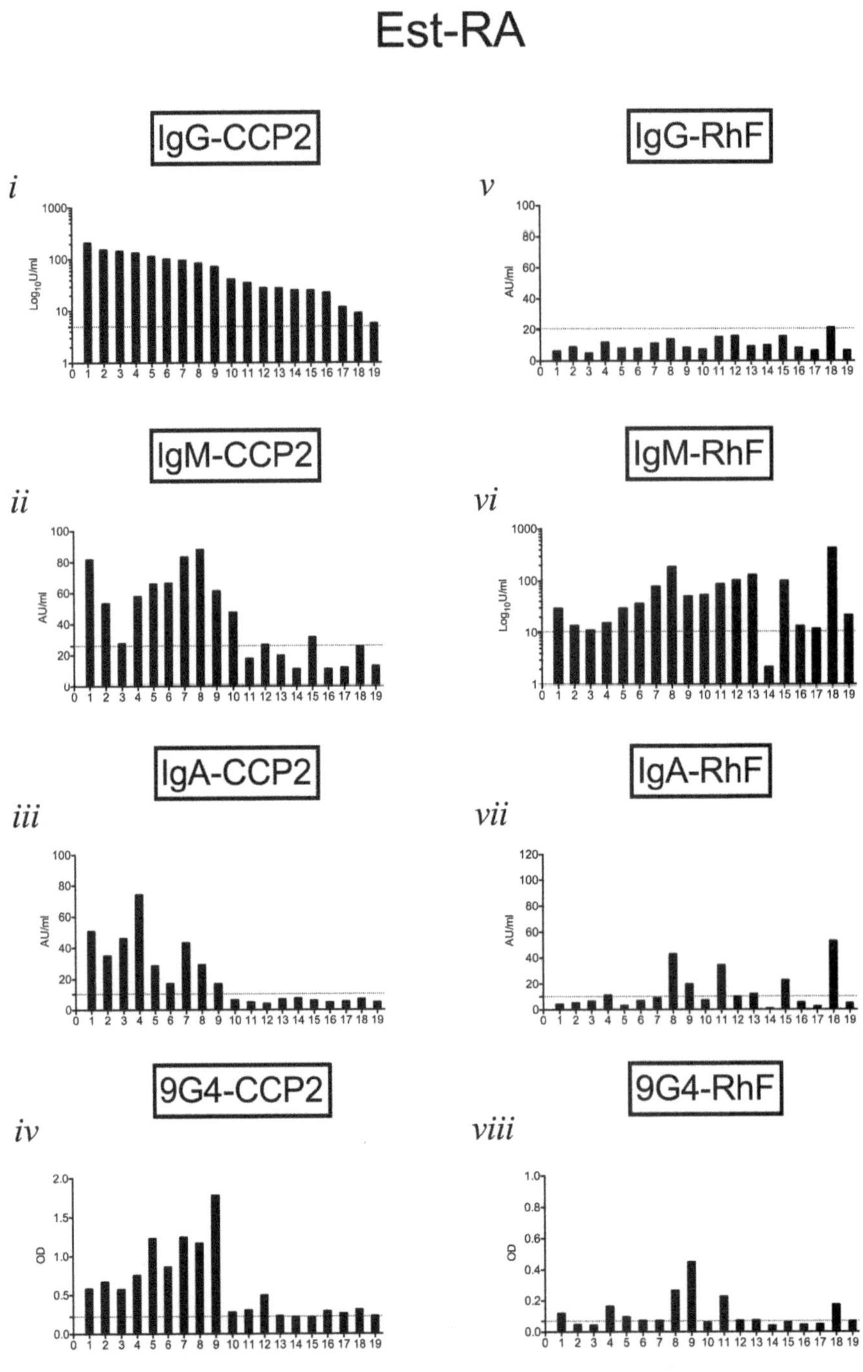

Figure 5. 9G4 expression and relative levels of autoantibodies in individual patients in the Est-RA cohort. Results for all autoantibody isotypes and for 9G4 expression were ranked in order of the relative levels of IgG-CCP2 in order to follow results for individual patients (as numbered on x-axis). Horizontal dotted lines show upper limit of normal ranges determined for each parameter as described in the text.

switched 9G4+Ig, 9G4+ B-cells are absent from tonsillar germinal centres in healthy individuals [35]. Following infections, such as with EBV, antibodies utilising VH4-34 show a transient increase, largely within the IgM pool. Expression of CD27 (expressed by most but not all memory-B-cells [36]) can only be detected on a small (<10%) sub-population of 9G4+ B-cells, but somewhat unusually such cells can co-express the naïve B cell marker, CD5 [37]. Taken together, these observations are consistent with the VH4-34 gene being utilised by naïve or pre-switch B-cells, which display a limited ability to undergo class switch [15]. The presence of such a high proportion of VH4-34-derived B-cells in the naïve compartment further suggest that this particular germ line sequence is preferentially selected for exit from the bone marrow into the periphery, regardless of CDR3 specificity.

In the context of autoimmunity, most notably SLE, class-switched (IgG) 9G4+ anti-dsDNA antibodies are present in serum and in involved renal tissue [25,34]. 9G4+ B-cells were also abundant in germinal centre (GC) reactions in tonsils from SLE patients but tonsils from RA patients resembled those of normal individuals with 9G4+ B-cells thus being excluded [35]. In another study, VH4-34 derived B-cells from normal human tonsils did show evidence of class switch [38], but the anatomical location of such B cells within the tonsil was not given. Somatic hypermutation was also detected before class switch in some clonally related transcripts, suggesting that VH4-34 (μ+) B-cells were indeed capable of undergoing both somatic mutation and class-switch, most likely outside a GC reaction [35].

We found that in samples from patients with the shortest history of polyarthritis (VERA), 9G4+CCP2 was most strongly associated with IgG-CCP2, particularly when co-existing in samples containing IgM-RhF. Although the relative contribution of different Ig isotypes to total 9G4-CCP2 binding was dificult to interpret due to probable interference with RhF, our results using Protein G columns (Figure S1) and pepsin digestion (data not shown) nevertheless suggested that both IgM- and IgG-CCP2 autoantibodies can express the 9G4+ idiotope, consistent with the possibility that class-switch of 9G4+CCP2 antibodies could occur.

9G4 expression on RhF in the RA cohorts was indeed found to be less common and somewhat lower than on CCP2-directed antibodies. In addition, the levels of 9G4 expression on antibodies to CCP2 and on RhF in individual samples (Figures 3–5) showed that the 9G4 idiotope was not necessarily present on both autoantibody specificities in the same sample and if present, relative expression usually differed. Expansion of 9G4+CCP2 autoreactivity was therefore both greater than that of 9G4+RhF, particularly in early RA patients, and therefore was not likely to be the result of a polyclonal expansion of all 'autoreactive' VH4-34-derived parent B-cells. In addition, we found that 9G4 expression was absent from antibodies to tetanus toxoid and pneumococcal capsular polysaccharides within serum samples positive for 9G4-CCP2 (Figure S2). This argues against a prior general expansion of VH4-34 encoded antibodies and further suggests that autoantigen specificity may play a role in the selection of particular 9G4+ B cell clones.

Intriguingly, the percentage of samples positive for IgM- and for IgA-CCP2 between VERA and ERA cohorts followed, rather than preceded positivity for IgG-class antibodies to CCP2 (Figure 2A; Figures 3 and 4). This supports the suggestion that the elicitation of IgG-CCP2 antibodies to a citrullinated protein may arise early in the underlying pathogenic process and also suggest a sequence of events not shared with conventional antibody responses to immunisation or infection [39]. In established RA, the persistence of multiple isotypes of anti-CCP2 over time, most notably in the IgM fraction, also indicates that there is a constant renewal of autoreactive (naïve) B-cells throughout the course of disease which then differentiate into plasmablasts, or long-lived plasma cells [40]. The kinetics of autoantibody production following B-cell depletion treatment with the anti-CD20 reagent, rituximab, have shown that at least a proportion of IgM-autoantibodies derive from early/naïve B-cells continuously exiting the bone marrow; a process interupted by this form of therapy [41]. Support for this scenario comes from the experiments of Samuels et al [42] who reported that VH regions cloned and translated from early naïve B-cells from RA patients contained a high proportion of transcripts with reactivity for citrullinated peptides. This would suggest that in RA, autoreactive B cell specificities escape deletion, receptor editing or anergy early in their development, ultimately giving rise to a population of B-cells which can also survive entry into the mature B cell compartment in the periphery.

The unique properties of B-cells expressing both the inherently autoreactive 9G4 epitope, coupled with specificity and high affinities for citrullinated residues through CDR3 may conceivably therefore be a key factor in the selection and possibly expansion of the immune response to citrullinated proteins in RA patients. Although B cell development in the bone marrow is largely antigen-independent, signaling through a functional B cell receptor complex (consisting of surface immunoglobulin, CD19 and co-receptors CD81, CD21), microenvironmental factors and also interaction between pre-B-cells, influences selection during differentiation towards entry into the peripheral pool. We have previously suggested that the expansion of autoreactive B cell clones in systemic autoimmune diseases relates to pro-survival properties imbued by certain B-cell receptors [43]. VH4-34 usage, combined with specificity for citrullinated residues, may therefore increase the probability of positive BCR signalling in parent B cells and contribute to the selection of auto-reactive B-cells either before their exit from the bone marrow and/or in the periphery of patients with RA.

Conclusion

In this cross-sectional study, seropositivity for autoantibodies expressing the 9G4 idiotope apparently increased with disease maturity in patients with RA. A higher proportion of patients with the earliest symptoms of polyarthritis whose disease resolved into Rheumatoid arthritis were also more likely to have 9G4+CCP2 than those with other diagnostic outcomes. The presence of 9G4+ antibodies of any isotype in the serum immunoglobulin pool is unusual and is here clearly associated with autoimmunity. 9G4+ autoantibodies were able to be detected in the circulation from the first weeks of resolution into RA and may thus represent a surrogate measure of selection of autoreactive B-cells into the periphery.

Supporting Information

Figure S1 9G4 binding to serum fractions separated by Protein G columns. IgM- and IgG- anti-CCP2 and 9G4+ CCP2 reactivity was measured in sera from 4 patients with established RA. Following separation on Protein G columns, flow through and eluted fractions were tested for IgM-, IgG- and 9G4-CCP2 activity.

Figure S2 9G4 binding to antibodies to microbial antigens. Antibodies to pneumococcal capsular polysaccharides (PCP – consisting of a combination of 23 serotypes of Streptococcus *pneumoniae* serotypes) and to tetanus toxoid (TT) were measured by ELISA using commercial kits. 9G4 expression on bound anti-microbial antibodies were then determined using methods described for autoantibodies.

Author Contributions

Conceived and designed the experiments: GC RAM TS AK. Performed the experiments: TS AK. Analyzed the data: GC TS AK MJL. Contributed reagents/materials/analysis tools: GC RAM AK JEF HC JP-P MJL. Contributed to the writing of the manuscript: GC TS RAM JP-P HC JEF MJL.

References

1. Schellekens GA, de Jong BA, van den Hoogen FH, van de Putte LB, van Venrooij WJ (1998) Citrulline is an essential constituent of antigenic determinants recognized by rheumatoid arthritis-specific autoantibodies. J Clin Invest 101: 273–281.

2. Verpoort KN, Jol-van der Zijde CM, Papendrecht-van der Voort EA, Ioan-Facsinay A, Drijfhout JW, et al. (2006) Isotype distribution of anti-cyclic citrullinated peptide antibodies in undifferentiated arthritis and rheumatoid arthritis reflects an ongoing immune response. Arthritis Rheum 54: 3799–3808.
3. Lakos G, Soos L, Fekete A, Szabo Z, Zeher M, et al. (2008) Anti-cyclic citrullinated peptide antibody isotypes in rheumatoid arthritis: association with disease duration, rheumatoid factor production and the presence of shared epitope. Clin Exp Rheumatol 26: 253–260.
4. Jansen AL, van der Horst-Bruinsma I, van Schaardenburg D, van de Stadt RJ, de Koning MH, et al. (2002) Rheumatoid factor and antibodies to cyclic citrullinated Peptide differentiate rheumatoid arthritis from undifferentiated polyarthritis in patients with early arthritis. J Rheumatol 29: 2074–2076.
5. Rantapaa-Dahlqvist S, de Jong BA, Berglin E, Hallmans G, Wadell G, et al. (2003) Antibodies against cyclic citrullinated peptide and IgA rheumatoid factor predict the development of rheumatoid arthritis. Arthritis Rheum 48: 2741–2749.
6. Nielen MM, van Schaardenburg D, Reesink HW, van de Stadt RJ, van der Horst-Bruinsma IE, et al. (2004) Specific autoantibodies precede the symptoms of rheumatoid arthritis: a study of serial measurements in blood donors. Arthritis Rheum 50: 380–386.
7. Sokolove J, Bromberg R, Deane KD, Lahey LJ, Derber LA, et al. (2012) Autoantibody epitope spreading in the pre-clinical phase predicts progression to rheumatoid arthritis. PLoS One 7: e35296.
8. van de Stadt LA, de Koning MH, van de Stadt RJ, Wolbink G, Dijkmans BA, et al. (2011) Development of the anti-citrullinated protein antibody repertoire prior to the onset of rheumatoid arthritis. Arthritis Rheum 63: 3226–3233.
9. Suwannalai P, van de Stadt LA, Radner H, Steiner G, El-Gabalawy HS, et al. (2012) Avidity maturation of anti-citrullinated protein antibodies in rheumatoid arthritis. Arthritis Rheum 64: 1323–1328.
10. Randen I, Brown D, Thompson KM, Hughes-Jones N, Pascual V, et al. (1992) Clonally related IgM rheumatoid factors undergo affinity maturation in the rheumatoid synovial tissue. J Immunol 148: 3296–3301.
11. Pascal V, Viktor K, Randen I, Thompson K, Steinitz M, et al. (1994) Nucleotide sequence analysis of rheumatoid factors and polyreactive antibodies derived from patients with rheumatoid arthritis reveals diverse use of VH and VL gene segments and extensive variability in CDR-3. Scand J Immunol 40: 125.
12. van der Woude D, Syversen SW, van der Voort EI, Verpoort KN, Goll GL, et al. (2010) The ACPA isotype profile reflects long-term radiographic progression in rheumatoid arthritis. Ann Rheum Dis 69: 1110–1116.
13. Rahman A, Latchman DS, Isenberg DA (1998) Immunoglobulin variable region sequences of human monoclonal anti-DNA antibodies. Semin Arthritis Rheum 28: 141–154.
14. Dorner T, Lipsky PE (2001) Immunoglobulin variable-region gene usage in systemic autoimmune diseases. Arthritis Rheum 44: 2715–2727.
15. Pugh-Bernard AE, Silverman GJ, Cappione AJ, Villano ME, Ryan DH, et al. (2001) Regulation of inherently autoreactive VH4-34 B cells in the maintenance of human B cell tolerance. J Clin Invest 108: 1061–1070.
16. Potter KN, Li YC, Capra JD (1994) The cross-reactive idiotopes recognized by the monoclonal antibodies 9G4 and LC1 are located in framework region 1 of two non-overlapping subsets of human VH4 family encoded antibodies. Scand J Immunol 40: 43–49.
17. Eda S, Yamanaka M, Beppu M (2004) Carbohydrate-mediated phagocytic recognition of early apoptotic cells undergoing transient capping of CD43 glycoprotein. J Biol Chem 279: 5967–5974.
18. Cappione AJ, Pugh-Bernard AE, Anolik JH, Sanz I (2004) Lupus IgG VH4.34 antibodies bind to a 220-kDa glycoform of CD45/B220 on the surface of human B lymphocytes. J Immunol 172: 4298–4307.
19. Mockridge CI, Rahman A, Buchan S, Hamblin T, Isenberg DA, et al. (2004) Common patterns of B cell perturbation and expanded V4-34 immunoglobulin gene usage in autoimmunity and infection. Autoimmunity 37: 9–15.
20. Kraj P, Friedman DF, Stevenson F, Silberstein LE (1995) Evidence for the overexpression of the VH4-34 (VH4.21) Ig gene segment in the normal adult human peripheral blood B cell repertoire. J Immunol 154: 6406–6420.
21. Chapman C, Spellerberg M, Hamblin T, Stevenson F (1995) Pattern of usage of the VH4-21 gene by B lymphocytes in a patient with EBV infection indicates ongoing mutation and class switching. Ann N Y Acad Sci 764: 195–197.
22. Milner EC, Anolik J, Cappione A, Sanz I (2005) Human innate B cells: a link between host defense and autoimmunity? Springer Semin Immunopathol 26: 433–452.
23. Kobie JJ, Alcena DC, Zheng B, Bryk P, Mattiacio JL, et al. (2012) 9G4 autoreactivity is increased in HIV-infected patients and correlates with HIV broadly neutralizing serum activity. PLoS One 7: e35356.
24. Roudier J, Silverman GJ, Chen, Carson DA, Kipps TJ (1990) Intraclonal diversity in the VH genes expressed by CD5- chronic lymphocytic leukemia-producing pathologic IgM rheumatoid factor. J Immunol 144: 1526–1530.
25. Isenberg D, Spellerberg M, Williams W, Griffiths M, Stevenson F (1993) Identification of the 9G4 idiotope in systemic lupus erythematosus. Br J Rheumatol 32: 876–882.
26. Locke IC, Leaker B, Cambridge G (1999) A comparison of the characteristics of circulating anti-myeloperoxidase autoantibodies in vasculitis with those in non-vasculitic conditions. Clin Exp Immunol 115: 369–376.
27. Pascual V, Victor K, Spellerberg M, Hamblin TJ, Stevenson FK, et al. (1992) VH restriction among human cold agglutinins. The VH4-21 gene segment is required to encode anti-I and anti-i specificities. J Immunol 149: 2337–2344.
28. Moura RA, de la Torre I, Leandro MJ, Edwards JCW, Fonseca JE, et al. (2012) 9g4 Expression on Autoantibodies to Citrullinated Peptides in Patients with Early Inflammatory Arthritis and Established Rheumatoid Arthritis. Annals of the Rheumatic Diseases 71.
29. Moura RA, Canhao H, Polido-Pereira J, Rodrigues AM, Navalho M, et al. (2013) BAFF and TACI gene expression are increased in patients with untreated very early rheumatoid arthritis. J Rheumatol 40: 1293–1302.
30. Cambridge G, Leandro MJ, Edwards JC, Ehrenstein MR, Salden M, et al. (2003) Serologic changes following B lymphocyte depletion therapy for rheumatoid arthritis. Arthritis Rheum 48: 2146–2154.
31. Weiblen BJ, Schumacher RT, Hoff R (1990) Detection of IgM and IgA HIV antibodies after removal of IgG with recombinant protein G. J Immunol Methods 126: 199–204.
32. Villeneuve E, Nam J, Emery P (2010) 2010 ACR-EULAR classification criteria for rheumatoid arthritis. Rev Bras Reumatol 50: 481–483.
33. Young KA, Deane KD, Derber LA, Hughes-Austin JM, Wagner CA, et al. (2013) Relatives without rheumatoid arthritis show reactivity to anti-citrullinated protein/peptide antibodies that are associated with arthritis-related traits: studies of the etiology of rheumatoid arthritis. Arthritis Rheum 65: 1995–2004.
34. van Vollenhoven RF, Bieber MM, Powell MJ, Gupta PK, Bhat NM, et al. (1999) VH4-34 encoded antibodies in systemic lupus erythematosus: a specific diagnostic marker that correlates with clinical disease characteristics. J Rheumatol 26: 1727–1733.
35. Cappione A 3rd, Anolik JH, Pugh-Bernard A, Barnard J, Dutcher P, et al. (2005) Germinal center exclusion of autoreactive B cells is defective in human systemic lupus erythematosus. J Clin Invest 115: 3205–3216.
36. Bohnhorst JO, Bjorgan MB, Thoen JE, Natvig JB, Thompson KM (2001) Bm1-Bm5 classification of peripheral blood B cells reveals circulating germinal center founder cells in healthy individuals and disturbance in the B cell subpopulations in patients with primary Sjogren's syndrome. J Immunol 167: 3610–3618.
37. Moura RA, de la Torre I, Leandro MJ, Cambridge G (2013) Effect of Rituximab on B Cell Subpopulations Expressing the 9g4 Idiotype in Patients with Rheumatoid Arthritis. Annals of the Rheumatic Diseases 72: A34–A35.
38. Chapman CJ, Mockridge CI, Hamblin TJ, Stevenson FK (1996) Tracking of the V4-34 (VH4-21) gene in human tonsil reveals clonal isotype switch events and a highly variable degree of somatic hypermutation. Clin Exp Immunol 105: 360–368.
39. Lundberg K, Kinloch A, Fisher BA, Wegner N, Wait R, et al. (2008) Antibodies to citrullinated alpha-enolase peptide 1 are specific for rheumatoid arthritis and cross-react with bacterial enolase. Arthritis Rheum 58: 3009–3019.
40. Weller S, Braun MC, Tan BK, Rosenwald A, Cordier C, et al. (2004) Human blood IgM "memory" B cells are circulating splenic marginal zone B cells harboring a prediversified immunoglobulin repertoire. Blood 104: 3647–3654.
41. Cambridge G, Perry HC, Nogueira L, Serre G, Parsons HM, et al. (2013) The effect of B-cell depletion therapy on serological evidence of B-cell and plasmablast activation in patients with rheumatoid arthritis over multiple cycles of rituximab treatment. J Autoimmun.
42. Samuels J, Ng YS, Coupillaud C, Paget D, Meffre E (2005) Impaired early B cell tolerance in patients with rheumatoid arthritis. J Exp Med 201: 1659–1667.
43. Edwards JC, Cambridge G (2006) B-cell targeting in rheumatoid arthritis and other autoimmune diseases. Nat Rev Immunol 6: 394–403.

11

Detection of Subclinical Synovial Inflammation by Microwave Radiometry

Evangelia Zampeli[1], Ioannis Raftakis[2], Archontoula Michelongona[3], Chara Nikolaou[3], Antonia Elezoglou[2], Konstantinos Toutouzas[3], Elias Siores[4], Petros P. Sfikakis[1]*

1 First Department of Propedeutic and Internal Medicine, Athens University Medical School, Athens, Greece, **2** Rheumatology Department, Asklepion General Hospital, Athens, Greece, **3** First Department of Cardiology, Athens University Medical School, Athens, Greece, **4** Institute for Materials Research and Innovation, University of Bolton, Bolton, United Kingdom

Abstract

Objective: Microwave Radiometry is a non-invasive method which determines within seconds the *in vivo* temperature of internal tissues at a depth of 3–7 cm with an accuracy of ±0.2°C. In this proof-of-concept study, we tested the hypothesis that, in absence of relevant clinical signs, increased local temperature detected by microwave radiometry reflects subclinical synovial inflammation, using ultrasound as reference method.

Methods: Knees of healthy controls, subjects with recent knee trauma and symptom-free patients with rheumatoid arthritis (RA) or osteoarthritis were examined by placing the microwave radiometry sensor, a) at the upper one third of the anterior surface of the thigh (control-point), and b) over the suprapatellar recess. Ultrasound was performed immediately after and the possible presence of fluid and/or synovitis was correlated with microwave radiometry findings.

Results: In 30 healthy and 10 injured knees the temperature was always lower than thigh (32.3±1.1 and 31.8±1.4 *versus* 34.1±0.9 and 33.6±1.2°C with a difference (ΔT) of −1.8±0.2 and −1.9±0.4°C respectively). Of 40 RA and 20 osteoarthritis knees examined, ultrasound findings indicative of subclinical inflammation (fluid effusion and/or Doppler signal) were found in 24 and 12, respectively, in which the temperature was higher than healthy knees and ΔT was lower (−0.9±0.7 in RA and −1.0±0.5 in osteoarthritis *versus* −1.8±0.2°C, $p<0.001$). The 5 RA knees with power Doppler findings indicative of grade 2 inflammation had a ΔT 3 times lower compared to healthy (−0.6±0.6, $p=0.007$), whereas the 9 RA and the 7 osteoarthritis knees with additionally fluid effusion, had even lower ΔT (−0.4±0.7, $p<0.001$).

Conclusion: Using a safe, rapid and easy-to-perform method, such as microwave radiometry, thermal changes within the knee joint may reflect non-clinically apparent joint inflammation. Refinement of this method, including production of sensors for small joints, could result to the development of the ideal objective tool to detect subclinical synovitis in clinical practice.

Editor: Stamatis-Nick Liossis, University of Patras Medical School, Greece

Funding: The authors have no support or funding to report.

Competing Interests: The authors have declared that no competing interests exist.

* E-mail: psfikakis@med.uoa.gr

Introduction

Rheumatoid arthritis, the most common systemic autoimmune disease, is characterised by the chronic inflammation in multiple joints which leads to cartilage damage and bone erosion. Joint inflammation is associated with peri-articular vasodilatation and synovial proliferation, which is accompanied by intra-articular angiogenesis [1]. Synovitis is not only the central characteristic of the pathophysiology of rheumatoid arthritis (RA), but also a key feature of osteoarthritis (OA) which affects hundreds of millions of people worldwide [2]. Since the activated synovium may produce proteases and cytokines that accelerate structural damage, the early and accurate detection of synovial inflammation, often localized and sometimes asymptomatic, is important [2].

Synovitis has traditionally been assessed by means of clinical and laboratory parameters suggestive of local inflammation. Modern imaging techniques, such as musculoskeletal ultrasound and magnetic resonance imaging (MRI), are playing an increasingly important role in the evaluation and monitoring of arthritis activity [3,4]. Use of ultrasound with power Doppler, a routinely available bedside imaging method, has become more sensitive and reproducible than clinical evaluation in assessing increased synovial vascularization in patients with arthritis, particularly in the early stages when X-rays are normal [1,4]. MRI, especially contrast-enhanced, has also proven to be more sensitive and reliable than clinical examination in the detection of synovial inflammatory activity and has the ability to quantify changes in synovial volumes and erosions [4]. At present, MRI involves substantial time and cost, exposure to contrast agents, and is not widely available for routine clinical use in many countries. Importantly, both ultrasound and MRI can detect subclinical synovial inflammation's presence which may explain the structural progression reported in RA patients who satisfy conventional criteria of disease remission [5].

Microwave radiometry (MR) detects non-invasively and accurately the relative changes of temperature in human tissues in depth [6,7]. MR measures natural electromagnetic radiation from internal tissues at microwave frequencies, based on the principle that the intensity of the radiation is proportional to the temperature of the tissue. Thermographic detection of human cancers by MR has been tried in early studies, albeit without considerable clinical implications [6]. Most recently, the safety and the effectiveness of MR to detect subclinical local inflammatory activation has been demonstrated in carotid atherosclerotic plaques [8,9]. No method is currently being employed for the *in vivo* measurement of joint temperature as an indicator of synovitis.

In initial studies we confirmed that the obtained *in vivo* temperature measurements by MR from joints with clinically overt inflammation was highly increased in patients with knee, ankle and carpal monoarthritis, when compared to the non-inflamed symmetrical joint. Therefore, the present proof-of-concept study was conducted to test the hypothesis that, in the absence of relevant clinical signs, MR may detect increased local temperature reflecting subclinical synovial inflammation which is, in parallel, diagnosed by joint ultrasound.

Patients and Methods

Ethics Statement

The study was approved by the Ethical/Scientific Committee of Laikon University Hospital and all subjects- patients and healthy controls- provided written informed consent according to the Declaration of Helsinki.

Protocol

Consecutive non-febrile patients with either RA (n = 20, aged 57.2±10.5 years) or OA (n = 10, aged 61.9±6.5 years) who fulfilled the respective American College of Rheumatology classification criteria were examined. In addition to their willingness to participate in the study, the only inclusion criterion was the absence of pain and any clinical sign of knee joint inflammation in physical examination performed by a rheumatologist. Healthy subjects without a history of knee trauma (n = 15, aged 32.1±6.9 years) served as controls. To further elaborate the hypothesis that increased local temperature detected by MR reflects subclinical synovial inflammation we also examined control subjects who had non-inflammatory unilateral knee pathology, either meniscal tear or cruciate ligament injury confirmed by MRI, in the past 3 months (n = 10, aged 45.6±6.5) All underwent evaluation by MR, followed immediately by knee ultrasound by an experienced operator who was blinded to MR measurements.

Microwave Radiometry Measurements

The MR measurements were performed with the RTM 01 RES microwave computer based system (Bolton, UK) that detects temperature from internal tissues at microwave frequencies. The basic principles of MR have been previously described [7]. Briefly, the essential basis for developing a microwave imaging technique is the significant contrast in the dielectric properties, at microwave frequencies, of different tissues. The depth of penetration depends on the wavelength, the dielectric properties and the water content of the tissue. The system of MR possesses an antenna with two sensors: a microwave and an infrared. The microwave sensor is 3.9 cm in diameter and detects microwave radiation at 2–5 GHz spectrum, which corresponds up to 7 cm in depth, with accuracy for temperature measurements of ±0.2°C. The sensor blocks all microwave signals from the environment. The 'volume under investigation' is a rectangular area of 3 cm in width, 2 cm in length, and 3–7 cm in depth depending on the dielectric properties of the underlying tissues. The second sensor is used for infrared measurements from the skin, for calibrating the microwave sensor readings [8,9].

All subjects were examined in a room with steady temperature (21–23°C) and before the temperature reading procedure they rested for 10 minutes to equilibrate to the ambient temperature. During measurements, with the individual in supine position, the microwave antenna of the device was placed in contact with the naked skin at 90° angle. The antenna was held at this position for 10 sec, required for the receiver to integrate the microwave emission and the conversion of the measured signal to temperature by a microprocessor. Measurements were taken at the upper one third of the anterior surface of the thigh, which was used as control point, and on the upper pole of the patella, by placing the antenna at the site over the suprapatellar recess (**Figure 1**). All measurements were performed 3 times at each of the 2 sites for every leg, in order to assess the reproducibility of the method (overall 12 measurements for each subject by each of 2 operators). The temperature of each site used for further analysis was the mean of the 3 temperatures. As the temperature of the knee was different than the temperature of the thigh, temperature differences (ΔT) were provided rather than absolute temperature values. ΔT for each leg was defined as the knee joint temperature (suprapatellar recess) minus the thigh temperature (control point). The mean value of the two ΔTs calculated by the two different operators was used for the analysis.

Ultrasound Imaging

Knee joint ultrasound was performed after the completion of MR measurements, to ensure that the water-based gel used for ultrasound will not influence the temperature distribution and the readings. All ultrasound assessments were performed using a 8–13 MHz linear transducer (Logiq P3, GE) by an experienced sonographer who was blinded to the subject's history and temperature readings. The scans were based on a protocol derived from EULAR guidelines [10] while the OMERACT guidelines for synovial effusion [11] were also met. Synovial effusion in grayscale was defined as an abnormal anechoic or hypoechoic area in the joint that is displaceable and compressible and lacks Doppler signal; as per the OMERACT guidelines [11].

The size of effusions was measured in the longitudinal suprapatellar position, with the knee in 30° of flexion. The maximum diameter of the effusion in the longitudinal view was used to quantify it and increased fluid in the suprapatellar recess was defined as >2.4 mm [10]. Synovial blood flow was evaluated by power Doppler ultrasound in the knee joint. Active synovitis was defined as the presence of intra-articular synovitis with power Doppler signal, which was graded on a semiquantitative scale from 0 to 3 (0 = absence, no intra-articular flow; 1 = mild, single-vessel signal or isolated signals; 2 = moderate, confluent vessels; 3 = marked, vessel signals in more than half of the intra-articular area) during the ultrasound examination [12].

Statistical Analysis

Statistical analysis was performed using Mann-Whitney U and significance was defined as $p<0.05$. Results are presented as the mean ± standard deviation.

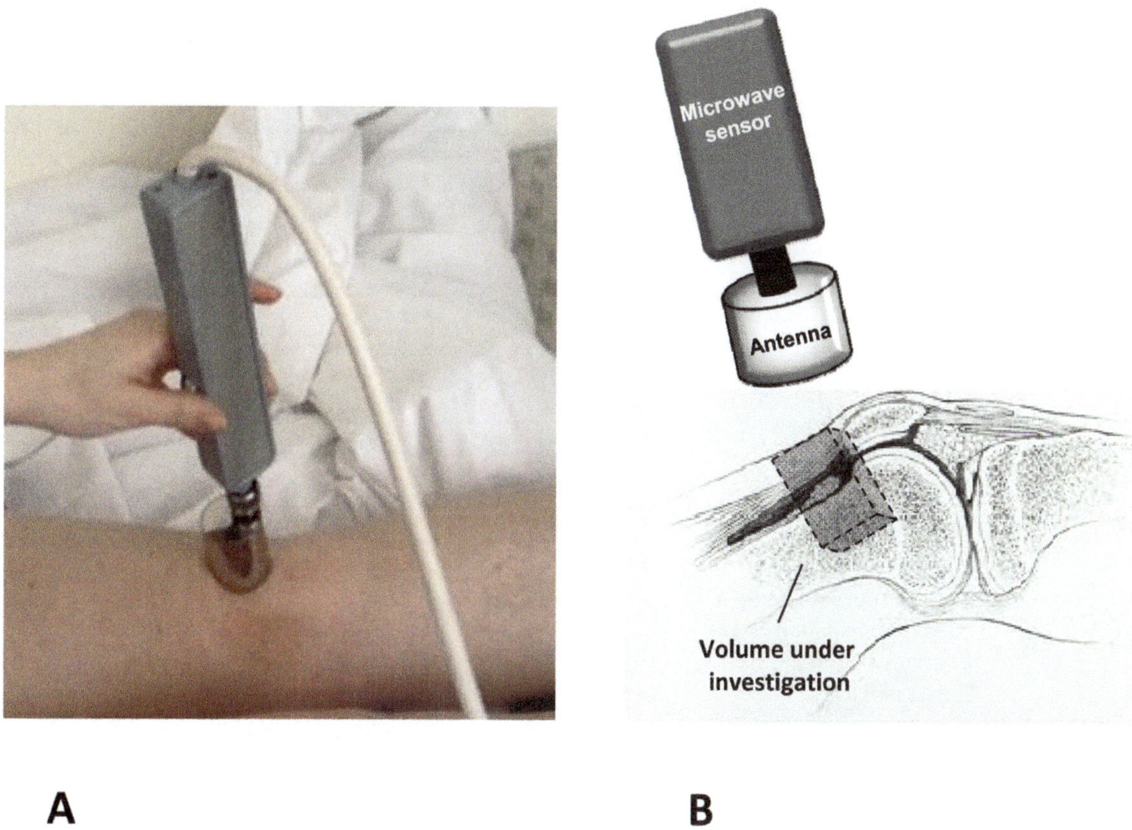

Figure 1. The microwave radiometry system. (A) The antenna for microwave radiometry device placed at 90° angle over the knee joint. (B) Schematic presentation of the system of microwave radiometry. The antenna of the microwave sensor is in contact to the skin above the volume under investigation, i.e. the knee joint.R.

Results

In the 15 healthy control subjects examined the obtained knee temperature by MR was always lower than thigh (32.3±1.1 *versus* 34.1±0.9°C, $p<0.001$ respectively), with a ΔT of −1.8±0.2°C. As expected, there were no abnormal findings in ultrasound examination. In the 10 control subjects with recent history of knee trauma, the obtained temperature from the injured knees was lower than the ipsilateral thigh (31.8±1.4 *versus* 33.6±1.2°C, $p<0.001$), with a ΔT of −1.9±0.2°C ($p=0.368$ *versus* healthy) and similar to the contralateral non-injured knee (32.3±0.7, $p=0.273$). Mild fluid effusion (2.6±0.3 mm) was detected in 6 knees, while power Doppler signal was not detected by ultrasound in any of the injured knees.

Forty RA and 20 OA asymptomatic knees were then examined. As shown in **Figure 2**, based on the ultrasonographic findings indicative of subclinical inflammation in at least one knee, the patients were further divided into subgroups. MR temperature readings of the thigh (control point) were similar to healthy subjects and comparable in all subgroups irrespectively of knee ultrasound findings. Namely, in the RA (N = 24) and OA (N = 12) knees with ultrasound findings indicative of subclinical inflammation the thigh temperature was 34.2±0.8°C ($p=0.969$) and 34.1±0.9°C ($p=0.897$) *versus* control thighs respectively. In addition, in the 16 RA and 8 OA knees without ultrasound findings indicative of subclinical inflammation the thigh temperature was 33.7±0.9°C ($p=0.418$) and 34.1±0.8°C ($p=0.904$) *versus* healthy thighs respectively. Asymptomatic RA and OA patients had comparable Erythrocyte Sedimentation Rate at 1h, whether or not knee ultrasound examination was positive for fluid and/or synovitis (*data not shown*).

In RA knees with ultrasound findings indicative of subclinical inflammation (fluid effusion and/or Doppler signal, N = 24) the temperature was higher than normal knees (33.1±1.0 *versus* 32.3±1.1°C, $p=0.058$) and the ΔT significantly lower (−0.9±0.7 *versus* −1.8±0.2°C, $p<0.001$), (**Figure 3A**). Similarly, OA knees with ultrasound findings indicative of inflammation (fluid effusion and/or Doppler signal, N = 12) had a significantly lower ΔT (−1.0±0.5 *versus* −1.8±0.2°C, $p<0.001$), (**Figure 3B**).

Intra-articular synovitis with power Doppler findings indicative of grade 2 inflammation was evident in 5 of 40 RA knees, 9 had additionally fluid effusion, while 10 had only fluid effusion. In these 5 knees the ΔT was 3 times lower compared to healthy (−0.6±0.6 *versus* −1.8±0.2°C, $p=0.007$), in the 9 knees the ΔT was even lower (−0.4±0.7, $p<0.001$), while in the 10 RA knees the ΔT was not significantly different than healthy knees (−1.6±0.7°C). Comparable results were found in 7 OA knees with power Doppler and fluid (ΔT = −0.6±0.8, $p<0.001$ *versus* healthy knees) and in 5 OA knees with only fluid (ΔT = −1.3±1.7) (**Table S1**). The mean size of the maximum diameter of effusion measured in the longitudinal view with the knee in 30° flexion was 2.8±0.3 mm in the RA group and 3.0±0.4 mm in the OA group. Intraobserver and interobserver differences of MR measurements were minimal (0.06±0.08°C and 0.08±0.11°C, respectively).

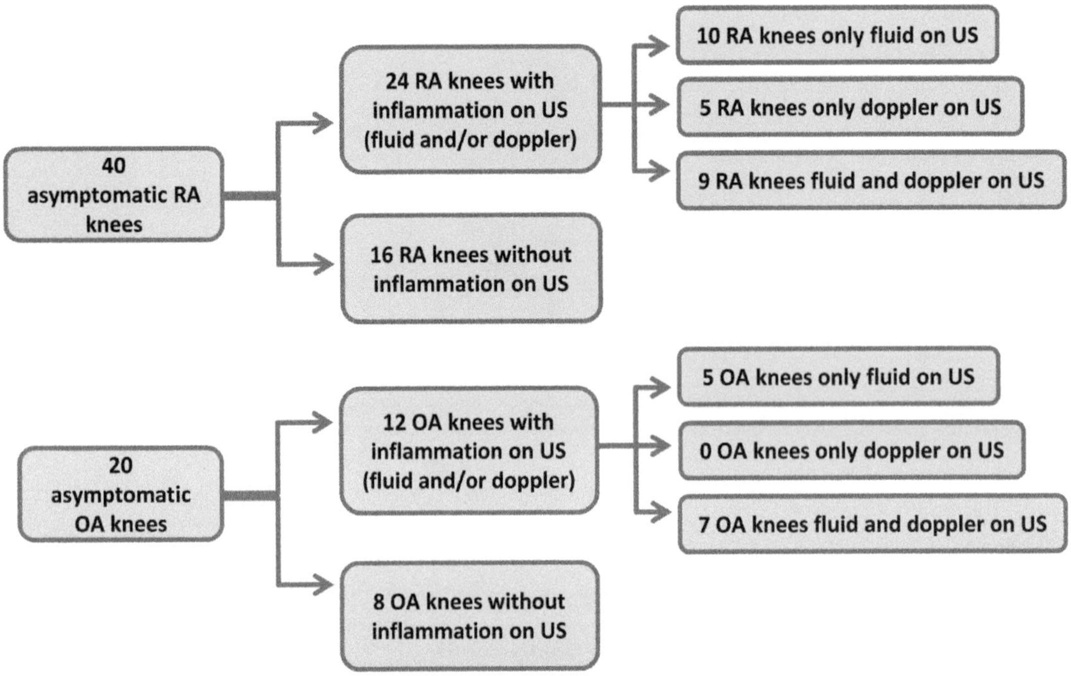

Figure 2. Subgroups of patients. Flow chart showing rheumatoid arthritis (RA) and osteoarthritis (OA) patients who were examined by microwave radiometry and the resulting subgroups based on findings indicative of subclinical inflammation in at least one knee, by ultrasound (US).

Discussion

In this proof-of-concept study the knee joint was elected for technical reasons related to the shape and the size of the currently available MR device. In patients with arthritis of inflammatory origin (RA or OA), compared to healthy controls and post-traumatic control knees, we found that: a) thermal changes within an asymptomatic knee joint can be indeed detected by MR, a safe, rapid and easy-to-perform, objective method b) higher temperatures detected by MR in RA or OA knees correlated with findings indicative of joint inflammation by ultrasound, used as reference method. Although, a limitation of the currently available MR technique is that it cannot clearly differentiate inflammatory arthritis of different aetiology and does not directly quantify functional or structural damage, this method appears to be an indirect indicator of joint inflammation, reflecting increased local (neo)vasculature content and low level inflammation which is not translated in clinical signs.

Swelling and temperature changes estimated during assessment of the number of joints with active arthritis are essential to determine inflammatory status in clinical practice. Imaging techniques (ultrasound, contrast-enhanced MRI) are increasingly used to improve the assessment of arthritis activity. On the other hand, radioisotopic and thermographic methods have been explored to quantify active arthritis with variable results. In addition to the fact that radioisotope use is a major limitation, correlations between thermographic indices and clinical assessment results have been conflicting [13]. Infrared thermography studies have shown that joints have normal thermal patterns based on the principle that a negative temperature gradient exists from the centre of a normal joint to the skin. The heat generated by increased vascularity in synovial inflammation distorts this gradient, and the normal thermal pattern is lost [14]. More recently, the ability of three-dimensional and thermal surface imaging to produce measures of joint volume, shape, and temperature to aid in the assessment of disease activity in arthritis has been reported, albeit with limitations related to joint deformities, when present, and with questionable inter- and intra-user variability [15]. MR can detect natural electromagnetic radiation from internal tissues at microwave frequencies, and the intensity of radiation is proportional to the temperature of the tissue. The main difference between the previously used infrared thermography and MR is that the former is a method of superficial screening, has only a very limited depth of penetration-approximately 2 mm- and thus allows to read and display skin temperature, whereas the latter detects signals at a much greater depth, up to 7 cm, reflecting the internal tissue temperature [6–9]. The possible impact of other adjacent tissues on the measurements of temperature in the current study seems limited, as the knees of patients without actual inflammation in ultrasound had comparable ΔT to healthy knees. It is known that although a positive power Doppler signal is indicative of active inflammation, negative signal does not necessarily mean absence of active synovitis [16]. Yet, as most recently shown, smoldering inflammation reflected by positive synovial vascularity (power Doppler) under low disease activity is linked to joint damage in RA [17]. Therefore, monitoring of synovial vascularity, as reflected by increased MR measurements, has the potential to provide useful joint information to tailor treatment strategies.

To conclude, the findings presented herein reinforce the utility of additional to physical examination methods for the accurate evaluation of disease status in patients with arthritis. MR may be potentially used to identify patients who might benefit from closer monitoring, early intervention, or more aggressive therapy. The combined prognostic value of MR with an imaging technique needs to be studied. Since thermal changes cannot be sensed by skin palpation in every joint, whereas they may precede inflammatory changes that can be detected by imaging methods, it is a challenge to refine MR methods and produce sensors for smaller joints that could detect increased temperature in precise

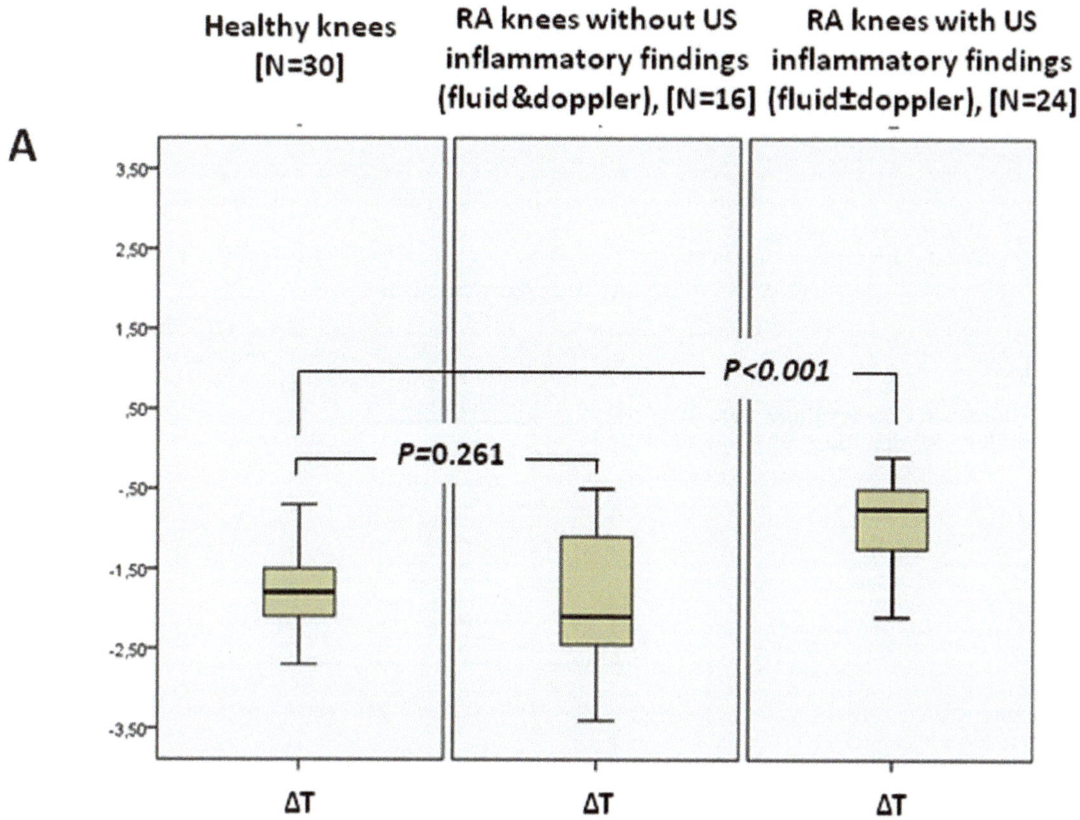
A
Healthy knees
[N=30]
RA knees without US
inflammatory findings
(fluid&doppler), [N=16]
RA knees with US
inflammatory findings
(fluid±doppler), [N=24]
3,50
2,50
1,50
,50
-,50
-1,50
-2,50
-3,50
P<0.001
P=0.261
ΔT
ΔT
ΔT

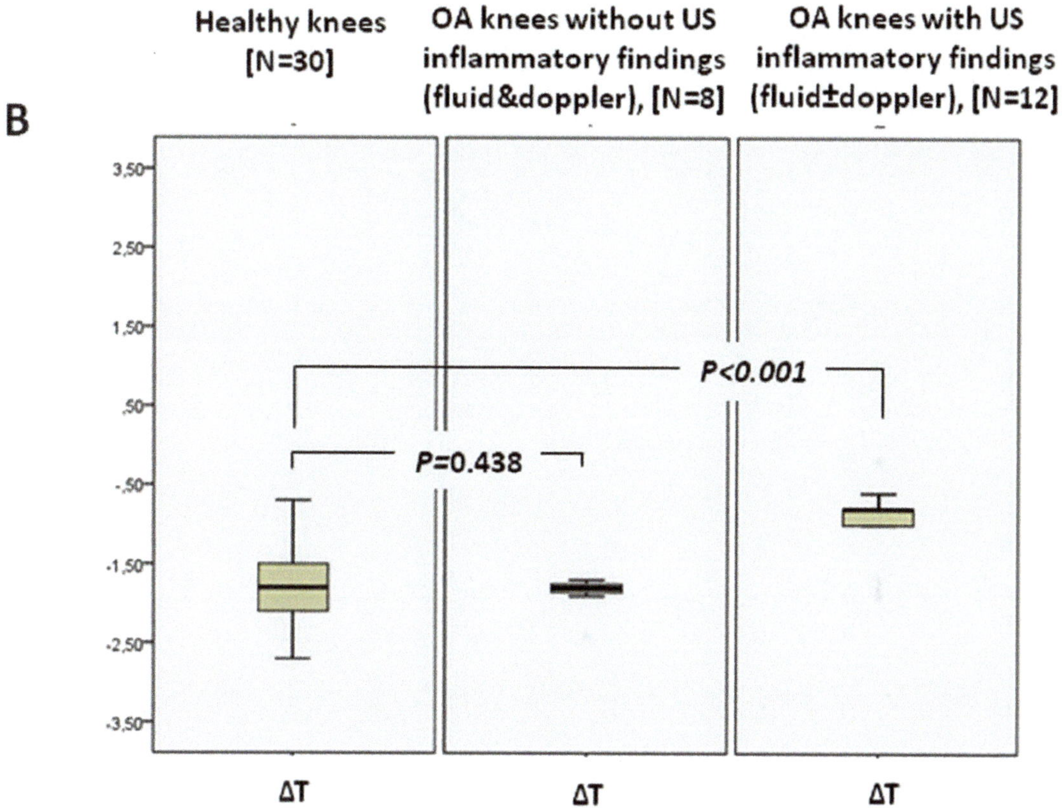
B
Healthy knees
[N=30]
OA knees without US
inflammatory findings
(fluid&doppler), [N=8]
OA knees with US
inflammatory findings
(fluid±doppler), [N=12]
3,50
2,50
1,50
,50
-,50
-1,50
-2,50
-3,50
P<0.001
P=0.438
ΔT
ΔT
ΔT

Figure 3. Temperature differences (ΔT) recorded by microwave radiometry device. Temperature differences (ΔT) between knee joint and thigh (control point) of healthy subjects and (A) patients with rheumatoid arthritis (RA) or (B) patients with osteoarthritis (OA) stratified by the presence of excess fluid and/or Doppler signal evidenced by knee joint ultrasound (US). Patients' knee joints with inflammatory US findings had smaller ΔT compared to healthy knees and patients' knees with normal US findings.

and/or targeted depths (i.e. specifically at synovium). This method may also provide additional information on the natural history of chronic arthritis. Prospective studies to reveal whether MR can serve as an objective tool to detect early and/or subclinical synovitis in the clinical setting, as well as its possible prognostic value are warranted.

Supporting Information

Table S1 Microwave radiometry recordings for all patients, stratified according to the knee ultrasound findings. Mean value ± standard deviation of absolute temperatures (T) and difference in temperature (ΔT) are given.

Author Contributions

Conceived and designed the experiments: KT PPS. Performed the experiments: EZ IR AM CN. Analyzed the data: EZ IR AE ES KT PPS. Contributed reagents/materials/analysis tools: AE ES. Wrote the paper: EZ ES KT PPS.

References

1. Naredo E, Collado P, Cruz A, Palop MJ, Cabero F, et al. (2007) Longitudinal power Doppler ultrasonographic assessment of joint inflammatory activity in early rheumatoid arthritis: predictive value in disease activity and radiologic progression. Arthritis Rheum 1: 116–24.
2. Sellam J, Berenbaum F (2010) The role of synovitis in pathophysiology and clinical symptoms of osteoarthritis. Nat Rev Rheumatol 6: 625–35.
3. Tamborrini G, Ciurea A, Bianchi S (2011) Musculoskeletal Ultrasound in Osteoarthritis and Rheumatoid Arthritis. US Musculoskeletal Review 1: 32–4.
4. Spalding SJ, Kwoh CK, Boudreau R, Enama J, Lunich J, et al. (2008) Three-dimensional and thermal surface imaging produces reliable measures of joint shape and temperature: a potential tool for quantifying arthritis. Arthritis Res Ther 1: R10.
5. Brown AK, Conaghan PG, Karim Z, Quinn MA, Ikeda K, et al. (2008) An explanation for the apparent dissociation between clinical remission and continued structural deterioration in rheumatoid arthritis. Arthritis Rheum 10: 2958–67.
6. Shaeffer J, El-Mahdi AM, Carr KL (1982) Thermographic detection of human cancers by microwave radiometry. Prog Clin Biol Res 107: 509–21.
7. Barrett AH, Myers PC (1975) Microwave thermography: a method of detecting subsurface thermal patterns. Bibl Radiol 6: 45–56.
8. Toutouzas K, Grassos H, Synetos A, Drakopoulou M, Tsiamis E, et al. (2011) A new non-invasive method for detection of local inflammation in atherosclerotic plaques: experimental application of microwave radiometry. Atherosclerosis 1: 82–9.
9. Toutouzas K, Grassos H, Drakopoulou M, Synetos A, Tsiamis E, et al. (2012) First in vivo application of microwave radiometry in human carotids: A new non-invasive method for detection of local inflammatory activation. J Am Coll Cardiol 59: 1645–53.
10. Backhaus M, Burmester G-R, Gerber T, Grassi W, Machold KP, et al. (2001) Guidelines for musculoskeletal ultrasound in rheumatology. Ann Rheum Dis 60: 641–9.
11. Wakefield RJ, Balint PV, Szkudlarek M, Filippucci E, Backhaus M, et al. (2005) Musculoskeletal ultrasound including definitions for ultrasonographic pathology. J Rheumatol 32: 2485–7.
12. Walther M, Harms H, Krenn V, Radke S, Faehndrich TP, et al. (2001) Correlation of power Doppler sonography with vascularity of the synovial tissue of the knee joint in patients with osteoarthritis and rheumatoid arthritis. Arthritis Rheum 44: 331–8.
13. de Silva M, Kyle V, Hazleman B, Salisbury R, Page-Thomas P, et al. (1986) Assessment of inflammation in the rheumatoid knee joint: correlation between clinical, radioisotopic, and thermographic methods. Ann Rheum Dis 45: 277–80.
14. Salisbury RS, Parr G, de Silva M, Hazleman BL, Page-Thomas DP (1983) Heat distribution over normal and abnormal joints: thermal pattern and quantification. Ann Rheum Dis 42: 494–9.
15. Spalding SJ, Kwoh CK, Boudreau R, Enama J, Lunich J, et al. (2008) Three-dimensional and thermal surface imaging produces reliable measures of joint shape and temperature: a potential tool for quantifying arthritis. Arthritis Res Ther 1: R10.
16. Koski JM, Saarakkala S, Helle M, Hakulinen U, Heikkinen JO, et al. (2006). Power Doppler ultrasonography and synovitis: correlating ultrasound imaging with histopathological findings and evaluating the performance of ultrasound equipments. Ann Rheum Dis 12: 1590–5.
17. Fukae J, Isobe M, Kitano A, Henmi M, Sakamoto F, et al. (2013) Positive synovial vascularity in patients with low disease activity indicates smouldering inflammation leading to joint damage in rheumatoid arthritis: time-integrated joint inflammation estimated by synovial vascularity in each finger joint. Rheumatology (Oxford) 3: 523–8.

12

The Coexistence of Antiphospholipid Syndrome and Systemic Lupus Erythematosus in Colombians

Juan-Sebastian Franco[1,2]*, Nicolás Molano-González[1], Monica Rodríguez-Jiménez[1], Yeny Acosta-Ampudia[1], Rubén D. Mantilla[1,2], Jenny Amaya-Amaya[1,2], Adriana Rojas-Villarraga[1,2], Juan-Manuel Anaya[1,2]*

1 Center for Autoimmune Diseases Research (CREA), School of Medicine and Health Sciences, Universidad del Rosario, Bogotá, Colombia, **2** Mederi, Hospital Universitario Mayor, Bogotá, Colombia

Abstract

Objectives: To examine the prevalence and associated factors related to the coexistence of antiphospholipid syndrome (APS) and systemic lupus erythematosus (SLE) in a cohort of Colombian patients with SLE, and to discuss the coexistence of APS with other autoimmune diseases (ADs).

Method: A total of 376 patients with SLE were assessed for the presence of the following: 1) confirmed APS; 2) positivity for antiphospholipid (aPL) antibodies without a prior thromboembolic nor obstetric event; and 3) SLE patients without APS nor positivity for aPL antibodies. Comparisons between groups 1 and 3 were evaluated by bivariate and multivariate analysis.

Results: Although the prevalence of aPL antibodies was 54%, APS was present in just 9.3% of SLE patients. In our series, besides cardiovascular disease (AOR 3.38, 95% CI 1.11–10.96, $p=0.035$), pulmonary involvement (AOR 5.06, 95% CI 1.56–16.74, $p=0.007$) and positivity for rheumatoid factor (AOR 4.68, 95%IC 1.63–14.98, $p=0.006$) were factors significantly associated with APS-SLE. APS also may coexist with rheumatoid arthritis, Sjögren's syndrome, autoimmune thyroid diseases, systemic sclerosis, systemic vasculitis, dermatopolymyositis, primary biliary cirrhosis and autoimmune hepatitis.

Conclusions: APS is a systemic AD that may coexist with other ADs, the most common being SLE. Awareness of this polyautoimmunity should be addressed promptly to establish strategies for controlling modifiable risk factors in those patients.

Editor: Jose Crispin, Beth Israel Deaconess Medical Center, United States of America

Funding: This work was supported by the School of Medicine and Health Sciences, Universidad del Rosario, Bogota, Colombia. The funders had no role in study design, data collection and analysis, decision to publish, or preparation of the manuscript.

Competing Interests: The authors have indicated that they have no conflicts of interest regarding the content of this article.

* Email: francoa.juan@gmail.com (JSF); juan.anaya@urosario.edu.co (JMA)

Introduction

Autoimmune diseases (ADs) are chronic conditions initiated by the loss of immunological tolerance to self-antigens, and they represent a heterogeneous group of disorders that affect specific target organs or multiple systems. Because of the chronic condition of these diseases, they constitute a significant burden on the health care system, with direct and indirect economic costs and quality of life impairment [1–4].

The fact that ADs share several subphenotypes, physiopathological mechanisms, environmental factors, and genetic factors has been called the "autoimmune tautology" and indicates that ADs share common physiopathological mechanisms and a common origin [1–9].

The clinical evidence of the autoimmune tautology highlights the coexistence of distinct ADs within an individual, which corresponds to polyautoimmunity, defined as the presence of more than one AD in a single patient [1,10]. When three or more ADs coexist, this condition is called multiple autoimmune syndrome (MAS) [11]. Factors significantly associated with polyautoimmunity include female gender and familial autoimmunity (i.e., the presence of diverse ADs in multiple members of a nuclear family) [10,12]. Polyautoimmunity represents the effect of a single genotype on diverse phenotypes [1].

Several subphenotypes are shared by ADs, including cutaneous involvement (i.e., photosensibility, alopecia, Raynaud's phenomenon), arthralgia and arthritis, fatigue, and even cardiovascular disease (CVD) [1,2]. Polyautoimmunity has been reported in most ADs, including systemic lupus erythematosus (SLE) [10,13], in which one of the most frequent coexistent disease is antiphospholipid syndrome (APS) [13]. Therefore, the purposes of this study were to examine the prevalence and associated factors of the coexistence of SLE and APS in a cohort of Colombian patients with SLE, as well as to discuss on the coexistence of APS with other ADs.

Patients and Methods

Study population

A cross-sectional analytical study was conducted in 376 Colombian patients with SLE. The subjects have been systematically followed at the Center for Autoimmune Diseases Research (CREA) in Bogota, Colombia. All of the subjects fulfilled the 1997 update of the American College of Rheumatology (ACR) classification criteria for SLE [14].

The patient socio-demographic and cumulative clinical and laboratory data, as well as a household description, were obtained by interview, standardized report form, physical examination and chart review as previously reported [15]. The data were collected in an electronic and secure database. The socio-demographic variables included age at SLE onset, disease duration, educational and socioeconomic status, current occupation, smoking habits, coffee consumption, expositional factors and physical activity. The age at onset (AOD) of the disease was defined as the first subjective experience of the symptom(s) and/or sign(s) described in any of the items of the classification criteria [16]. The duration of disease was considered as the difference between the AOD and the date of the first participation in the study. The educational level was recorded as the number of years of education and was divided into two groups (equal to or more than 9 years and less than 9 years of education) based on the "General Law of Education" in Colombia [17,18]. The socioeconomic status was categorized on the basis of national legislation and was divided into low (1 and 2), intermediate (3) and high (4–6) status [19]. The smoking habits were assessed as never smoking; 1–6, 6–15, and >15 packages/year; or cessation of cigarette consumption. Coffee intake was asked as yes or not and measured in cups per day (i.e., 1–2, 2–4, >4).

Ethics statement

This study was performed in compliance with Act 008430/1993 of the Ministry of Health of the Republic of Colombia, which classified it as minimal-risk research. All of the patients voluntarily accepted to participate in the study by reading and signing the informed consent. The institutional review board of the Universidad del Rosario approved the study design.

Clinical variables

Clinical and laboratory variables were registered as present or absent at any time during the course of the disease as previously reported [15,20]. In particular, lupus nephritis was defined as active urinary sediment, or proteinuria >500 mg/24 h or positive renal biopsy (ISN/RNP). Pulmonary compromise was considered in the presence of pulmonary hypertension, or pulmonary embolism or diffuse alveolar hemorrhage. Pleuritis was defined as the presence of pleural rub and/or effusion and/or typical pleuritic pain, and confirmed by chest X-ray or computed tomography. Neurologic involvement included the presence of seizures without any other definable cause, or psychosis lacking any other definable cause, or other conditions such as peripheral neuropathy, stroke, transverse myelitis, chorea, or other central nervous system lesions directly attributable to SLE in the absence of other causes. Autoimmune hemolytic anemia (hematocrit <35%, reticulocyte count >4%, and positive Coombs test), leukopenia (white cells <4000/mm3) and thrombocytopenia (platelets <100000/mm3) were also assessed. Other manifestations such as polyautoimmunity [1,10], MAS [11], familial autoimmunity, and familial autoimmune disease [12] were also included.

CVD represents a broad spectrum of manifestations (i.e., subphenotypes) such as hypertension (HTN), myocardial infarction (MI), peripheral vascular disease (PVD), and cerebrovascular accidents (i.e., stroke). Since atherosclerosis (AT), the usual cause of CVD, starts when the endothelium becomes damaged, and is considered to be an autoimmune-inflammatory disease, CVD was assessed by characterizing the following five subphenotypes: HTN, defined as having blood pressure ≥140/90 mm Hg recorded as an average of two measurements, with at least a 15-minute interval between the measurements or the use of any antihypertensive medication [21]; a history of stroke; a coronary event [i.e., unstable angina, MI]; a thrombotic event (other than MI and carotid involvement, requiring anticoagulant treatment); and carotid disease (by the Doppler criteria or intima-media thickness ≥0.9). The traditional risk factors assessed and included were smoking [22], type 2 diabetes mellitus [23] and dyslipidemia [24].

Concerning pharmacological treatment, the current or past use of steroid therapy (i.e., prednisolone, methylprednisolone, deflazacort), antimalarials (i.e., cloroquine, hydroxychloroquine), immunosupressors (i.e., azathioprine, mycophenolate mofetil and cyclophosphamide) and biological therapy (i.e., rituximab) were also recorded.

APS polyautoimmunity assessment

All of the patients were systematically assessed and classified for the presence of the following: 1) confirmed APS according to the 2006 update of the classification criteria [i.e., a thromboembolic event and positivity for anti-cardiolipin (aCL) IgG/IgM in medium or high titer, anti-beta 2-glycoprotein 1 (B2GPI) IgG/IgM antibodies or lupus anticoagulant (LAC), on two or more occasions] [25]; 2) positivity for antiphospholipid (aPL) antibodies (i.e., aCL IgG/IgM, B2GPI IgG/IgM or LAC) without a prior thromboembolic nor obstetric event; and 3) SLE patients without APS nor positivity for aPL antibodies.

Laboratory measurements

The relevant laboratory variables associated with SLE were registered. Patients underwent measurement of the following antibodies by ELISA using commercial kits (QUANTA Lite, INOVA Diagnostics, San Diego, CA, USA): anti-double strand DNA antibodies (anti-dsDNA), precipitating antibodies to extractable nuclear antigens (ENAs: Sm, U1-RNP, Ro/SS-A, La/SS-B), aCL IgG and IgM, B2GPI IgG and IgM antibodies and rheumatoid factor (RF) IgM. The positive cut-off values were >300 UI for anti-dsDNA; >40 UI aCL (IgG and IgM), and B2GPI (IgG and IgM); >20 UI ENAs; and >6 UI for RF. Additionally, the antinuclear antibodies (ANAs) were measured by indirect immunofluorescence on HEp-2 cell (NOVA Lite™ Hep-2 ANA kit, INOVA Diagnostics, San Diego, CA, USA), according to the manufacturer's instructions. Other autoantibodies, including lupus anticoagulant, anti-Scl 70, -centromere, -mitochondrial, and -smooth muscle antibodies, were recorded. White blood cell and platelet count, hemoglobin levels, mean corpuscular volume, complement (i.e., C3 and C4 levels), venereal disease research laboratory results, and creatinine levels were extracted from each patient's clinical record.

Statistical analysis

First, univariate descriptive statistics were performed. The categorical variables were described by the frequencies. The quantitative continuous variables were described as the mean and standard deviation, as well as the median and interquartile range. The comparisons between group 1 (i.e., confirmed APS) and 3 (i.e., SLE patients with neither APS nor positive aPL autoantibodies) in

Table 1. Demographic and clinical characteristics of 376 patients with SLE.

Characteristic	*Median, range*
Age(y)	36, 25–46
Age at SLE onset (y)	27, 19–38
Duration of disease (y)	5, 2–11
Sociodemographic characteristics	***%(n/N)***
Female	91.8 (345/376)
LEL	13.8 (51/369)
Low SES	24.2 (86/355)
Ever smoking	36.3 (134/369)
Coffee intake	61.8 (225/364)
Clinical variables	***%(n/N)***
Female	91.8 (345/376)
Arthritis	74.7 (281/376)
Malar rash	44.4 (167/376)
Photosensitivity	57.2 (215/376)
Oral ucers	30.6 (115/376)
Alopecia	49.7 (187/376)
Serositis	30 (113/376)
Renal involvement	44.9 (168/376)
Neurological involvement	40.9 (154/376)
Pulmonary involvement	10.4 (39/376)
Haematological involvement	79.1 (295/376)
CVD	38.5(145/376)
Pregnancy loss	20.5 (70/342)
Poliautoimmunity	31.1 (112/376)
AITD	11.97 (45/376)
SS	9.04 (34/376)
RA	6.12 (23/376)
MAS	7.98 (30/376)
Familial autoimmunity	19.68 (74/376)
APS assessment	***%(n/N)***
Group 1 (APS)	9.3 (35/376)
Group 2 (aPL antibodies)	30.8 (116/376)
Group 3 (SLE without APS nor aPL)	59.8 (225/376)
Medication	***%(n/N)***
Steroid therapy	87.3 (281/322)
Antimalarials	86 (277/322)
Immunosupressors[a]	51.1 (164/321)
Laboratory findings	***%(n/N)***
ANA (+)	100 (376/376)
Anti dsDNA (+)	66.1 (236/357)
Anti Sm (+)	39.9 (144/361)
Anti Ro (+)	49.45 (180/364)
Anti La (+)	25.6 (93/363)
Anti RNP (+)	44.5 (161/362)
LAC (+)	51.45 (71/158)
aCL IgG (+)	33.3 (120/360)
aCL IgM (+)	39.8 (140/352)
B2GPI IgG (+)	11.3 (33/293)
B2GPI IgM (+)	13.5 (39/288)
RF IgM (+)	42.1 (120/285)

Table 1. Cont.

Characteristic	*Median, range*
Hypocomplementemia[b]	66.4 (209/315)

APS: antiphospholipid syndrome; aCL: anticardiolipin antibodies; AITD: autoimmune thyroid disease; ANA: antinuclear antibodies; B2GPI: anti-β2 glycoprotein I antibodies; CVD: cardiovascular disease; LAC: lupus anticoagulant; LEL: low educational level; MAS: multiple autoimmune syndrome; RA: rheumatoid arthritis; RF: rheumatoid factor; SS: Sjögren's síndrome; SES: socioeconomic status; y: years.
[a]Immunosupressors based on treatment with mycophenolate mophetil and/or cyclophosphamide and/or azathioprine.
[b]Hypocomplementemia defined as the presence of low C3 or C4.

relation to the other categorical variables, were assessed by chi square tests or Fisher's exact tests when facing small sample sizes. The comparisons between the two groups in relation to the continuous variables were performed with the Kruskal-Wallis test. A logistic regression model with APS and SLE polyautoimmunity as the dependent variable was fit (group 1 vs. group 3). As the independent factors, the model included the variables that were statistically significant in the bivariate analyses and those variables that were biologically plausible. The model was adjusted by gender and duration of the disease. The adequacies of the logistic models were assessed using the Hosmer–Lemeshow goodness-of-fit test. The Nagelkerke R2 (i.e., the pseudo-R2) was used to estimate the percentage of variance explained by the models. The adjusted odds ratios (AOR) were calculated with 95% confidence intervals (CI). The Wald statistical test was used to evaluate the significance of the individual logistic regression coefficients for each independent variable. The statistical analyses were performed in R 3.0.2 [26].

Results

Of the 376 patients with SLE, 91.8% were women. Thirty-five patients fulfilled the classification criteria for APS, with a prevalence of 9.3%, representing the second most common polyautoimmunity, preceded by autoimmune thyroid disease, which disclosed a prevalence of 12%. The range of time elapsed from the SLE onset to the diagnosis of APS was 1 to 7 years. All of the patients had SLE prior to the diagnosis of APS. Out of the 35 patients with APS-SLE, 51.4% had a prior thromboembolic event, 40% pregnancy loss and 8.5% had both. Among the non-criteria manifestations, 9 (26%) patients had pulmonary involvement, of whom 6 had pulmonary hypertension and 3 pulmonary embolism, 6 (17%) patients had thrombocytopenia, and 5 (14%) livedo reticularis. Regarding CVD, this was present in 22 (63%) patients, of whom 18 had thrombosis and 10 hypertension (29%). There were 2 additional patients with prior thromboembolic and/or obstetric manifestations and positivity for aPL below medium or high titers that were excluded from further analysis, but in whom a "seronegative" APS could not be rule out. The most frequently found aPL antibody was LAC, with a prevalence rate of 51.5%, followed by aCL IgM with 40% and IgG with 33%. B2GPI IgG and IgM were positive in 11% and 13% of the patients, respectively. Of the SLE patients, 60% had neither APS nor positivity for aPL antibodies. The characteristics of the cohort are illustrated in Table 1. Socioeconomic status, smoking and coffee intake had no significant influence of the coexistence of SLE-APS. Although SLE disease activity index (SLEDAI) was calculated upon study entry, this variable was not included in the analysis.

Factors associated with APS polyautoimmunity

There was no difference in the patient age, AOD or duration of SLE. CVD, Sjögren's syndrome (SS), pulmonary involvement and positivity for RF were risk factors significantly associated with APS. The presence of alopecia was negatively associated with APS (Table 2).

The adjusted effects of the risk factors for APS polyautoimmunity

As expected, CVD was associated with APS-SLE. The main subphenotypes associated with CVD in APS-SLE were thrombosis and hypertension. Additional variables influencing this condition were pulmonary involvement and positivity for RF, regardless of gender and duration of the disease. Alopecia was confirmed to be negatively associated with APS (Table 3). A second logistic regression model was fit to evaluate the effect of aPL alone (i.e.,

Table 2. Factors associated with APS in SLE (bivariate analysis).

Variable	*SLE + APS* %(n/N)	*SLE* %(n/N)	*OR (95% CI)*	*p*
Gender	91.4 (32/35)	92.9 (211/227)	0.81 (0.22–2.9)	0.746
CVD	62.2 (23/37)	36.1 (82/227)	2.74 (1.42–6.1)	0.002
Abortion	46.8 (15/32)	13.9 (29/308)	4.97 (2.45–11.83)	<0.001
SS	25.7 (9/35)	7.5 (17/227)	3.88 (1.77–10.47)	<0.001
Alopecia	28.6 (10/35)	55.5 (126/227)	0.30 (0.15–0.70)	0.003
Pulmonary involvement	25.7 (9/35)	9.7 (22/227)	2.97 (1.38–7.73)	0.006
RF IgM (+)	57.1 (16/28)	34.5 (59/171)	2.29 (1.12–5.55)	0.02

APS: antiphospholipid syndrome; OR: odds ratio; 95% CI: 95% confidence interval; CVD: cardiovascular disease; RF: rheumatoid factor; SLE: systemic lupus erythematosus; SS: Sjögren's syndrome.

Table 3. Adjusted factors associated with APS in SLE polyautoimmunity (multivariate analysis).

Characteristics	*β*	*AOR*	*95% CI*	*p**
CVD	1.218	3.38	1.11–10.96	0.035
Alopecia	−1.556	0.21	0.06–0.64	0.009
Pulmonary involvement	1.62	5.06	1.56–16.74	0.007
RF IgM (+)	1.543	4.68	1.63–14.98	0.006

AOR: adjusted odds ratio; 95% CI: 95% confidence interval; CVD: cardiovascular disease; RF: rheumatoid factor.
*Variables statistically significant are shown.

group 2) on the expression of SLE without APS nor positivity for aPL antibodies (i.e., group 3). An association between aPL and RF was observed, but not with clinical features.

Discussion

In our series, the coexistence of APS with SLE was 9.3% and was associated with a distinctive subphenotype characterized by a higher risk of CVD, pulmonary involvement and positivity for RF.

The interplay between SLE and APS has been analyzed over the years, since APS was initially not considered to be a systemic AD and was thought to occur only in patients with SLE [27–29]. Furthermore, APS has been found to be associated with systemic manifestations (e.g., non-thrombotic renal disease, migraine, livedo reticularis, pulmonary hypertension, MI) and laboratory features (e.g., positive ANAs, hypocomplementemia) also present in patients with SLE, complicating the clear differentiation between these entities [27–29]. However, rather than being the spectrum of the same disease, the coexistence of APS and SLE is a reflection of complex disease traits and highlights the common mechanisms shared by ADs [1,4].

The association between CVD and SLE mortality was first established by Urowitz et al. [30], with the description of the bimodal pattern of mortality in SLE patients, with an early death due to active disease and infections, and a late death secondary to CVD. Despite a reduction in SLE mortality over the years, CVD remains prevalent among these patients, affecting up to 28% of patients after four decades of disease duration [31,32]. Traditional risk factors have been described for CVD in SLE (e.g., HTN, dyslipidemia) [33]. However, Esdaile et al. [34] demonstrated that these factors do not fully account for the accelerated AT in these patients, suggesting that there are factors related with the disease involved in the development of CVD. Among the novel risk factors described, polyautoimmunity with APS has been associated with CVD. In fact, APS has been reported as a non-traditional risk factor for CVD in SLE [15]. Other studies have reported similar results, as well as an increased accrual of damage measured by the SLE Damage Index [35–38]. Different mechanisms involving the role of aPL in the process of AT have been described, and these include overexpression of tissue factor, annexin I and II, cytokines and other mediators of endothelial dysfunction [39–41]; oxidative perturbations and mitochondrial dysfunction [42]; and cross-reactivity with oxidized low-density lipoproteins, accelerating their influx into macrophage and AT development [43]. Recently, Perez-Sanchez et al. [44] found a close relationship between patients with APS and those with polyautoimmunity of SLE and APS in the groups of genes belonging to the cluster of AT, highlighting the role of novel risk factors in the development of CVD among these patients.

The pulmonary involvement described in SLE and APS may be similar, and include pulmonary hypertension, pulmonary embolism and diffuse alveolar hemorrhage [45–47]. In our results, the association with pulmonary involvement was driven by the presence of pulmonary hypertension. aPL has been associated with the development of pulmonary hypertension in patients with SLE [48–51]. The positivity for RF seem to have a dual role in autoimmunity with a protective effect by interfering with the binding complement system to immune complexes, or a harmful effect by enhancing immune mediated tissue damage [52]. In SLE, positivity for RF has been found to have a protective role in the development of lupus nephritis [53–55]. In our results, we found that the positivity for FR IgM was associated with the coexistence of APS and SLE, as well as with the positivity for aPL antibodies. Similarly, Spadaro et al. [52] previously reported the relationship between different isotypes of RF in patients with APS and SLE polyautoimmunity. Positivity for RF IgG was negatively associated with serosal and hematological involvement, and negatively correlated with aCL IgG titer, suggesting that RF IgG is related with the absence of APS; on the other hand, RF IgM was associated with aCL IgM positivity, implying a possible relation with APS [52]. The interplay of RF isotypes in ADs and polyautoimmunity requires further investigation.

As already mentioned, APS was primarily recognized in patients with SLE and was, therefore, considered to be an overlap syndrome (i.e., "secondary" APS). The major difference between polyautoimmunity and overlap syndrome is that the former is the presence of two or more well-defined autoimmune conditions (i.e., overt clinical manifestations mediated by T or B cell responses) fulfilling the validated classification criteria whereas the latter is the partial presence of signs and symptoms of diverse ADs [1]. An overlap syndrome may evolve towards a well-defined phenotype or remain as an undifferentiated AD for years (i.e., the presence of some subphenotypes) [1]. The international consensus statement on an update of the classification criteria for definite APS advised against using the term "secondary" APS because no difference was found in the clinical consequences of aPL antibodies among the patients in this category (Evidence Level I) [25]. The consensus is that, rather than distinguishing patients by "primary" and "secondary" APS, documenting the coexistence of SLE (or other ADs) is more advantageous for classification [25]. In agreement with this argument, we have proposed the term "polyautoimmunity" instead of secondary AD to refer to the coexistence of two or more ADs [10].

Besides SLE, APS has been described in most ADs, including rheumatoid arthritis, SS, autoimmune thyroid diseases, systemic sclerosis (SSc), systemic vasculitis, dermatopolymyositis, primary biliary cirrhosis (PBC) and autoimmune hepatitis (AIH) [35–37,56–89]. Moreover, the coexistence of APS with other ADs may be associated with a modified clinical course, especially in SSc (i.e., associated with pulmonary arterial hypertension and MI), PBC (i.e., higher Mayo risk score) and AIH (i.e., associated with

Table 4. Polyautoimmunity in APS.

AD	*APS*	*aCL % (n/N)*		*LAC*	*B2GPI*	*Commentary*	*Ref.*
	% (n/N)	*IgG*	*IgM*	*% (n/N)*	*% (n/N)*		
SLE	6.5 (44/679)	-	-	-	-	The patients with SLE/APS polyautoimmunity were more likely to die from cardiovascular disease (i.e., myocardial infarction, acute coronary syndrome). These patients had a higher SDI score and poorer survival, which did not reach statistical significance.	[35]
	19.2 (5/26)	25 (5/20)		27.8 (5/18)	-	The SLE patients with intracranial hemorrhage had polyautoimmunity, including APS, more frequently than did the controls. Thrombocytopenia was found to be an independent risk factor for intracranial hemorrhage.	[56]
	19 (19/100)	53 (53/100)		2 (2/100)	84 (84/100)	IgG aCL and B2GPI correlated with a previous history of arthritis.	[57]
	8.4 (8/95)	13.4 (13/95)	2.1 (2/85)	-	-	The occurrence of aCL positivity was significantly associated with venous/arterial thrombosis and abortion. Thrombocytopenia was more frequent among the aCL positive patients; however, it did not reach statistical significance.	[58]
	12.4 (16/129)	15.5 (20/129)	13.9 (18/129)	-	10.1 (13/129)	In a mestizo cohort of SLE patients, aCL positivity was significantly associated with venous/arterial thrombosis and fetal loss.	[59]
	9.2 (12/130)	18.5 (24/130)		-	-	The occurrence of aCL positivity was present before the diagnosis of SLE and prior to the development of the clinical features of APS. The aCL positivity was associated with a higher number of the ACR criteria and early AOD of SLE as well as cutaneous, serosal, neuropsychiatric and renal involvement.	[60]
	12 (20/166)*	-	-	-	-	Polyautoimmunity with APS increased the risk of pregnancy loss, especially after week 20 of gestation.	[61]
	28.4 (50/176)	-	-	-	-	APS and damage (measured by SDI) were significantly associated with higher mortality in SLE patients.	[36]
	14.1 (28/198)	36.9 (73/198)	17.7 (35/198)	21.7 (43/198)	-	The independent predictor factors for diminished survival with SLE duration of 15 years were AOD, renal involvement and APS polyautoimmunity.	[37]
RA	3.6 (3/84)	8.3 (7/84)	2.4 (2/84)	-	7.1 (6/84)	The prevalence of aPL antibodies in RA was reported. No correlation was found with the clinical features.	[62]
	-	12.4 (12/97)	11.3 (11/97)	1 (1/97)	12.4 (12/97)	There was a negative association between aPL antibodies and anti-CCP antibodies.	[63]
	-	20.2 (35/173)	15.6 (27/173)	-	-	The presence of aCL antibodies was associated with rheumatoid nodules. The patients with aCL antibodies had more cutaneous manifestations (e.g., livedo reticularis, purpura, cutaneous ulcers); however, this association was not significant.	[64]
	-	8.9 (15/168)	4.2 (7/168)	5.9 (10/168)	-	The RA patients with positivity for aPL antibodies and high levels of homocysteine might be at a higher risk for thrombotic events.	[65]

Table 4. Cont.

AD	APS	aCL % (n/N)		LAC	B2GPI	Commentary	Ref.
	% (n/N)	IgG	IgM	% (n/N)	% (n/N)		
	-	6.8 (7/102)	0.9 (1/102)	-	-	A significant correlation was found between the aCL and anti-CCP antibody levels.	[66]
	-	11.9 (22/184)	4.3 (8/184)	3.8 (7/184)	-	The RA patients with positivity for aCL and a history of arterial/venous thrombosis were found to have lower levels of free protein S.	[67]
SS	4.1 (3/74)	32.4 (24/74)	6.8 (5/74)	10.8 (8/74)	4.1 (3/74)	The aPL-antibody positive patients were associated with polyautoimmunity. They had peripheral neuropathy and the presence of hypergammaglobulinemia.	[68]
	3 (3/100)	1 (1/100)	3 (3/100)	9 (9/100)	5 (5/100)	LAC was associated with a significantly higher risk for deep venous thrombosis, stroke and/or myocardial infarction. No significant association was found with the clinical features.	[69]
	3.1 (4/130)	10.8 (14/130)	6.2 (8/130)	9.2 (12/130)	-	The presence of aPL antibodies was associated with a higher prevalence of ANAs positivity.	[70]
	1.0 (4/402)	4.7 (19/402)	1.5 (6/402)	4.7 (19/402)	-	APS is an infrequent, but not exceptional, polyautoimmunity in SS.	[71]
	-	12.7 (8/63)	6.3 (4/63)	-	-	The presence of aCL antibodies was associated with RNP positivity. No relationship was found with the clinical features or extra glandular manifestations.	[72]
AITD	-	35.5 (11/31)	35.5 (11/31)	-	-	There was an increased incidence of aCL in patients with AITD. None of the patients had clinical features of APS.	[73]
	-	43.8 (57/130)	10 (13/130)	-	-	The prevalence of aPL is increased in AITD. There was no correlation between aPL titer and the titer of thyroid autoantibodies.	[74]
	-	10.1 (7/69)	5.8 (4/69)	-	-	The patients with aCL did not exhibit a higher titer of thyroid autoantibodies.	[75]
	-	10.5 (2/19)	10.5 (2/19)	-	-	The patients with Hashimoto's thyroiditis had an increased incidence of aCL. There was no correlation with thyroid autoantibodies titer.	[76]
SSc	2.7 (3/108)	11.1 (12/108)	2.7 (3/108)	-	6.5 (7/108)	The SSc patients with aCL positivity were associated with pulmonary hypertension. The patients with PAH had higher titers of aCL; however, this association was not significant.	[77]
	-	19.1 (13/68)	20.6 (14/68)	-	-	Anticentromere antibodies, anti-ScL-70 and smoking were significantly associated with severe ischemia and amputation in SSc, whereas no relationship was found with aCL.	[78]
	-	12.2 (10/82)	3.7 (3/82)	-	-	No association was found between aCL and the clinical features of SSc.	[79]

Table 4. Cont.

AD	*APS*	*aCL % (n/N)*		*LAC*	*B2GPI*	*Commentary*	*Ref.*
	% (n/N)	*IgG*	*IgM*	*% (n/N)*	*% (n/N)*		
	-	20.8 (10/48)	35 (17/48)	23.8 (5/21)	-	The presence of IgM aCL was significantly associated with higher cutaneous involvement (e.g., the number of lesions, plaques and body areas affected) and ANA and RF positivity in the patients with localized SSc compared to the controls.	[80]
	-	17.5 (20/40)	5 (2/40)	5 (2/40)	50 (20/40)	The aPL-antibody patients had a tendency to Raynaud's phenomenon, cutaneous ulcerations and pulmonary hypertension; however, this correlation was not significant.	[81]
	-	8.6 (9/105)	11.4 (12/105)	-	-	The SSc patients with aCL were significantly associated with ischemia or myocardial necrosis (i.e., on the electrocardiogram and/or scintigraphic findings). There was a higher prevalence of digital pitting scars, acroosteolysis and pulmonary involvement; however, it did not reach statistical significance.	[82]
	1.4 (1/72)	9.7 (7/72)		-	-	No correlation was found between aPL antibodies and the clinical features of SSc.	[83]
Systemic vasculitis	6.3 (12/144)	8 (12/144)		5.6 (8/144)	-	The presence of aPL antibodies might influence the clinical course for systemic vascularity.	[84]
DM/PM	3.1 (3/97)	-	-	-	-	The prevalence of polyautoimmunity with APS was reported in a cohort of DM/PM.	[85]
	-	2.7 (1/36)	5.6 (2/36)	-	-	The prevalence of aCL in ADs was reported	[86]
PBC	1.4 (1/31)	-	-	-	-	The prevalence of MAS in the patients with AIH/PBC polyautoimmunity was evaluated. AITD was found to be the most prevalent AD. There was no correlation with the therapy response.	[87]
	-	27.3 (27/99)	27.3 (27/99)	-	2 (2/99)	IgG aCL were significantly associated with the presence of cirrhosis, a higher Mayo risk score and thrombocytopenia.	[88]
AIH	-	38.9 (23/59)	23.7 (14/59)	-	3.4 (2/59)	IgG aCL were significantly associated with the presence of cirrhosis and disease activity (in the clinical features and the laboratory).	[89]

AD: autoimmune disease; aCL: anticardiolipin antibodies; AIH: autoimmune hepatitis; AITD: autoimmune thyroid disease; anti-CCP: anti-cyclic citrullinated peptides antibodies; AOD: age at onset of disease; APS: antiphospholipid syndrome; B2GPI: anti-beta 2 glycoprotein I antibodies; DM/PM: dermatopolymyositis; LAC: lupus anticoagulant; MAS: multiple autoimmune syndrome; PBC: primary biliary cirrhosis; SDI: systemic lupus erythematosus damage index; SLE: systemic lupus erythematosus; SS: Sjögren's syndrome; SSc: scleroderma; RA: rheumatoid arthritis; RF: rheumatoid factor.

*Correspond to 166 pregnancies in 125 women followed in the Hopkins Lupus Cohort.

cirrhosis and disease activity) (Table 4). Therefore, APS should be addressed in patients with the aforementioned ADs.

Although our study sample size was not negligible, as a cross-sectional study, it would have been more valuable to have had an appropriate follow up to address the association of APS and SLE polyautoimmunity by the inclusion of other measurements such as antibodies isotypes (e.g., B2GPI IgA [90], RF IgG), serologic biomarkers and genetic markers.

Conclusions

APS is considered a systemic AD, and may coexist with other ADs, SLE being the most frequent. The coexistence of APS and SLE is associated with a more severe subphenotype characterized by a higher CVD rate and pulmonary involvement. CVD is a major cause of morbidity and mortality in SLE patients. Novel risk factors related to autoimmunity are recognized because the traditional risk factors do not completely explain the high CVD rates. APS polyautoimmunity should be addressed in every SLE patient to identify the higher risk population and encourage prevention strategies and early therapeutic intervention. APS should be included as a non-traditional risk factor for CVD in SLE and other ADs in further studies.

Acknowledgments

We thank all patients for their participation in the study, and colleagues at the Center for Autoimmune Diseases Research (CREA) for their fruitful discussions and contributions.

Author Contributions

Conceived and designed the experiments: JMA. Performed the experiments: JSF NMG YAA MRJ JMA. Analyzed the data: JSF NMG MRJ JAA JMA. Contributed reagents/materials/analysis tools: JMA JSF NMG YAA MRJ RDM ARV. Wrote the paper: JSF NMG MRJ YAA RDM JAA ARV JMA.

References

1. Anaya JM (2014) The diagnosis and clinical significance of polyautoimmunity. Autoimmun Rev 4–5: 4–7.
2. Anaya JM, Rojas-Villarraga A, Shoenfeld Y (2013) From the mosaic of autoimmunity to the autoimmune tautology. In: Anaya JM, Rojas-Villarraga A, Shoenfeld Y, Levy R, Cervera R, editors. Autoimunity From bench to bedside. Bogotá: Editorial Universidad del Rosario. pp. 237–245.
3. Anaya JM, Rojas-Villarraga A, García-Carrasco M (2012) The autoimmune tautology: from polyautoimmunity and familial autoimmunity to the autoimmune genes. Autoimmune Dis 2012.
4. Anaya JM (2010) The autoimmune tautology. Arthritis Res Ther 12: 147.
5. Shoenfeld Y, Isenberg DA (1989) The mosaic of autoimmunity. Immunol Today 10: 123–6.
6. Anaya JM, Corena R, Castiblanco J, Rojas-Villarraga A, Shoenfeld Y (2007) The kaleidoscope of autoimmunity: multiple autoimmune syndromes and familial autoimmunity. Expert Rev Clin Immunol 3: 623–35.
7. Anaya JM (2012) Common mechanisms of autoimmune diseases (the autoimmune tautology). Autoimmun Rev 11: 781–4.
8. Cifuentes RA, Restrepo-Montoya D, Anaya JM (2012) The autoimmune tautology: an in silico approach. Autoimmune Dis 2012: 792106.
9. Rojas-Villarraga A, Castellanos-delahoz J, Perez-Fernandez O, Amaya-Amaya J, Franco JS, et al. (2013) The autoimmune ecology. In: Anaya JM, Shoenfeld Y, Rojas-Villarraga A, Levy R, Cervera R, editors. Autoimunity From bench to bedside. Bogotá: Editorial Universidad del Rosario. pp. 322–41.
10. Rojas-Villarraga A, Amaya-Amaya J, Rodriguez-Rodriguez A, Mantilla RD, Anaya J-M (2012) Introducing polyautoimmunity: secondary autoimmune diseases no longer exist. Autoimmune Dis 2012: 254319.
11. Anaya J-M, Castiblanco J, Rojas-Villarraga A, Pineda-Tamayo R, Levy RA, et al. (2012) The multiple autoimmune syndromes. A clue for the autoimmune tautology. Clin Rev Allergy Immunol 43: 256–64.
12. Cárdenas-Roldán J, Rojas-Villarraga A, Anaya JM (2013) How do autoimmune diseases cluster in families? A systematic review and meta-analysis. BMC Med 11: 73.
13. Rojas-Villarraga A, Toro C-E, Espinosa G, Rodríguez-Velosa Y, Duarte-Rey C, et al. (2010) Factors influencing polyautoimmunity in systemic lupus erythematosus. Autoimmun Rev 9: 229–32.
14. Klippel J, Lahita R, Esdaile JM, Hahn BH, Urowitz MB, et al. (1999) Guidelines for referral and management of systemic lupus erythematosus in adults. American College of Rheumatology Ad Hoc Committee on Systemic Lupus Erythematosus Guidelines. Arthritis Rheum 42: 1785–96.
15. Amaya-Amaya J, Sarmiento-Monroy JC, Caro-Moreno J, Molano-González N, Mantilla RD, et al. (2013) Cardiovascular disease in latin american patients with systemic lupus erythematosus: a cross-sectional study and a systematic review. Autoimmune Dis 2013: 794383.
16. Hochberg MC (1997) Updating the American College of Rheumatology revised criteria for the classification of systemic lupus erythematosus. Arthritis Rheum 40: 1725.
17. Ministry of Education (1992) Law of Higher Education – Law 30 of 1992. Government of Colombia. Available: http://www.mineducacion.gov.co/1621/articles-86437_Archivo_pdf.pdf. Accessed 2014 Jul 10.
18. Ministry of Education (1994) Law 115 of 1994. Government of Colombia. Available: http://www.mineducacion.gov.co/1621/articles-85906_archivo_pdf.pdf. Accessed 2014 Jul 10.
19. Calixto OJ, Anaya JM (2014) Socioeconomic status. The relationship with health and autoimmune diseases. Autoimmun Rev 13: 641–54.
20. Anaya JM, Cañas C, Mantilla RD, Pineda-Tamayo R, Tobón GJ, et al. (2011) Lupus nephritis in Colombians: contrasts and comparisons with other populations. Clin Rev Allergy Immunol 40: 199–207.
21. Jones DW, Hall JE (2004) Seventh report of the Joint National Committee on Prevention, Detection, Evaluation, and Treatment of High Blood Pressure and evidence from new hypertension trials. Hypertension 43: 1–3.
22. Toloza SMA, Uribe AG, McGwin G, Alarcón GS, Fessler BJ, et al. (2004) Systemic lupus erythematosus in a multiethnic US cohort (LUMINA). XXIII. Baseline predictors of vascular events. Arthritis Rheum 50: 3947–57.
23. American Diabetes Association (2014) Diagnosis and classification of diabetes mellitus. Diabetes Care 37 (Suppl 1): S81–90.
24. Stone NJ, Bilek S, Rosenbaum S (2005) Recent National Cholesterol Education Program Adult Treatment Panel III update: adjustments and options. Am J Cardiol 96: 53E–59E.
25. Miyakis S, Lockshin MD, Atsumi T, Branch DW, Brey RL, et al. (2006) International consensus statement on an update of the classification criteria for definite antiphospholipid syndrome (APS). J Thromb Haemost 4: 295–306.
26. Team RC (2013) R: A language and environment for statistical computing.
27. Agmon-Levin N, Shoenfeld Y (2014) The spectrum between antiphospholipid syndrome and systemic lupus erythematosus. Clin Rheumatol 33: 293–5.
28. Taraborelli M, Andreoli L, Tincani A (2012) Much more than thrombosis and pregnancy loss: the antiphospholipid syndrome as a "systemic disease". Best Pract Res Clin Rheumatol 26: 79–90.
29. Agmon-Levin N, Mosca M, Petri M, Shoenfeld Y (2012) Systemic lupus erythematosus one disease or many? Autoimmun Rev 11: 593–5.
30. Urowitz MB, Bookman AA, Koehler BE, Gordon DA, Smythe HA, et al. (1976) The bimodal mortality pattern of systemic lupus erythematosus. Am J Med 60: 221–5.
31. Nikpour M, Gladman DD, Urowitz MB (2013) Premature coronary heart disease in systemic lupus erythematosus: what risk factors do we understand? Lupus 22: 1243–50.
32. Urowitz MB, Gladman DD, Tom BDM, Ibañez D, Farewell VT (2008) Changing Patterns in Mortality and Disease Outcomes for Patients with Systemic Lupus Erythematosus. J Rheumatol 35: 2152.
33. Nikpour M, Urowitz MB, Gladman DD (2009) Epidemiology of atherosclerosis in systemic lupus erythematosus. Curr Rheumatol Rep 11: 248–54.
34. Esdaile JM, Abrahamowicz M, Grodzicky T, Li Y, Panaritis C, et al. (2001) Traditional Framingham risk factors fail to fully account for accelerated atherosclerosis in systemic lupus erythematosus. Arthritis Rheum 44: 2331–7.
35. Mok CC, Chan PT, Ho LY, Yu KL, To CH (2013) Prevalence of the antiphospholipid syndrome and its effect on survival in 679 Chinese patients with systemic lupus erythematosus: a cohort study. Medicine (Baltimore) 92: 217–22.
36. Signorelli FV, Salles GF, Papi JA (2011) Antiphospholipid syndrome as predictor of mortality in Brazilian patients with systemic lupus erythematosus. Lupus 20: article 419.
37. Ruiz-Irastorza G, Egurbide M-V, Ugalde J, Aguirre C (2004) High impact of antiphospholipid syndrome on irreversible organ damage and survival of patients with systemic lupus erythematosus. Arch Intern Med 164: 77–82.
38. Soares M, Reis L, Papi JAS, Cardoso CRL (2003) Rate, pattern and factors related to damage in Brazilian systemic lupus erythematosus patients. Lupus 12: 788–94.
39. Cuadrado MJ, López-Pedrera C, Khamashta MA, Camps MT, Tinahones F, et al. (1997) Thrombosis in primary antiphospholipid syndrome: a pivotal role for monocyte tissue factor expression. Arthritis Rheum 40: 834–41.
40. Cugno M, Borghi MO, Lonati LM, Ghiadoni L, Gerosa M, et al. (2010) Patients with antiphospholipid syndrome display endothelial perturbation. J Autoimmun 34: 105–10.
41. López-Pedrera C, Cuadrado MJ, Herández V, Buendia P, Aguirre MA, et al. (2008) Proteomic analysis in monocytes of antiphospholipid syndrome patients:

deregulation of proteins related to the development of thrombosis. Arthritis Rheum 58: 2835–44.
42. Perez-Sanchez C, Ruiz-Limon P, Aguirre MA, Bertolaccini ML, Khamashta MA, et al. (2012) Mitochondrial dysfunction in antiphospholipid syndrome: implications in the pathogenesis of the disease and effects of coenzyme Q(10) treatment. Blood 119: 5859–70.
43. Hasunuma Y, Matsuura E, Makita Z, Katahira T, Nishi S, et al. (1997) Involvement of beta 2-glycoprotein I and anticardiolipin antibodies in oxidatively modified low-density lipoprotein uptake by macrophages. Clin Exp Immunol 107: 569–73.
44. Perez-Sanchez C, Barbarroja N, Messineo S, Ruiz-Limon P, Rodriguez-Ariza A, et al. (2014) Gene profiling reveals specific molecular pathways in the pathogenesis of atherosclerosis and cardiovascular disease in antiphospholipid syndrome, systemic lupus erythematosus and antiphospholipid syndrome with lupus. Ann Rheum Dis DOI: 10.1136/annrheumdis-2013-204600.
45. Paran D, Fireman E, Elkayam O (2004) Pulmonary disease in systemic lupus erythematosus and the antiphospholpid syndrome. Autoimmun Rev 3: 70–5.
46. Pego-Reigosa JM, Medeiros DA, Isenberg DA (2009) Respiratory manifestations of systemic lupus erythematosus: old and new concepts. Best Pract Res Clin Rheumatol 23: 469–80.
47. Stojanovich L (2006) Pulmonary manifestations in antiphospholipid syndrome. Autoimmun Rev 5: 344–8.
48. Cefle A, Inanc M, Sayarlioglu M, Kamali S, Gul A, et al. (2011) Pulmonary hypertension in systemic lupus erythematosus: relationship with antiphospholipid antibodies and severe disease outcome. Rheumatol Int 31: 183–9.
49. Asherson RA, Higenbottam TW, Dinh Xuan AT, Khamashta MA, Hughes GR (1990) Pulmonary hypertension in a lupus clinic: experience with twenty-four patients. J Rheumatol 17: 1292–8.
50. Alarcón-Segovia D, Pérez-Vázquez ME, Villa AR, Drenkard C, Cabiedes J (1992) Preliminary classification criteria for the antiphospholipid syndrome within systemic lupus erythematosus. Semin Arthritis Rheum 21: 275–86.
51. Alarcón-Segovia D, Delezé M, Oria CV, Sánchez-Guerrero J, Gómez-Pacheco L, et al. (1989) Antiphospholipid antibodies and the antiphospholipid syndrome in systemic lupus erythematosus. A prospective analysis of 500 consecutive patients. Medicine (Baltimore) 68: 353–65.
52. Spadaro A, Riccieri V, Terracina S, Rinaldi T, Taccari E, et al. (2000) Class specific rheumatoid factors and antiphospholipid syndrome in systemic lupus erythematosus. Lupus 9: 56–60.
53. Skare TL, Silva MBG, Holler AP, Chavez PA (2009) Protective role of rheumatoid factor in lupus nephritis. Clin Exp Rheumatol 27: 895.
54. Feldman D, Ginzler E, Kaplan D (1989) Rheumatoid factor in patients with systemic lupus erythematosus. J Rheumatol 16: 618–22.
55. Hill GS, Hinglais N, Tron F, Bach JF (1978) Systemic lupus erythematosus. Morphologic correlations with immunologic and clinical data at the time of biopsy. Am J Med 64: 61–79.
56. Gao N, Wang ZL, Li MT, Han SM, Dang YQ, et al. (2013) Clinical characteristics and risk factors of intracranial hemorrhage in systemic lupus erythematosus. Lupus 22: 453–60.
57. Gould T, Tikly M, Asherson R, Loizou S, Singh S (2006) Prevalence and clinical correlates of anti-phospholipid antibodies in South Africans with systemic lupus erythematosus. Scand J Rheumatol 35: 29–34.
58. Vianna JL, Haga HJ, Tripathi P, Cervera R, Khamashta MA, et al. (1992) Reassessing the status of antiphospholipid syndrome in systemic lupus erythematosus. Ann Rheum Dis 51: 160–1.
59. Aguirre V, Cuchacovich R, Barria L, Aris H, Trejo C, et al. (2001) Prevalence and isotype distribution of antiphospholipid antibodies in Chilean patients with systemic lupus erythematosus (SLE). Lupus 10: 75–80.
60. McClain MT, Arbuckle MR, Heinlen LD, Dennis GJ, Roebuck J, et al. (2004) The prevalence, onset, and clinical significance of antiphospholipid antibodies prior to diagnosis of systemic lupus erythematosus. Arthritis Rheum 50: 1226–32.
61. Clowse ME, Magder LS, Witter F, Petri M (2006) Early risk factors for pregnancy loss in lupus. Obstet Gynecol 107: 293–9.
62. Palomo I, Pinochet C, Alarcón M, Sandoval R, Gonzalez J, et al. (2006) Prevalence of antiphospholipid antibodies in Chilean patients with rheumatoid arthritis. J Clin Lab Anal 20: 190–4.
63. Jeleniewicz R, Majdan M, Targońska-Stępniak B, Dryglewska M (2012) Prevalence of antiphospholipid antibodies in rheumatoid arthritis patients and relationship with disease activity. Pol Arch Med Wewn 122: 480–6.
64. Wolf P, Gretler J, Aglas F, Auer-Grumbach P, Rainer F (1994) Anticardiolipin antibodies in rheumatoid arthritis: their relation to rheumatoid nodules and cutaneous vascular manifestations. Br J Dermatol 131: 48–51.
65. Seriolo B, Fasciolo D, Sulli A, Cutolo M (2001) Homocysteine and antiphospholipid antibodies in rheumatoid arthritis patients: relationships with thrombotic events. Clin Exp Rheumatol 19: 561–4.
66. Vittecoq O, Jouen-Beades F, Krzanowska K, Bichon-Tauvel I, Menard JF, et al. (2000) Prospective evaluation of the frequency and clinical significance of antineutrophil cytoplasmic and anticardiolipin antibodies in community cases of patients with rheumatoid arthritis. Rheumatology (Oxford) 39: 481–9.
67. Seriolo B, Accardo S, Garnero A, Fasciolo D, Cutolo M (1999) Anticardiolipin antibodies, free protein S levels and thrombosis: a survey in a selected population of rheumatoid arthritis patients. Rheumatology (Oxford) 38: 675–8.
68. Fauchais A, Lambert M, Launay D, Queyrel V, Nguyen N, et al. (2004) Antiphospholipid antibodies in primary Sjögren's syndrome: prevalence and clinical significance in a series of 74 patients. Lupus 13: 245–8.
69. Pasoto SG, Chakkour HP, Natalino RR, Viana VST, Bueno C, et al. (2012) Lupus anticoagulant: a marker for stroke and venous thrombosis in primary Sjögren's syndrome. Clin Rheumatol 31: 1331–8.
70. Cervera R, García-Carrasco M, Font J, Ramos M, Reverter JC, et al. (1997) Antiphospholipid antibodies in primary Sjögren's syndrome: prevalence and clinical significance in a series of 80 patients. Clin Exp Rheumatol 15: 361–5.
71. Ramos-Casals M, Nardi N, Brito-Zerón P, Aguiló S, Gil V, et al. (2006) Atypical autoantibodies in patients with primary Sjögren syndrome: clinical characteristics and follow-up of 82 cases. Semin Arthritis Rheum 35: 312–21.
72. Jedryka-Goral A, Jagiello P, D'Cruz DP, Maldykowa H, Khamashta MA, et al. (1992) Isotype profile and clinical relevance of anticardiolipin antibodies in Sjogren's syndrome. Ann Rheum Dis 51: 889–91.
73. Paggi A, Caccavo D, Ferri GM, Di Prima MA, Amoroso A, et al. (1994) Anticardiolipin antibodies in autoimmune thyroid diseases. Clin Endocrinol (Oxf) 40: 329–33.
74. Nabriski D, Ellis M, Ness-Abramof R, Shapiro M, Shenkman L (2000) Autoimmune thyroid disease and antiphospholipid antibodies. Am J Hematol 64: 73–5.
75. Díez JJ, Doforno RA, Iglesias P, Sastre J, Gómez-Pan A, et al. (1993) Anticardiolipin antibodies in autoimmune thyroid disease. J Clin Lab Immunol 40: 125–34.
76. Osundeko O, Hasinski S, Rose LI (2001) Anticardiolipin antibodies in Hashimoto's disease. Endocr Pract 7: 181–3.
77. Assous N, Allanore Y, Batteux F, Meune C, Toulon P, et al. (2005) Prevalence of antiphospholipid antibodies in systemic sclerosis and association with primitive pulmonary arterial hypertension and endothelial injury. Clin Exp Rheumatol 23: 199–204.
78. Herrick AL, Heaney M, Hollis S, Jayson MI (1994) Anticardiolipin, anticentromere and anti-Scl-70 antibodies in patients with systemic sclerosis and severe digital ischaemia. Ann Rheum Dis 53: 540–2.
79. Enzenauer RJ, Collier DH, Lopez LR (2006) Anticardiolipin antibodies in scleroderma. J Clin Rheumatol 12: 324–6.
80. Sato S, Fujimoto M, Hasegawa M, Takehara K (2003) Antiphospholipid antibody in localised scleroderma. Ann Rheum Dis 62: 771–4.
81. Touré AO, Ly F, Sall A, Diatta A, Gadji M, et al. (2013) Antiphospholipid antibodies and systemic scleroderma. Turkish J Haematol 30: 32–6.
82. Picillo U, Migliaresi S, Marcialis MR, Ferruzzi AM, Tirri G (1997) Clinical setting of patients with systemic sclerosis by serum autoantibodies. Clin Rheumatol 16: 378–83.
83. Gupta R, Thabah MM, Gupta S, Shankar S, Kumar A (2009) Clinical significance of antiphospholipid antibodies in Indian scleroderma patients. Rheumatol Int 30: 277–9.
84. Rees JD, Lança S, Marques PV, Gómez-Puerta JA, Moco R, et al. (2006) Prevalence of the antiphospholipid syndrome in primary systemic vasculitis. Ann Rheum Dis 65: 109–11.
85. Sherer Y, Livneh A, Levy Y, Shoenfeld Y, Langevitz P (2000) Dermatomyositis and polymyositis associated with the antiphospholipid syndrome-a novel overlap syndrome. Lupus 9: 42–6.
86. Merkel PA, Chang Y, Pierangeli SS, Convery K, Harris EN, et al. (1996) The prevalence and clinical associations of anticardiolipin antibodies in a large inception cohort of patients with connective tissue diseases. Am J Med 101: 576–83.
87. Efe C, Wahlin S, Ozaslan E, Berlot AH, Purnak T, et al. (2012) Autoimmune hepatitis/primary biliary cirrhosis overlap syndrome and associated extrahepatic autoimmune diseases. Eur J Gastroenterol Hepatol 24: 531–4.
88. Zachou K, Liaskos C, Rigopoulou E, Gabeta S, Papamichalis P, et al. (2006) Presence of high avidity anticardiolipin antibodies in patients with autoimmune cholestatic liver diseases. Clin Immunol 119: 203–12.
89. Liaskos C, Rigopoulou E, Zachou K, Georgiadou S, Gatselis N, et al. (2005) Prevalence and clinical significance of anticardiolipin antibodies in patients with type 1 autoimmune hepatitis. J Autoimmun 24: 251–60.
90. Murthy V, Willis R, Romay-Penabad Z, Ruiz-Limón P, Martínez-Martínez LA, et al. (2013) Value of isolated IgA anti-β2 -glycoprotein I positivity in the diagnosis of the antiphospholipid syndrome. Arthritis Rheum 65: 3186–93.

13

Simultaneous Automated Screening and Confirmatory Testing for Vasculitis-Specific ANCA

Mandy Sowa[1], Kai Grossmann[1], Ilka Knütter[1], Rico Hiemann[2], Nadja Röber[3], Ursula Anderer[2], Elena Csernok[4], Dimitrios P. Bogdanos[5], Maria Orietta Borghi[6], Pier Luigi Meroni[6], Peter Schierack[2], Dirk Reinhold[7], Karsten Conrad[3¶], Dirk Roggenbuck[1,2*¶]

1 Research and Development Department, GA Generic Assays GmbH, Dahlewitz/Berlin, Germany, **2** Faculty of Science, Brandenburg University of Technology Cottbus-Senftenberg, Senftenberg, Germany, **3** Institute of Immunology, Technical University of Dresden, Dresden, Germany, **4** Department of Rheumatology, University of Schleswig-Holstein Campus Lübeck and Rheumaklinik Bad Bramstedt, Bad Bramstedt, Germany, **5** Division of Transplantation, Immunology and Mucosal Biology, King's University College, London, United Kingdom, **6** Department of Rheumatology, University of Milan, Milan, Italy, **7** Institute of Molecular and Clinical Immunology, Otto-von-Guericke University Magdeburg, Magdeburg, Germany

Abstract

Anti-neutrophil cytoplasmic antibodies (ANCA) are the serological hallmark of small vessel vasculitis, so called ANCA-associated vasculitis. The international consensus requires testing by indirect immunofluorescence (IIF) on human ethanol-fixed neutrophils (ethN) as screening followed by confirmation with enzyme-linked immunosorbent assays (ELISAs). This study evaluates the combination of cell- and microbead-based digital IIF analysis of ANCA in one reaction environment by the novel multiplexing CytoBead technology for simultaneous screening and confirmatory ANCA testing. Sera of 592 individuals including 118 patients with ANCA-associated vasculitis, 133 with rheumatoid arthritis, 49 with infectious diseases, 77 with inflammatory bowel syndrome, 20 with autoimmune liver diseases, 70 with primary sclerosing cholangitis and 125 blood donors were tested for cytoplasmic ANCA (C-ANCA) and perinuclear ANCA (P-ANCA) by classical IIF and ANCA to proteinase 3 (PR3) and myeloperoxidase (MPO) by ELISA. These findings were compared to respective ANCA results determined by automated multiplex CytoBead technology using ethN and antigen-coated microbeads for microbead immunoassays. There was a good agreement for PR3- and MPO-ANCA and a very good one for P-ANCA and C-ANCA by classical and multiplex analysis (Cohen's kappa [κ] = 0.775, 0.720, 0.876, 0.820, respectively). The differences between classical testing and CytoBead analysis were not significant for PR3-ANCA, P-ANCA, and C-ANCA ($p<0.05$, respectively). The prevalence of confirmed positive ANCA findings by classical testing (IIF and ELISA) compared with multiplex CytoBead analysis (IIF and microbead immunoassay positive) resulted in a very good agreement ($\kappa = 0.831$) with no significant difference of both methods ($p = 0.735$). Automated endpoint-ANCA titer detection in one dilution demonstrated a very good agreement with classical analysis requiring dilution of samples ($\kappa = 0.985$). Multiplexing by CytoBead technology can be employed for simultaneous screening and quantitative confirmation of ANCA. This novel technique provides fast and cost-effective ANCA analysis by automated digital IIF for the first time.

Editor: Massimo Pietropaolo, University of Michigan Medical School, United States of America

Funding: This work was supported by the Federal Ministry of Economics and Technology Central Innovation Programme SME ZIM-KOOP (grants KF2379003AJ0, KF2379004AJ1) and the Federal Ministry of Education (Research projects InnoProfile 03IP611, InnoProfile-Transfer 03IPT611A and InnoProfile-Transfer 03IP611X). The funders had no role in study design, data collection and analysis, decision to publish, or preparation of the manuscript.

Competing Interests: Dirk Roggenbuck has a management role and is a shareholder of GA Generic Assays GmbH and Medipan GmbH. Both companies are diagnostic manufacturers. All other authors declare that they have no competing financial interests.

* Email: dirk.roggenbuck@hs-lausitz.de

¶ These authors are joint senior authors on this work.

Introduction

Autoimmune vascular disorders comprising granulomatosis with polyangiitis (GPA, formerly Wegener's granulomatosis), microscopic polyangiitis (MPA), and eosinophilic granulomatosis with polyangiitis (EGPA, formerly Churg-Strauss syndrome) are characterized by microvascular inflammation, tissue necrosis, and the appearance of anti-neutrophil cytoplasmic antibody (ANCA) [1–6]. Thus, the term ANCA-associated vasculitis has been coined for this distinct disease group characterized by loss of tolerance to neutrophilic targets. According to the international consensus statement for ANCA testing, indirect immunofluorescence (IIF) findings on ethanol-fixed human neutrophils (ethN) are recommended to be confirmed with antigen-specific enzyme-linked immunosorbent assays (ELISAs) [2,4,7,8]. ANCA IIF reveals two main patterns on ethN sub-classifying ANCAs into cytoplasmic ANCA (C-ANCA) and perinuclear ANCA (P-ANCA). The C- and P-ANCA in human patients with ANCA-associated vasculitis are mainly directed against proteinase 3 (PR3) and myeloperoxidase (MPO), respectively, and seem to be associated with disease activity [9,10]. However, ANCA IIF patterns as well as PR3- and MPO-ANCA can be observed in other inflammatory conditions and several ANCA-specific targets apart from MPO and PR3 have been reported which lowers the specificity of ANCA testing by IIF [11,12]. Thus, a C-ANCA pattern confirmed by PR3-ANCA ELISA positivity is indicative for GPA [1,3], whereas a P-ANCA pattern confirmed by a positive MPO-ANCA ELISA finding supports the diagnosis of MPA and EGPA [11]. Furthermore, the corresponding ANCA titers are often associated with activity of disease in patients with GPA and MPA.

Consequently, appropriate ANCA testing requires two independent assay techniques to be run currently. Thus, the combination of both IIF and antigen-specific assays was confirmed in several studies to be the optimal strategy for ANCA detection [13].

Recently, IIF microscopy employing fluorescent microbeads as solid phase has been reported offering the opportunity to multiplex autoantibody analysis [14,15]. For the first time, we employed this novel multiplexing technique along with ethN-based IIF for the development of one reaction environment to combine screening and confirmatory ANCA testing. Thus, pattern recognition of P-ANCA and C-ANCA on ethN was aligned with the quantitative determination of PR3- and MPO-ANCA by the means of a novel software module for the automated pattern recognition system Aklides. Existing multiplex ANCA testing such as the mosaic technique does not offer these benefits [16].

Automated digital IIF has been used in HEp2-cell based assays for analysis of antinuclear (ANA) and dsDNA antibodies. Moreover, analysis of respective autoantibody endpoint titers without serial dilution became available by the introduction of calibration tools for digital immunofluorescence [17–22]. We developed a similar technique for ANCA-endpoint titer determination by the novel combined ANCA test. Thus, the novel CytoBead test system presents a unique combination of a classical cell-based assay with multiplexing microbead technology for the simultaneous quantitative analysis of ANCA and their specificities to PR3 and MPO.

In the present study, we evaluated the performance of the novel CytoBead ANCA assay and compared it with classical ANCA testing by independent techniques. Furthermore, we compared the quantitative assessment of PR3- and MPO-ANCA as well as the ANCA-endpoint-titer analysis of the CytoBead ANCA assay on the automated interpretation system Aklides with classical ELISA and IIF methods.

Materials and Methods

Patients and controls

Sera of 592 individuals including 118 patients with ANCA-associated vasculitis, 300 with autoimmune and gastrointestinal diseases, 49 with infectious diseases, and 125 blood donors (BD) were enrolled for the present evaluation (Table 1; patient sera are non-consecutive). Patients with ANCA-associated vasculitis were diagnosed based on typical disease history, characteristic clinical findings, and confirmed clinical histology according to the criteria of the 1994 Chapel Hill Consensus Conference, the consensus statement of 1999, 2012 and the 1990 American College of Rheumatology [2,4,23]. Serum samples were obtained from patients with a confirmed clinical diagnosis of GPA or MPA irrespective of serology.

Serum samples from patients with rheumatoid arthritis (RA), primary sclerosing cholangitis (PSC), autoimmune hepatitis type1 and 2, ulcerative colitis (UC), Crohn's disease (CD) were used as disease controls (Table 1). In total, 49 sera from patients with infectious disease (cytomegalovirus [CMV], rubella virus, Toxoplasma gondii, Epstein-Barr virus [EBV]) were included as further disease controls. In particular, patients with herpes viral infections have the potential to induce ANCA production due to overall B cell stimulation and, thus, could demonstrate false-positive results.

The study received approval from the ethical committee of the Technical University of Dresden (EK56022014) and fulfilled the ethical guidelines of the most recent declaration of Helsinki. An approval of the donors was not necessary because fully anonymized probes used as quality controls in routine diagnostics were selected for this study only. The ethical committee waived the need for written informed consent from the participants accordingly.

Detection of PR3- and MPO-ANCA with antigen-specific ELISA

PR3- and MPO-ANCA were detected using commercially available antigen-specific ELISAs according to instructions of the manufacturers (GA Generic Assays GmbH, Dahlewitz, Germany; Orgentec GmbH, Wiesbaden, Germany) as described elsewhere [24,25]. The PR3- and MPO-ANCA ELISAs of GA Generic Assays GmbH revealed intra-assay variabilities of 5.2% each and inter-assay variabilities of 6.2% each for a serum with 20.0 U/mL PR3-ANCA and 20.0 U/mL MPO-ANCA, respectively. The PR3- and MPO-ANCA ELISAs of Orgentec GmbH revealed intra-assay variabilities of 3.3% and 4.1% for sera with 14.0 U/mL PR3-ANCA and 30.2 U/mL MPO-ANCA and inter-assay variabilities of 6.8% and 4.9% for sera with 51.7 U/mL PR3-ANCA and 33.8 U/mL MPO-ANCA, respectively.

Determination of ANCA by indirect immunofluorescence

PR3- and MPO-ANCA have been analyzed by IIF employing a commercial kit with ethN (GA Generic Assays GmbH). Patient sera and control sera were diluted 1/20 and 50 µl per well were used. The sera were incubated for 30 minutes on the slides and afterwards washed five times each two minutes with phosphate buffered saline (PBS). Subsequently an AlexaFluor 488 conjugated polyclonal anti-human IgG antibody (Dianova GmbH, Hamburg, Germany) was used as secondary antibody and incubated again 30 minutes. After incubation the slides were washed accordingly and the wells were covered with a specific covering solution. The slides were evaluated automatically using the Aklides platform (Medipan, Berlin/Dahlewitz, Germany) as described elsewhere [26]. Briefly, images were assessed automatically using a motorized inverse microscope (IX81, Olympus Corporation, Tokyo, Japan) with a motorized scanning stage (IM120, Märzhäuser, Wetzlar, Germany); 400 nm and 490 nm light-emitting diodes (LED) (PrecisExcite, CoolLED, Andover, UK), and a charge-coupled device grey-scale camera (DX4, Kappa, Gleichen, Germany). The interpretation system is controlled by the Aklides software consisting of modules for device and autofocus control, image analysis, and pattern recognition algorithms. The novel autofocus based on Haralick's image characterization of objects through grey-scale transition using DAPI as fluorescent dye for focusing, quality evaluation, and object recognition. Two-dimensional images were acquired using an objective with 40-fold magnification (Olympus semiapochromat LUCPLFLN 40X, 0.60 NA, W.D. 2.7–4.0 mm). Fluorescence detection was performed using LED excitation with appropriate multiband filter for the DAPI and FITC dyes (DA/FI-A, Semrock, Rochester, USA). Single DAPI and FITC image were serially captured and stored in lossless compressed Tagged Image File (TIF) format.

Table 1. Characteristics of patients and controls: 118 patients with anti-neutrophil cytoplasmic antibody (ANCA)-associated vasculitis, 300 with autoimmune and gastrointestinal diseases, 49 with infectious disorders, and 125 blood donors (BD) were enrolled in the study.

Diagnosis	N	Gender	Age	Age
		f/m	median	interquartile range
ANCA-associated vasculitis				
GPA	90	51/39	65	56–89
MPA	28	14/14	67	51–72
Autoimmune disease controls				
RA	133	99/34	62	56–69
PSC	70	21/49	45	35–57
AIH I	10	8/2	13	12–15
AIH II	10	10/0	11	8–14
UC	57	31/26	49	38–57
CD	20	15/5	40	32–54
Infectious disease controls				
Toxoplasmosis	16	15/1	34	27–43
CMV	25	23/2	38	33–41
Rubella	5	5/0	36	31–37
EBV	3	2/1	10	7–23
Blood Donors	125	64/61	21	21–26

AIH, autoimmune hepatitis; CMV, Cytomegalovirus; CD, Crohn's disease; EBV, Epstein-Barr virus; f, female; GPA, granulomatosis with polyangiitis; m, male; MPA, microscopic polyangiits; N, number; PSC, primary sclerosing cholangitis; RA, rheumatoid arthritis; UC, ulcerative colitis.

Multiplex detection of ANCA by CytoBead ANCA

CytoBead ANCA (GA Generic Assays GmbH) is a multiplex IIF test in one reaction environment combining the screening of ANCA on ethN and their confirmation with multiplex microbead immunoassays, using 9 µm and 15 µm red fluorescent microbeads (excitation 610 nm/emission 690 nm) coated with recombinant antigens PR3 and MPO, respectively. Triple parted wells on microscopic glass slides were employed for the fixation of neutrophils in the middle compartment as well as PR3- and MPO-coated microbeads in the right compartment (Fig. 1). The left compartment was not used and can be employed for further antibody determinations in the framework of an autoantibody profiling [27,28]. Furthermore, a reference microbead population of 12 µm labelled by a green emitting fluorescence dye filling the entire microbead is immobilized on the right compartment. Thus, the differently sized green fluorescence halos of positively stained PR3- and MPO-coated microbeads can be distinguished. In general, PR3-ANCA positive sera show cytoplasmic fluorescence patterns on ethN and a green fluorescence halo on the surface of PR3-coated microbeads only. In contrast, MPO-ANCA positive sera show perinuclear fluorescence patterns on ethN and a green fluorescence halo on the surface of MPO-coated microbeads. For automation, the fluorescence intensities of the fluorescence halos can be quantified and simultaneously located to the appropriate microbead population by the Aklides system.

Fully automated interpretation and pattern recognition of ANCA

The concept of the fully automated interpretation system Aklides for evaluation of ANCA IIF patterns is based on novel mathematical software algorithms for pattern recognition [25,26]. To obtain a reproducible IIF read out signal, the excitation light intensity was calibrated employing a recently developed calibration tool [20]. Novel fluorescent calibration microbeads employed guarantee satisfactory inter-laboratory reproducibility for the calibration process.

Cells and microbeads were characterized by regional, topological, and texture/surface descriptors by employing image data of DAPI and FITC for cells and Cy5 for microbeads. A minimum of 20 stained ethN and 50 microbeads were counted at each sample. The obtained mean fluorescence intensities (MFI) reflect the specific ANCA reactivity of the serum sample. The final read out is expressed as arbitrary units.

Automated endpoint-titer ANCA determination with Aklides

Automated ANCA endpoint-titer determination avoiding serial dilution of samples was developed using analysis algorithms for endpoint-titers of antinuclear antibodies described recently. In order to compensate the different MFI of the two ANCA patterns, the Aklides software harmonizes the fluorescence intensity measurement by including several object description characteristics for MFI analysis. Nevertheless, ANCA positive sera with differing classical end-point titers diluted at 1 to 20 revealed differing MFI values in particular for higher titers depending on the ANCA pattern. Thus, the novel software module for ANCA end-point titer determination employs different algorithms depending on the ANCA IIF pattern analysed by the Aklides system.

Quantification of ANCA with lot-specific standard curves

For the quantification of ANCA by microbead immunoassays of CytoBead testing, computer-stored lot-specific standard master curves were established. Stable microbead reactivity permitted the use of a single lot-specific standard curve to quantify ANCA

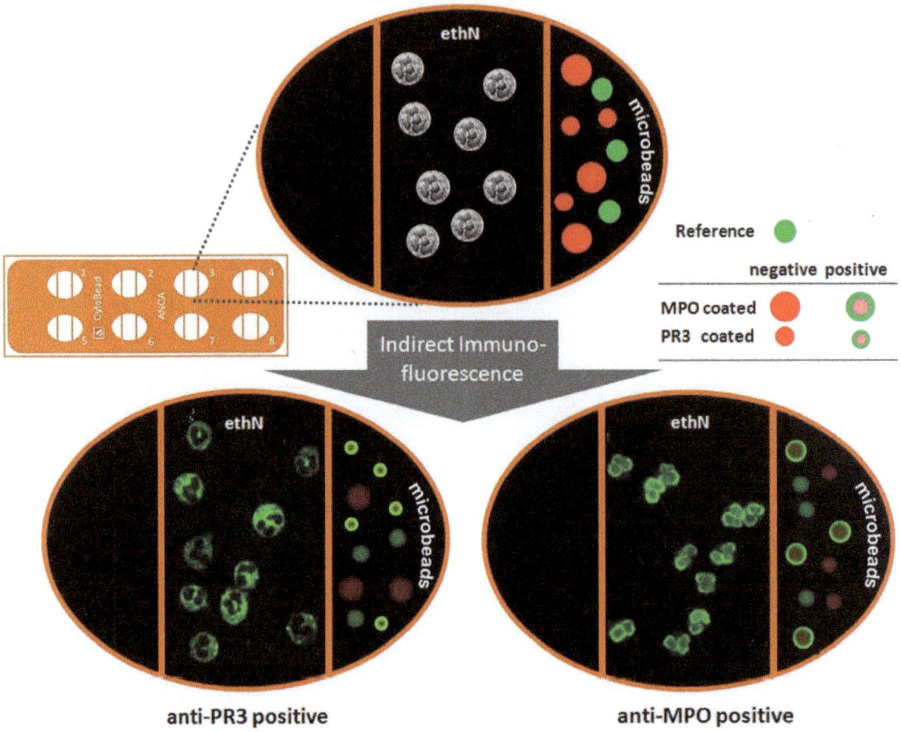

Figure 1. CytoBead ANCA assay principle. Microscopic glass slides with ethanol-fixed human neutrophils (ethN; middle compartment of the well) and proteinase 3 (PR3) as well as myeloperoxidase (MPO) coated microbeads (right compartment of the well) are used for detection of anti-neutrophil cytoplasmic antibodies (ANCAs) by ethN-based indirect immunofluorescence and simultaneous analysis of PR3- and MPO-ANCA by microbead immunoassay. PR3-ANCA positive sera show cytoplasmic fluorescence patterns on ethN and a green fluorescence halo on the surface of PR3-coated microbeads (9 μm). In contrast, MPO-ANCA positive sera show perinuclear fluorescence patterns on ethN and a green fluorescence halo on the surface of MPO-coated microbeads (15 μm).

concentrations. Thus, these standard master curves were obtained by assaying dilutions (1/20 to 1/2560) of reference sera for MPO-ANCA (human reference serum #15) and PR3-ANCA (human reference serum #16) of the International Center for Disease Control and Prevention (CDC).

After acquisition by the Aklides system, PR3- and MPO-ANCA standard curves were fitted using a 5-parameter logistic-fitting curve model [29]. Curve fit parameters were then stored in a post-analysis charge certificate and provided for each assay run to analyze the obtained MFI data. Quantitative data are processed after recalibration of initial stored lot-specific master curves by a two-point recalibration using adjuster signal levels of the current run.

For assay performance assessment, intra- and inter-assay coefficients of variations (CV) were calculated by a eight-fold measurement of serum samples within one run (intra-assay) and further by measurement on 3 different days (inter-assay). The functional assay sensitivity (limit of quantification), being the lowest detectable concentration with an inter-assay CV lower or equal than 20%, for PR3- and MPO-ANCA was determined as described previously [30].

Data standardisation

For the data comparison, ELISA findings in units per millilitre (U/ml) and CytoBead ANCA assay data in international units (IU) were standardized. The highest standard curve concentration points of the ELISA and CytoBead ANCA assay were referred to as 100% and results converted respectively.

Statistical analysis

Inter-rater agreement statistics (Cohen's kappa, κ) and McNemar's test were used for group comparison. P values below 0.05 were considered to be significant. Receiver operating characteristics (ROC) curve analysis was performed using MedCalc software (MedCalc, Mariakerke, Belgium; Version 12.4.0).

Results

CytoBead ANCA cut-off determination

To determine the cut-off of the novel CytoBead ANCA for PR3- and MPO-ANCA, 465 human sera of patients and controls including 118 patients with ANCA-associated vasculitis, 133 with RA, 49 with ID, 20 with CD, 20 with AIH and 125 BD were run with the Aklides IIF interpretation system. Patients with PSC and UC were excluded from the ROC curve analysis due to the known frequent number of positive ANCA (especially PR3-ANCA) findings in these patient groups. The obtained MFIs were standardised as described in Material and Methods and subjected to ROC curve analysis to obtain the respective cut-off values for each ANCA specificity (Fig. 2). For PR3-ANCA the calculated cut-off was 8.4% (0.9 IU/mL) and for MPO-ANCA 19.3% (3.0 IU/mL). The area under curve (AUC) was determined for PR3-ANCA employing 90 sera of patients with GPA as positive criterion at 0.896 (95% confidence interval [CI]: 0.864–0.923) and for MPO-ANCA using 28 patients with MPA as positive criterion at 0.934 (95% CI: 0.904–0.957); $p<0.0001$, respectively.

The PR3- and MPO-ANCA microbead immunoassays of the multiplex CytoBead testing displayed an intra-assay variability of

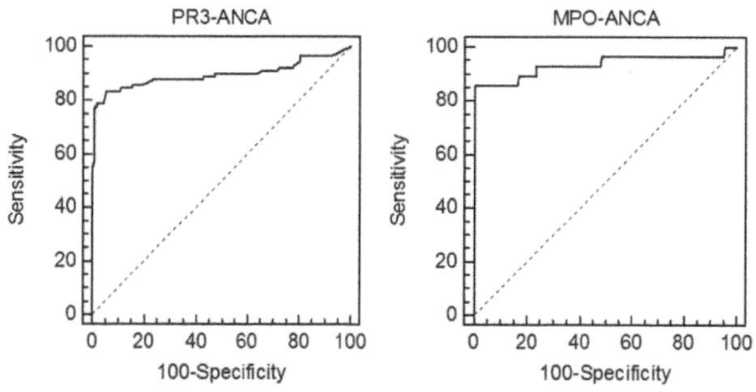

Figure 2. Receiver-operating characteristic curve analysis of anti-neutrophil cytoplasmic antibodies (ANCAs) to proteinase 3 (PR3) and myeloperoxidase (MPO) by CytoBead ANCA. 465 sera from 118 patients with ANCA-associated vasculitis, 133 with rheumatoid arthritis, 49 with infectious diseases, 20 with Crohn's disease, 20 with autoimmune hepatitis and 125 blood donors were included. PR3- and MPO-ANCA were determined simultaneously by microbead immunoassay employing 90 patients with granulomatosis with polyangiitis and 28 patients with microscopic polyangiitis as positive criterion, respectively.

7.1% and 7.7% and an inter-assay variability of 7.2% and 7.6% for sera with 25 IU/mL PR3-ANCA and 100 IU/mL MPO-ANCA, respectively.

The functional assay sensitivity for PR3-ANCA and MPO-ANCA were analyzed as 5.8% (0.6 IU/ml) and 16.1% (2.5 IU/ml), respectively.

Comparison of ANCA prevalences determined by classical and multiplex CytoBead assays

ANCA immunofluorescence pattern as well as PR3- and MPO-ANCA were determined by classical ELISA and IIF and compared with respective findings by automated IIF and microbead immunoassay employing the CytoBead technology (Table 2). According to inter-rater agreement statistics, there was a good agreement for PR3- and MPO-ANCA ($\kappa = 0.775$, 95% CI: 0.710–0.839; 0.720, 95% CI: 0.596–0.843, respectively, Table 3). The agreement for P-ANCA and C-ANCA between classical IIF and CytoBead analysis was very good ($\kappa = 0.876$, 95% CI: 0.812–0.940; 0.820, 95% CI: 0.755–0.844, respectively).

The CytoBead technique determined one C-ANCA and one P-ANCA positives more in patients with GPA and MPA, respectively, compared with the classical method.

However, according to McNemar's test, the differences between classical testing and CytoBead analysis were not significant for PR3-ANCA, P-ANCA, and C-ANCA (1.18%, 95% CI: −1.14%–3.34%; 0.17%, 95% CI: −0.41%–0.50%; 0.34%, 95% CI: −1.25%–1.82%; $p<0.05$, respectively).

In contrast, MPO-ANCA demonstrated a significant difference for both methods (1.69%, 95% CI: 0.14%–2.65%; $p = 0.031$). Whereas there was no significant difference for positive MPO-ANCA findings obtained by both methods in controls, a tendency for a higher prevalence of positive MPO-ANCA detected by CytoBead microbead immunoassay (35/118, 29.7%) compared to those by EIA (23/118, 19.5%) was found in patients with ANCA-associated vasculitis. The CytoBead microbead immunoassay detected significantly more MPO-ANCA positives in patients with GPA in contrast to the classical ELISA (11/90, 12.2% *vs* 3/90. 3.3%, $p = 0.048$).

For the serological diagnosis of ANCA-associated vasculitis, a positive ANCA finding by IIF should be confirmed by a positive PR3- or MPO-ANCA result. Thus, we compared the prevalences of confirmed positive ANCA findings by classical testing (IIF and ELISA positive) with multiplex CytoBead analysis (IIF and microbead immunoassay positive) resulting in a very good agreement for both techniques ($\kappa = 0.831$, 95% CI: 0.777–0.885). McNemars test did not reveal a significant difference for confirmed positive ANCA findings obtained by classical and multiplex analysis (0.51%, 95% CI: −1.58%–2.50%; $p = 0.735$).

Furthermore, we compared the prevalences of positive C-ANCA findings by classical IIF testing confirmed by PR3 ANCA ELISA with respective multiplex CytoBead analysis (PR3 ANCA IIF and PR3 ANCA microbead immunoassay positive). There was a very good agreement for both techniques ($\kappa = 0.937$, 95% CI: 0.893–0.980) and McNemar's test did not reveal a significant difference (1.01%, 95% CI: −0.07%–1.34%; $p = 0.070$). The respective comparison of the prevalences for positive P-ANCA findings by classical IIF testing confirmed by MPO ANCA ELISA with multiplex CytoBead analysis (MPO ANCA IIF and MPO ANCA microbead immunoassay positive) revealed also a very good agreement for both techniques ($\kappa = 0.884$, 95% CI: 0.792–0.976). McNemar's test did not demonstrate a significant difference (0.34%, 95% CI: −0.56%–0.92%; $p = 0.688$).

Comparison of ANCA levels determined by classical and multiplex CytoBead assays

For the sake of comparison of ANCA levels by classical and multiplex testing, concentrations obtained by the different PR3- and MPO-ANCA assays were harmonized by standardizing values to the cut-offs of the respective assays and reporting them in % (Fig. 3). Standardized data of classical ELISA and multiplex testing by CytoBead microbead immunoassay were subjected to ROC curve analysis using 118 samples of patients with ANCA-associated vasculitis as disease criterion for ANCA *vs* 474 controls (Fig. 4). The AUC for PR3-ANCA by ELISA and microbead immunoassay did not demonstrate a statistical difference ($p>0.05$). In contrast, there was a significant higher AUC for MPO-ANCA levels by microbead immunoassay compared with those by ELISA ($p = 0.016$).

Automated endpoint-ANCA titer evaluation

Employing a test set of 34 sera from patients with GPA (n = 8), MPA (n = 10), RA (n = 6), and BD (n = 10), respective MFI values obtained by 1 to 20 diluted samples by CytoBead technology were compared with classical ANCA-endpoint titers determined by serial dilution in classical IIF. The resulting interdependence of classical P-ANCA and C-ANCA endpoint titers with quantitative MFI obtained by digital IIF were used to establish an automated method for the determination of endpoint ANCA titers in one dilution. Inter-rater agreement statistics revealed a very good agreement comparing both methods for endpoint ANCA titer analysis including all data pairs of titers equal or higher than 10 and combining titers equal or higher than 320 in a 6×6 frequency table (weighted $\kappa = 0.985$, 95% CI 0.980–0.991). In routine IIF autoantibody testing, a difference of one titer is not considered significant [31]. Accordingly, automated endpoint ANCA titer analysis of 586 (99.0%) out of the 592 samples investigated did not reveal different titers compared to those detected by the classical method (Table 4). Only 6 (0.1%) sera demonstrated differences of more than one ANCA titer level.

Discussion

For more than 25 years, ANCA serology has been an essential diagnostic tool for the differential diagnosis of vasculitic disorders and IIF is still considered the gold standard for ANCA screening

Table 2. Assessment of anti-neutrophil cytoplasmic antibodies (ANCA) and ANCA against proteinase 3 (PR3) and myeloperoxidase (MPO) by classical and automated multiplex analysis in one reaction environment.

	Classical testing					CytoBead assay				
	ELISA		*IIF*	*ELISA or IIF*	*ELISA and IIF*	*MIA*		*IIF*	*MIA or IIF*	*MIA and IIF*
samples (N)	*PR3-ANCA*	*MPO-ANCA*	*C/P-ANCA*			*PR3-ANCA*	*MPO-ANCA*	*C/P-ANCA*		
GPA (90)	78 (86.7%)	3* (3.3%)	77 (85.6%)	81 (90.0%)	77 (85.6%)	70 (77.8%)	11* (12.2%)	83 (92.2%)	85 (94.4%)	72 (80.0%)
MPA (28)	0 (0.0%)	20 (71.4%)	26 (92.9%)	26 (92.9%)	20 (71.4%)	0 (0.0%)	24 (85.7%)	28 (100.0%)	28 (100.0%)	24 (85.7%)
RA (133)	0 (0.0%)	0 (0.0%)	47 (35.3%)	47 (35.3%)	0 (0.0%)	0 (0.0%)	0 (0.0%)	47 (35.3%)	47 (35.3%)	0 (0.0%)
PSC (70)	31 (44.3%)	3 (4.3%)	49 (70.0%)	53 (75.7%)	27 (38.6%)	24 (34.3%)	1 (1.4%)	49 (70.0%)	52 (74.3%)	21 (30.0%)
AIH1 (10)	3 (30.0%)	1 (10.0%)	9 (90.0%)	9 (90.0%)	1 (10.0%)	1 (10.0%)	1 (10.0%)	9 (90.0%)	9 (90.0%)	2 (20.0%)
AIH2 (10)	1 (10.0%)	1 (10.0%)	3 (30.0%)	3 (30.0%)	2 (20.0%)	2 (20.0%)	1 (10.0%)	3 (30.0%)	3 (30.0%)	3 (30.0%)
UC (57)	10 (17.5%)	1 (1.8%)	26 (45.6%)	29 (50.9%)	8 (14.0%)	18 (31.6%)	1 (1.8%)	26 (45.6%)	33 (57.9%)	10 (17.5%)
CD (20)	0 (0.0%)	0 (0.0%)	2 (10.0%)	2 (10.0%)	0 (0.0%)	0 (0.0%)	0 (0.0%)	2 (10.0%)	2 (10.0%)	0 (0.0%)
ID (49)	0 (0.0%)	0 (0.0%)	0 (0.0%)	0 (0.0%)	0 (0.0%)	0 (0.0%)	0 (0.0%)	0 (0.0%)	0 (0.0%)	0 (0.0%)
BD (125)	0 (0.0%)	0 (0.0%)	7 (5.6%)	7 (5.6%)	0 (0.0%)	0 (0.0%)	0 (0.0%)	13 (10.4%)	13 (10.4%)	0 (0.0%)

ANCA were determined by enzyme-linked immunosorbent assay (ELISA), classical indirect immunofluorescence (IIF) on ethanol-fixed neutrophils and multiplex CytoBead assay in patients and controls: 118 patients with ANCA-associated vasculitis, 300 with autoimmune and gastrointestinal diseases, 49 with infectious disorders, and 125 blood donors (BD).

* $p<0.05$.

AIH, autoimmune hepatitis; BD, blood donors; CD, Crohn's disease; c/p ANCA, cytoplasmic/perinuclear ANCA; GPA, granulomatosis with polyangiitis; ID, infectious diseases; MIA, microbead immunoassay; MPA, microscopic polyangiitis; N, number; PSC, primary sclerosing cholangitis; RA, rheumatoid arthritis; UC, ulcerative colitis.

Table 3. Comparison of perinuclear (P-ANCA) and cytoplasmic (C-ANCA) anti-neutrophil cytoplasmic antibodies and ANCA against proteinase 3 (PR3) and myeloperoxidase (MPO) levels by classical and automated multiplex microbead assay analysis in one reaction environment.

PR3-ANCA		**CytoBead**			**C-ANCA**		**CytoBead**		
		positive	**negative**	**N**			**positive**	**negative**	**N**
ELISA	Positive	98	25	123	**Classical IIF**	positive	80	9	89
	Negative	18	451	469		negative	10	493	503
	N	116	476	592		N	90	502	592
MPO-ANCA		**CytoBead**			**P-ANCA**		**CytoBead**		
		positive	**negative**	**N**			**positive**	**negative**	**N**
ELISA	Positive	25	4	29	**Classical IIF**	positive	75	1	76
	Negative	14	549	563		negative	2	514	516
	N	39	553	592		N	77	515	592
		CytoBead (MIA or IIF)					**CytoBead (MIA and IIF)**		
		positive	**negative**	**N**			**positive**	**negative**	**N**
Classical testing	Positive	249	9	258	**Classical testing**	positive	116	19	457
(ELISA or IIF)	Negative	25	309	334	**(ELISA and IIF)**	negative	16	441	135
	N	274	318	592		N	460	132	592
PR3 ANCA		**CytoBead (PR3 ANCA MIA and C-ANCA IIF)**			**MPO ANCA**		**CytoBead (MPO ANCA MIA and P-ANCA IIF)**		
		positive	**negative**	**N**			**positive**	**negative**	**N**
Classical testing	Positive	68	7	75	**Classical testing**	positive	24	2	26
(PR3 ANCA ELISA and C-ANCA IIF)	Negative	1	516	517	**(MPO ANCA ELISA and P-ANCA IIF)**	negative	4	562	566
	N	69	523	592		N	28	564	592

PR3- and MPO-ANCA were determined by enzyme-linked immunosorbent assay (ELISA) and multiplex CytoBead microbead assay in 118 patients with ANCA-associated vasculitis, 300 with autoimmune and gastrointestinal diseases, 49 with infectious disorders, and 125 blood donors (BD).

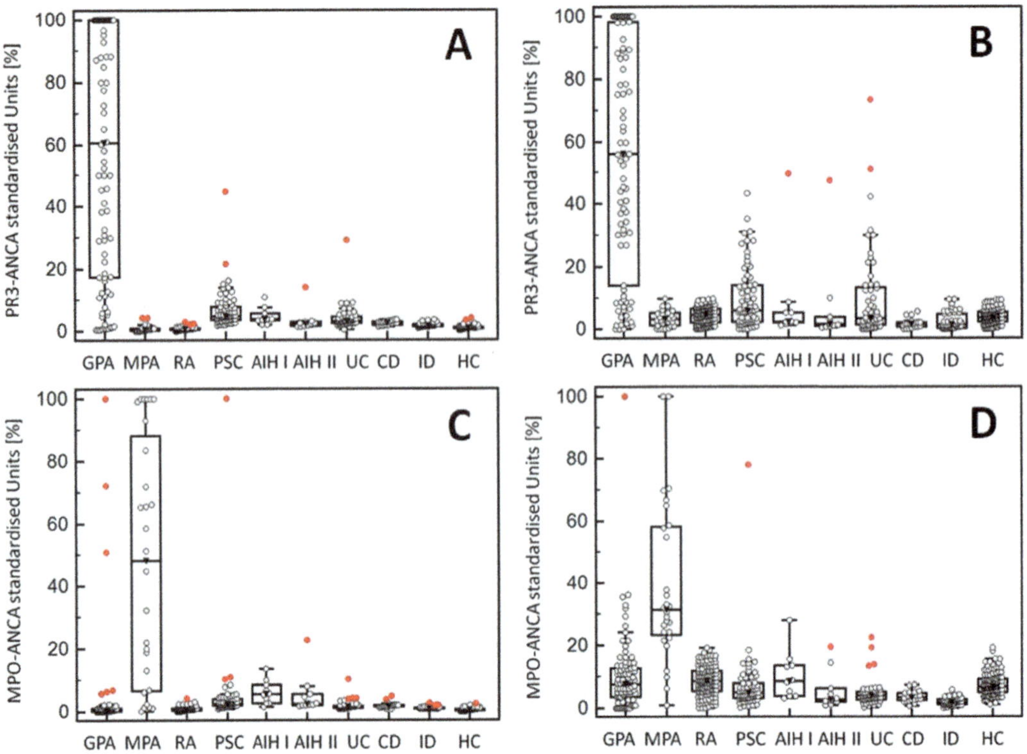

Figure 3. Anti-neutrophil cytoplasmic antibodies (ANCA) against proteinase 3 (PR3) and myeloperoxidase (MPO) levels by classical and automated multiplex microbead assay analysis in one reaction environment. PR3- and MPO-ANCA were determined by enzyme-linked immunosorbent assay (ELISA) (A, C, respectively) and multiplex CytoBead microbead assay (B, D, respectively) in 118 patients with ANCA-associated vasculitis, 300 with autoimmune and gastrointestinal diseases, 49 with infectious disorders, and 125 blood donors (BD). (Data are displayed in Box-and-Whisker plots with *far out* values, defined as values that are smaller than the lower quartile minus 3 times the interquartile range, or larger than the upper quartile plus 3 times the interquartile range, displayed as red circles.). AIH, autoimmune hepatitis; CD, Crohn's disease; GPA, granulomatosis with polyangiitis; ID, infectious diseases; MPA, microscopic polyangiitis; PSC, primary sclerosing cholangitis; RA, rheumatoid arthritis; UC, ulcerative colitis.

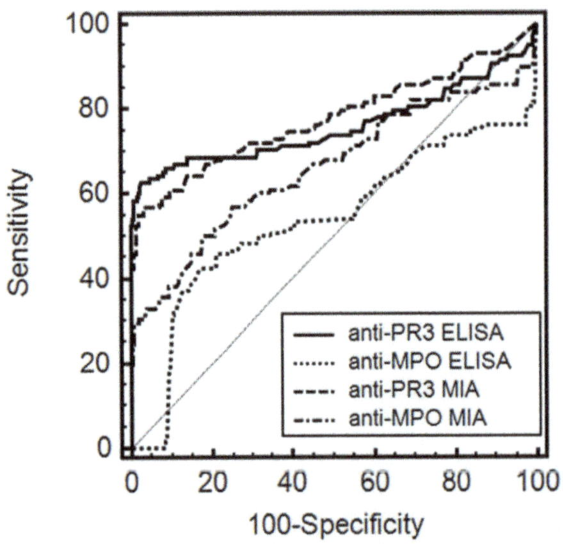

		ELISA	MIA
PR3-ANCA	AUC	0.758	0.776
	95% CI	0.722- 0.792	0.74- 0.809
	p-value	0.438	
MPO-ANCA	AUC	0.577	0.661
	95% CI	0.495- 0.577	0.621- 0.699
	p-value	0.016	

Figure 4. Receiver-operating characteristic curve analysis of anti-neutrophil cytoplasmic antibodies (ANCA) against proteinase 3 (PR3) and myeloperoxidase (MPO) levels by classical and automated multiplex microbead assay testing. PR3- and MPO-ANCA were determined by enzyme-linked immunosorbent assay (ELISA) and multiplex CytoBead microbead assay (MIA) in 118 patients with ANCA-associated vasculitis as disease criterion and in 300 patients with autoimmune and gastrointestinal diseases, 49 with infectious disorders, and 125 blood donors (BD) as control criterion. MPO-ANCA detected by MIA demonstrated a significantly higher AUC compared with those determined by ELISA. AUC, area under the curve; CI, confidence interval.

Table 4. Comparison of classical with automated anti-neutrophil cytoplasmic antibody (ANCA) endpoint-titer analysis.

Classical (1/titer)	Automated (1/titer)										
	=<10	20	40	80	160	320	640	1280	2560	5120	N
=<10	402 (99.3%)	2 (0.5%)	1 (0.2%)	0	0	0	0	0	0	0	405
20	8 (12.3%)	55 (84.6%)	1 (1.5%)	1 (1.5%)	0	0	0	0	0	0	65
40	0	6 (27.3%)	13 (59.1%)	3 (13.6%)	0	0	0	0	0	0	22
80	0	0	5 (26.3%)	12 (63.2%)	2 (10.5%)	0	0	0	0	0	19
160	0	0	0	4 (33.3%)	6 (50.0%)	1 (8.3%)	0	1 (8.3%)	0	0	12
320	0	0	0	0	6 (24.0%)	12 (48.0%)	7 (28.0%)	0	0	0	25
640	0	0	0	0	2 (8.3%)	6 (25.0%)	11 (45.8%)	5 (20.8%)	0	0	24
1280	0	0	0	0	0	1 (7.7%)	4 (30.8%)	7 (53.8%)	1 (7.7%)	0	13
2560	0	0	0	0	0	0	0	0	1 (50.0%)	1 (50.0%)	2
5120	0	0	0	0	0	0	0	0	2 (40.0%)	3 (60.0%)	5
	410	63	20	20	16	20	22	13	4	4	592

ANCA endpoint titers were determined by serial dilution of the 592 samples included in the study by classical indirect immunofluorescence (IIF) and compared to those detected by automated CytoBead IIF on the digital IIF interpretation system Aklides using a 1 to 20 serum dilution only.

[1,7,13]. However, so called obligatory second-line testing to confirm ANCA reactivity by molecular solid-phase immunoassays have been recommended for various reasons [32]. Indeed, IIF is the simplest multiparametric test available allowing the contemporary sensitive detection of C- and P-ANCA. However, its specificity for GPA is obviously lower than that of the antigen-specific PR3-ANCA assays. Thus, the combination of both IIF and antigen-specific assays was confirmed in several studies to be the optimal strategy for ANCA detection [33].

Currently, such tests such as ELISAs, microbead-based or line immunoassays are well established [13,34,35]. Their over the past years continuously improved performance, particularly regarding the analysis of PR3-ANCA, have questioned the usefulness of IIF for ANCA testing [24,25,36]. Indeed, the need to run two different assay techniques in the recommended two-tier algorithm increases the workload in an already limited in capacity autoimmune laboratory. However, IIF seems to be an indispensable technique in autoimmune diagnostics due to its unsurpassed sensitivity [37]. Apart from ANCA testing, this has been also decisively demonstrated for the assessment of antinuclear antibodies as confirmed by other groups [38,39].

Hence, combination of the advantages of IIF regarding cell-based assays and its potential for multiplexing by microbead immunoassay within on reaction environment could revolutionize autoimmune diagnostics [15,40]. Indeed, combining screening and confirmatory testing for disease-specific autoantibodies will generate many benefits ranging from shorter hands-on times, better reproducibility of results to more cost-effectiveness in particular for larger series of samples due the opportunity of using automation and modern data management. We and others could already proved the usefulness of automated ethN-based ANCA testing employing digital immunofluorescence and pattern recognition on novel automated IIF interpretation systems such as Aklides [26,41–44]. Furthermore, we have shown the usefulness of this new IIF technique for multiplexing analysis of autoantibodies [14,15,45]. Therefore, we attempted to combine both approaches for effective ANCA testing by IIF in one test environment and to develop additionally an automated interpretation method for the simultaneous pattern interpretation of P- as well as C-ANCA on the one hand and quantitative assessment of PR3- and MPO-ANCA on the other. An earlier attempt by the so called mosaic technique employing several tissue- and cell-based assay sets in one reaction environment did not provide quantitative ANCA interpretation [16].

We could demonstrate a very good to good agreement for P- and C-ANCA as well as PR3- and MPO-ANCA testing by classical and novel multiplex CytoBead analysis. As a matter of fact, the prevalences of positive ANCA confirmed by PR3- or MPO-ANCA showed a very good agreement for both methods. To the best of our knowledge, this is the first report of a combined quantitative screening and confirmatory testing for the serology of ANCA-associated vasculitis. The use of a lower dilution (1 to 20) for PR3- and MPO-ANCA analysis by microbead immunoassay within the reaction environment of the CytoBead technology did not result in a poorer assay performance compared with even third-generation assays for PR3-ANCA. The lower dilution seems to provide a better reaction environment resulting in higher sensitivity mainly for MPO-ANCA. We detected a significantly higher MPO-ANCA prevalence in patients with GPA by the microbead immunoassay compared with ELISA. However, this elevated prevalence of MPO-ANCA could be due to false positive results and needs to be confirmed by further studies. Furthermore, the CytoBead analysis has a greater dynamic range by employing fluorescence instead of optical density measurement in ELISA subjected to the Lambert–Beer law.

The combination of IIF and autoantigen-specific microbead immunoassay resulted in an improvement of the specificity of ANCA testing. In particular patients with RA and AIH type 1 demonstrated a high prevalence of ANCA on ethN not confirmed by molecular PR3- or MPO-ANCA analysis. This phenomenon could be observed for classical as well as multiplex testing in this study and classical ANCA particularly atypical ANCA on ethN have been found in various other diseases than ANCA-associated vasculitis [11,46–48].

The different median ages of the patient cohorts could have an influence on the ANCA assessment. Elevated titers of antinuclear antibodies have been reported in aging individuals leading to a lower specificity of antinuclear antibody testing regarding this population. Since antinuclear antibody positivity could lead to false positive P-ANCA results, a lower false positive rate could be expected in the control groups with lower median ages such as AIH 1, AIH 2, CD, PSC, and UC. However, this was not the case in this study except for patients suffering from UC and PSC regarding PR3-ANCA in particular. Furthermore, our data confirmed recent data of PR3-ANCA positive patients suffering from UC and PSC detected by sensitive assay techniques [49,50]. Thus, PR3-ANCA might be even proposed as diagnostic parameter for these clinical entities [51]. However, the majority of positive ANCA detected by ethN-based IIF employing both classical and automated IIF were not confirmed by PR3- or MPO-ANCA in these patient cohorts hinting to the presence of other neutrophilic autoantigenic targets.

Quantitative PR3- and MPO-ANCA analysis by multiplex CytoBead technology was at least equal or better compared to classical ELISA testing according to ROC curve analysis. Furthermore, automated endpoint ANCA titer analysis by only one serum dilution using automated IIF interpretation demonstrated a very good agreement with the classical one. Damoiseaux and colleagues could also demonstrate efficient endpoint ANCA titer analysis without serial dilution of samples using digital IIF [51,52]. We and others have shown the usefulness of automated endpoint titer analysis for other autoantibodies such as ANA [20,21,43,44]. Thus, automated IIF combining screening and confirmatory ANCA analysis simultaneously in one reaction environment appears to be a unique opportunity to replace the time-consuming classical two-tier ANCA testing by a one-step analysis. This is especially important for the emergency diagnostics of rapid progressive glomerulonephritis as an oligosymptomatic manifestation of ANCA-associated vasculitis.

Conclusions

The CytoBead technology combining screening and confirmatory PR3- and MPO-ANCA testing simultaneously is an alternative to the conventional two-tier ANCA analysis algorithm, which comprises the screening on ethN and confirmation with molecular solid-phase immunoassays. It can be employed for the sensitive and specific detection of ANCA in patients with ANCA-associated vasculitides and probably in patients with UC and PSC as shown elsewhere previously.

The use of digital IIF interpretation systems provides the opportunity to perform automated and standardized quantitative ANCA testing which meets with the demand of modern autoimmune diagnostics in particular for emergency ANCA analysis.

The novel CytoBead technology enables the simultaneous detection of autoantibodies by cell- and microbead-based immunoassays in one reaction environment and, thus, represents an ideal platform for multiplexing of other autoimmune disease-specific antibodies.

Author Contributions

Performed the experiments: MS IK KG NR RH. Analyzed the data: KC D. Reinhold UA EC PS D. Roggenbuck. Contributed reagents/materials/analysis tools: KC PLM MOB DPB EC. Contributed to the writing of the manuscript: MS D. Roggenbuck. Developed the CytoBead ANCA assay: MS KG. Carried out indirect immunofluorescence assays: MS KG NR. Developed the pattern recognition algorithms: RH.

References

1. Bosch X, Guilabert A, Font J (2006) Antineutrophil cytoplasmic antibodies. Lancet 368: 404–418. S0140-6736(06)69114-9 [pii]; doi: 10.1016/S0140-6736(06)69114-9
2. Jennette JC, Falk RJ, Andrassy K, Bacon PA, Churg J, et al. (1994) Nomenclature of systemic vasculitides. Proposal of an international consensus conference. Arthritis Rheum 37: 187–192.
3. Falk RJ, Gross WL, Guillevin L, Hoffman GS, Jayne DR, et al. (2011) Granulomatosis with polyangiitis (Wegener's): an alternative name for Wegener's granulomatosis. Arthritis Rheum 63: 863–864. doi: 10.1002/art.30286
4. Savige J, Gillis D, Benson E, Davies D, Esnault V, et al. (1999) International Consensus Statement on Testing and Reporting of Antineutrophil Cytoplasmic Antibodies (ANCA). Am J Clin Pathol 111: 507–513.
5. Wiik A (2003) Autoantibodies in vasculitis. Arthritis Res Ther 5: 147–152. DA - 20030501.
6. van der Woude FJ, Rasmussen N, Lobatto S, Wiik A, Permin H, et al. (1985) Autoantibodies against neutrophils and monocytes: tool for diagnosis and marker of disease activity in Wegener's granulomatosis. Lancet 1: 425–429. S0140-6736(85)91147-X [pii].
7. Savige J, Dimech W, Fritzler M, Goeken J, Hagen EC, et al. (2003) Addendum to the International Consensus Statement on testing and reporting of antineutrophil cytoplasmic antibodies. Quality control guidelines, comments, and recommendations for testing in other autoimmune diseases. Am J Clin Pathol 120: 312–318. doi: 10.1309/WAEP-ADW0-K4LP-UHFN
8. Jennette JC, Falk RJ, Hu P, Xiao H (2013) Pathogenesis of antineutrophil cytoplasmic autoantibody-associated small-vessel vasculitis. Annu Rev Pathol 8: 139–160. doi: 10.1146/annurev-pathol-011811-132453
9. Gou SJ, Xu PC, Chen M, Zhao MH (2013) Epitope analysis of anti-myeloperoxidase antibodies in patients with ANCA-associated vasculitis. PLoS One 8: e60530. doi: 10.1371/journal.pone.0060530; PONE-D-12-38469 [pii].
10. Muller A, Voswinkel J, Gottschlich S, Csernok E (2007) Human proteinase 3 (PR3) and its binding molecules: implications for inflammatory and PR3-related autoimmune responses. Ann N Y Acad Sci 1109: 84–92. DA - 20070905.
11. Merkel PA, Polisson RP, Chang Y, Skates SJ, Niles JL (1997) Prevalence of antineutrophil cytoplasmic antibodies in a large inception cohort of patients with connective tissue disease. Ann Intern Med 126: 866–873.
12. Ruffatti A, Sinico RA, Radice A, Ossi E, Cozzi F, et al. (2002) Autoantibodies to proteinase 3 and myeloperoxidase in systemic sclerosis. J Rheumatol 29: 918–923.
13. Csernok E, Holle JU (2010) Twenty-eight years with antineutrophil cytoplasmic antibodies (ANCA): how to test for ANCA - evidence-based immunology? Autoimmun Highlights 1: 39–43. doi: 10.1007/s13317-010-0007-3
14. Grossmann K, Roggenbuck D, Schroder C, Conrad K, Schierack P, et al. (2011) Multiplex assessment of non-organ-specific autoantibodies with a novel microbead-based immunoassay. Cytometry A 79: 118–125. doi: 10.1002/cyto.a.21009
15. Willitzki A, Hiemann R, Peters V, Sack U, Schierack P, et al. (2012) New platform technology for comprehensive serological diagnostics of autoimmune diseases. Clinical and Developmental Immunology 2012: 284740.
16. Damoiseaux J, Steller U, Buschtez M, Vaessen M, Rosemann A, et al. (2009) EUROPLUS ANCA BIOCHIP mosaic: PR3 and MPO antigen microdots improve the laboratory diagnostics of ANCA-associated vasculitis. J Immunol Methods 348: 67–73. S0022-1759(09)00201-4 [pii]; doi: 10.1016/j.jim.2009.07.001
17. Hiemann R, Buttner T, Krieger T, Roggenbuck D, Sack U, et al. (2009) Challenges of automated screening and differentiation of non-organ specific autoantibodies on HEp-2 cells. Autoimmun Rev 9: 17–22. DA - 20090911.
18. Egerer K, Roggenbuck D, Hiemann R, Weyer MG, Buttner T, et al. (2010) Automated evaluation of autoantibodies on human epithelial-2 cells as an approach to standardize cell-based immunofluorescence tests. Arthritis Res Ther 12: R40. DA - 20100402.

19. Kivity S, Gilburd B, Agmon-Levin N, Carrasco MG, Tzafrir Y, et al. (2011) A novel automated indirect immunofluorescence autoantibody evaluation. Clin Rheumatol 31: 503–509. doi: 10.1007/s10067-011-1884-1
20. Roggenbuck D, Hiemann R, Bogdanos D, Reinhold D, Conrad K (2013) Standardization of automated interpretation of immunofluorescence tests. Clin Chim Acta 421C: 168–169. S0009-8981(13)00110-1 [pii]; doi: 10.1016/j.cca.2013.03.019
21. Roggenbuck D, Hiemann R, Schierack P, Reinhold D, Conrad K (2014) Digital immunofluorescence enables automated detection of antinuclear antibody endpoint titers avoiding serial dilution. Clin Chem Lab Med 52: e9–e11. doi: 10.1515/cclm-2013-0543; /j/cclm.ahead-of-print/cclm-2013-0543/cclm-2013-0543.xml [pii].
22. Roggenbuck D, Reinhold D, Hiemann R, Anderer U, Conrad K (2011) Standardized detection of anti-ds DNA antibodies by indirect immunofluorescence - A new age for confirmatory tests in SLE diagnostics. Clin Chim Acta 412: 2011–2012. S0009-8981(11)00382-2 [pii]; doi: 10.1016/j.cca.2011.07.005
23. Jennette JC (2013) Overview of the 2012 revised International Chapel Hill Consensus Conference nomenclature of vasculitides. Clin Exp Nephrol 17: 603–606. doi: 10.1007/s10157-013-0869-6
24. Roggenbuck D, Buettner T, Hoffmann L, Schmechta H, Reinhold D, et al. (2009) High-sensitivity detection of autoantibodies against proteinase-3 by a novel third-generation enzyme-linked immunosorbent assay. Ann N Y Acad Sci 1173: 41–46. DA - 20090917.
25. Holle JU, Csernok E, Fredenhagen G, Backes M, Bremer JP, et al. (2010) Clinical evaluation of hsPR3-ANCA ELISA for detection of antineutrophil cytoplasmatic antibodies directed against proteinase 3. Ann Rheum Dis 69: 468–469. DA - 20100128.
26. Knutter I, Hiemann R, Brumma T, Buttner T, Grossmann K, et al. (2012) Automated interpretation of ANCA patterns - a new approach in the serology of ANCA-associated vasculitis. Arthritis Res Ther 14: R271. ar4119 [pii]; doi: 10.1186/ar4119
27. Conrad K, Roggenbuck D, Reinhold D, Dorner T (2009) Profiling of rheumatoid arthritis associated autoantibodies. Autoimmun Rev 9: 431–435. DA - 20091216.
28. Roggenbuck D, Egerer K, von Landenberg P, Hiemann R, Feist E, et al. (2012) Antiphospholipid antibody profiling - Time for a new technical approach. Autoimmun Rev 11: 821–826.
29. Giraldo J, Vivas NM, Vila E, Badia A (2002) Assessing the (a)symmetry of concentration-effect curves: empirical versus mechanistic models. Pharmacol Ther 95: 21–45. S0163725802002231 [pii].
30. Zöphel K, Wunderlich G, Kotzerke J, von Landenberg P, Roggenbuck D (2009) M22 based (manual) ELISA for TSH-receptor antibody (TRAb) measurement is more sensitive than 2nd generation TRAb assays. Clin Chim Acta 403: 266. DA - 20090427.
31. Sack U, Conrad K, Csernok E, Frank I, Hiepe F, et al. (2009) Autoantibody Detection Using Indirect Immunofluorescence on HEp-2 Cells. Ann N Y Acad Sci 1173: 166–173. doi: 10.1111
32. Conrad K, Roggenbuck D, Reinhold D, Sack U (2011) Autoantibody diagnostics in clinical practice. Autoimmun Rev 207–211. S1568-9972(11)00116-9 [pii]; doi: 10.1016/j.autrev.2011.05.014
33. Radice A, Bianchi L, Maggiore U, Vaglio A, Sinico RA (2013) Comparison of PR3-ANCA specific assay performance for the diagnosis of granulomatosis with polyangiitis (Wegener's). Clin Chem Lab Med 1–9. doi: 10.1515/cclm-2013-0308; /j/cclm.ahead-of-print/cclm-2013-0308/cclm-2013-0308.xml [pii].
34. Csernok E, Ahlquist D, Ullrich S, Gross WL (2002) A critical evaluation of commercial immunoassays for antineutrophil cytoplasmic antibodies directed against proteinase 3 and myeloperoxidase in Wegener's granulomatosis and microscopic polyangiitis. Rheumatology (Oxford) 41: 1313–1317. DA - 20021107.
35. Holle JU, Herrmann K, Gross WL, Csernok E (2012) Comparative analysis of different commercial ELISA systems for the detection of anti-neutrophil cytoplasm antibodies in ANCA - associated vasculitides. Experimental Rheumatol 1–4.
36. Damoiseaux J, Dahnrich C, Rosemann A, Probst C, Komorowski L, et al. (2009) A novel enzyme-linked immunosorbent assay using a mixture of human native and recombinant proteinase-3 significantly improves the diagnostic potential for antineutrophil cytoplasmic antibody-associated vasculitis. Ann Rheum Dis 68: 228–233. DA - 20090113.
37. Tozzoli R, Bonaguri C, Melegari A, Antico A, Bassetti D, et al. (2012) Current state of diagnostic technologies in the autoimmunology laboratory. Clin Chem Lab Med 51(1): 1–10.
38. Meroni PL, Schur PH (2010) ANA screening: an old test with new recommendations. Ann Rheum Dis 69: 1420–1422. ard.2009.127100 [pii]; doi: 10.1136/ard.2009.127100
39. Agmon-Levin N, Damoiseaux J, Kallenberg C, Sack U, Witte T, et al. (2014) International recommendations for the assessment of autoantibodies to cellular antigens referred to as anti-nuclear antibodies. Ann Rheum Dis 73: 17–23. annrheumdis-2013-203863 [pii]; doi: 10.1136/annrheumdis-2013-203863
40. Rodiger S, Schierack P, Bohm A, Nitschke J, Berger I, et al. (2013) A Highly Versatile Microscope Imaging Technology Platform for the Multiplex Real-Time Detection of Biomolecules and Autoimmune Antibodies. Adv Biochem Eng Biotechnol 133: 35–74. doi: 10.1007/10_2011_132
41. Damoiseaux J, Mallet K, Vaessen M, Austen J, Tervaert JWC (2012) Automatic reading of anca-slides: evaluation of the aklides system. Clin Dev Immunol 2012: 762874.
42. Melegari A, Bonaguri C, Russo A, Luisita B, Trenti T, et al. (2012) A comparative study on the reliability of an automated system for the evaluation of cell-based indirect immunofluorescence. Autoimmun Rev 11: 713–716. S1568-9972(12)00002-X [pii]; doi: 10.1016/j.autrev.2011.12.010
43. Bonroy C, Verfaillie C, Smith V, Persijn L, De Witte E, et al. (2013) Automated indirect immunofluorescence antinuclear antibody analysis is a standardized alternative for visual microscope interpretation. Clin Chem Lab Med 1–9. doi: 10.1515/cclm-2013-0016; /j/cclm.ahead-of-print/cclm-2013-0016/cclm-2013-0016.xml [pii].
44. Bossuyt X, Cooreman S, De Baere H, Verschueren P, Westhovens R, et al. (2013) Detection of antinuclear antibodies by automated indirect immunofluorescence analysis. Clin Chim Acta 415: 101–106. S0009-8981(12)00456-1 [pii]; doi: 10.1016/j.cca.2012.09.021
45. George S, Paulick S, Knutter I, Rober N, Hiemann R, et al. (2014) Stable Expression of Human Muscle-Specific Kinase in HEp-2 M4 Cells for Automatic Immunofluorescence Diagnostics of Myasthenia Gravis. PLoS One 9: e83924. doi: 10.1371/journal.pone.0083924; PONE-D-13-32944 [pii].
46. Savige J, Davies D, Falk RJ, Jennette JC, Wiik A (2000) Antineutrophil cytoplasmic antibodies and associated diseases: a review of the clinical and laboratory features. Kidney Int 57: 846–862. kid901 [pii]; doi: 10.1046/j.1523-1755.2000.057003846.x
47. Tsiveriotis K, Tsirogianni A, Pipi E, Soufleros K, Papasteriades C (2011) Antineutrophil cytoplasmic antibodies testing in a large cohort of unselected greek patients. Autoimmune Dis 2011: 626495. doi: 10.4061/2011/626495
48. Ying CM, Yao DT, Ding HH, Yang CD (2014) Infective endocarditis with antineutrophil cytoplasmic antibody: report of 13 cases and literature review. PLoS One 9: e89777. doi: 10.1371/journal.pone.0089777; PONE-D-13-26829 [pii].
49. Arias-Loste MT, Bonilla G, Moraleja I, Mahler M, Mieses MA, et al. (2013) Presence of anti-proteinase 3 antineutrophil cytoplasmic antibodies (anti-PR3 ANCA) as serologic markers in inflammatory bowel disease. Clin Rev Allergy Immunol 45: 109–116. doi: 10.1007/s12016-012-8349-4
50. Van Biervliet S, Bonroy C, Vande Velde S, De Bruyne R, Van Winckel M, et al. (2013) C-ANCA/proteinase 3-positive colitis in children: a distinctive form of inflammatory bowel disease or vasculitis with colitis as initial presentation? J Pediatr Gastroenterol Nutr 57: 489–492. doi: 10.1097/MPG.0b013e31829d4e9e
51. Conrad K, Roggenbuck D, Laass MW (2014) Diagnosis and classification of ulcerative colitis. Autoimmun Rev. S1568-9972(14)00040-8 [pii]; doi: 10.1016/j.autrev.2014.01.028
52. Boomsma MM, Damoiseaux JG, Stegeman CA, Kallenberg CG, Patnaik M, et al. (2003) Image analysis: a novel approach for the quantification of antineutrophil cytoplasmic antibody levels in patients with Wegener's granulomatosis. J Immunol Methods 274: 27–35. S0022175902002739 [pii].

Assessment of Activity Limitations with the Health Assessment Questionnaire Predicts the Need for Support Measures in Patients with Rheumatoid Arthritis: A Multicenter Observational Study

Xavier Janssens[1]*, Saskia Decuman[1,2], Filip De Keyser[1], and the Belgian Rheumatoid Arthritis Disability Assessment study group

1 Department of Rheumatology, Ghent University Hospital, Ghent, Belgium, 2 Department of Internal Medicine, Ghent University, Ghent, Belgium

Abstract

Objective: This study investigated whether the Health Assessment Questionnaire (HAQ) can be used as an instrument to assess the need for social support measures that address activity limitations and participation issues in patients with rheumatoid arthritis (RA).

Methods: This multicenter observational study included patients with RA and disease duration of at least one year, consulting their rheumatologist for routine evaluation of disease activity. In the single study visit data on demographics, disease history and current treatment were collected. DAS28 values were collected to evaluate current RA disease activity. Patients were asked to fill out the HAQ and SF-36 questionnaires. Receiver Operator Characteristics (ROC) curves were constructed to evaluate the performance of the HAQ, SF-36 and DAS28 in predicting the need for nine supporting measures available for chronically ill patients in the Belgian social security system. The expert opinion of the treating rheumatologist was used as a reference.

Results: The study included 316 patients with a mean age of 59.8±12.6 years, disease duration of 11.4±9.3 years, mean DAS28 values of 2.83±1.17. Mean HAQ score was 0.95±0.73, mean SF-36 score 56.5±21.3. HAQ scores >1 were observed in 39.4% of patients. The area under the HAQ ROC curve was consistently >0.7 and higher for the HAQ than for SF-36 or DAS28 for all support measures. Rheumatologists on average recommended 3.67 support measures.

Conclusion: The HAQ score was found to be a good predictor of the need for social support measures in patients with RA.

Editor: Arvind Chopra, Center for Rheumatic Diseases, India

Funding: This work was supported by an unrestricted educational grant from Roche, by the 'Fonds de la Recherche de l'Association Polyarthrite-FRAP' and by the 'Fonds voor Wetenschappelijk Reuma Onderzoek/Fonds pour la Recherche Scientifique en Rhumatologie'. The funders had no role in study design, data collection and analysis,decision to publish, or preparation of the manuscript.

Competing Interests: F. De Keyser received research support from Roche, UCB, Actelion; served as consultant for MSD/Schering Plough, Abbott, UCB, Roche, GSK. Funding from Roche was received for this specific study. X. Janssens and S. Decuman declare that they have no conflicts of interest. There are no patents, products in development or marketed products to declare.

* Email: janssens.reuma@skynet.be

Introduction

As a chronic inflammatory disease, rheumatoid arthritis (RA) can lead to impairment of physical functioning and mobility, loss of productivity, and difficulties in performing normal daily activities. Patients with RA are confronted with extra costs to compensate for these difficulties, as well as with extra health care costs, often in combination with loss of income [1,2].

To limit the impact of RA on functioning and quality of life, support measures addressing activity limitations and participation issues are an important complement to the medical treatment. In order to promote equitable allocation of supporting measures and determine the level and type of supporting measures needed, objective and reliable evaluation of the level and area of activity limitations in patients is essential.

The Health Assessment Questionnaire (HAQ) was developed three decades ago at Stanford University by Fries and colleagues as a patient-reported outcome instrument designed to measure health status and health-related quality of life. It is a 20-item questionnaire covering activities of daily living in 8 domains. Respondents indicate for every item whether they can do the activity 'without any difficulty', with 'some' or 'much difficulty' or are 'unable to do' the activity. The HAQ yields a disability index (HAQ-DI) score between 0 and 3, where 0 means no disability and 3 represents total dependence on others [3–5]. HAQ scores >1 are considered to indicate the presence of disability.

The HAQ is one of the most important patient-reported outcome measures in RA clinical trials, but is also commonly used by rheumatologists in daily practice [6,7], to assess the functional status of their patients. The HAQ has been translated in many languages [8] and has proven validity and reliability in patients with RA [9,10].

In the Belgian social security system, nine different social support measures are currently available for persons with chronic daily activity limitations and loss of autonomy, to promote their reintegration and participation. These support measures comprise financial benefits, disease cost reduction measures, tax benefits and social benefits (see Table 1). There is no validated score for allocation of these benefits.

In this study, we investigated whether the HAQ can predict the need for such social support measures in patients with RA, with the expert opinion of the treating rheumatologist as a reference and compared the performance of HAQ, DAS28 and SF-36.

Patients and Methods

Ethics Statement

All patients gave written informed consent and the study was approved by the Ethics Committee of the University Hospital Ghent (ref. 2010-094) and the ethical committees of the participating clinical centers.

Study Design

Patients eligible for inclusion in this multicenter observational study were at least 18 years of age, met the American College of Rheumatology (ACR) classification criteria for RA [11], had a disease duration of at least one year and consulted their rheumatologist for routine half-yearly outpatient evaluation (according to nomenclature number 478030 of the Belgian social security system). No specific exclusion criteria were defined.

To obtain a representative population of patients with RA, participating rheumatologists asked the first eligible patient in every consultation time block to participate in the study. Patients who gave their written informed consent were included in the study and proceeded with the study data collection in the same visit.

Data collected comprised patient demographics, disease history, current treatment, DAS28, HAQ and SF-36 questionnaires. The treating rheumatologists scored the need for each of 9 different supporting measures (Table 1) available for chronically ill patients in the Belgian social security system on a four item categorical scale as: certainly needed, probably needed, probably not needed or certainly not needed. HAQ and SF-36 questionnaires were filled out independently by the patient; the rheumatologists were unaware of the SF-36 or HAQ scores, which were only calculated during data analysis.

Data analysis and statistics

Data are presented as mean ± standard deviation for normally distributed variables, as median (range) for variables not following a normal distribution or as percentages. Statistical analysis was performed with SPSS version 20 software (IBM Corporation, Armonk, New York, USA). A p-value <0.05 was considered statistically significant.

The Kolmogorov-Smirnov test was used to assess the normal distribution of variables. To compare age groups <65 y versus ≥ 65 y, unpaired t-test or Mann-Whitney U-test was used for continuous variables, and chi-square test for categorical variables.

To evaluate the performance of the HAQ, SF-36 and DAS28 as tests to predict the need for social support measures by patients with RA, Receiver Operator Characteristics (ROC) curves were constructed and the area under the ROC curve (AUC) was calculated [12], with the recommendation of the treating rheumatologist for all nine support measures (Table 1) as the reference. To this end, the scores 'certainly needed' and 'probably needed' were considered as a positive recommendation for a particular support measure, unless otherwise stated. For the purpose of constructing the ROC-curve with sensitivity and specificity for the outcome that at least one support measure is considered necessary by the treating rheumatologist, only the score 'certainly needed' was considered as a positive score. The relevance of such exercise is that a cut-off for this criterium could define a subpopulation of RA patients who would certainly need at least one support measure and a complimentary subpopulation in which no essential support measures apply.

The AUCs of the ROC curves for HAQ, SF-36 and DAS28 were compared using ANOVA.

Table 1. Social support measures for chronically ill patients in Belgium.

Support measure	Type	Description
Integration allowance	Financial benefit (<65 years)	To compensate extra costs due to diminished autonomy and to enhance social participation of person with special needs.
Allowance for help to the aged	Financial benefit (>65 years)	For seniors with chronic health disorders confronted with supplementary costs due to loss of autonomy, in order to enhance their social participation.
Tax reduction	Tax benefit	Income tax exemption for families with one or more disabled persons.
Parking card	Promotion of mobility	For persons with mobility restrictions. Allows parking in parking places reserved for disabled persons and parking without time limit in areas of time restricted parking.
Vehicle tax waiver	Tax benefit	Exemption of car tax for disabled persons
Free public transportation for attendant	Promotion of mobility	Free public transportation access for companions of people with mobility restrictions who can't travel alone
Social telephone rate	Cost reduction	Reduced telephone connection rate, subscription fee and call charges for people with functional limitations.
Social rate utility services	Cost reduction	Exemption of regular allowance and free delivery of a fixed amount of gas and electricity for disabled persons.
Allowance for chronic illness	Financial benefit (<65 years)	Premium for persons with a chronic disease confronted with high medical costs.

Table 2. Population characteristics.

Population characteristics		Overall	<65 y	≥65 y
Nr of patients		316	200	116
% of patients		100	63.3	36.7
Age (y)		59.8±12.6	52.6±9.9	72.31±5.4
Gender ratio (% female)		69.9	73.5	63.8
RA characteristics				
Disease duration (y)		11.4±9.3	10.8±8.98	12.2±9.8
RF (% positive)		72.9	71.5	75.2
Anti-CCP (% positive)		58.7	60.5	55.6
Erosions (% positive)		65.5	65.3	66.0
DAS 28		2.83±1.17	2.89±1.16	2.71±1.18
HAQ		0.95±0.73	0.91±0.68	1.01±0.81
	% HAQ >1	39.4	37.0	42.2
SF-36	Total	56.5±21.3	54.0±20.8	60.9±21.6
	MCS	60.6±21.6	58.2±21.4	64.7±21.2
	PCS	49.4±21.4	47.02±20.9	53.6±21.6
Treatment (% of patients)				
DMARDs		86.4	86.0	87.1
DMARDs – no biologicals		51.6	45.5	62.1
Biologicals		45.9	52.5	34.5
Corticosteroids		44.6	56.5	46.6
NSAIDs		42.2	44.5	38.4

Data are expressed as mean ± standard error or as percentages. *Abbreviations: CRP: C-reactive protein, DAS28: disease activity score using 28 joint counts, DMARDs: Disease-modifying anti-rheumatic drugs, HAQ: Health Assessment Questionnaire, MCS: mental component summary, NSAIDs: non-steroidal anti-inflammatory drugs, PCS: physical component summary, SF-36: Short Form-36.*

The Youden index (sensitivity + specificity − 1) was used to provide a single statistic to capture the performance of the predictive tests [13].

Results

Population characteristics

Table 2 summarizes the study population characteristics. The study included 316 patients with RA. Patients were on average 59.8±12.6 years old, with 36.7% (n = 116) of patients aged 65 or older, 69.9% were female. Mean disease duration was 11.4±9.3 years, rheumatoid factor was present in 72.9% of patients and anti-CCP in 58.7%. DAS28 values were 2.83±1.17, HAQ scores were 0.95±0.73 and 39.4% of patients had a HAQ score >1. SF-36 scores were 56.5±21.3, with lower scores on the physical than on the mental subscale, suggesting a larger impact of RA on physical than on mental functioning. HAQ scores and DAS28 values did not differ significantly between patients below 65 years of age and older patients, but patients aged 65 or older had significantly higher SF-36 scores (Figure 1A).

Current RA treatment included DMARDs in 86.4% of patients, 45.9% of patients were on biologicals. Corticosteroids were used by 44.6% and NSAIDs by 42.2% of patients.

Assessment of the need for social support measures by the rheumatologist

The need for the social support measures listed in Table 1 was scored for every patient by the rheumatologist as certainly or probably needed or certainly or probably not needed. Rheumatologists on average recommended 3.67 support measures per patient.

The most frequently recommended support measures were the allowance for chronic illness (62.2%), tax reduction (51.5%) and social telephone rate (49.5%). Integration allowance was recommended for 43.6% of patients <65 years of age, allowance for help to the aged was recommended for 48.6% of patients older than 65. Rheumatologists recommended the social rate for utility services in 42.2% of patients. Vehicle tax waiver, parking card and free public transportation for an attendant were recommended for respectively 45.6%, 37.8% and 26.9% of patients. (Figure 2).

Predicting the need for social support measures

The number of benefits recommended by the rheumatologist clearly increased with increasing HAQ scores, but not with increasing DAS28 values. Likewise, the number of benefits recommended did not increase with decreasing SF-36 scores (Figure 1B).

In order to assess whether measures of disease activity or functioning can predict the need for social support measures, ROC curve analysis was performed with HAQ, SF-36 and DAS28 for each of the social support measures, with the recommendation of the rheumatologist as reference or gold standard.

The AUC of these ROC curves are presented in Table 3. For all support measures, AUCs were significantly higher for the HAQ than for either SF-36 or DAS28, with AUC values for HAQ of at least 0.7 for all measures (ANOVA, $p = 0.001$), indicating that the HAQ score is a valuable predictor of the need for social support measures in patients with RA and is superior in that function to

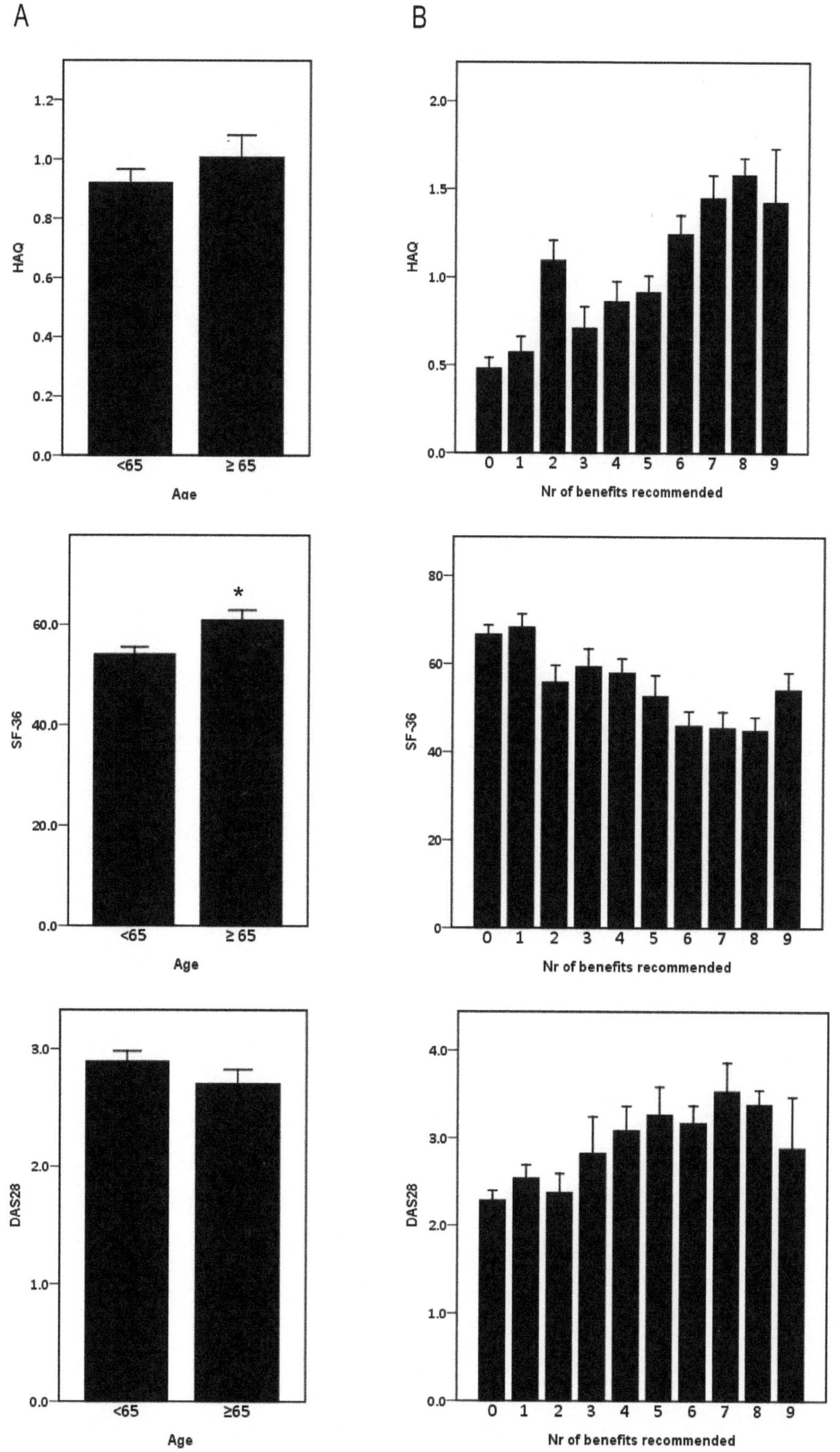

Figure 1. HAQ, SF-36 and DAS 28. A. In function of patient age category. Means for HAQ and DAS28 did not differ between patients below 65 y of age and patients of 65 or older, but patients in the latter age category had significantly higher SF-36 scores *: $p<0.05$ (t-test, error bars represent standard error of the mean). B. In function of number of benefits recommended by the rheumatologist. (Error bars represent standard error of the mean).

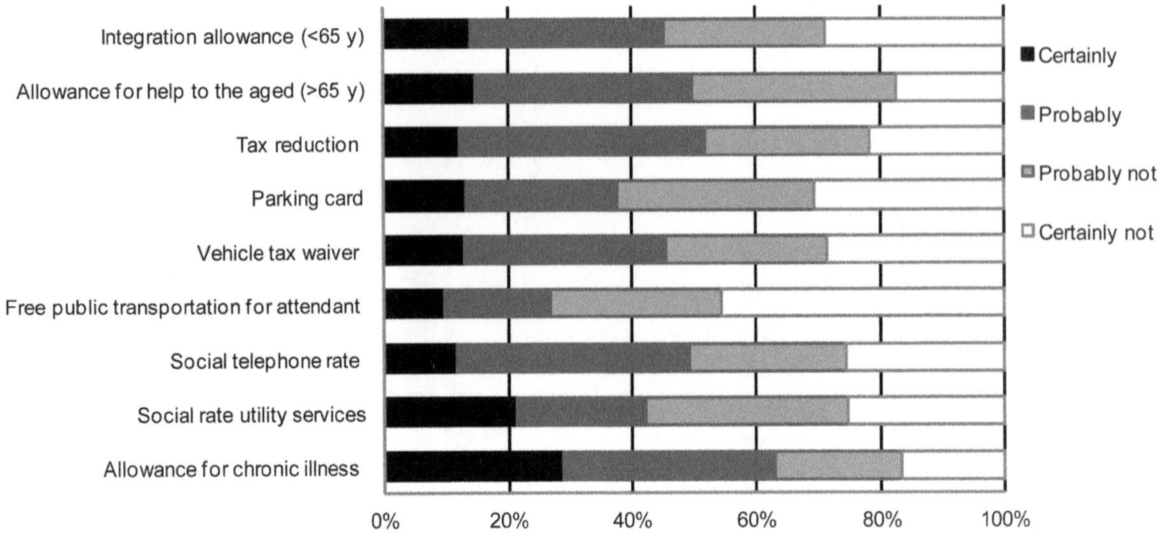

Figure 2. Assessment of need for social support measures by the rheumatologist. Data are expressed as percentage of patients. For support measures with age limits, the patient percentage refers only to the patients in the age category eligible to receive the benefit.

DAS28 and SF-36. Figure 3 shows the ROC curves of the HAQ as predictor for the need for support measures. See File S1 for the raw data for these ROC curves.

An additional purpose was to create a ROC-curve with sensitivity and specificity for the outcome that at least one support measure is considered certainly necessary by the treating rheumatologist. In this way, one can propose a cut-off to define a subpopulation of RA patients who would certainly need at least one support measure and a complimentary subpopulation in which no essential support measures apply. Thus, in the latter subpopulation with a score beneath such cut-off, one would not miss any essential support measure. The AUC for such ROC-curve with HAQ, SF-36 and DAS28 was respectively 0.750, 0.698 and 0.656. For the HAQ, the Youden Index for this analysis reached a maximum of 0.391 for a HAQ cut-off of 0.69 (sensitivity 80.8% and specificity 58.3%). In our study population, 133 patients (42.1%) had a HAQ score below 0.69.

No support measures were recommended by the rheumatologist in 24.4% of patients overall and in 43.3% of patients with a HAQ score below 0.69.

Discussion

Optimal care for patients with RA needs to include support measures to compensate for difficulties in performing daily activities and participation issues. Together, they may alleviate the substantial impact this disease may have.

In this study we evaluated whether disease activity parameters such as DAS28, indicators of functioning such as HAQ, or a measure of health status like SF-36 can predict the need for social support measures, since equitable allocation of benefits requires a reliable measure to evaluate activity limitation.

In this representative, unselected population of patients with longstanding RA, the HAQ score was found to be the best predictor for the need of social support measures, with AUC of the ROC curve of at least 0.7 for all support measures investigated.

Table 3. AUC of ROC- curves for HAQ, SF-36 and DAS28.

	HAQ	SF-36	SF-36 PCS	DAS28
Integration allowance (<65 y)	0.806	0.725	0.779	0.695
Allowance for help to the aged (>65 y)	0.798	0.798	0.776	0.785
Tax reduction	0.766	0.727	0.748	0.713
Parking card	0.831	0.728	0.750	0.703
Vehicle tax waiver	0.778	0.710	0.715	0.632
Free public transportation for attendant	0.700	0.642	0.650	0.660
Social telephone rate	0.775	0.708	0.721	0.665
Social rate utility services	0.755	0.735	0.748	0.647
Allowance for chronic illness	0.707	0.639	0.657	0.641

Areas under the curve (AUC) of the ROC curve analysis performed with HAQ, SF-36, SF-36 physical component score (PCS) and DAS28 for the social support measures available in Belgium in order to assess whether these instruments can be used to predict the need for social support measures in patients with RA. The recommendation of the rheumatologist was used as reference.

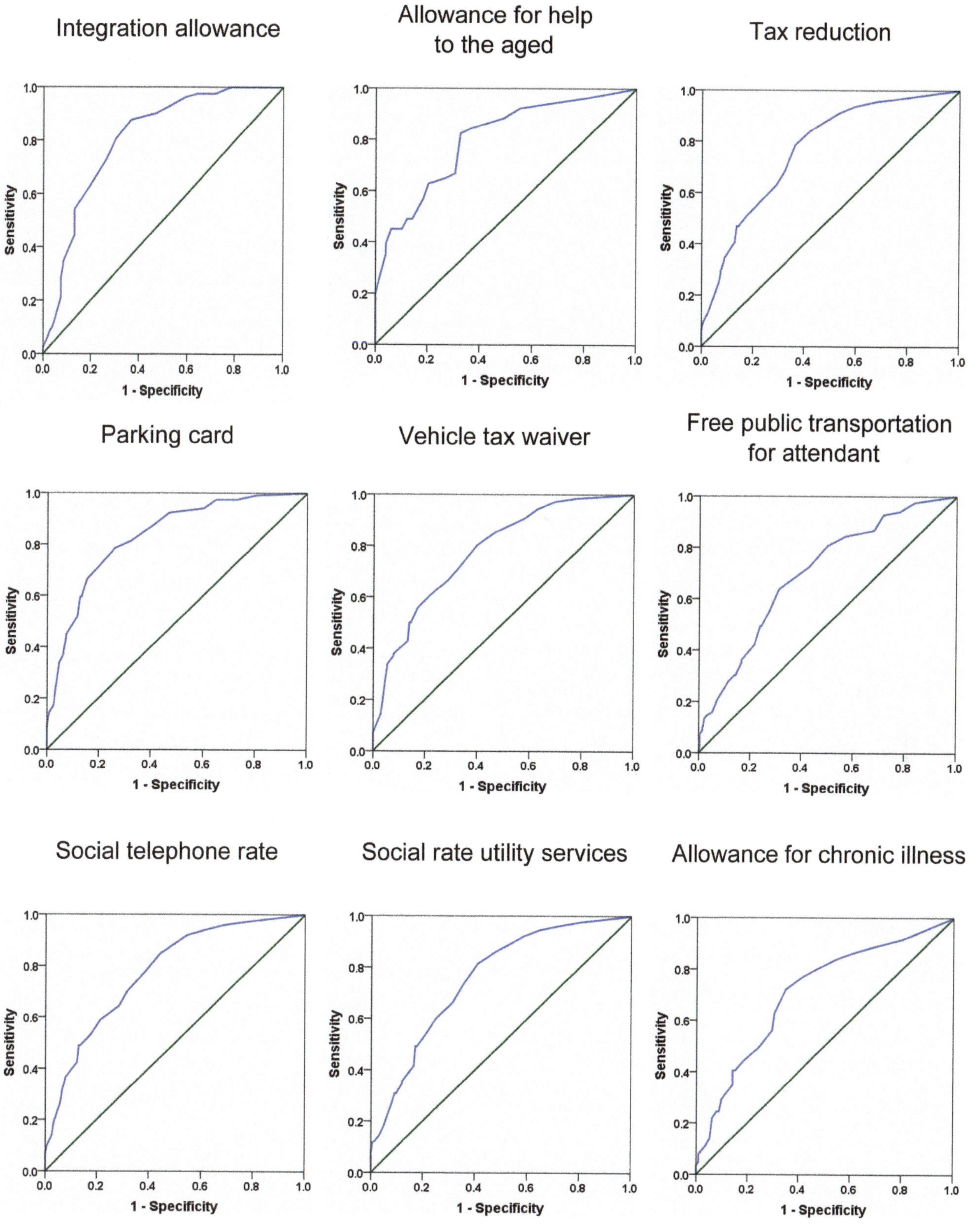

Figure 3. ROC curves for HAQ predicting the need for different social support measures. Receiver operator characteristic analysis (ROC) demonstrates that the Health Assessment Questionnaire (HAQ) performs well as a tool to predict the need for social support measures in patients with RA. The recommendation by the treating rheumatologist was used as reference.

Previous studies in the United Kingdom (UK) showed that the HAQ can be used to predict successful application for access to benefits and financial support [14–16]. In the UK, 69% of the patients with RA or osteoarthritis of hip or knee and a HAQ score >1.5 who applied were awarded the benefit [15].

In our study, no data were collected on actual applications to receive the social support measures studied, nor on actual allocation of these benefits, so that the results of our study solely represent the expert opinion of the treating rheumatologists on their patients' needs. We did not attempt to calculate HAQ cut-off values for the different support measures investigated, but instead chose to include the raw data of the ROC curves as supplementary data (File S1). Consequently, the data from this study can be used to calculate HAQ cut-offs to suit the sensitivity or specificity limits one wishes to use or to fit the budget available for these benefits.

Based upon our analysis, we propose a HAQ cut-off value of 0.69 to define two RA subpopulations according to whether or not these patients absolutely require at least one of the described support measures. The relevance of this cut-off could be that in case the HAQ score is lower than this cut-off, one could justify not pursuing further efforts for allocation of support measures.

Functioning may be further impaired by factors such as age and comorbidity. It is an important strength of the HAQ to provide a comprehensive assessment of a patient's functioning, not only determined by RA, but also by old age or limitations as a consequence of superimposed comorbidity. The need of support measures will increase with this global loss of functioning and not just with the functional limitations of RA.

We did not collect socioeconomic parameters or educational status in this study. The impact of these parameters on functioning are still controversial: a Swedish cross sectional study reported no influence of socioeconomic factors and education on disability in RA patients [17] but a number of studies have found RA disease activity and severity to be more pronounced in patients with lower socio-economic status [18,19].

Our findings indicate that it would be feasible to expand the scope of application of the HAQ to include its use as an instrument for allocating access to financial or social support measures or to tax benefits for patients with RA. Such an approach would have the added benefit of reducing the administrative burden involved with benefit allocation by using the results of a test that is widely used and accepted for clinical monitoring of patients with RA.

Additional research is needed to investigate whether the use of HAQ score to determine the need of support can be generalized to other regions, with other types of support measures available, and to determine what the impact would be of using the HAQ for the actual allocation of social support measures. A follow-up study investigating which domains of the HAQ determine best the need for which kind of support measures is currently ongoing.

In summary, the HAQ score was found to be a good predictor (better than DAS28 and SF-36) for the need for social support measures in patients with RA, as assessed by the rheumatologist.

Supporting Information

File S1 ROC curve data tables for the HAQ. Tables with coordinates of the ROC curve analysis investigating the performance of the Health Assessment Questionnaire (HAQ) as an instrument to evaluate the need for social support measures in patients with RA. The expert opinion of the treating rheumatologist on the need for social support measures was used as a reference.

Acknowledgments

The Belgian Rheumatoid Arthritis Disability Assessment study group: Ackerman C (Lead author, AZ St Lucas, Gent, christine.ackerman@azstlucas.be), André B (CHU Sart Tilman Liège), Brasseur J-P (Clinique Saint-Pierre, Ottignies), Cremer D (Hôpital Saint-Joseph, Liège), De Brabanter G (AZ St-Lucas, Brugge), De Keyser F (AZ Alma, Sijsele), Durez P (Cliniques Universitaires Saint-Luc, Bruxelles), Fontaine M-A (Hôpital Saint-Joseph, Liège), Gyselbrecht L (ASZ, Aalst), Houssiau F (Cliniques Universitaires Saint-Luc, Bruxelles), Lauwerys B (Cliniques Universitaires Saint-Luc, Bruxelles), Maeyaert B (AZ St-Lucas, Brugge), Stubbe M (ULB, Erasme), Vandenberghe M (ASZ, Aalst), Vanden Berghe M (GHDC Hôpital Saint-Joseph, Gilly), Van Mullem X (GHDC Hôpital Saint-Joseph, Gilly), Verschueren P (UZ Gasthuisberg, Leuven), Westhovens R (UZ Gasthuisberg, Leuven).

The authors acknowledge the contribution of Veerle Persy, MD, PhD as an independent medical writer on behalf of Hugin Mugin Research.

Author Contributions

Conceived and designed the experiments: XJ FDK. Performed the experiments: XJ SD FDK. Analyzed the data: XJ SD FDK. Contributed reagents/materials/analysis tools: FDK. Wrote the paper: XJ.

References

1. Yelin E, Wanke L (1999) An assessment of the annual and long-term direct costs of rheumatoid arthritis: the impact of poor function and functional decline. Arthritis Rheum 42: 1209–1218. doi:10.1002/1529-0131(199906)42:6<1209::AID-ANR18>3.0.CO;2-M.
2. Huscher D, Merkesdal S, Thiele K, Zeidler H, Schneider M, et al. (2006) Cost of illness in rheumatoid arthritis, ankylosing spondylitis, psoriatic arthritis and systemic lupus erythematosus in Germany. Ann Rheum Dis 65: 1175–1183. doi:10.1136/ard.2005.046367.
3. Bruce B, Fries JF (2003) The Stanford Health Assessment Questionnaire: a review of its history, issues, progress, and documentation. J Rheumatol 30: 167–178.
4. Bruce B, Fries JF (2003) The Stanford Health Assessment Questionnaire: dimensions and practical applications. Health Qual Life Outcomes 1: 20. doi:10.1186/1477-7525-1-20.
5. Bruce B, Fries JF (2005) The Health Assessment Questionnaire (HAQ). Clin Exp Rheumatol 23: S14–8.
6. Wolfe F, Kleinheksel SM, Cathey MA, Hawley DJ, Spitz PW, et al. (1988) The clinical value of the Stanford Health Assessment Questionnaire Functional Disability Index in patients with rheumatoid arthritis. J Rheumatol 15: 1480–1488.
7. Pincus T (2006) The DAS is the most specific measure, but a patient questionnaire is the most informative measure to assess rheumatoid arthritis. J Rheumatol 33: 834–837.
8. Zandbelt MM, Welsing PM, van Gestel a M, van Riel PL (2001) Health Assessment Questionnaire modifications: is standardisation needed? Ann Rheum Dis 60: 841–845.
9. Linde L, Sørensen J, Ostergaard M, Hørslev-Petersen K, Hetland ML (2008) Health-related quality of life: validity, reliability, and responsiveness of SF-36, 15D, EQ-5D [corrected] RAQoL, and HAQ in patients with rheumatoid arthritis. J Rheumatol 35: 1528–1537.
10. Sokka T, Kautiainen H, Hannonen P, Pincus T (2006) Changes in Health Assessment Questionnaire disability scores over five years in patients with rheumatoid arthritis compared with the general population. Arthritis Rheum 54: 3113–3118. doi:10.1002/art.22130.
11. Arnett FC, Edworthy SM, Bloch DA, McShane DJ, Fries JF, et al. (1988) The American Rheumatism Association 1987 revised criteria for the classification of rheumatoid arthritis. Arthritis Rheum 31: 315–324.
12. Bewick V, Cheek L, Ball J (2004) Statistics review 13: receiver operating characteristic curves. Crit Care 8: 508–512. doi:10.1186/cc3000.
13. Youden WJ (1950) Index for rating diagnostic tests. Cancer 3: 32–35.
14. Memel DS, Kirwan JR, Langley C, Hewlett S, Hehir M (2002) Prediction of successful application for disability benefits for people with arthritis using the Health Assessment Questionnaire. Rheumatology (Oxford) 41: 100–102.
15. Langley C, Memel DS, Kirwan JR, Pollock J, Hewlett S, et al. (2004) Using the Health Assessment Questionnaire and welfare benefits advice to help people disabled through arthritis to access financial support. Rheumatology (Oxford) 43: 863–868. doi:10.1093/rheumatology/keh184.

16. Fruin C, Pitt PI (2008) Welfare benefit promotion within a district general hospital rheumatology centre: a joint project with the local Citizens Advice Bureau. Musculoskeletal Care 6: 211–219. doi:10.1002/msc.133.
17. Bendtsen P, Bjurulf P, Trell E, Lindström F, Larsson JE (n.d.) Cross-sectional assessment and subgroup comparison of functional disability in patients with rheumatoid arthritis in a Swedish health-care district. Disabil Rehabil 17: 94–99.
18. Harrison MJ, Farragher TM, Clarke AM, Manning SC, Bunn DK, et al. (2009) Association of functional outcome with both personal- and area-level socioeconomic inequalities in patients with inflammatory polyarthritis. Arthritis Rheum 61: 1297–1304. doi:10.1002/art.24830.
19. Massardo L, Pons-Estel BA, Wojdyla D, Cardiel MH, Galarza-Maldonado CM, et al. (2012) Early rheumatoid arthritis in Latin America: low socioeconomic status related to high disease activity at baseline. Arthritis Care Res (Hoboken) 64: 1135–1143. doi:10.1002/acr.21680.

15

Role of Key *TYMS* Polymorphisms on Methotrexate Therapeutic Outcome in Portuguese Rheumatoid Arthritis Patients

Aurea Lima[1,2,3]*, Vítor Seabra[1], Miguel Bernardes[4,5], Rita Azevedo[2,4], Hugo Sousa[2,4,6], Rui Medeiros[2,3,6,7]

1 CESPU, Institute of Research and Advanced Training in Health Sciences and Technologies, Department of Pharmaceutical Sciences, Higher Institute of Health Sciences-North (ISCS-N), Gandra PRD, Portugal, **2** Molecular Oncology Group CI, Portuguese Institute of Oncology of Porto (IPO-Porto), Porto, Portugal, **3** Abel Salazar Institute for the Biomedical Sciences (ICBAS) of University of Porto, Porto, Portugal, **4** Faculty of Medicine of University of Porto (FMUP), Porto, Portugal, **5** Rheumatology Department of São João Hospital Center, Porto, Portugal, **6** Virology Service, Portuguese Institute of Oncology of Porto (IPO-Porto), Porto, Portugal, **7** Research Department-Portuguese League Against Cancer (LPCC-NRNorte), Porto, Portugal

Abstract

Background: Therapeutic outcome of rheumatoid arthritis (RA) patients treated with methotrexate (MTX) can be modulated by thymidylate synthase (TS) levels, which may be altered by genetic polymorphisms in TS gene (*TYMS*). This study aims to elucidate the influence of *TYMS* polymorphisms in MTX therapeutic outcome (regarding both clinical response and toxicity) in Portuguese RA patients.

Methods: Clinicopathological data from 233 Caucasian RA patients treated with MTX were collected, outcomes were defined and patients were genotyped for the following *TYMS* polymorphisms: 1) 28 base pairs (bp) variable number tandem repeat (rs34743033); 2) single nucleotide polymorphism C>G (rs2853542); and 3) 6 bp sequence deletion (1494del6, rs34489327). Chi-square and binary logistic regression analyses were performed, using genotype and haplotype-based approaches.

Results: Considering *TYMS* genotypes, 3R3R ($p = 0.005$, OR = 2.34), 3RC3RG ($p = 0.016$, OR = 3.52) and 6bp− carriers ($p = 0.011$, OR = 1.96) were associated with non-response to MTX. Multivariate analysis confirmed the increased risk for non-response to MTX in 6bp− carriers ($p = 0.016$, OR = 2.74). Data demonstrated that *TYMS* polymorphisms were in linkage disequilibrium ($p < 0.00001$). Haplotype multivariate analysis revealed that haplotypes harboring both 3R and 6bp− alleles were associated with non-response to MTX. Regarding MTX-related toxicity, no statistically significant differences were observed in relation to *TYMS* genotypes and haplotypes.

Conclusion: Our study reveals that *TYMS* polymorphisms could be important to help predicting clinical response to MTX in RA patients. Despite the potential of these findings, translation into clinical practice needs larger studies to confirm these evidences.

Editor: Yue Wang, National Institute for Viral Disease Control and Prevention, CDC, China, China

Funding: Funding support from a Doctoral Grant (SFRH/BD/64441/2009) for Aurea Lima - Fundação para a Ciência e Tecnologia (FCT). The funders had no role in study design, data collection and analysis, decision to publish, or preparation of the manuscript.

Competing Interests: The authors have declared that no competing interests exist.

* Email: aurea.lima@iscsn.cespu.pt

Introduction

Methotrexate (MTX) is the cornerstone for rheumatoid arthritis (RA) treatment and is the most widely used disease-modifying antirheumatic drug (DMARD) in newly diagnosed patients [1,2]. Despite its cost-effectiveness, therapeutic outcome is variable mainly concerning to MTX clinical response and/or development of MTX-related toxicity [3–7]. MTX is an antifolate drug with important anti-inflammatory and antiproliferative effects, partly achieved by the intracellular inhibition of thymidylate synthase (TS) [8–10]. TS is a key protein for the *de novo* pyrimidine synthesis and is responsible for the simultaneous conversion of deoxyuridine monophosphate (dUMP) and 5,10-methylenetetrahydrofolate (5,10-MTHF) to deoxythymidine monophosphate (dTMP) and dihydrofolate (DHF). Subsequently, the dTMP is phosphorylated to deoxythymidine triphosphate (dTTP) and used for the deoxyribonucleic acid (DNA) synthesis and repair [6,11,12] (Figure 1A). Since TS levels were found to be predictive of MTX therapeutic outcome [13,14] and genetic polymorphisms in TS gene (*TYMS*) have been associated with TS levels [15,16], pharmacogenomics has raised great interest and, in fact, some studies have attempted to clarify the influence of genetic variations on clinical response to MTX in RA [17]. The most studied polymorphisms (rs34743033, rs2853542 and rs34489327) are represented on Figure 1B. Polymorphism rs34743033 is a 28 base pairs (bp) variable number tandem repeat (VNTR), located on 5′

untranslated region (UTR) [18]. Is characterized by exhibiting a putative Enhancer box (E-box) sequence on the first 28 bp repeat of 2R allele and on the two first repeats of 3R allele [15,19]. Therefore, a higher number of repeats should increase the amount of E-box binding sites for the upstream stimulating factors (USF), leading to an increased transcription of *TYMS* and, consequently, to higher TS levels [20]. In addition, a single nucleotide polymorphism (SNP) characterized by a cytosine to guanine (C>G) transition on the twelfth nucleotide of the second repeat of VNTR 3R allele (rs2853542) has been described [15]. In the presence of cytosine (3RC) the E-box seems to be disrupted, reducing the stimulation of transcription in comparison to 3RG, thereby decreasing TS levels [15]. Since this SNP occurs within the *TYMS* 28 bp VNTR polymorphism, several studies have been performed combining the information from both *TYMS* enhancer region (TSER) polymorphisms [6,21]. Another important polymorphism is a 6 bp sequence (TTAAAG) deletion (1494del6, rs34489327) at 3′UTR, which seems to affect a region of TS pre-messenger ribonucleic acid (mRNA) that contains *cis* adenylate-uridylate-rich elements (AREs) [22,23]. These elements bind to a *trans* AU-rich factor 1 (AUF1), preferentially in the presence of deletion allele (6bp−), diminishing mRNA stability and, consequently, decreasing TS levels [16,22,23]. Therefore, the aim of this study was to elucidate the clinical relevance of these *TYMS* polymorphisms, by genotype and haplotype-based approaches, in MTX therapeutic outcome of Portuguese RA patients.

Methods

Patients and study design

A retrospective study was performed between January 2009 and December 2012 at São João Hospital Center (Porto, Portugal) in a cohort of consecutive Caucasian patients (≥18 years) with RA treated with MTX. Patients were excluded from the study if there was history of drug abuse, recent pregnancy or desire to become pregnant. The study was approved by the Ethical Committee of São João Hospital Center (reference 33/2009), procedures were considered to be according to the standards of the Helsinki Declaration and all patients provided an informed written consent.

After diagnosis, patients were classified according the 1987 criteria of the American College of Rheumatology (ACR) and reclassified according the 2010 criteria of the ACR and the European League Against Rheumatism (EULAR) [24]. All patients were initially treated with 10 mg *per os* (PO)/week of MTX in monotherapy. This dose was increased 5 mg at each three weeks if the patients did not meet the EULAR criteria for response, i.e., if presented a Disease Activity Score in 28 joints (DAS28) >3.2. Every 3 months treatment response was evaluated and, on the: 1) first evaluation, if patients have no response or show gastrointestinal toxicity, administration route was changed to subcutaneous (SC); 2) second evaluation, if maximum tolerable dose was used without response, MTX therapy was discontinued or associated with other synthetic DMARD; and 3) third evaluation, in patients without response and other contraindication, therapy was changed by associating a biological DMARD. The occurrence of MTX-related toxicity was registered at each visit and, according to severity, MTX dose was adjusted or discontinued. Folic acid supplementation was prescribed to all patients for the prevention of toxicity occurrence and their regular compliance was registered [7,25,26]. Other concomitant drugs, such as corticosteroids and non-steroidal anti-inflammatories (NSAIDs) were allowed during the study.

Outcome definition

Non-response. MTX clinical response was recorded at time of each visit. Non-response was defined when patients presented a DAS28>3.2, calculated and defined as described by Prevoo *et al.* [27], in two consecutive evaluations. Therefore, non-response to MTX had a minimum period of MTX therapy, at least, of six months.

Toxicity. The occurrence of MTX-related toxicity, defined when patients presented any adverse drug reaction (ADR) related to MTX, was recorded upon each visit. The type of ADR was classified in System Organ Class (SOC) disorders, in accordance with Common Terminology Criteria for Adverse Events (CTCAE) [28].

Samples handling and *TYMS* genotyping

Whole blood samples from each patient were obtained with standard venipuncture technique in ethylenediaminetetraacetic acid (EDTA) containing tubes. Genomic DNA was extracted with QIAamp DNA Blood Mini Kit (QIAGEN, Hilden, Germany) according to manufacturer instructions and total genomic DNA was quantified, and its purity analyzed, using the NanoDrop 1000 Spectrophotometer v3.7 (Thermo Scientific, Wilmington DE, USA).

TSER polymorphisms. 28 bp VNTR polymorphism (rs34743033) and SNP C>G (rs2853542) at the twelfth nucleotide of the second repeat of 3R allele were genotyped as described by Lima *et al.* [29]. For quality control, 10% of the samples were randomly selected for a second analysis and 10% percent of cases were confirmed by automated sequencing in a 3130×l Genetic Analyzer using the Kit BigDye Terminator v3.1 (Life Technologies, Foster City, CA, USA). Results were 100% concordant.

TYMS 1494del6 polymorphism. 1494del6 polymorphism (rs34489327) was genotyped as described by Lima *et al.* [29] with slight modifications. PCR products were purified with USB ExoSAP-IT (Affymetrix, Santa Clara, CA, USA) before cycle sequencing. Sequence reactions were carried out using the sequencing Kit BigDye Terminator v.3.1 (Life Technologies, Foster City, CA, USA) according to manufacturer's specifications. The sequencing profile was 30 cycles at 96°C for 10 seconds, 55°C for 10 seconds and 60° for 60 seconds, followed by an extension cycle at 60°C for 10 minutes. The sequence products were purified with illustra Sephadex G-50 Fine DNA Grade (GE Healthcare, Fairfield, CT, EUA) columns, denatured with Hi-Di Formamide and run in an 3130×l Genetic Analyzer (Life Technologies, Foster City, CA, USA). For quality control, 10% of the samples were randomly selected for a second analysis and results were 100% concordant.

Polymorphisms classification and linkage disequilibrium measure

TSER polymorphisms were classified according to their theoretical TS functional *status* as previously described [6] and grouped by predicted expression levels, as follow: low expression genotypes (2R2R, 2R3RC and 3RC3RC), median expression genotypes (2R3RG and 3RC3RG) and high expression genotype (3RG3RG). Haplotype analysis was performed using a two-stage iterative method named expectation maximization algorithm (SNPStats software) [30]. In order to estimate LD between pairs of alleles at TSER and *TYMS* 1494del6 *loci*, D' coefficients were calculated in Arlequin for Windows, Version 3.11 (University of Berne, Bern, Switzerland) [31] with 100,000 number of steps in Markov chain. The measure was interpretable as the proportion of maximum possible level of association between two *loci*, given the allele frequencies, ranging from 0 (linkage equilibrium) to 1

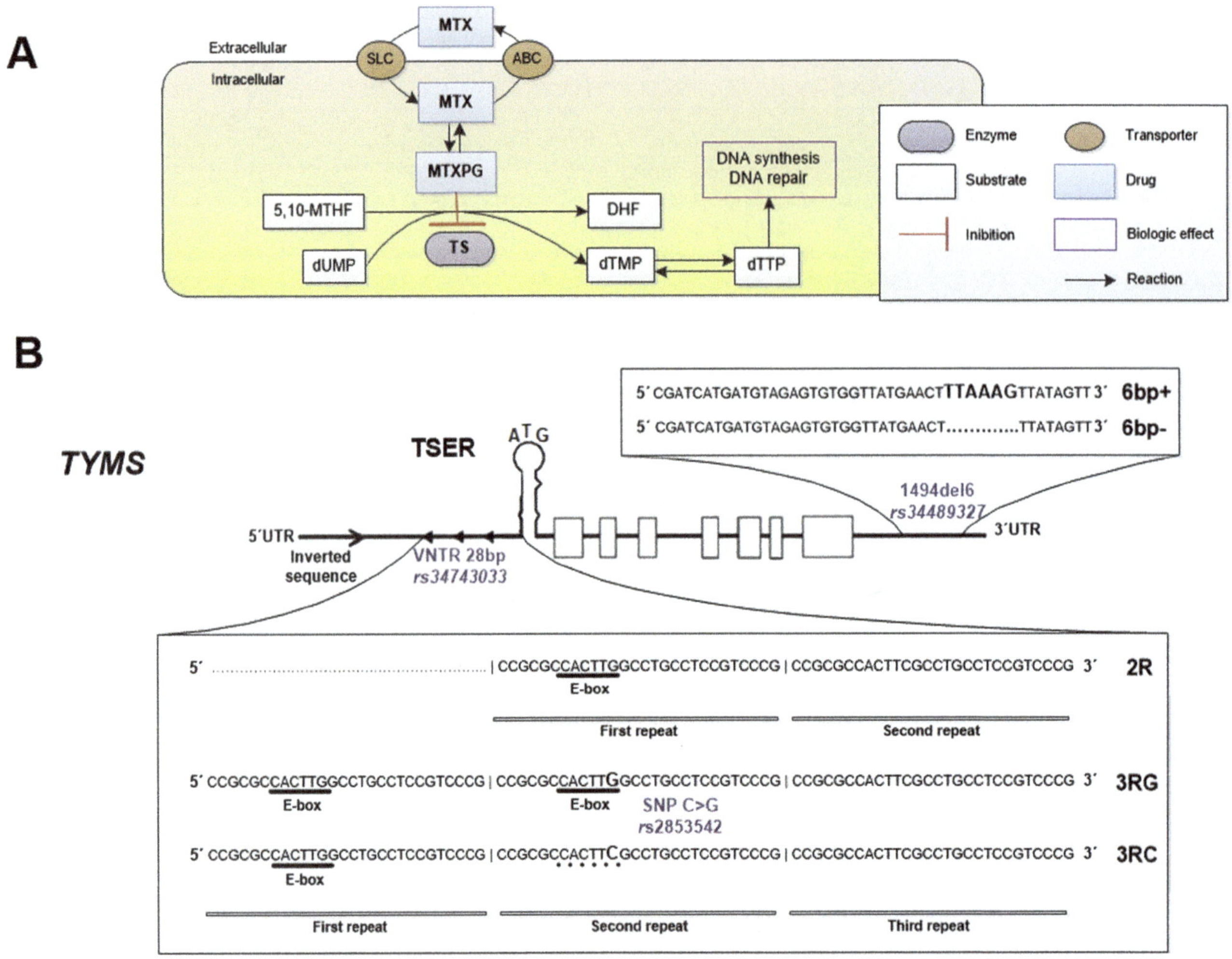

Figure 1. Part of MTX action mechanism in which thymidylate synthase (TS) is involved (A). MTX enters the cell after binding to folate transporters, mainly by solute carriers (SLC), and can be exported by members of the ATP-binding cassette (ABC) transporters family. To prevent MTX rapid efflux from cells and enhance its intracellular retention, MTX is polyglutamated by the enzyme folylpolyglutamyl synthase into MTX polyglutamates (MTXPGs) which inhibit TS activity. TS is a key protein for the *de novo* pyrimidine synthesis and is responsible for the simultaneous conversion of deoxyuridine monophosphate (dUMP) and 5,10-methylenetetrahydrofolate (5,10-MTHF) to deoxythymidine monophosphate (dTMP) and dihydrofolate (DHF). Subsequently, the dTMP is phosphorylated to deoxythymidine triphosphate (dTTP) and used for the DNA synthesis and repair. *TYMS* structure and location of VNTR 28 bp (rs34743033), SNP C>G (rs2853542) and 1494del6 (rs34489327) polymorphisms (B). 5,10-MTHF: 5,10-methylenetetrahydrofolate; A: adenine; ABC: ATP-binding cassette; bp: base pairs; C: cytosine; del: deletion; DHF: dihydrofolate; dTMP: deoxythymidine monophosphate; dTTP: deoxythymidine triphosphate; dUMP: deoxyuridine monophosphate; E-box: enhancer box; G: guanine; MTXPG: methotrexate polyglutamates; R: repeat; SLC: solute carrier; SNP: single nucleotide polymorphism; TS: thymidylate synthase (protein); TSER: thymidylate synthase enhancer region; T: thymine; *TYMS*: thymidylate synthase (gene); UTR: untranslated region; VNTR: variable number tandem repeat.

(complete LD) [32]. Possible haplotypes were tested for association with risk for non-response to MTX and for MTX-related toxicity by taking the most frequent haplotype as reference.

Statistical analysis

Statistical analyses were performed with either IBM SPSS Statistics for Windows, Version 20.0 (IBM Corp, Armonk, NY, USA), OpenEpi for Windows, Version 2.3.1 [33] and SNPStats software [30]. Genotype and allele frequencies were assessed and tested for Hardy-Weinberg equilibrium (HWE). All statistical tests were two-sided and a probability (p) value of 5% or less was considered as statistically significant. The Pearson Chi-square test or Fisher's exact test were used to compare the outcome variables and *TYMS* polymorphisms. The odds ratio (OR) and the correspondent 95% confidence intervals (CI) were calculated as a measure of the association between the categorical variables. To correct for multiple comparisons, Bonferroni's method was applied in order to control the false positive rate, and a significance level of $\alpha = 0.05/(n \text{ comparisons})$ was used [34]. Forest plot was performed using MedCalc software for Windows, Version 13.1.2 [35]. Multivariate analysis with binary logistic regression was used to identify which *TYMS* genotypes or haplotypes could predict the occurrence of non-response to MTX and MTX-related toxicity. This analysis was performed adjusting to potential confounding clinicopathological variables in three steps. In the first step patient-related variables (age, gender and smoking) were considered; in a second step, beyond patient-related variables, disease-related variables (diagnosis age and disease duration) were added; and in a third step, beyond patient and disease-related variables,

Table 1. *Thymidylate synthase* polymorphisms and methotrexate therapeutic outcome.

	MTX Response				MTX Toxicity			
	Response	Non-Response	p	OR (95% CI)	Non-Toxicity	Toxicity	p	OR (95% CI)
***TYMS* 28 bp VNTR (rs34743033)[#]**								
2R2R	19 (54.3)	16 (45.7)		Reference	25 (71.4)	10 (28.6)		Reference
2R3R	62 (49.6)	63 (50.4)	0.624	1.21 (0.57–2.56)	78 (62.4)	47 (37.6)	0.324	1.51 (0.67–3.41)
3R3R	21 (30.4)	48 (69.6)	**0.018**[¥]	2.71 (1.17–6.29)	50 (72.5)	19 (27.5)	0.911	0.95 (0.39–2.35)
2R carriers	81 (50.6)	79 (49.4)		Reference	103 (64.4)	57 (35.6)		Reference
3R3R	21 (30.4)	48 (69.6)	**0.005**[¥]	2.34 (1.29–4.27)	50 (72.5)	19 (27.5)	0.233	0.69 (0.37–1.28)
2R2R	19 (54.3)	16 (45.7)		Reference	25 (71.4)	10 (28.6)		Reference
3R carriers	83 (42.8)	111 (57.2)	0.208	1.59 (0.77–3.27)	128 (66.0)	66 (34.0)	0.529	1.29 (0.58–2.84)
2R allele	100 (51.3)	95 (48.7)		Reference	128 (65.6)	67 (34.4)		Reference
3R allele	104 (39.5)	159 (60.5)	**0.012**[¥]	1.61 (1.09–2.38)	178 (67.7)	85 (32.3)	0.647	0.91 (0.60–1.38)
TSER polymorphisms (rs2853542* and rs34743033)								
Functional 2R								
2R2R	19 (54.3)	16 (45.7)		Reference	25 (71.4)	10 (28.6)		Reference
2R3RC	32 (47.1)	36 (52.9)	0.487	1.34 (0.59–3.03)	44 (64.7)	24 (35.3)	0.492	1.36 (0.56–3.31)
3RC3RC	9 (31.0)	20 (69.0)	0.062	2.64 (0.94–7.39)	23 (79.3)	6 (20.7)	0.469	0.65 (0.20–2.08)
Functional 3R								
2R3RG	30 (52.6)	27 (47.4)		Reference	34 (59.6)	23 (40.4)		Reference
3RC3RG	6 (24.0)	19 (76.0)	**0.016**[¥]	3.52 (1.23–10.10)	16 (64.0)	9 (36.0)	0.710	0.83 (0.31–2.20)
3RG3RG	6 (40.0)	9 (60.0)	0.384	1.67 (0.52–5.30)	11 (73.3)	4 (26.7)	0.384[$]	0.54 (0.15–1.90)
2R allele	100 (51.3)	95 (48.7)		Reference	128 (65.6)	67 (34.4)		Reference
3RC allele	56 (37.1)	95 (62.9)	**0.008**[¥]	1.79 (1.13–2.82)	106 (70.2)	45 (29.8)	0.369	0.81 (0.50–1.31)
3RG allele	48 (42.9)	64 (57.1)	0.155	1.40 (0.86–2.30)	72 (64.3)	40 (35.7)	0.810	1.06 (0.63–1.78)
TSER polymorphisms grouped according to theoretically TS expression levels**								
Low expression	60 (45.5)	72 (54.5)		Reference	92 (69.7)	40 (30.3)		Reference
Median expression	36 (43.9)	46 (56.1)	0.824	1.07 (0.61–1.85)	50 (61.0)	32 (39.0)	0.189	1.47 (0.83–2.63)
High expression	6 (40.0)	9 (60.0)	0.687	1.25 (0.42–3.71)	11 (73.3)	4 (26.7)	1.000[$]	0.84 (0.25–2.79)
Low+Median expression	96 (44.9)	118 (55.1)		Reference	142 (66.4)	72 (33.6)		Reference
High expression	6 (40.0)	9 (60.0)	0.714	1.22 (0.42–3.55)	11 (73.3)	4 (26.7)	0.778[$]	0.72 (0.22–2.33)
Low expression	60 (45.5.)	72 (54.5)		Reference	92 (69.7)	40 (30.3)		Reference
Median+High expression	42 (43.4)	55 (56.7)	0.746	1.09 (0.64–1.85)	61 (62.9)	36 (37.1)	0.279	1.36 (0.78–2.36)
***TYMS* 1494del6 (rs34489327)**								
6bp+6bp+	61 (53.5)	53 (46.5)		Reference	78 (68.4)	36 (31.6)		Reference
6bp+6bp−	38 (39.2)	59 (60.8)	**0.038**	1.79 (1.03–3.10)	59 (60.8)	38 (39.2)	0.249	1.40 (0.79–2.46)
6bp−6bp−	6 (27.3)	16 (72.7)	**0.024**[¥]	3.07 (1.12–8.41)	19 (86.4)	3 (13.6)	0.122[$]	0.34 (0.10–1.23)

Table 1. Cont.

	MTX Response				MTX Toxicity			
	Response	Non-Response	*p*	OR (95% CI)	Non-Toxicity	Toxicity	*p*	OR (95% CI)
6bp+6bp+	61 (53.5)	53 (46.5)		Reference	78 (68.4)	36 (31.6)		Reference
6bp− carriers	44 (37.0)	75 (63.0)	**0.011**¥	1.96 (1.16–3.31)	78 (65.5)	41 (34.5)	0.641	1.14 (0.66–1.97)
6bp+ carriers	99 (46.9)	112 (53.1)		Reference	137 (64.9)	74 (35.1)		Reference
6bp−6bp−	6 (27.3)	16 (72.7)	0.078	2.36 (0.89–6.26)	19 (86.4)	3 (13.6)	0.055$	0.29 (0.08–1.02)
6bp+ allele	160 (49.2)	165 (50.8)		Reference	215 (66.2)	110 (33.8)		Reference
6bp− allele	50 (35.5)	91 (64.5)	**0.006**¥	1.76 (1.15–2.71)	97 (68.8)	44 (31.2)	0.578	0.89 (0.57–1.38)

Results are expressed in n (%). *p* value<0.05 was considered to be of statistical significance (highlighted in bold).
$Fisher's exact test used when number of cases of one cell was less than 5.
¥Statistically significant when *p* values were adjusted for multiple comparisons correction using Bonferroni's method (α = 0.05/n comparisons).
#3R4R genotype (n = 4) was excluded from analyses due to the low frequency.
*rs2853542 - *TYMS* SNP C>G on 3R allele.
**Genotypes theoretically associated with TS expression: a) high: 3RG3RG; b) median: 2R3RG and 3RC3RG; c) low: 2R2R, 2R3RC and 3RC3RC.
bp: base pairs; C: cytosine; del: deletion; G: guanine; OR: odds ratio; R: repeat; SNP: single nucleotide polymorphism; TS: thymidylate synthase (protein); TSER: *TYMS* enhancer region; *TYMS*: thymidylate synthase (gene); VNTR: variable number tandem repeat.

treatment-related variables (folic acid supplementation, corticosteroids therapy, use of NSAIDs, other concomitant DMARDs used and MTX administration characteristics - dose, treatment duration and administration route) were also considered.

Results

Population description

This study included follow-up data of 233 patients, 196 (84.1%) females and 37 (15.9%) males, with a mean age of 51±11.6 years old, of which 32 (13.7%) were smokers. Considering the disease-related variables, the mean age at diagnosis was 40.3±13.2 years old and the median disease duration was 7.0 years (0.3–51.0). All 233 (100.0%) patients were treated with MTX with a median dose of 15.0 mg/week (2.5–25.0), 118 (50.6%) complied regularly to folic acid supplementation, 188 (80.7%) were under corticosteroid therapy and 170 (73.0%) used NSAIDs.

Non-response to MTX (DAS28 >3.2 in two consecutive evaluations) was observed in 128 (54.9%) patients. Regarding disease activity, the mean for DAS28 was 4.2±1.3. MTX-related toxicity was registered in 77 (33.0%) patients. The observed ADRs were classified in SOCs disorders as follow: 58 (75.3%) gastrointestinal disorders (abdominal distension, diarrhea, dyspepsia, nauseas, stomach pain and/or vomiting); 9 (11.7%) skin and subcutaneous tissue disorders (alopecia, rash maculo-papular and rheumatoid nodulosis exacerbation); 5 (6.5%) hepatobiliary disorders (determined by transaminases serum elevation); and 5 (6.5%) respiratory, thoracic and mediastinal disorders (hypersensitivity pneumonitis). Since the number of cases in each SOCs disorders were small, the evaluation of *TYMS* polymorphisms with clinical relevance as possible biomarkers of MTX-related toxicity was performed for MTX-related overall toxicity.

TYMS genotype and haplotype analyses

Genotypes distribution of *TYMS* polymorphisms was in HWE (p>0.050) in the studied population. Frequencies of 28 bp VNTR alleles and genotypes were: 2R allele 41.8%; 3R allele 57.3%; 4R allele 0.9%; 2R2R 15.0% (n = 35); 2R3R 53.7% (n = 125); 3R3R 29.6% (n = 69); and 3R4R 1.7% (n = 4). Due to the low frequency of 3R4R genotype, it was excluded from the analyses. Considering TSER polymorphisms, genotypes distribution was: 2R allele 42.6%; 3RC allele 33.0%; 3RG allele 24.4%; 2R2R 15.3% (n = 35); 2R3RC 29.7% (n = 68); 2R3RG 24.9% (n = 57); 3RC3RC 12.6% (n = 29); 3RC3RG 10.9% (n = 25); and 3RG3RG 6.6% (n = 15). According to TS theoretical functional *status*, genotypes frequencies were: low expression 57.6% (n = 132); median expression 35.8% (n = 82); and high expression 6.6% (n = 15). Frequencies of 1494del6 alleles and genotypes were: 6pb+ allele 70.0%; 6bp− allele 30.0%; 6bp+6bp+ 48.9% (n = 114); 6bp+6bp− 41.6% (n = 97); and 6bp−6bp− 9.5% (n = 22).

Haplotype analysis revealed that 28 bp VNTR and 1494del6 polymorphisms were in LD (p<0.00001). Alleles 2R and 6bp+, and alleles 3R and 6bp− were the most linked ones (D' = 0.67 for both). The analysis demonstrated four haplotypes: 2R6bp+ 38.4%; 2R6bp− 4.1%; 3R6bp+ 31.7% and 3R6bp− 25.8%. TSER and 1494del6 polymorphisms were also in LD (p<0.00001). Alleles 2R and 6bp+ (D' = 0.67) and 3RG and 6bp− (D' = 0.48) demonstrated to be the most linked ones. This analysis showed six haplotypes: 2R6bp+ 38.4%; 2R6bp− 4.1%; 3RC6bp+ 22.7%; 3RG6bp+ 9.0%; 3RC6bp− 10.3%; and 3RG6bp− 15.5%.

Table 2. *Thymidylate synthase* haplotypes and methotrexate therapeutic outcome.

	MTX Response				MTX Toxicity			
TYMS Haplotypes	Response	Non-Response	p	OR (95% CI)	Non-Toxicity	Toxicity	p	OR (95% CI)
Based on *TYMS* 28 bp VNTR and *TYMS* 1494del6 polymorphisms								
2R6bp+	43.0	30.0		Reference	36.2	33.9		Reference
2R6bp−	6.0	7.4	0.360	1.70 (0.54–5.32)	5.7	10.2	0.190	2.20 (0.69–7.03)
3R6bp+	33.9	34.5	0.100	1.55 (0.92–2.60)	33.1	37.8	0.490	1.23 (0.69–2.20)
3R6bp−	17.1	28.1	**0.001**	2.54 (1.46–4.43)	25.0	18.1	0.320	0.74 (0.41–1.34)
Based on TSER and *TYMS* 1494del6 polymorphisms								
2R6bp+	43.2	30.2		Reference	36.2	34.8		Reference
2R6bp−	5.8	7.2	0.360	1.70 (0.55–5.24)	5.6	9.3	0.220	2.02 (0.66–6.20)
3RC6bp+	21.2	25.6	**0.041**	1.79 (1.03–3.12)	23.8	23.6	0.820	1.07 (0.59–1.95)
3RC6bp−	6.2	11.8	**0.013**	2.80 (1.25–6.25)	10.9	6.0	0.240	0.55(0.21–1.47)
3RG6bp+	12.5	8.7	0.880	1.06 (0.50–2.24)	9.3	13.3	0.300	1.53 (0.69–3.38)
3RG6bp−	11.1	16.5	**0.009**	2.39 (1.24–4.59)	14.2	13.0	0.810	0.92 (0.46–1.82)

Results are expressed in estimated frequencies (%) under linkage disequilibrium. p value<0.05 was considered to be of statistical significance (highlighted in bold).
bp: base pairs; C: cytosine; del: deletion; G: guanine; OR: odds ratio; R: repeat; TSER: *TYMS* enhancer region; *TYMS*: thymidylate synthase (gene); VNTR: variable number tandem repeat.

Table 3. Multivariate analysis of *thymidylate synthase* polymorphisms and clinical response to methotrexate.

	Patient-related		Patient+Disease-related		Patient+Disease+Treatment-related	
	p	OR (95% CI)	*p*	OR (95% CI)	*p*	OR (95% CI)
***TYMS* genotypes**						
***TYMS* 28 bp VNTR (rs34743033)**						
2R carriers		Reference		Reference		Reference
3R3R	**0.013**	2.23 (1.19–4.17)	**0.013**	2.24 (1.19–4.21)	0.135	1.99 (0.81–4.91)
TSER polymorphisms						
Functional 3R						
2R3RG		Reference		Reference		Reference
3RC3RG	0.069	2.90 (0.92–9.13)	0.071	2.91 (0.91–9.25)	0.203	2.70 (0.59–12.47)
***TYMS* 1494del6 (rs34489327)**						
6bp+6bp+		Reference		Reference		Reference
6bp− carriers	**0.003**	2.33 (1.32–4.10)	**0.003**	2.38 (1.34–4.23)	**0.016**	2.74 (1.21–6.23)
***TYMS* haplotypes**						
Based on *TYMS* 28 bp VNTR and *TYMS* 1494del6 polymorphisms						
2R6bp+		Reference		Reference		Reference
3R6bp−	**<0.001**	2.87 (1.59–5.19)	**<0.001**	2.92 (1.60–5.32)	**0.012**	2.68 (1.25–5.75)
Based on TSER and *TYMS* 1494del6 polymorphisms						
2R6bp+		Reference		Reference		Reference
3RC6bp+	**0.041**	1.81 (1.03–3.20)	**0.035**	1.86 (1.05–3.31)	0.090	1.85 (0.91–3.76)
3RC6bp−	**0.012**	2.97 (1.28–6.93)	**0.018**	2.75 (1.19–6.32)	**0.048**	2.89 (1.01–8.21)
3RG6bp−	**0.004**	2.78 (1.39–5.56)	**0.003**	3.06 (1.49–6.31)	**0.043**	2.60 (1.04–6.49)

P value<0.05 is considered to be of statistical significance (highlighted in bold).
Adjusted variables include: 1) patient-related variables (age, gender and smoking); 2) disease-related variables (diagnosis age and disease duration); and 3) treatment-related variables (folic acid supplementation, corticosteroids, non-steroidal anti-inflammatories, other concomitant disease-modifying antirheumatic drugs and methotrexate administration characteristics - dose, treatment duration and administration route). Genetic variables include: *TYMS* genotypes and *TYMS* haplotypes.
bp: base pairs; C: cytosine; del: deletion; G: guanine; OR: odds ratio; R: repeat; TSER: *TYMS* enhancer region; *TYMS*: thymidylate synthase (gene); VNTR: variable number tandem repeat.

TYMS genotypes and MTX therapeutic outcome

Table 1 reports the relation between *TYMS* polymorphisms and MTX therapeutic outcome both regarding MTX non-response and toxicity.

Non-response. In relation to 28 bp VNTR polymorphism, 3R allele was significantly associated with non-response to MTX when compared to 2R allele ($p = 0.012$, OR = 1.61). In addition, 3R homozygotes were associated with more than 2-fold increased risk for non-response to MTX when compared to 2R homozygotes ($p = 0.018$, OR = 2.71) and 2R carriers ($p = 0.005$, OR = 2.34) and remained significant after corrected for multiple comparisons. For TSER polymorphisms, 3RC allele shown to be associated with non-response to MTX when compared to 2R allele ($p = 0.008$, OR = 1.79). Furthermore, and attending to functional 3R, 3RC3RG was related with more than 3-fold increased risk for non-response to MTX when compared to 2R3RG ($p = 0.016$, OR − 3.52), which remained significant after multiple comparisons correction. Considering the 1494del6 polymorphism, 6bp− allele was significantly associated with non-response to MTX when compared to 6bp+ allele ($p = 0.006$, OR = 1.76). Moreover, and compared to 6bp+ homozygotes, 6bp+6bp− ($p = 0.038$, OR = 1.79), 6bp−6bp− ($p = 0.024$, OR = 3.07) and 6bp− carriers ($p = 0.011$, OR = 1.96) presented a statistically significant increased risk for non-response to MTX and, excepting for 6bp+ 6bp−, continued significant after correcting for multiple comparisons.

Toxicity. No statistically significant differences were observed in relation to *TYMS* genotypes and MTX-related overall toxicity.

TYMS haplotypes and MTX therapeutic outcome

Table 2 represents the relationship between *TYMS* haplotypes and MTX therapeutic outcome both regarding MTX non-response and toxicity.

Non-response. 3R6bp− haplotype was found significantly associated with non-response to MTX when compared to 2R6bp+ haplotype ($p = 0.001$, OR = 2.54). Moreover, 3RC6bp+, 3RC6bp− and 3RG6bp− haplotypes were statistically significant associated with non-response to MTX when compared to 2R6bp+ haplotype ($p = 0.041$, OR = 1.79; $p = 0.013$, OR = 2.80; and $p = 0.009$, OR = 2.39, respectively).

Toxicity. No statistically significant differences were observed in relation to *TYMS* haplotypes and MTX-related overall toxicity.

Multivariate analysis

Multivariate analysis was performed in three steps adjusting to potential confounding variables. Table 3 shows multivariate analysis results of *TYMS* genotypes and haplotypes and clinical response to MTX. Figure 2 resumes the impact of all potential confounding variables in the association of *TYMS* genotypes and haplotypes with clinical response to MTX. Regarding *TYMS* genotypes, results demonstrated that 6bp− carriers were statistically significant associated with more than 2-fold increased risk for

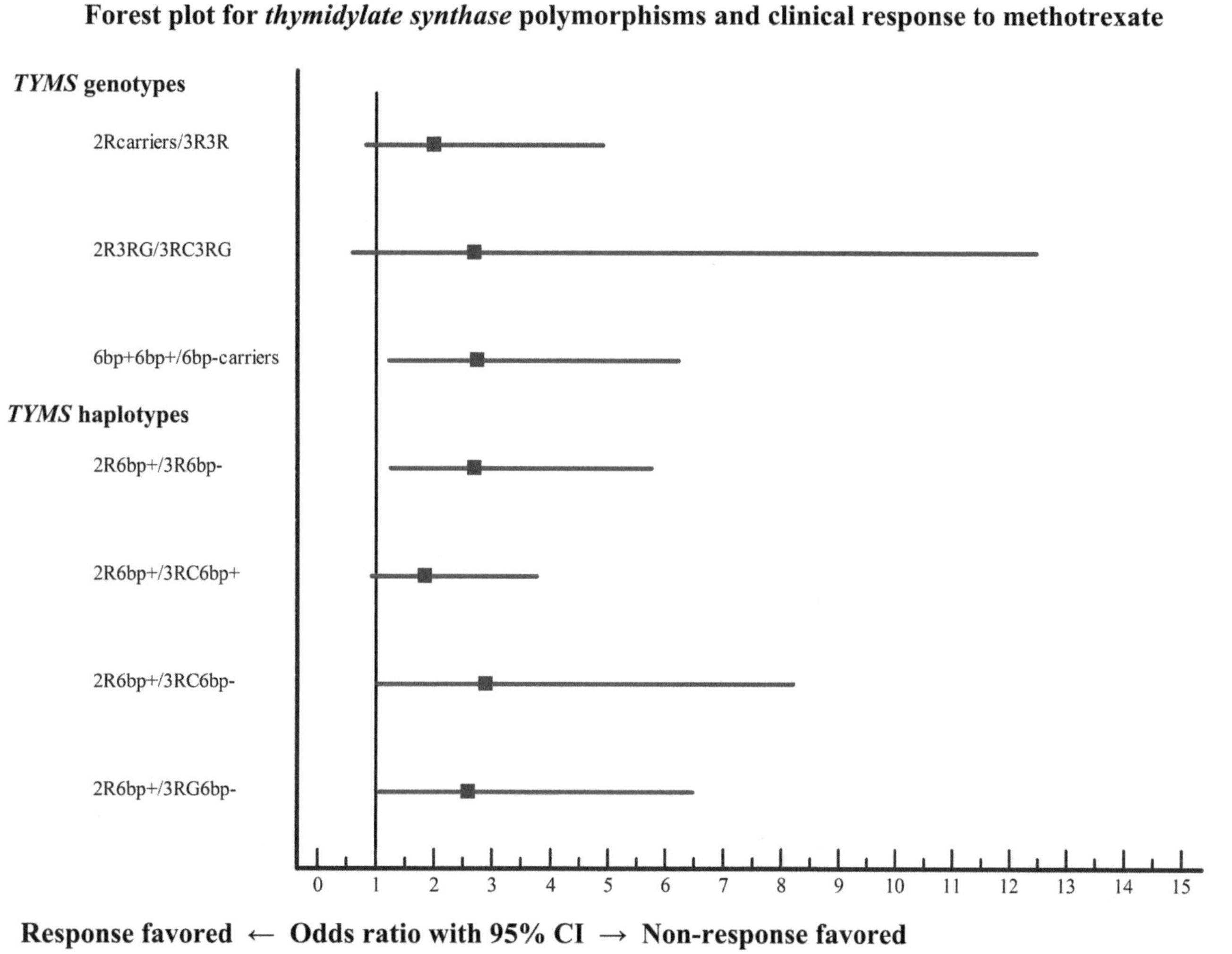

Figure 2. Forest plot of multivariate analysis in the association of *thymidylate synthase* genotypes and haplotypes with clinical response to methotrexate. Odds ratio and 95% confidence intervals are reported for clinical response to methotrexate. bp: base pairs; C: cytosine; CI: confidence interval; del: deletion; G: guanine; R: repeat; TYMS: thymidylate synthase (gene).

non-response to MTX when compared to 6bp+ homozygotes ($p = 0.016$, OR = 2.74). According to *TYMS* haplotypes, our results shown that haplotypes harboring simultaneously 3R and 6bp− alleles were statistically significant associated with almost 3-fold increased risk for non-response to MTX when compared to 2R6bp+ haplotype.

Discussion

Thymidylate synthase is a key enzyme for DNA synthesis and repair [11,12] inhibited by MTXPGs and, therefore, contributes for MTX antiproliferative and anti-inflammatory effects [10]. In fact, TS levels were found to be predictive of MTX therapeutic outcome [13,14]. Since genetic polymorphisms in *TYMS* have been associated with TS levels [6], in this study we aimed to elucidate the influence of *TYMS* polymorphisms (28 bp VNTR, SNP C>G and 1494del6) in MTX therapeutic outcome of Portuguese RA patients.

All patients enrolled in this study were recruited within a well-defined geographical area and were of Caucasian ethnicity, with gender and age at time of diagnosis distributions similar to other reported populations [36,37]. Genotypes distribution of *TYMS* polymorphisms was in HWE and was similar to those found for other Caucasian populations [21,38,39]. Nevertheless, and despite the potential of our results, possible study limitations include: 1) relatively reduced population size; 2) presence of other *TYMS* polymorphisms that possibly could alter TS expression or functionality; 3) limited screen of some important genes that codify other enzymes involved in MTX action mechanism.

TYMS genotypes and MTX therapeutic outcome

Non-response. Among our population and regarding 28 bp VNTR polymorphism, 3R allele was associated with risk for non-response to MTX, which increases in the presence of both 3R alleles, in accordance to previous studies [13,40]. Literature describes 3R allele as associated with higher TS levels [19,20] and TS levels as predictive of clinical response to MTX [13,40]. Moreover, 3R allele has been associated with higher MTX doses required [13] and higher RA disease activity [40]. Despite the significant univariate analysis results, multivariate analysis did not confirm them. Additionally, other studies demonstrated associations between 3R homozygotes and response to MTX [39] or showed no association [21,41–43]. It has been suggested by some authors that it is of greater importance to consider the SNP C>G on 3R allele and analyze the TSER polymorphisms instead of studying 28 bp VNTR polymorphism alone. 3RG allele was associated with higher transcriptional activity and translation efficiency due to its increased ability to complex with the USF protein [15,44]. Accordingly, the number of functional E-box in both 2R and 3RC alleles should be the same [6,15], which should reveal that patients with these genotypes would have similar TS expression and, consequently, a resembling clinical response. However, our results seem to demonstrate that 2R and 3RC alleles are different since 3RC3RG genotype was associated with over 3-fold increased risk for non-response to MTX when compared to 2R3RG. In addition, our results showed that 3RC allele was associated with non-response to MTX, when compared to 2R allele, and 3RC3RC genotype has a non-significant trend for non-response to MTX when compared to 2R2R genotype. Nevertheless, no statistically significant differences were observed attending to TSER polymorphisms grouped according to theoretically TS expression levels and to multivariate analysis. Moreover, a previous study demonstrated that non-response to MTX was associated to 3RG3RG patients [21]. Therefore, the putative relationship between TSER polymorphisms and clinical response to MTX outcome needs further clarification.

In relation to 1494del6 polymorphism, our results demonstrated that 6bp− allele was associated with non-response to MTX. Additionally, multivariate analysis showed that 6bp− carriers were associated with about 3-fold increased risk for non-response to MTX. *In vitro* studies have demonstrated that 6bp− allele has decreased mRNA stability and, thereby reduced TS expression [22,23], however, in other previously reported studies in RA Caucasian patients no association was observed [41]. Moreover, one study in Psoriasis, a disease where MTX is used in similar doses than RA, 6bp− allele demonstrated a trend for non-response, however, this study included Caucasian and non-Caucasian patients [45]. Studies in Asiatic patients have reported different results, some of them reported an association between 6bp− allele and response [13,43], while others reported no associations [42,46]. From all of these results it seems that ethnicity could be an important factor to predict the clinical response to MTX.

Toxicity. Regarding the occurrence of MTX-related overall toxicity, our results did not reach significance pertaining to TSER and 1494del6 polymorphisms, in accordance with previously reported studies [21,41,42,46,47]. Nevertheless, other studies reported significant associations of 28 bp VNTR polymorphism with MTX-related toxicity [38,48]. To the best of our knowledge this is the first report evaluating the influence of TSER polymorphisms in MTX-related toxicity in RA.

TYMS haplotypes and MTX therapeutic outcome

Non-response. Haplotypes may have a particular significance in regard to functionality or as genetic markers for unknown functional variants. Therefore, haplotype analysis was performed, to assess of possible consequences on the phenotype in the copresence of several variants of the same gene. As reported by others [6,39,49,50], *TYMS* polymorphisms were in LD, especially 2R6bp+ and 3RG6bp− haplotypes. Univariate haplotype analysis demonstrated that 3R6bp−, 3RC6bp+, 3RC6bp− and 3RG6bp− haplotypes (haplotypes harboring 3R allele for 28 bp VNTR, 3RC allele for TSER and 6bp− allele for 1494del6) were associated with almost 3-fold increased risk for non-response to MTX. Nevertheless, multivariate analysis showed that haplotypes harboring simultaneously 3R and 6bp− alleles (3R6bp−, 3RC6bp− and 3RG6bp−) were associated with non-response to MTX. This suggests a prominent role of the 3′-UTR polymorphism in predicting the clinical response to MTX and it seems that 6bp− allele can interact differently with 2R and 3R alleles, in agreement with Lurje *et al.* [51]. Additionally, our results suggested that the haplotype revealing more risk for non-response to MTX was 3RC6bp−, which combines the major risk alleles from the 5′UTR (3RC) and from the 3′UTR (6bp−). Only one study in RA has performed haplotype analysis, where an association between 3R6bp− haplotype and response to MTX was demonstrated [39]. Nevertheless, there are some important differences: no reference to SNP C>G; studied population included patients with early RA; and the study evaluated the impact in clinical response to MTX combined therapy with sulfasalazine. Thus, we propose that *TYMS* haplotype analysis should be used in future studies to elucidate the influence of *TYMS* in MTX therapeutic outcome, which could help to interpret these preliminary conflicting data.

Toxicity. Regarding MTX-related toxicity, no differences were observed attending to *TYMS* haplotypes. Despite it was expected that *TYMS* haplotypes follow the same tendency as *TYMS* genotypes, to the best of our knowledge no studies analyzed the *TYMS* haplotypes and the development of toxicity arising from MTX in RA.

The observed discrepancies among different studies could be explained by inter-study variability, ethnicity variability, samples sizes, variety of methods used to measure the MTX therapeutic outcome, different treatment regimens, and different genotyping protocols with limited quality of results. Therefore, functional TS studies in RA should be conducted to better understanding TS expression regulation mechanism and its putative importance in establishing more effective clinical therapeutic strategies when MTX is used in RA patients. To the best of our knowledge, this is the first report regarding the study of the association of *TYMS* polymorphisms with MTX therapeutic outcome in Portuguese RA patients. This study concluded that *TYMS* polymorphisms seem to be important to predict clinical response to MTX in RA patients; *TYMS* genotypes and haplotypes harboring 6bp− allele were associated with non-response to MTX; *TYMS* haplotypes harboring simultaneously 3R and 6bp− alleles seem to be predictors of non-response to MTX; and, to elucidate the role of *TYMS* on MTX therapeutic outcome full haplotypic information should be exploited. Despite the potential of our findings, translation into clinical practice requires larger and multicentric studies in order to clearly endorse the utility of these polymorphisms.

Acknowledgments

The authors wish to acknowledge to *Fundação para a Ciência e Tecnologia* (FCT) for the Doctoral Grant (SFRH/BD/64441/2009) for Aurea Lima and also to the nursing service of Rheumatology Day Hospital of São João Hospital Center and the physicians from the Rheumatology Department of São João Hospital Center, especially to Lucia Costa (MD.) and Francisco Ventura (MD. Ph.D.).

Author Contributions

Conceived and designed the experiments: AL VS MB RM. Performed the experiments: AL RA. Analyzed the data: AL VS. Contributed reagents/materials/analysis tools: AL HS RM. Wrote the paper: AL VS MB RA HS RM.

References

1. O'Dell JR (2004) Therapeutic strategies for rheumatoid arthritis. N Engl J Med 350: 2591–2602.
2. Mikuls TR, O'Dell J (2000) The changing face of rheumatoid arthritis therapy: results of serial surveys. Arthritis Rheum 43: 464–465.
3. Ranganathan P, McLeod HL (2006) Methotrexate pharmacogenetics: the first step toward individualized therapy in rheumatoid arthritis. Arthritis Rheum 54: 1366–1377.
4. Benucci M, Saviola G, Manfredi M, Sarzi-Puttini P, Atzeni F (2011) Cost effectiveness analysis of disease-modifying antirheumatic drugs in rheumatoid arthritis. A systematic review literature. Int J Rheumatol 2011: 845496.
5. Finckh A, Liang MH, van Herckenrode CM, de Pablo P (2006) Long-term impact of early treatment on radiographic progression in rheumatoid arthritis: A meta-analysis. Arthritis Rheum 55: 864–872.
6. Lima A, Azevedo R, Sousa H, Seabra V, Medeiros R (2013) Current approaches for TYMS polymorphisms and their importance in molecular epidemiology and pharmacogenetics. Pharmacogenomics 14: 1337–1351.
7. Lima A, Bernardes M, Sousa H, Azevedo R, Costa L, et al. (2013) SLC19A1 80G allele as a biomarker of methotrexate-related gastrointestinal toxicity in Portuguese rheumatoid arthritis patients. Pharmacogenomics.
8. Chan ES, Cronstein BN (2002) Molecular action of methotrexate in inflammatory diseases. Arthritis Res 4: 266–273.
9. Swierkot J, Szechinski J (2006) Methotrexate in rheumatoid arthritis. Pharmacol Rep 58: 473–492.
10. Kremer JM (2004) Toward a better understanding of methotrexate. Arthritis Rheum 50: 1370–1382.
11. Krajinovic M, Costea I, Primeau M, Dulucq S, Moghrabi A (2005) Combining several polymorphisms of thymidylate synthase gene for pharmacogenetic analysis. Pharmacogenomics J 5: 374–380.
12. Touroutoglou N, Pazdur R (1996) Thymidylate synthase inhibitors. Clin Cancer Res 2: 227–243.
13. Kumagai K, Hiyama K, Oyama T, Maeda H, Kohno N (2003) Polymorphisms in the thymidylate synthase and methylenetetrahydrofolate reductase genes and sensitivity to the low-dose methotrexate therapy in patients with rheumatoid arthritis. Int J Mol Med 11: 593–600.
14. Krajinovic M, Costea I, Chiasson S (2002) Polymorphism of the thymidylate synthase gene and outcome of acute lymphoblastic leukaemia. Lancet 359: 1033–1034.
15. Mandola MV, Stoehlmacher J, Muller-Weeks S, Cesarone G, Yu MC, et al. (2003) A novel single nucleotide polymorphism within the 5′ tandem repeat polymorphism of the thymidylate synthase gene abolishes USF-1 binding and alters transcriptional activity. Cancer Res 63: 2898–2904.
16. Mandola MV, Stoehlmacher J, Zhang W, Groshen S, Yu MC, et al. (2004) A 6 bp polymorphism in the thymidylate synthase gene causes message instability and is associated with decreased intratumoral TS mRNA levels. Pharmacogenetics 14: 319–327.
17. Zhu H, Deng FY, Mo XB, Qiu YH, Lei SF (2014) Pharmacogenetics and pharmacogenomics for rheumatoid arthritis responsiveness to methotrexate treatment: the 2013 update. Pharmacogenomics 15: 551–566.
18. Marsh S, McKay JA, Cassidy J, McLeod HL (2001) Polymorphism in the thymidylate synthase promoter enhancer region in colorectal cancer. Int J Oncol 19: 383–386.
19. Corre S, Galibert MD (2005) Upstream stimulating factors: highly versatile stress-responsive transcription factors. Pigment Cell Res 18: 337–348.
20. Marsh S (2005) Thymidylate synthase pharmacogenetics. Invest New Drugs 23: 533–537.
21. Jekic B, Lukovic L, Bunjevacki V, Milic V, Novakovic I, et al. (2013) Association of the TYMS 3G/3G genotype with poor response and GGH 354GG genotype with the bone marrow toxicity of the methotrexate in RA patients. Eur J Clin Pharmacol 69: 377–383.
22. Pullmann R Jr, Abdelmohsen K, Lal A, Martindale JL, Ladner RD, et al. (2006) Differential stability of thymidylate synthase 3′-untranslated region polymorphic variants regulated by AUF1. J Biol Chem 281: 23456–23463.
23. Zhang Z, Shi Q, Sturgis EM, Spitz MR, Hong WK, et al. (2004) Thymidylate synthase 5′- and 3′-untranslated region polymorphisms associated with risk and progression of squamous cell carcinoma of the head and neck. Clin Cancer Res 10: 7903–7910.
24. Aletaha D, Neogi T, Silman AJ, Funovits J, Felson DT, et al. (2010) 2010 rheumatoid arthritis classification criteria: an American College of Rheumatology/European League Against Rheumatism collaborative initiative. Ann Rheum Dis 69: 1580–1588.
25. Ortiz Z, Shea B, Suarez Almazor M, Moher D, Wells G, et al. (2000) Folic acid and folinic acid for reducing side effects in patients receiving methotrexate for rheumatoid arthritis. Cochrane Database Syst Rev: CD000951.
26. Ortiz Z, Shea B, Suarez-Almazor ME, Moher D, Wells GA, et al. (1998) The efficacy of folic acid and folinic acid in reducing methotrexate gastrointestinal toxicity in rheumatoid arthritis. A metaanalysis of randomized controlled trials. J Rheumatol 25: 36–43.
27. Prevoo ML, van 't Hof MA, Kuper HH, van Leeuwen MA, van de Putte LB, et al. (1995) Modified disease activity scores that include twenty-eight-joint counts. Development and validation in a prospective longitudinal study of patients with rheumatoid arthritis. Arthritis Rheum 38: 44–48.
28. U.S. department of health and human services (2010) Common Terminology Criteria for Adverse Events (CTCAE) Version 4.03. National Institutes of Health and National Cancer Institute.
29. Lima A, Seabra V, Martins S, Coelho A, Araujo A, et al. (2014) Thymidylate synthase polymorphisms are associated to therapeutic outcome of advanced non-small cell lung cancer patients treated with platinum-based chemotherapy. Mol Biol Rep.
30. Sole X, Guino E, Valls J, Iniesta R, Moreno V (2006) SNPStats: a web tool for the analysis of association studies. Bioinformatics 22: 1928–1929.
31. Excoffier L, Laval G, Schneider S (2005) Arlequin (version 3.0): an integrated software package for population genetics data analysis. Evol Bioinform Online 1: 47–50.
32. Schaid DJ, Rowland CM, Tines DE, Jacobson RM, Poland GA (2002) Score tests for association between traits and haplotypes when linkage phase is ambiguous. Am J Hum Genet 70: 425–434.
33. Sullivan KM, Dean A, Soe MM (2009) OpenEpi: a web-based epidemiologic and statistical calculator for public health. Public Health Rep 124: 471–474.
34. Bland JM, Altman DG (1995) Multiple significance tests: the Bonferroni method. BMJ 310: 170.
35. Schoonjans F, Zalata A, Depuydt CE, Comhaire FH (1995) MedCalc: a new computer program for medical statistics. Comput Methods Programs Biomed 48: 257–262.
36. Gibofsky A (2012) Overview of epidemiology, pathophysiology, and diagnosis of rheumatoid arthritis. Am J Manag Care 18: S295–302.
37. Rindfleisch JA, Muller D (2005) Diagnosis and management of rheumatoid arthritis. Am Fam Physician 72: 1037–1047.
38. Bohanec Grabar P, Logar D, Lestan B, Dolzan V (2008) Genetic determinants of methotrexate toxicity in rheumatoid arthritis patients: a study of polymorphisms affecting methotrexate transport and folate metabolism. Eur J Clin Pharmacol 64: 1057–1068.
39. James HM, Gillis D, Hissaria P, Lester S, Somogyi AA, et al. (2008) Common polymorphisms in the folate pathway predict efficacy of combination regimens containing methotrexate and sulfasalazine in early rheumatoid arthritis. J Rheumatol 35: 562–571.
40. Dervieux T, Furst D, Lein DO, Capps R, Smith K, et al. (2004) Polyglutamation of methotrexate with common polymorphisms in reduced folate carrier, aminoimidazole carboxamide ribonucleotide transformylase, and thymidylate synthase are associated with methotrexate effects in rheumatoid arthritis. Arthritis Rheum 50: 2766–2774.
41. Owen SA, Hider SL, Martin P, Bruce IN, Barton A, et al. (2012) Genetic polymorphisms in key methotrexate pathway genes are associated with response to treatment in rheumatoid arthritis patients. Pharmacogenomics J 13: 227–234.
42. Ghodke Y, Chopra A, Joshi K, Patwardhan B (2008) Are Thymidylate synthase and Methylene tetrahydrofolate reductase genes linked with methotrexate response (efficacy, toxicity) in Indian (Asian) rheumatoid arthritis patients? Clin Rheumatol 27: 787–789.
43. Inoue S, Hashiguchi M, Takagi K, Kawai S, Mochizuki M (2009) Preliminary study to identify the predictive factors for the response to methotrexate therapy in patients with rheumatoid arthritis. Yakugaku Zasshi 129: 843–849.
44. Kawakami K, Watanabe G (2003) Identification and functional analysis of single nucleotide polymorphism in the tandem repeat sequence of thymidylate synthase gene. Cancer Res 63: 6004–6007.
45. Campalani E, Arenas M, Marinaki AM, Lewis CM, Barker JN, et al. (2007) Polymorphisms in folate, pyrimidine, and purine metabolism are associated with efficacy and toxicity of methotrexate in psoriasis. J Invest Dermatol 127: 1860–1867.
46. Takatori R, Takahashi KA, Tokunaga D, Hojo T, Fujioka M, et al. (2006) ABCB1 C3435T polymorphism influences methotrexate sensitivity in rheumatoid arthritis patients. Clin Exp Rheumatol 24: 546–554.
47. Ranganathan P, Culverhouse R, Marsh S, Mody A, Scott-Horton TJ, et al. (2008) Methotrexate (MTX) pathway gene polymorphisms and their effects on MTX toxicity in Caucasian and African American patients with rheumatoid arthritis. J Rheumatol 35: 572–579.
48. Weisman MH, Furst DE, Park GS, Kremer JM, Smith KM, et al. (2006) Risk genotypes in folate-dependent enzymes and their association with methotrexate-related side effects in rheumatoid arthritis. Arthritis Rheum 54: 607–612.
49. Dotor E, Cuatrecases M, Martinez-Iniesta M, Navarro M, Vilardell F, et al. (2006) Tumor thymidylate synthase 1494del6 genotype as a prognostic factor in colorectal cancer patients receiving fluorouracil-based adjuvant treatment. J Clin Oncol 24: 1603–1611.
50. Lima A, Seabra V, Martins S, Coelho A, Araújo A, et al. (2014) Thymidylate synthase polymorphisms are associated to therapeutic outcome of advanced non-small cell lung cancer patients treated with platinum-based chemotherapy. Molecular Biology Reports: 1–9.
51. Lurje G, Zhang W, Yang D, Groshen S, Hendifar AE, et al. (2008) Thymidylate synthase haplotype is associated with tumor recurrence in stage II and stage III colon cancer. Pharmacogenet Genomics 18: 161–168.

Osteoprotegerin CGA Haplotype Protection against Cerebrovascular Complications in Anti-CCP Negative Patients with Rheumatoid Arthritis

Fernanda Genre[1☯], Raquel López-Mejías[1☯], Mercedes García-Bermúdez[2☯], Santos Castañeda[3], Carlos González-Juanatey[4], Javier Llorca[5], Alfonso Corrales[1], Begoña Ubilla[1], José A. Miranda-Filloy[6], Trinitario Pina[1], Carmen Gómez-Vaquero[7], Luis Rodríguez-Rodríguez[8], Benjamín Fernández-Gutiérrez[8], Alejandro Balsa[9], Dora Pascual-Salcedo[9], Francisco J. López-Longo[10], Patricia Carreira[11], Ricardo Blanco[1], Isidoro González-Álvaro[3], Javier Martín[2¶], Miguel A. González-Gay[1*¶]

1 Epidemiology, Genetics and Atherosclerosis Research Group on Systemic Inflammatory Diseases, Rheumatology Division, IDIVAL, Santander, Spain, **2** Instituto de Parasitología y Biomedicina López-Neyra, IPBLN-CSIC, Granada, Spain, **3** Department of Rheumatology, Hospital Universitario la Princesa, IIS-Princesa, Madrid, Spain, **4** Cardiology Division, Hospital Universitario Lucus Augusti, Lugo, Spain, **5** Department of Epidemiology and Computational Biology, School of Medicine, University of Cantabria, and CIBER Epidemiología y Salud Pública (CIBERESP), IDIVAL, Santander, Spain, **6** Division of Rheumatology, Hospital Universitario Lucus Augusti, Lugo, Spain, **7** Department of Rheumatology, Hospital Universitario Bellvitge, Barcelona, Spain, **8** Department of Rheumatology, Hospital Clínico San Carlos, Madrid, Spain, **9** Department of Rheumatology, Hospital Universitario La Paz, Madrid, Spain, **10** Department of Rheumatology, Hospital General Universitario Gregorio Marañón, Madrid, Spain, **11** Department of Rheumatology, Hospital Universitario 12 de Octubre, Madrid, Spain

Abstract

Introduction: Rheumatoid arthritis is an inflammatory disease with high incidence of cardiovascular disease due to accelerated atherosclerosis. Osteoprotegerin (OPG) has been associated with increased risk of atherosclerotic disease in the general population. Several polymorphisms in the *OPG* gene with functional effects on cardiovascular disease in non-rheumatic individuals have been described. Therefore, we aimed to analyze the effect of three of these functional *OPG* polymorphisms on the risk of cardiovascular disease in a large and well-characterized cohort of Spanish patients with rheumatoid arthritis.

Methods: Three *OPG* gene variants (rs3134063, rs2073618 and rs3134069) were genotyped by TaqMan assays in 2027 Spanish patients with rheumatoid arthritis. Anti-cyclic citrullinated peptide (anti-CCP) antibody testing was positive in 997 of 1714 tested. Also, 18.3% of the whole series had experienced cardiovascular events, including 5.4% with cerebrovascular accidents. The relationship between *OPG* variants and cardiovascular events was assessed using Cox regression.

Results: No association between *OPG* gene variants and cardiovascular disease was observed in the whole group of rheumatoid arthritis patients or in anti-CCP positive patients. Nevertheless, a protective effect of CGA haplotype on the risk of cardiovascular disease in general, and specifically in the risk of cerebrovascular complications after adjusting for sex, age at disease diagnosis and traditional cardiovascular risk factors was disclosed in anti-CCP negative patients (HR = 0.54; 95%CI: 0.31–0.95; p = 0.032 and HR = 0.17; 95%CI: 0.04–0.78; p = 0.022, respectively).

Conclusion: Our results indicate a protective effect of the *OPG* CGA haplotype on cardiovascular risk, mainly due to a protective effect against cerebrovascular events in anti-CCP negative rheumatoid arthritis patients.

Editor: Francesc Palau, Centro de Investigación Príncipe Felipe – CIPF, Spain

Funding: This study was supported by European Union FEDER funds and "Fondo de Investigación Sanitaria" (grants PI06/0024, PS09/00748 and PI12/00060) (Spain). This work was also partially supported by RETICS Programs RD12/0009 (RIER) from "Instituto de Salud Carlos III" (ISCIII) (Spain), and in part by grants from the European IMI BTCure Program. FG and BU are supported by funds from the RETICS Program (RIER) (RD12/0009/0013). RLM is a recipient of a Sara Borrell postdoctoral fellowship from the "Instituto de Salud Carlos III" at the Spanish Ministry of Health (Spain). The funders had no role in study design, data collection and analysis, decision to publish, or preparation of the manuscript.

Competing Interests: This study was funded in part by grants from the European IMI BTCure Program.

* Email: miguelaggay@hotmail.com

☯ These authors contributed equally to this work.

¶ MAGG and JM are co-senior authors on this work.

Introduction

Rheumatoid arthritis (RA) is a chronic inflammatory rheumatic disease associated with high incidence of cardiovascular (CV) morbidity and mortality compared to the general population [1–4], similarly to what occurs in type 2 diabetes [5,6]. Specifically, it has been shown a high incidence of coronary heart disease and a high rate of CV events in RA [7,8] due to accelerated atherosclerosis [9]. Besides traditional CV risk factors [4,10] and the magnitude and severity of the chronic inflammatory response [8], genetic factors located inside [8] and outside the Human Leukocyte Antigen (HLA) region [11,12] play a pivotal role in the development of atherogenesis in RA [13–15].

Osteoprotegerin (OPG) belongs to the TNF receptor superfamily and is implicated in bone remodeling and in the atherosclerotic process. This molecule acts as a decoy receptor for the receptor activator of nuclear factor-κB ligand (RANKL), inhibiting binding of RANKL to its receptor, RANK [16,17]. Binding of RANKL to OPG inhibits osteoclastogenesis, although it is also well known that both molecules are involved in vascular wall mineralization [16]. Additionally, OPG acts as a soluble neutralizing receptor of TNF-related apoptosis-inducing ligand (TRAIL), an anti-inflammatory molecule with anti-atherosclerotic properties [18–20]. Despite having a paradoxically protective effect on vascular calcification [21,22], OPG has been associated with increased risk of atherosclerotic disease in the general population [23].

The human *OPG* gene (also called *TNFRSF11B*) is located on chromosome 8q24. This gene is affected by genetic polymorphisms with functional consequences on CV disease and bone metabolism [24,25]. Recently, several groups have reported that a single-nucleotide OPG polymorphism (SNP) located in the 5′ UTR region (rs2073617), as well as one in exon 1 (rs2073618) and another in the promoter region (rs3134069) were associated with atherosclerosis and risk of cerebrovascular disease in non-rheumatic individuals [26,27].

Considering the functional involvement of the above mentioned *OPG* polymorphisms in the CV disease, in the present study we aimed to analyze the potential association of these gene variations on the risk of developing CV disease in a large and well-characterized cohort of patients with RA, also evaluating their combined effect on this risk.

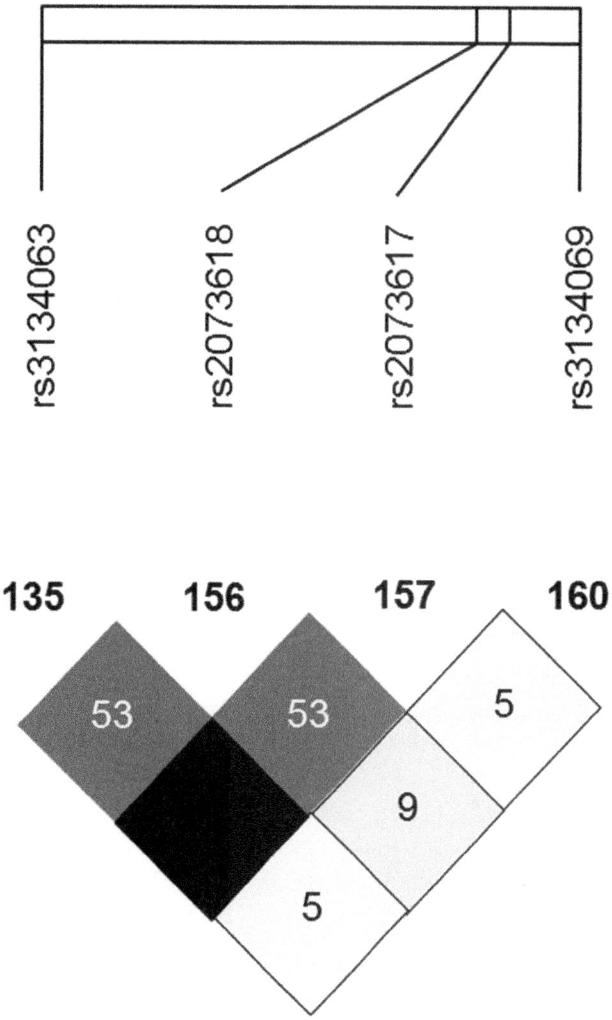

Figure 1. Linkage disequilibrium (LD) pattern of the OPG polymorphisms analyzed in our study (in European population). Data obtained by HapMap Project phase I, II and III and HAPLOVIEW (v.4.2) software. The LD between the OPG polymorphisms studied is shown in a scale from minimum (white) to maximum (black).

Materials and Methods

Patients and Study Protocol

A set of 2027 Spanish patients with RA were included in the present study. Blood samples were obtained from patients recruited from Hospital Lucus Augusti (Lugo), Hospital Marqués de Valdecilla (Santander), Hospital de Bellvitge (Barcelona), and Hospital Clínico San Carlos, Hospital La Paz, Hospital La Princesa, Hospital Gregorio Marañón and Hospital 12 de Octubre (Madrid). A subject's written consent was obtained according to the declaration of Helsinki, and the study was approved by the Ethics Committee of Galicia for Hospital Lucus Augusti, of Cantabria for Hospital Universitario Marqués de Valdecilla, of Cataluña for Hospital de Bellvitge and of Madrid for Hospital Clínico San Carlos, Hospital La Paz, Hospital La Princesa, Hospital Gregorio Marañón and Hospital 12 de Octubre. All the patients fulfilled the 1987 American College of Rheumatology (ACR) and also the 2010 classification criteria for RA [28,29]. In all the cases, the samples were assessed for *OPG* rs2073618 and rs3134069 polymorphisms. Additionally, rs2073617 polymorphism was assessed with a pre-designed Taqman probe for the rs3134063 polymorphism, which is in complete linkage disequilibrium with rs2073617 ($r^2 = 1$, http://hapmap.ncbi.nlm.nih.gov/). The linkage disequilibrium (LD) pattern of the *OPG* polymorphisms analyzed in our study obtained by HapMap Project phase I, II and III (in the European population) and HAPLOVIEW (v.4.2) software is displayed in **Figure 1**.

Information on the main demographic data, clinical characteristics, CV risk factors and CV events of patients enrolled in the study is shown in **Table 1**. Anti-cyclic citrullinated peptide (anti-CCP) antibody testing were positive in 997 (58.2%) of 1714 RA patients in whom this result was available. Three hundred and seventy (18.3%) of these 2027 patients had experienced CV events. One-hundred and nine (5.4%) of the 2027 patients had suffered cerebrovascular accidents. Definitions of CV events and traditional CV risk factors were established as previously described [8,30].

Genotyping

DNA from patients was obtained from peripheral blood using standard methods. The *OPG* rs3134063, rs2073618 and

Table 1. Demographic and clinical characteristics of the Spanish patients with RA included in the study.

Clinical Feature		**% (n/N)**
Patients		2027
Main characteristics	Age at the time of disease onset (years, mean ± SD)	51.2±14.9
	Follow-up (years, mean ± SD)	11.7±8.4
	Female gender	75.3 (1527/2027)
	Rheumatoid factor positive*	68.6 (1344/1958)
	Anti-CCP antibodies positive	58.2 (997/1714)
	Shared epitope positive	63.7 (726/1139)
Cardiovascular risk factors	Hypertension	38.2 (763/1996)
	Diabetes mellitus	12.3 (246/1995)
	Dyslipidemia	35.9 (713/1984)
	Obesity	18.8 (345/1840)
	Smoking habit	24.9 (491/1974)
Patients with cardiovascular events		18.3 (370/2027)
	Ischemic heart disease	8.9 (180/2020)
	Heart failure	5.6 (113/2027)
	Cerebrovascular accident	5.4 (109/2027)
	Peripheral arteriopathy	2.6 (52/2025)

CCP: cyclic citrullinated protein/peptide antibodies; RA: rheumatoid arthritis; SD: standard deviation.
*At least two determinations at different times were required.

rs3134069 polymorphisms were genotyped with TaqMan SNP pre-designed genotyping assays (C__32324439_10, C___1971047_1_, and C__27464534_10, respectively) in a 7900 HT real-time polymerase chain reaction (PCR) system, according to the conditions recommended by the manufacturer (Applied Biosystem, Foster City, CA, USA). Negative controls and duplicate samples were included to check the accuracy of genotyping.

Statistical analysis

The genotype data were checked for deviation from Hardy-Weinberg equilibrium (HWE) using http://ihg.gsf.de/cgi-bin/hw/hwa1.pl.

The relationship between alleles, genotypes and haplotypes, and CV events that occurred in the follow-up was tested using Cox regression adjusting for sex, age at RA diagnosis and traditional CV risk factors. For that purpose, we used the most frequent allele, genotype and haplotype as reference; the end of follow-up was the first date among the end of the study, date of death or date of CV event. Follow-up time was estimated as the difference between the

Table 2. Results of haplotype analysis in anti-CCP negative RA patients in association with CV events.

Variable		*HR (95% CI)*	p
	Age at RA diagnosis (by each year)	**1.08 (1.06–1.10)**	**<0.001**
	Hypertension	0.98 (0.63–1.51)	0.929
	Diabetes mellitus	**1.58 (1.01–2.45)**	**0.043**
	Obesity	1.22 (0.78–1.89)	0.390
	Dyslipidemia	1.27 (0.84–1.93)	0.254
	Smoking	1.12 (0.85–1.48)	0.417
Haplotypes (rs3134063, rs2073618, rs3134069)		*HR (95% CI)**	*p**
	TCA	1 (reference)	-
	TGA	0.94 (0.55–1.60)	0.825
	CCA	1.09 (0.68–1.76)	0.724
	CGA	**0.54 (0.31–0.95)**	**0.032**

CCP: cyclic citrullinated protein/peptide antibodies; CI: confidence interval; CV: cardiovascular; HR: hazard ratios; RA: rheumatoid arthritis.
*Adjusted for sex, age at RA diagnosis and traditional CV risk factors (hypertension, diabetes mellitus, dyslipidemia, obesity, and smoking habit).

Table 3. Association between *OPG* polymorphisms and the risk to develop cerebrovascular events in anti-CCP negative RA patients.

SNP	*Genotype/Allele*	*HR (95%CI)*	*p**
rs3134063	TT	1 (reference)	-
	CT	0.61 (0.21–1.76)	0.362
	CC	0.14 (0.02–1.23)	0.077
	T	1 (reference)	-
	C	0.52 (0.26–1.06)	0.072
rs2073618	CC	1 (reference)	-
	CG	0.60 (0.20–1.82)	0.368
	GG	**0.17 (0.03–0.89)**	**0.035**
	C	1 (reference)	-
	G	**0.45 (0.22–0.91)**	**0.025**
rs3134069	AA	1 (reference)	-
	AC	1.20 (0.26–5.64)	0.814
	CC	-	-
	A	1 (reference)	-
	C	1.18 (0.27–5.09)	0.823

CCP: cyclic citrullinated protein/peptide antibodies; CI: confidence interval; HR: hazard ratios; RA: rheumatoid arthritis.
*Adjusted for sex, age at RA diagnosis and traditional CV risk factors (hypertension, diabetes mellitus, dyslipidemia, obesity, and smoking habit).

RA diagnosis date and the end of follow-up. Patients without CV events in the follow-up time or dying by any non-CV cause were considered as censored. Results were expressed as hazard ratios (HR) with 95% confidence interval (CI). Statistical significance was defined as $p \leq 0.05$, and all analyses were performed using STATA statistical software 12/SE (Stata Corp., College Station, TX, USA).

Results

OPG rs3134063, rs2073618 and rs3134069 genotype distribution was in Hardy-Weinberg equilibrium ($p > 0.05$). Genotyping success was greater than 96% in all the cases. Genotype and allele frequencies of the *OPG* rs3134063, rs2073618 and rs3134069 polymorphisms were in agreement with the data of the HapMap project (http://hapmap.ncbi.nlm.nih.gov/).

There was no association between *OPG* gene variants and CV disease when all the RA patients were assessed as a whole. It was also the case for the group of anti-CCP positive patients (data not shown). Nevertheless, an association between *OPG* gene polymorphisms and CV disease was observed in those who were anti-CCP negative (**Table 2**). In this regard, even if no association was observed between allelic and genotypic *OPG* variants and CV disease (not shown), in the haplotype analysis, a protective effect of

Table 4. Results of haplotype analysis in anti-CCP negative RA patients in association with cerebrovascular events.

Variable		*HR (95% CI)*	p
	Age at RA diagnosis (by each year)	**1.09 (1.05–1.13)**	**<0.001**
	Hypertension	1.13 (0.51–2.48)	0.769
	Diabetes mellitus	**3.71 (1.78–7.70)**	**<0.001**
	Obesity	1.28 (0.58–2.83)	0.547
	Dyslipidemia	0.80 (0.39–1.66)	0.556
	Smoking	1.13 (0.68–1.88)	0.632
Haplotypes (rs3134063, rs2073618, rs3134069)		*HR (95% CI)**	*p**
	TCA	1 (reference)	-
	TGA	1.38 (0.56–3.42)	0.487
	CCA	1.16 (0.49–2.76)	0.740
	CGA	**0.17 (0.04–0.78)**	**0.022**

CCP: cyclic citrullinated protein/peptide antibodies; CI: confidence interval; CV: cardiovascular; HR: hazard ratios; RA: rheumatoid arthritis.
*Adjusted for sex, age at RA diagnosis and traditional CV risk factors (hypertension, diabetes mellitus, dyslipidemia, obesity, and smoking habit).

the CGA haplotype on the risk of CV disease after adjusting for sex, age at RA diagnosis and traditional CV risk factors was disclosed in the group of anti-CCP negative RA patients (HR = 0.54; 95% CI: 0.31–0.95; p = 0.032) (**Table 2**).

In a further step, we aimed to determine the type of CV event associated with *OPG* gene variants in the group of anti-CCP negative patients. Whereas no association was observed with ischemic heart disease (data not shown), we found an association of cerebrovascular complications with rs2073618 *OPG* polymorphism in this group of patients. In this respect, the risk of cerebrovascular complications was statistically decreased in the group of anti-CCP negative patients who carried the *OPG* rs2073618 GG genotype after adjusting the results for potential confounder factors (HR = 0.17; 95% CI: 0.03–0.89; p = 0.035) (**Table 3**). In accordance with these results, a protective effect of the CGA haplotype on the risk of cerebrovascular events after adjusting for sex, age at RA diagnosis and traditional CV risk factors was observed in the anti-CCP negative RA patients (HR = 0.17; 95% CI: 0.04–0.78; p = 0.022) (**Table 4**).

Discussion

RA is associated with increased morbidity and mortality attributable to accelerated atherosclerosis and CV events [7,9], in a similar fashion to what is observed in other autoimmune diseases such as diabetes [6]. Therefore, the search of new genetic markers which could help physicians to stratify RA patients according to their CV risk, leading thus to an improved and more personalized treatment, has become a main goal for several groups of research.

OPG has been proposed as a potential biomarker of CV risk since increased levels of this protein have been associated with CV disease [23]. In this regard, OPG levels were associated with biomarkers of endothelial activation (intercellular adhesion molecule-1), carotid intima-media wall thickness and carotid plaques in RA patients with severe disease [31]. In keeping with these results, an independent correlation of OPG levels with asymmetric dimethylarginine (ADMA), another biomarker of endothelial cell activation, has been disclosed in ankylosing spondylitis patients undergoing anti-TNF-α therapy [32]. Increasing concentrations of OPG have also been associated with the severity of CV complications in diabetic patients [33–37], reinforcing the idea that OPG could be used as a prognostic factor of CV disease in the clinic.

Several groups have described sequence variations in the gene that codifies OPG [24–26]. As elegantly proposed by Soufi et al., variations in the different regions of the *OPG* gene could combine to affect its transcription, intracellular trafficking or secretion [24]. To the best of our knowledge, our study constitutes the first attempt to assess the potential effect of rs3134063, rs2073618 and rs3134069 on the risk to develop CV disease in a large and well-characterized cohort of RA patients.

When we studied the influence of the different *OPG* polymorphisms on the risk of CV disease, we found a protective effect of the CGA haplotype on the risk of CV events in the subgroup of RA patients who were anti-CCP negative. Interestingly, further analyses disclosed that this protective effect was specifically focused on the risk of developing cerebrovascular accidents. In this regard, anti-CCP negative RA patients who carried an *OPG* rs20730618 GG genotype had a lower risk of developing cerebrovascular complications. Additionally, when we combined the different genetic variants to create haplotypes, our results also revealed a protective effect of the CGA haplotype (that carries the G allele of the *OPG* rs2073618) against the risk of cerebrovascular events in the subgroup of anti-CCP negative RA patients. These results are in line with those obtained by Biscetti et al., who found a synergistic effect of rs3134069, rs2073617 and rs2073618 associated with cerebral ischemic events in a cohort of diabetic patients [27]. Likewise, our results are in accordance with those obtained by Mankoč Ramuš et al., who also found an association between a combination of two of the *OPG* gene variants studied by our group and diabetic retinopathy [38].

Interestingly, the protective effect of the *OPG* CGA haplotype was found in anti-CCP negative but not anti-CCP positive RA patients. This could be explained by the fact that anti-CCP positive and anti-CCP negative RA are considered different disease entities [39]. Several pieces of evidence disclose that anti-CCP antibodies are markers of severe disease, and that risk factors such as HLA class II alleles associate with anti-CCP status and a more severe disease course [40]. In this regard, anti-CCP positive RA patients display a more severe radiological destruction and elevated DAS28 and CRP values than anti-CCP negative patients [39,41].

Taken all these considerations together, our results and those previously mentioned support the idea that, in an attempt to establish the potential association between multiple genetic markers in a chromosomal region and traits of interest in complex diseases, haplotype analyses appear to provide more useful information than the separate assessment of individual gene variants [27,38,42–45]. Hence, combination analyses often help to disclose hidden signals and may tag other regional polymorphic sites.

Conclusion

Our results indicate a protective effect of the *OPG* CGA haplotype on CV risk, mainly due to a protective effect against cerebrovascular events in anti-CCP negative RA patients.

Acknowledgments

We wish to thank all the patients with RA that participated to make this study possible.

We want to specially thank Rodrigo Ochoa, Sofía Vargas, M. Luisa López, M. Jesús Ibañez and Sara Olavarria for their technical assistance.

Author Contributions

Conceived and designed the experiments: FG RLM MGB JM MAGG. Performed the experiments: FG RLM MGB BU. Analyzed the data: FG RLM MGB JL. Contributed reagents/materials/analysis tools: FG RLM MGB SC CGJ JL AC BU JAMF TP CGV LRR BFG AB DPS FJLL PC RB IGA JM MAGG. Contributed to the writing of the manuscript: FG RLM MGB JM MAGG. Involved in the acquisition and interpretation of data and in revising it critically for important intellectual content: SC BFG.

References

1. Avina-Zubieta JA, Thomas J, Sadatsafavi M, Lehman AJ, Lacaille D (2012) Risk of incident cardiovascular events in patients with rheumatoid arthritis: a meta-analysis of observational studies. Ann Rheum Dis 71: 1524–1529.
2. Goodson N, Marks J, Lunt M, Symmons D (2005) Cardiovascular admissions and mortality in an inception cohort of patients with rheumatoid arthritis with onset in the 1980s and 1990s. Ann Rheum Dis 64: 1595–1601.
3. Solomon DH, Karlson EW, Rimm EB, Cannuscio CC, Mandl LA, et al. (2003) Cardiovascular morbidity and mortality in women diagnosed with rheumatoid arthritis. Circulation 107: 1303–1307.
4. Del Rincon ID, Williams K, Stern MP, Freeman GL, Escalante A (2001) High incidence of cardiovascular events in a rheumatoid arthritis cohort not explained by traditional cardiac risk factors. Arthritis Rheum 44: 2737–2745.

5. Peters MJ, van Halm VP, Voskuyl AE, Smulders YM, Boers M, et al. (2009) Does rheumatoid arthritis equal diabetes mellitus as an independent risk factor for cardiovascular disease? A prospective study. Arthritis Rheum 61: 1571–1579.
6. van Halm VP, Peters MJ, Voskuyl AE, Boers M, Lems WF, et al. (2009) Rheumatoid arthritis versus diabetes as a risk factor for cardiovascular disease: a cross-sectional study, the CARRE Investigation. Ann Rheum Dis 68: 1395–1400.
7. Wolfe F, Freundlich B, Straus WL (2003) Increase in cardiovascular and cerebrovascular disease prevalence in rheumatoid arthritis. J Rheumatol 30: 36–40.
8. Gonzalez-Gay MA, Gonzalez-Juanatey C, Lopez-Diaz MJ, Piñeiro A, Garcia-Porrua C, et al. (2007) HLA-DRB1 and persistent chronic inflammation contribute to cardiovascular events and cardiovascular mortality in patients with rheumatoid arthritis. Arthritis Rheum 57: 125–132.
9. Gonzalez-Gay MA, Gonzalez-Juanatey C, Martin J (2005) Rheumatoid arthritis: a disease associated with accelerated atherogenesis. Semin Arthritis Rheum 35: 8–17.
10. Dessein PH, Joffe BI, Veller MG, Stevens BA, Tobias M, et al. (2005) Traditional and nontraditional cardiovascular risk factors are associated with atherosclerosis in rheumatoid arthritis. J Rheumatol 32: 435–442.
11. García-Bermúdez M, López-Mejías R, Genre F, Castañeda S, González-Juanatey C, et al. (2013) SMAD3 rs17228212 gene polymorphism is associated with reduced risk to cerebrovascular accidents and subclinical atherosclerosis in anti-CCP negative Spanish rheumatoid arthritis patients. PLoS One 8: e77695.
12. López-Mejías R, García-Bermúdez M, González-Juanatey C, Castañeda S, Miranda-Filloy JA, et al. (2012) NFKB1-94ATTG ins/del polymorphism (rs28362491) is associated with cardiovascular disease in patients with rheumatoid arthritis. Atherosclerosis 224: 426–429.
13. Gonzalez-Gay MA, Gonzalez-Juanatey C, Piñeiro A, Garcia-Porrua C, Testa A, et al. (2005) High-grade C-reactive protein elevation correlates with accelerated atherogenesis in patients with rheumatoid arthritis. J Rheumatol 32: 1219–1223.
14. Del Rincón I, Williams K, Stern MP, Freeman GL, O'Leary DH, et al. (2003) Association between carotid atherosclerosis and markers of inflammation in rheumatoid arthritis patients and healthy subjects. Arthritis Rheum 48: 1833–1840.
15. Rodríguez-Rodríguez L, López-Mejías R, García-Bermúdez M, González-Juanatey C, González-Gay MA, et al. (2012) Genetic markers of cardiovascular disease in rheumatoid arthritis. Mediators Inflamm 2012: 574817.
16. Hofbauer LC, Schoppet M (2004) Clinical implications of the osteoprotegerin/RANKL/RANK system for bone and vascular diseases. JAMA 292: 490–495.
17. Van Campenhout A, Golledge J (2009) Osteoprotegerin, vascular calcification and atherosclerosis. Atherosclerosis 204: 321–329.
18. Secchiero P, Corallini F, Beltrami AP, Ceconi C, Bonasia V, et al. (2010) An imbalanced OPG/TRAIL ratio is associated to severe acute myocardial infarction. Atherosclerosis 210: 274–277.
19. Secchiero P, Rimondi E, di Iasio MG, Agnoletto C, Melloni E, et al. (2013) C-reactive protein downregulates TRAIL expression in human peripheral monocytes via an Egr-1-dependent pathway. Clin Cancer Res 19: 1949–1959.
20. Di Bartolo BA, Cartland SP, Harith HH, Bobryshev YV, Schoppet M, et al. (2013) TRAIL-deficiency accelerates vascular calcification in atherosclerosis via modulation of RANKL. PLoS One 8: e74211.
21. Callegari A, Coons ML, Ricks JL, Yang HL, Gross TS, et al. (2013) Bone marrow- or vessel wall-derived osteoprotegerin is sufficient to reduce atherosclerotic lesion size and vascular calcification. Arterioscler Thromb Vasc Biol 33: 2491–2500.
22. Morony S, Tintut Y, Zhang Z, Cattley RC, Van G, et al. (2008) Osteoprotegerin inhibits vascular calcification without affecting atherosclerosis in ldlr (−/−) mice. Circulation 117: 411–420.
23. Kiechl S, Schett G, Wenning G, Redlich K, Oberhollenzer M, et al. (2004) Osteoprotegerin is a risk factor for progressive atherosclerosis and cardiovascular disease. Circulation 109: 2175–2180.
24. Soufi M, Schoppet M, Sattler AM, Herzum M, Maisch B, et al. (2004) Osteoprotegerin gene polymorphisms in men with coronary artery disease. J Clin Endocrinol Metab 89: 3764–3768.
25. Roshandel D, Holliday KL, Pye SR, Ward KA, Boonen S, et al. (2011) Influence of polymorphisms in the RANKL/RANK/OPG signaling pathway on volumetric bone mineral density and bone geometry at the forearm in men. Calcif Tissue Int 89: 446–455.
26. Straface G, Biscetti F, Pitocco D, Bertoletti G, Misuraca M, et al. (2011) Assessment of the genetic effects of polymorphisms in the osteoprotegerin gene, TNFRSF11B, on serum osteoprotegerin levels and carotid plaque vulnerability. Stroke 42: 3022–3028.
27. Biscetti F, Straface G, Giovannini S, Santoliquido A, Angelini F, et al. (2013) Association between TNFRSF11B gene polymorphisms and history of ischemic stroke in Italian diabetic patients. Hum Genet 132: 49–55.
28. Arnett FC, Edworthy SM, Bloch DA, McShane DJ, Fries JF, et al. (1988) The American Rheumatism Association 1987 revised criteria for the classification of rheumatoid arthritis. Arthritis Rheum 31: 315–324.
29. Aletaha D, Neogi T, Silman AJ, Funovits J, Felson DT, et al. (2010) 2010 Rheumatoid arthritis classification criteria: an American College of Rheumatology/European League Against Rheumatism collaborative initiative. Arthritis Rheum 62: 2569–2581.
30. Gonzalez-Juanatey C, Llorca J, Martin J, Gonzalez-Gay MA (2009) Carotid intima-media thickness predicts the development of cardiovascular events in patients with rheumatoid arthritis. Semin Arthritis Rheum 38: 366–371.
31. Dessein PH, López-Mejias R, González-Juanatey C, Genre F, Miranda-Filloy JA, et al. (2014) Independent Relationship of Osteoprotegerin Concentrations with Endothelial Activation and Carotid Atherosclerosis in Patients with Severe Rheumatoid Arthritis. J Rheumatol 41: 429–436.
32. Genre F, López-Mejías R, Miranda-Filloy JA, Ubilla B, Carnero-López B, et al. (2014) Osteoprotegerin correlates with disease activity and endothelial activation in non-diabetic ankylosing spondylitis patients undergoing TNF-α antagonist therapy. Clin Exp Rheumatol: In press.
33. Chen WJ, Rijzewijk LJ, van der Meer RW, Heymans MW, van Duinkerken E, et al. (2011) Association of plasma osteoprotegerin and adiponectin with arterial function, cardiac function and metabolism in asymptomatic type 2 diabetic men. Cardiovasc Diabetol 10: 67.
34. Jorsal A, Tarnow L, Flyvbjerg A, Parving HH, Rossing P, et al. (2008) Plasma osteoprotegerin levels predict cardiovascular and all-cause mortality and deterioration of kidney function in type 1 diabetic patients with nephropathy. Diabetologia 51: 2100–2107.
35. Anand DV, Lahiri A, Lim E, Hopkins D, Corder R (2006) The relationship between plasma osteoprotegerin levels and coronary artery calcification in uncomplicated type 2 diabetic subjects. J Am Coll Cardiol 47: 1850–1857.
36. Rasmussen LM, Tarnow L, Hansen TK, Parving HH, Flyvbjerg A (2006) Plasma osteoprotegerin levels are associated with glycaemic status, systolic blood pressure, kidney function and cardiovascular morbidity in type 1 diabetic patients. Eur J Endocrinol 154: 75–81.
37. Bjerre M (2013) Osteoprotegerin (OPG) as a biomarker for diabetic cardiovascular complications. Springerplus 2: 658.
38. Mankoč Ramuš S, Kumše T, Globočnik Petrovič M, Petrovič D, Cilenšek I (2013) SNP rs2073618 of the osteoprotegerin gene is associated with diabetic retinopathy in Slovenian patients with type 2 diabetes. Biomed Res Int 2013: 364073.
39. van der Helm-van Mil AH, Verpoort KN, Breedveld FC, Toes RE, Huizinga TW (2005) Antibodies to citrullinated proteins and differences in clinical progression of rheumatoid arthritis. Arthritis Res Ther 7(5): R949–958.
40. van Gaalen FA, van Aken J, Huizinga TW, Schreuder GM, Breedveld FC, et al. (2004) Association between HLA class II genes and autoantibodies to cyclic citrullinated peptides (CCPs) influences the severity of rheumatoid arthritis. Arthritis Rheum 50(7): 2113–2121.
41. del Val del Amo N, Ibanez Bosch R, Fito Manteca C, Gutierrez Polo R, Loza Cortina E (2006) Anti-cyclic citrullinated peptide antibody in rheumatoid arthritis: relation with disease aggressiveness. Clin Exp Rheumatol 24(3): 281–286.
42. Zhao H, Pfeiffer R, Gail MH (2003) Haplotype analysis in population genetics and association studies. Pharmacogenomics 4: 171–178.
43. Morris RW, Kaplan NL (2002) On the advantage of haplotype analysis in the presence of multiple disease susceptibility alleles. Genet Epidemiol 23: 221–233.
44. Martin ER, Lai EH, Gilbert JR, Rogala AR, Afshari AJ, et al. (2000) SNPing away at complex diseases: analysis of single-nucleotide polymorphisms around APOE in Alzheimer disease. Am J Hum Genet 67: 383–394.
45. Drysdale CM, McGraw DW, Stack CB, Stephens JC, Judson RS, et al. (2000) Complex promoter and coding region beta 2-adrenergic receptor haplotypes alter receptor expression and predict in vivo responsiveness. Proc Natl Acad Sci USA 97: 10483–10488.

Divergent Gene Activation in Peripheral Blood and Tissues of Patients with Rheumatoid Arthritis, Psoriatic Arthritis and Psoriasis following Infliximab Therapy

Alexander Rosenberg[1], Hongtao Fan[3], Yahui G. Chiu[1], Rebecca Bolce[3], Darren Tabechian[1], Rick Barrett[1], Sharon Moorehead[1], Frédéric Baribaud[3], Hao Liu[3], Nancy Peffer[3], David Shealy[3], Edward M. Schwarz[2], Christopher T. Ritchlin[1,2]*

1 Division of Allergy, Immunology and Rheumatology, University of Rochester Medical Center, Rochester, NY, United States of America, **2** The Center for Musculoskeletal Research, University of Rochester Medical Center, Rochester, NY, United States of America, **3** Janssen Research and Development LLC, Spring House, PA, United States of America

Abstract

Objective: The immune inflammatory disorders rheumatoid arthritis (RA), psoriatic arthritis (PsA) and psoriasis (Ps) share common pathologic features and show responsiveness to anti-tumor necrosis factor (TNF) agents yet they are phenotypically distinct. The aim of this study was to examine if anti-TNF therapy is associated with divergent gene expression profiles in circulating cells and target tissues of patients with these diseases.

Methods: Peripheral blood $CD14^+$ and $CD14^-$ cells were isolated from 9 RA, 12 PsA and 10 Ps patients before and after infliximab (IFX) treatment. Paired synovial (n = 3, RA, PsA) and skin biopsies (n = 5, Ps) were also collected. Gene expression was analyzed by microarrays.

Results: 26 out of 31 subjects responded to IFX. The transcriptional response of $CD14^+$ cells to IFX was unique for the three diseases, with little overlap (<25%) in significantly changed gene lists (with PsA having the largest number of changed genes). In Ps, altered gene expression was more pronounced in lesional skin (relative to paired, healthy skin) compared to blood (relative to healthy controls). Marked suppression of up-regulated genes in affected skin was noted 2 weeks after therapy but the expression patterns differed from uninvolved skin. Divergent patterns of expression were noted between the blood cells and skin or synovial tissues in individual patients. Functions that promote cell differentiation, proliferation and apoptosis in all three diseases were enriched. RA was enriched in functions in $CD14^-$ cells, PsA in $CD14^+$ cells and Ps in both $CD14^+$ and $CD14^-$ cells, however, the specific functions showed little overlap in the 3 disorders.

Conclusion: Divergent patterns of altered gene expression are observed in RA, PsA and Ps patients in blood cells and target organs in IFX responders. Differential gene expression profiles in the blood do not correlate with those in target organs.

Editor: Paul Proost, University of Leuven, Rega Institute, Belgium

Funding: This work was funded by Janssen R&D, LLC. Authors who were employed by Janssen R&D, LLC generated the microarray data and contributed to study design, data analysis and manuscript preparation.

Competing Interests: FB, HL, NP and DS are employees of Janssen R&D Johnson & Johnson, (JNJ) and own stock in JNJ. R. Bolce and HF were employees of Janssen R&D and held stock in JNJ. AR holds stock in JNJ. R. Barrett is now employed by JNJ. CTR is a consultant for Janssen and was the first author on a recent trial that they sponsored. DT, SM, EMS, YGC and have no additional competing interests.

* Email: Christopher_Ritchlin@urmc.rochester.edu

Introduction

Immune mediated inflammatory disorders are a group of diseases that share several common features including pathologic mechanisms characterized by proliferation and accumulation of immune cells, increased release of TNF and other cytokines and altered tissue remodeling. Other common features include cardiovascular and metabolic comorbidities and responsiveness to anti-Tumor Necrosis Factor (TNF) agents [1–3]. While TNF blockade has proven to be a highly effective treatment for rheumatoid arthritis (RA), psoriatic arthritis (PsA) and psoriasis (Ps), three of the most prevalent immune mediated inflammatory disorders, recent evidence indicate that each disease arises by distinct pathophysiologic mechanisms. For example, RA is strongly linked to MHC class II genes and citrullinated autoantibodies with pathogenic potential whereas PsA and Ps share strong MHC Class I associations and disease-specific antibodies have not been identified [4–6]. From a therapeutic perspective, agents that target B and T cells are highly effective in RA [7] but not in PsA or Ps [8,9], and methotrexate, a cornerstone drug in RA and Ps, is not effective in PsA [8–10]. Lastly, molecules in the IL-23/Th17 pathway are important targets in Ps [11,12] and PsA [13] but do not show great promise in RA [14].

A central question that remains to be addressed is whether TNF inhibition has divergent effects on key gene networks in these three diseases. Over the past decade, investigators have turned to microarray analytic techniques of peripheral blood cells and target tissues (synovium, skin) to examine cross-sectional (compared to control samples) and longitudinal (before and after therapy) gene expression [15]. From these studies, several fundamental insights emerged. First, the molecular network in the immune mediated inflammatory disorders is far more complex than expected [16]. Second, cross-sectional differential gene expression is much lower in blood cells and in specific cell lineages compared to whole tissues [15]. Third, gene expression signatures in blood cells and synovial biopsies are heterogeneous and very patient-specific [17]. Fourth, to date, no pre-treatment gene expression profile in blood or tissue can accurately and reliably predict response to anti-TNF therapy in any of these three diseases [18–20]. Despite these caveats, microarray studies in autoimmune disorders (multiple sclerosis, SLE, Crohn's disease, ulcerative colitis, juvenile rheumatoid arthritis and type 1 diabetes) reveal shared perturbations of common cellular processes, particularly apoptosis, regulation of cytokines and T cell activation [21].

Taken together, microarray studies reveal a complex, heterogeneous immune inflammatory response in the immune mediated inflammatory diseases yet common signatures, as outlined above, are characteristic of specific autoimmune diseases. Given the marked effects of TNF inhibition on patient reported outcomes, systemic inflammation and tissue remodeling in RA, PsA and Ps, genomic analysis of cells and tissues before and after treatment has the potential to unveil pivotal overlapping and disease-specific transcriptional events in disease pathogenesis. We hypothesize that TNF inhibition will result in differential effects on gene expression in the blood cells and target tissues that will be specific to each disorder-RA, PsA and Ps. To examine this hypothesis, we analyzed cells associated with innate immunity ($CD14^+$ monocytes) and cells primarily associated with acquired immune responses ($CD14^-$ T and B lymphocytes) separately and compared gene expression in the blood to profiles observed in target tissues (synovium, skin) before and after IFX therapy.

Patients and Methods

Patients

Between April 2007 and June 2009, 31 patients with active RA, PsA and Ps who were naïve to anti-TNF agents, were recruited from the Faculty Rheumatology Clinics at the University of Rochester Medical Center after informed, written consent was obtained in a protocol approved by the Research Subjects Review Board at the University of Rochester Medical Center. Of the 31 subjects, 9 had active RA [22] and 12 had PsA [23] despite treatment with Disease Modifying Anti-Rheumatic Drugs (DMARDs). Also, 10 patients with extensive Ps (>5% Body Surface Area, BSA) documented by a dermatologist, were enrolled and they were examined by a rheumatologist to exclude the presence of inflammatory arthritis (see Table 1 and Figure 1). Nineteen healthy controls were also recruited.

A Disease Activity-C Reactive Protein (DAS-CRP) score was calculated based on a 28-joint count performed on the RA and PsA patients at baseline, week 2 and week 10 [24] and a Psoriasis Area and Severity Index (PASI) score [25] was obtained on the Ps subjects at the same time points; baseline and 10 week scores are shown in Figure 1. Patients were considered non-responders if the improvement in DAS28<1.2 (if the endpoint DAS28>5.1) or if the improvement in DAS28<0.6 (if the endpoint DAS28<5.1). In a similar fashion, we used the PASI50 (<50% reduction in PASI) to determine non-responders in our Ps subjects.

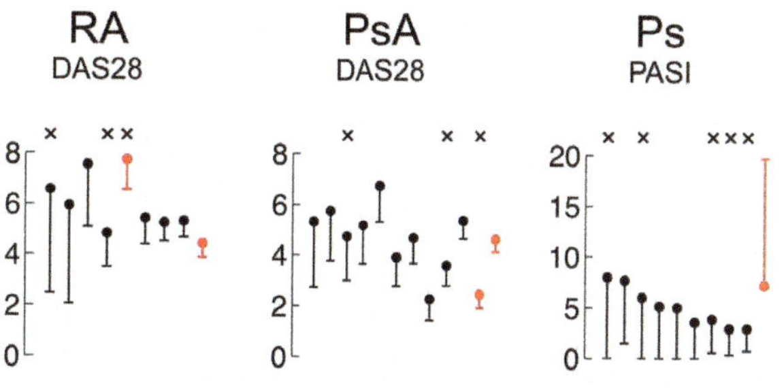

Figure 1. Disease activity before and after IFX for all RA, PsA and Ps subjects in study. Closed circles and horizontal line segments represent disease activity at baseline and 10 weeks post IFX, respectively. For RA and PsA, x's above the plots indicate patients that donated knee biopsy at baseline and 10 weeks post IFX. For Ps, they indicate patients that donated lesional and non-lesional skin at baseline as well as lesional skin 2 weeks post IFX. Red indicates IFX non-responders. For RA and PsA, a non-responder had an improvement in DAS28 of less than 1.2 (if the endpoint DAS28>5.1) or less than 0.6 (if the endpoint DAS28<5.1). For Ps, a non-responder had <50% reduction in PASI due to the treatment.

Skin and synovial biopsies

4 mm punch biopsies were performed on involved and uninvolved skin at baseline in 5 Ps patients. A repeat biopsy was performed at week 2 after IFX therapy at a site adjacent to the baseline biopsy of involved skin. Synovial biopsies were performed on the knee of 3 RA and 3 PsA subjects with a Parker Pearson biopsy needle (Dyna Medical, London, Canada) under ultrasound guidance at baseline and repeated on the same knee at week 10. Several synovial biopsy specimens (6–10) were retrieved in each knee from areas of inflamed synovium and the samples were pooled for transcriptome analysis from each patient.

Blood Sampling for RNA isolation

20 mL of blood was collected from registered subjects at baseline, week 2 and week 10 and purified by ficol gradient. $CD14^+$ cells were positively selected by Miltenyi, anti-CD14 magnetic beads following manufacturer's instructions. Briefly, ficol-purified PBMC were incubated with anti-CD14 beads (Miltenyi Biotech, Cambridge, Mass) and added into a Miltenyi column under the field of magnetic force. The unbound cells ($CD14^-$) were collected and considered as flow through. Bound $CD14^+$ cells were flushed out and purity (>90%) was checked by flow cytometry. Additionally, CD14 gene expression assessed by microarrays was consistently high (~12 in $\log_2$ units) in every patient sample derived from $CD14^+$ cells.

RNA Isolation and quantification

Total RNA was isolated from $CD14^+$ monocytes and $CD14^-$ cells using the RNeasy Mini Kit with DNase digestion on the column (Qiagen, Inc. Valencia, CA, USA) as per the manufacturer's instructions. Total RNA was isolated from biopsy samples using the RNeasy Lipid Tissue Mini Kit with DNase digestion on the column (Qiagen, Inc. Valencia, CA, USA) as per the manufacturer's instructions. The quality and quantity of RNA was assessed using the Agilent 2100 Bioanalyzer (South Plainfield, NJ, USA) or the Caliper LabChip GX (PerkinElmer, Inc. Waltham, MA, USA). Only those RNAs with a RNA Integrity Number (RIN, Agilent) or RNA Quality Score (RQS, PerkinEl-

Table 1. Patient demographics.

	RA	PsA	Ps	HC
n	9	12	10	19
Age (mean ± s.d.)	51.6±10.9	52.7±13.3	40.9±15.1	42±13.3
Gender (m/f)	1/8	6/6	4/6	6/13
Dx Duration (mean ± s.d.)	9.8±5.7	8.1±6.0	10.1±7.0	
Baseline Methotrexate	6	8	0	
Baseline Hydroxychloroquine	1	0	0	
Baseline Leflunomide	1	0	0	
Baseline topicals	0	0	10	
No Baseline Meds	1	4	0	
Activity Measure	DAS28	DAS28	PASI	
Baseline Activity (mean ± s.d.)	6.03±1.23	4.54±1.73	5.26±1.92	

mer) of greater than 4.0 (out of 10) were submitted for microarray. $CD14^+$ depleted PBMC and $CD14^+$ monocyte RNAs had an average RQS of 9.4, and biopsy RNAs had an average RQS/RIN of 6.7.

Microarray data analysis

RNA samples were processed using the High Throughput HG133plus2 PM microarray platform (Affymetrix Inc., Santa Clara CA) at the Janssen R&D microarray core facility in La Jolla, CA. Arrays were processed in an order random with respect to sample groups in order to minimize the intrusion of batch effects. The CEL files were normalized using RMA algorithm implemented in ArrayStudio version 4.1 (OmicSoft, Durham, NC.). The MAS5 QC report and principal component analysis (PCA) were used for outlier detection before proceeding to analysis. A General Linear Model (GLM) implemented in ArrayStudio was used to detect significantly differentially expressed genes. Significant genes were based on the following 3 criteria: 1. A fold change in the comparison greater than 1.5; 2. A raw P value less than 0.05; 3. A mean expression value equal or higher than 5 (log_2 value) in either control or disease samples. For biopsy specimens, differential gene expression was analyzed using paired t-tests and genes were selected based on p-value (affymetrix probe sets with no associated gene annotation were not included). For heat maps, when multiple probe sets for a single gene were available in statistical lists, the one with the lowest p value was chosen as a representative for visualization. Gene list relationships were analyzed using hive plots. Ingenuity Pathway Analysis (IPA, Ingenuity Systems, Redwood City, CA) was used to find enriched annotations and predicted transcription factors [26]. Clustering, additional statistical tests and visualizations were performed using Matlab (MathWorks, Natick, MA). The microarray data discussed in this publication have been deposited in NCBI's Gene Expression Omnibus [27]and are available through GEO Series accession number GSE57386 (http://www.ncbi.nlm.nih.gov/geo/query/acc.cgi?acc=GSE57386).

RT-PCR validation of microarray data

Validation of microarray results from cells and biopsy samples by real-time polymerase chain reaction (RT-PCR) was performed on a subset of genes that met significance criteria described above, and were of biological interest. RNA from $CD14^+$ and $CD14^-$ cells was reverse transcribed using the High-capacity cDNA Reverse Transcription kit (Life Technologies, Grand Island, NY). RNA from biopsies was amplified using the Ovation RNA Amplification System V2 (NuGen Technologies, San Carlos, CA) RT-PCR reactions were performed using TaqMan Gene Expression Assays (Life Technologies, Grand Island, NY) and run on an Applied Biosystems ViiA7 instrument under standard cycling conditions. TaqMan Gene Expression Assays are listed in Tables S2–S5. Statistical analysis of RT-PCR data was conducted using Prism version 6.05 (GraphPad Software, La Jolla CA) and ArrayStudio. TaqMan data (after normalization to GAPDH), was first log2 transformed and paired T test (if paired samples) was used to determine the significance and fold change of gene expression change; when there were no paired samples, GLM (General Linear Model) implemented in ArrayStudio was used to conduct the statistical tests.

Results

Patient Characteristics

The demographics and baseline medications for the patients in the 3 groups are outlined in Table 1. The Ps patients were younger than the RA or PsA patients and the RA patients were almost all female. The average disease duration ranged between 8 and 10 years and most of the patients with RA and PsA were inadequate responders to disease modifying anti-rheumatic agents (DMARDs) and the most commonly prescribed medication was methotrexate. Eight of the 9 RA patients were positive for anti-CCP antibodies. Patients had active skin and joint disease as measured by the Psoriasis Area and Severity Index (PASI) and BSA (>5%), and Disease DAS28-CRP scores, respectively.

Treatment Response

The baseline DAS28-CRP scores in RA and PsA were 6.03 and 4.54 and the baseline PASI score in the Ps subjects was 5.26. The mean change following IFX therapy in the DAS28 in RA was 1.90 ($p<.007$), in PsA was 1.19, ($p<.001$) and the mean change in PASI for the nine responders was 4.6±1.8 ($p<.008$). The DAS28 and PASI scores for individual subjects are depicted in Figure 1. All patients in the RA and PsA groups had lower DAS28 scores at week 10. One Ps patient had an increase in the PASI score at week 10. In all other Ps patients, the scores improved.

General transcriptomic changes

In general, transcriptomic changes in the peripheral blood subsets for all diseases were less striking than those found in Ps biopsy samples, and did not maintain their significance when accounting for multiple comparisons. Tables 2 and 3 summarize the results of various group comparisons. In Table 2, numbers of significant genes found within each cell type for cross-sectional comparisons with healthy controls, or longitudinal comparisons to baseline are shown. Note that for all diseases, for both $CD14^+$ and $CD14^-$, greater transcriptomic changes were observed in the baseline disease samples relative to healthy controls than in the treated disease samples relative to baseline disease, with the exception of PsA at 10 weeks (see Figures S1 and S2 for cross-sectional disease comparisons). For the treatment effect comparisons, the RA samples revealed a similar degree of changes at both time points, whereas in PsA and Ps, most of the significant gene changes were at the 10 week time point for $CD14^+$ cells. For $CD14^-$, RA had more changes at 2 weeks whereas PsA and Ps had more changes at 10 weeks. The results for the biopsy comparisons are shown in Table 3. The most dramatic response was seen in Ps with the most significant genes found when comparing non-lesional and psoriatic skin from the same patients. Far fewer significant genes were found in the knee biopsy samples but the sample size for those comparisons was very small.

Validation of gene expression

Genes with significant changes in expression and of biological interest were selected for validation with RT-PCR assays and are shown in Tables S2–S4. The correlation between expression on microarray and RT-PCR for the $CD14^+$ cells was 100% (fold-change in same direction) or 67% (fold-change in same direction and significant $p \leq 0.05$) based on the group comparisons. The agreement between expression change by microarray and by RT-PCR for the biopsies was 97% in terms of direction of change. In addition to having the same direction of change, 78% were also significant by both measures ($p \leq 0.05$). Furthermore, we compared the top 50 genes for paired lesional vs. non-lesional Ps samples in a recent meta-study [28] to our data (a subset of microarrays in this study) and found remarkable consistency (see Figure S5), indicating that the microarray measurements we report are capable of reproducing published results.

IFX response in $CD14^+$ cells

The number of significant annotated genes for either 2 or 10 week relative to baseline whose corresponding probe sets met our statistical criteria (see Methods) for RA, PsA and Ps in $CD14^+$ and $CD14^-$ cells are shown in Table 2. These lists of significant genes that changed in response to IFX had limited overlap, and thus were fairly distinct. Figure 2 illustrates this finding for $CD14^+$ cells as a hive plot which reveals more information about the overlap than a Venn diagram. Each shaded bar emanating from the center represents an ordered arrangement of probe sets color-coded according to fold-change relative to baseline. Arcs connecting the bars indicate probe sets present in two lists (green if in all three). The small number of arcs as compared to the lengths of the gene lists (indicated within each bar) reflects the low overlap between pairs of lists. Furthermore, when there is overlap, it tends to be concentrated for genes with large fold changes.

Figure 3 is a heat map showing the response to IFX at both time points in all three diseases for a more stringent subset of the significant genes, although note that outliers are present in each group. For all diseases, most genes shown are different at either 2 or 10 weeks, with a minority significant at both time points. Additionally, for all diseases, most of the significant genes are up-

Table 2. Numbers of significant genes in PBMC comparisons.

		RA (n = 9)			PsA (n = 12)			Ps (n = 10)		
Comparison	Cell	Total	Up	Down	Total	Up	Down	Total	Up	Down
Disease (Dx vs. HC at BL)	$CD14^+$	349	170	179	81	14	67	125	76	49
	$CD14^-$	371	259	112	197	53	144	441	184	257
Treatment (2 wk vs. BL)	$CD14^+$	77	42	35	75	62	13	29	15	14
	$CD14^-$	141	90	51	4	4	0	9	6	3
Treatment (10 wk vs. BL)	$CD14^+$	69	56	13	140	71	69	102	85	17
	$CD14^-$	76	32	44	225	53	172	67	59	8

Numbers reflect total number of genes as well as the number up- and down-regulated. These numbers were derived from a slightly larger number of probe sets. Unannotated probe sets are not included in this tabulation. BL = baseline, HC = healthy control (n = 19), Dx = disease. Numbers are based on general linear model with $p < .05$ and fold change at least 1.5.

Table 3. Numbers of significant genes in biopsy comparisons.

Comparison	RA (n = 3)			PsA (n = 3)			Ps (n = 5)		
	Total	Up	Down	Total	Up	Down	Total	Up	Down
L skin at BL vs. NL skin at BL	–	–	–	–	–	–	1417	850	567
L tissue at 2 or 10 wk vs. L tissue at BL	64	32	32	52	26	26	326	74	252
L skin at 2 wk vs. NL skin at BL	–	–	–	–	–	–	203	102	101

Numbers reflect total number of genes as well as the number up- and down-regulated. These numbers were derived from a slightly larger number of probe sets. Unannotated probe sets are not included in this tabulation.
BL = baseline, L = lesional, NL = non-lesional. Numbers are based on paired t-test with p<.01 and fold change at least 1.5.

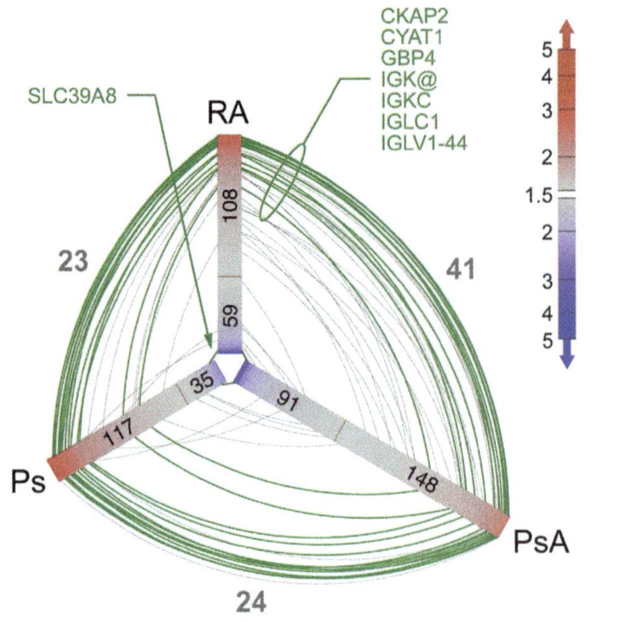

Figure 2. Venn/hive plots showing genes that changed following IFX treatment in three diseases in CD14⁺ cells. The three shaded bars emanating from the center each represent a list of significant probe sets where their members are distributed along the bar sorted by fold-change (indicated by color). The numbers of probe sets up- and down-regulated are shown on the red and blue portions of the bars, respectively. For example, in PsA,148 genes were up-regulated and 91 down-regulated following IFX therapy. Arcs that connect pairs of shaded bars represent genes that are common between two comparisons (in the same fashion, the intersect of two circles in a Venn diagram); the gray numbers indicate the numbers of arcs. Probe sets that are common to all three lists are represented by green arcs (15 probe sets representing eight genes). Probe set lists were obtained using a general linear model with p<.05, with the requirement that the $\log_2$ signal was required to be >5 for at least one of the sample groups and the absolute fold change was required to be greater than 1.5. Only annotated probe sets are depicted. For this figure, the larger fold change was used for the two time points after baseline.
doi:10.1371/journal.pone.0110657.g002

regulated in response to IFX (see also Figure 2). A similar display of data is shown for $CD14^-$ cells in Figure S3. For these cells, PsA had substantially more changed genes, mostly at 10 weeks and down-regulated.

IFX response in biopsy samples

Gene expression data from biopsy samples were available in a limited set of patients and is shown in Figure 4. Three gene lists are depicted: Ps genes (n = 127) which are the union of significant genes from the three possible pairwise comparisons, and PsA genes (n = 6) and RA genes (n = 9) derived from the respective knee biopsy samples. Each columnar block in the heat map represents the five possible paired comparisons (one each for RA and PsA, three for Ps, as noted in Figure 4). Large significant differences were observed in genes from Ps biopsy samples as indicated by the darker shades of red/blue. Responses are shown as insets for five selected genes significant for Ps that are relevant because they have established associations with Ps based on genome wide studies or transcriptome analyses [29–32]. Responses of these genes for all samples are shown in Figure S4. Note that Ps genes did not appear to have consistent expression patterns for the individuals in RA or PsA. Similarly, the PsA and RA genes, which appeared to have much weaker effects in the PsA and RA comparisons, respectively,

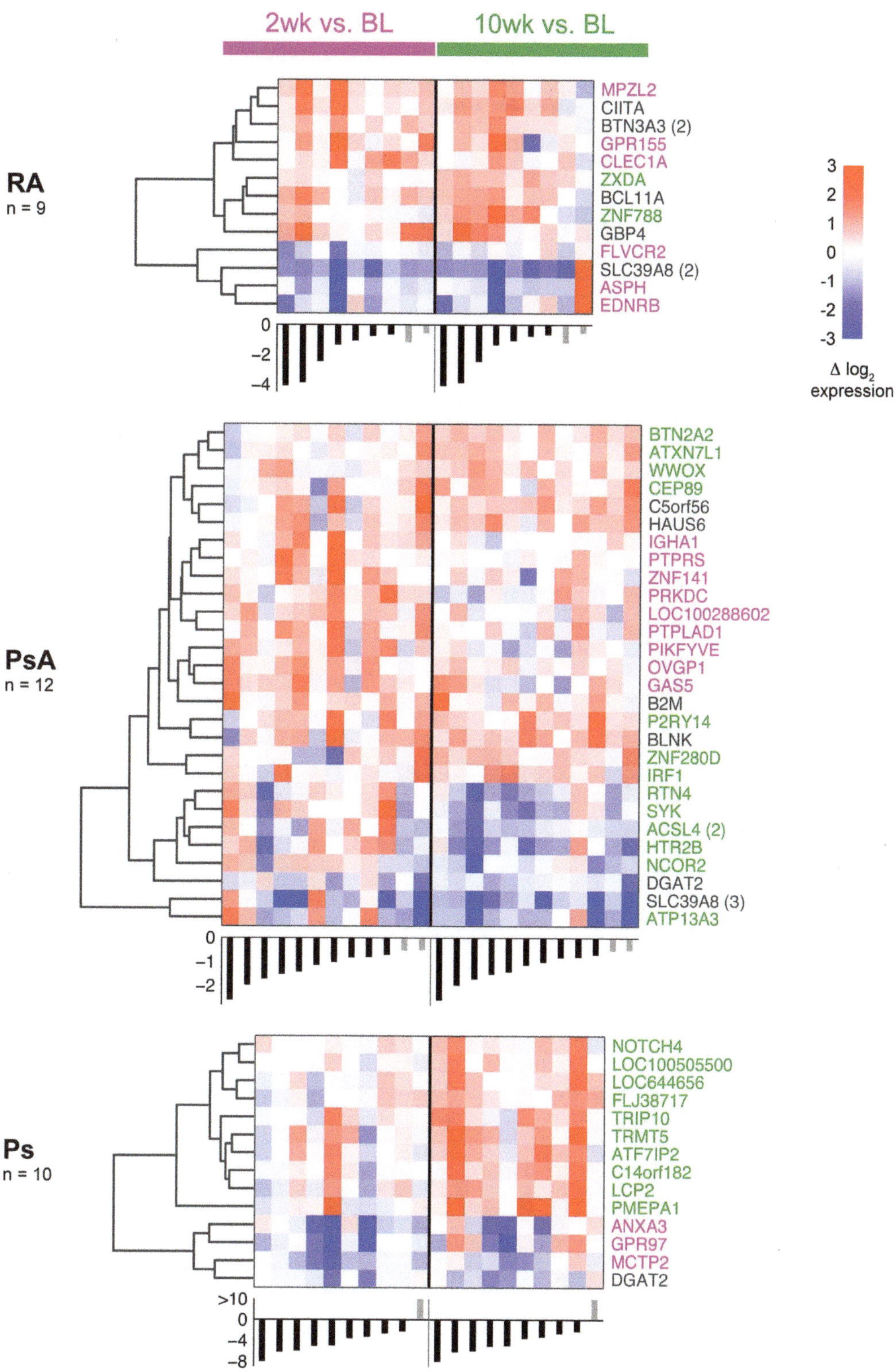

Figure 3. Heat map of IFX treatment effect for CD14+ cells in different diseases. In each heat map, columns correspond to patients and rows to probe sets. Separate heat maps are shown for three diseases and two cell types as indicated. Color is the log_2 difference in expression at 2 or 10 weeks relative to baseline as specified by the blue and gold bars, respectively (patients are in same order for each set of columns for each disease). Probe set clustering was accomplished using Euclidean distance and complete linkage. Only genes for which $p<.005$ for one of the time points are shown. BL = baseline. Font color for gene names indicate whether the probe set was significant at $p<.05$ at 2 weeks (purple), 10 weeks (green) or both (gray). For all heat maps, the columns (patients) are sorted first by responders/non-responders, and then by change in disease activity at 10 weeks relative to baseline (DAS28 for RA and PsA, PASI for Ps), which is shown beneath each heat map (responders are black bars, non-responders are gray bars).

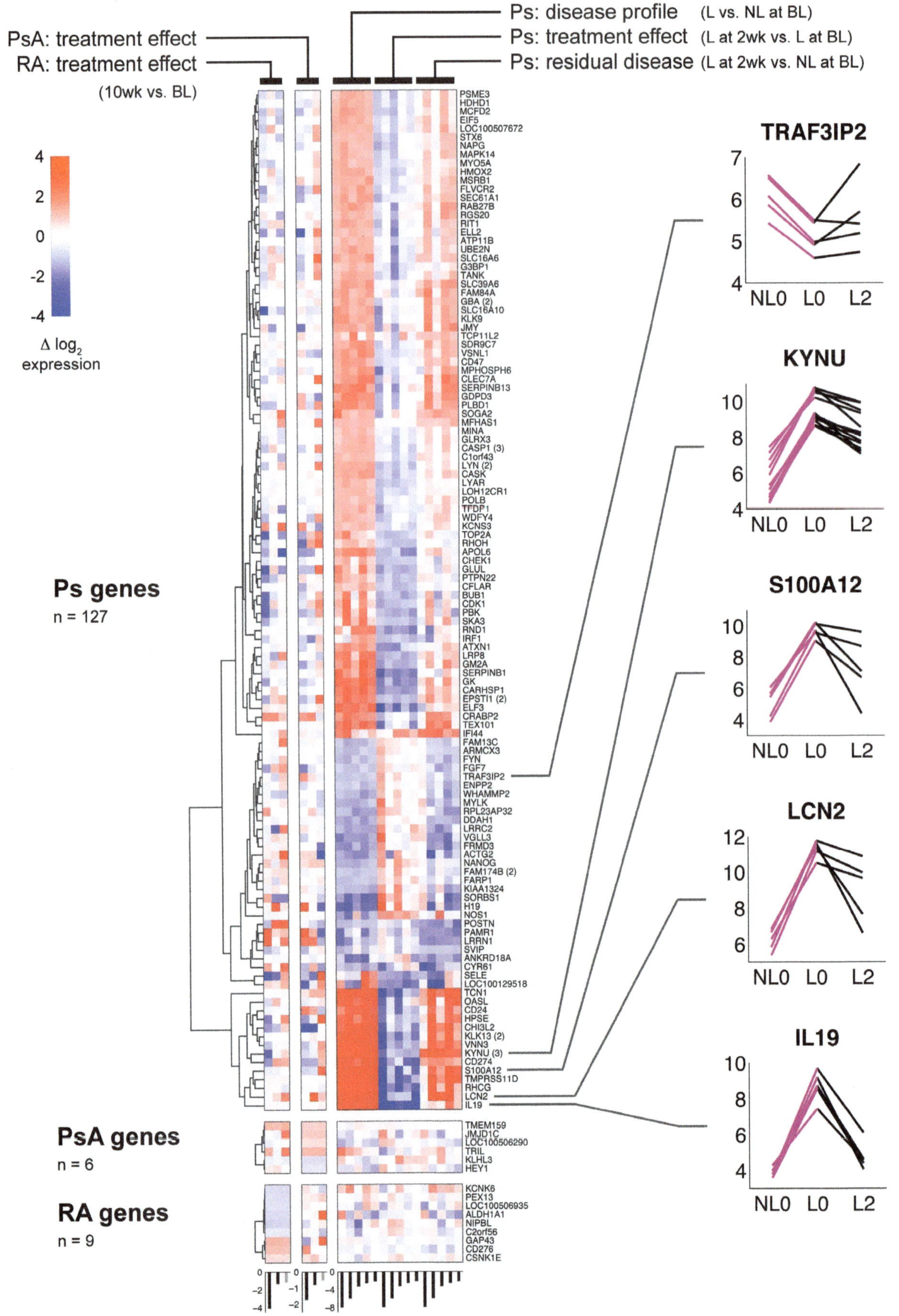
PsA: treatment effect
RA: treatment effect
(10wk vs. BL)
Ps: disease profile (L vs. NL at BL)
Ps: treatment effect (L at 2wk vs. L at BL)
Ps: residual disease (L at 2wk vs. NL at BL)
4
2
0
-2
-4
Δ $\log_2$ expression
Ps genes
n = 127
PsA genes
n = 6
RA genes
n = 9
PSME3
HDHD1
MCFD2
EIF5
LOC100507672
STX6
NAPG
MAPK14
MYO5A
HMOX2
MSRB1
FLVCR2
SEC61A1
RAB27B
RGS20
RIT1
ELL2
ATP11B
UBE2N
SLC16A6
G3BP1
TANK
SLC39A6
FAM84A
GBA (2)
SLC16A10
KLK9
JMY
TCP11L2
SDR9C7
VSNL1
CD47
MPHOSPH6
CLEC7A
SERPINB13
GDPD3
PLBD1
SOGA2
MFHAS1
MINA
GLRX3
CASP1 (3)
C1orf43
LYN (2)
CASK
LYAR
LOH12CR1
POLB
TFDP1
WDFY4
KCNS3
TOP2A
RHOH
APOL6
CHEK1
GLUL
PTPN22
CFLAR
BUB1
CDK1
PBK
SKA3
RND1
IRF1
ATXN1
LRP8
GM2A
SERPINB1
GK
CARHSP1
EPSTI1 (2)
ELF3
CRABP2
TEX101
IFI44
FAM13C
ARMCX3
FYN
FGF7
TRAF3IP2
ENPP2
WHAMMP2
MYLK
RPL23AP32
DDAH1
LRRC2
VGLL3
FRMD3
ACTG2
NANOG
FAM174B (2)
FARP1
KIAA1324
SORBS1
H19
NOS1
POSTN
PAMR1
LRRN1
SVIP
ANKRD18A
CYR61
SELE
LOC100129518
TCN1
OASL
CD24
HPSE
CHI3L2
KLK13 (2)
VNN3
KYNU (3)
CD274
S100A12
TMPRSS11D
RHCG
LCN2
IL19
TMEM159
JMJD1C
LOC100506290
TRIL
KLHL3
HEY1
KCNK6
PEX13
LOC100506935
ALDH1A1
NIPBL
C2orf56
GAP43
CD276
CSNK1E
TRAF3IP2
KYNU
S100A12
LCN2
IL19
NL0 L0 L2

Figure 4. Heat map of IFX treatment effect in tissues. Paired t-tests were used to identify significant probe sets in different tissues. For Ps, comparisons, probe sets were selected where $p<0.0005$ and there was at least a 2-fold change in expression. For RA and PsA, paired t-tests were used and probe sets were selected where $p<0.001$ with at least a 1.5-fold change. Ps, PsA and RA probe set lists comprise the sets of rows, and RA, PsA and Ps samples comprise sets of columns. Color is the log_2 difference in expression. Probe set clustering (Euclidean distance, complete linkage) was based on the corresponding sample type. BL: baseline, L: lesional, NL: non-lesional skin. Five genes are highlighted: each line is a patient; violet, black segments are cross-sectional, longitudinal comparisons, respectively. Within each of the five groups of columns corresponding to the five comparisons at the top, patients (individual heat map columns) are sorted by change in disease activity. See legend for Figure 3 for details.

showed no consistent pattern in Ps; the end-organ responses to the diseases were distinct.

The overlap of Ps genes for biopsy comparisons are shown as a hive plot in Figure 5A at a more permissive statistical threshold than in Figure 4. Unlike the $CD14^+$ or $CD14^-$ comparisons which did not show strong statistical changes when accounting for multiple comparisons, the Ps biopsy comparisons at $p<.01$ had estimated false discovery rates of up to approximately 5% (disease effect, 3 O'clock), 27% (treatment effect, 10 O'clock) and 35% (residual disease effect, 7 O'clock). Note that all probe sets ($n = 155$) that are in both the disease profile list ($n = 1672$) and the treatment effect list ($n = 379$) have reciprocal directions of change; those that are up-regulated in lesional tissue relative to non-lesional tissue before treatment are down-regulated in lesional tissue following treatment, and vice-versa. When comparing the disease profile ($n = 1672$) with the residual disease effect ($n = 228$) which are genes that are different between treated, lesional tissue and pre-treated, non-lesional tissue (7 O'clock), overlapping probe sets ($n = 85$) always are changed in the same direction. These genes do not appear to return to a non-lesion pattern of expression. Figure 5B shows the overlap of significant probe sets for both circulating cells ($CD14^+$ and $CD14^-$) as well as the end organ (lesional skin) for Ps in response to IFX. The transcriptomic response to IFX appears to be unique to each compartment. These data demonstrate that peripheral blood profiles do not provide a valid assessment of gene response changes in psoriatic skin.

Distinct enriched functions in cells and tissue in response to IFX

Enriched functions derived from IPA for the IFX transcriptomic response in the three diseases are shown in Figure 6. In Ps lesional skin, the most enriched functions were Ps, segregation of chromosomes, arthritis and necrosis with many other functions related to cell death and cell movement. For Ps, in $CD14^-$ cells, enriched functions are related to cell maturation and cell death, whereas in $CD14^+$ cells, functions related to cell migration and blood vessel development appear to be enriched. For genes involved in the IFX response in PsA, only $CD14^+$ cells showed enriched functions, largely related to inflammatory response, migration and apoptosis. In contrast, only RA $CD14^-$ cells showed enriched functions following IFX treatment for immune response, activation, proliferation and autoimmune disease. Taken together, these diverse patterns of enriched function parallel the divergent transcriptomic response in the three diseases.

Key upstream regulator involvement following IFX therapy in psoriatic skin and peripheral blood

The predicted involvement of IFX transcriptional regulators based on 379 probe sets that were significantly changed in psoriatic skin following treatment is shown in Table 4 (and with the target genes in Table S1). This analysis identifies a potential upstream regulator if the list of genes is enriched for targets of the regulator in question, and if the pattern of up- and down-regulation is consistent with an activation state [26]. Eight transcription factors whose targets overlapped with genes represented by the input probe set list with $p<.0001$ (based on IPA upstream regulator analysis) are listed, and those whose targets changed in directions consistent with an activated or inhibited state are shaded orange or pink, respectively. Targets that correspond to probe sets in the input list are shown as well, along with their direction of change in response to IFX. With the exception of STAT3, none of the predicted regulators themselves were changed, although, of the target genes represented in the significant gene list, the vast majority were down-regulated. Note that FOX01 [33], STAT3 [34], RELA [35] and JUN [36], transcriptional regulators important in cell proliferation and differentiation, show inhibition in contrast to KDM5B, a histone demethylase that blocks terminal differentiation [37] and TP53, an inducer of cell death [38] which show activation.

Evidence for upstream regulator involvement was weaker in peripheral blood, and in no case was there predicted activation or inhibition. For the following results, a more permissive threshold of $p<.001$ was used. In RA, $CD14^+$ cells showed enrichment for interferon regulatory factor IRF4 and SMARCA4 [39] a chromatin remodeling protein while $CD14^-$ cells were enriched for CEBPE [40], which regulates myeloid differentiation and musculin (MSC) [41], a transcription factor expressed in skeletal muscle. In PsA, $CD14^+$ cells were enriched for CEBPA, a transcription factor critical for granulocyte differentiation [42], while $CD14^-$ cells showed no suggested involvement for a particular transcription factor. In Ps, $CD14^+$ cells, AR met the significance threshold while in $CD14^-$ cells, RORC, a transcription factor in Th17 cells [43], NR3C1, a glucocorticoid gene with polymorphisms linked to obesity, hypertension, elevated lipid levels and increased cardiovascular risk [44], and PYCARD-an adaptor protein for NLRP3 the inflammasome forming protein [45] had the lowest p values. Note that none of these regulators found in Ps blood were in common with those listed in Table 4.

Discussion

The immune mediated inflammatory diseases RA, PsA and Ps have divergent phenotypes but share several pathologic features that include overproduction of TNF and other cytokines, along with cellular proliferation and tissue remodeling. They also have overlapping metabolic and cardiovascular comorbidities and demonstrate, on average, good to excellent responses to anti-TNF agents. We hypothesized that the genomic response to anti-TNF agents in these three diseases would be distinct and would vary in the different cell types and target tissues. To our knowledge, this is the first study of differential gene expression in discrete populations of monocytes and immune cells that also examined expression in target tissues following treatment with IFX. We found the effect of IFX on the number of genes expressed by $CD14^+$ and $CD14^-$ cells more striking in PsA compared to RA and Ps. Moreover, the response in RA was clustered around the 2 week time point whereas the most notable effect on gene expression in PsA and Ps was at 10 weeks. In Ps biopsies, a large number of genes were dramatically down-regulated by IFX at 2 weeks but the gene expression profile in skin from patients with

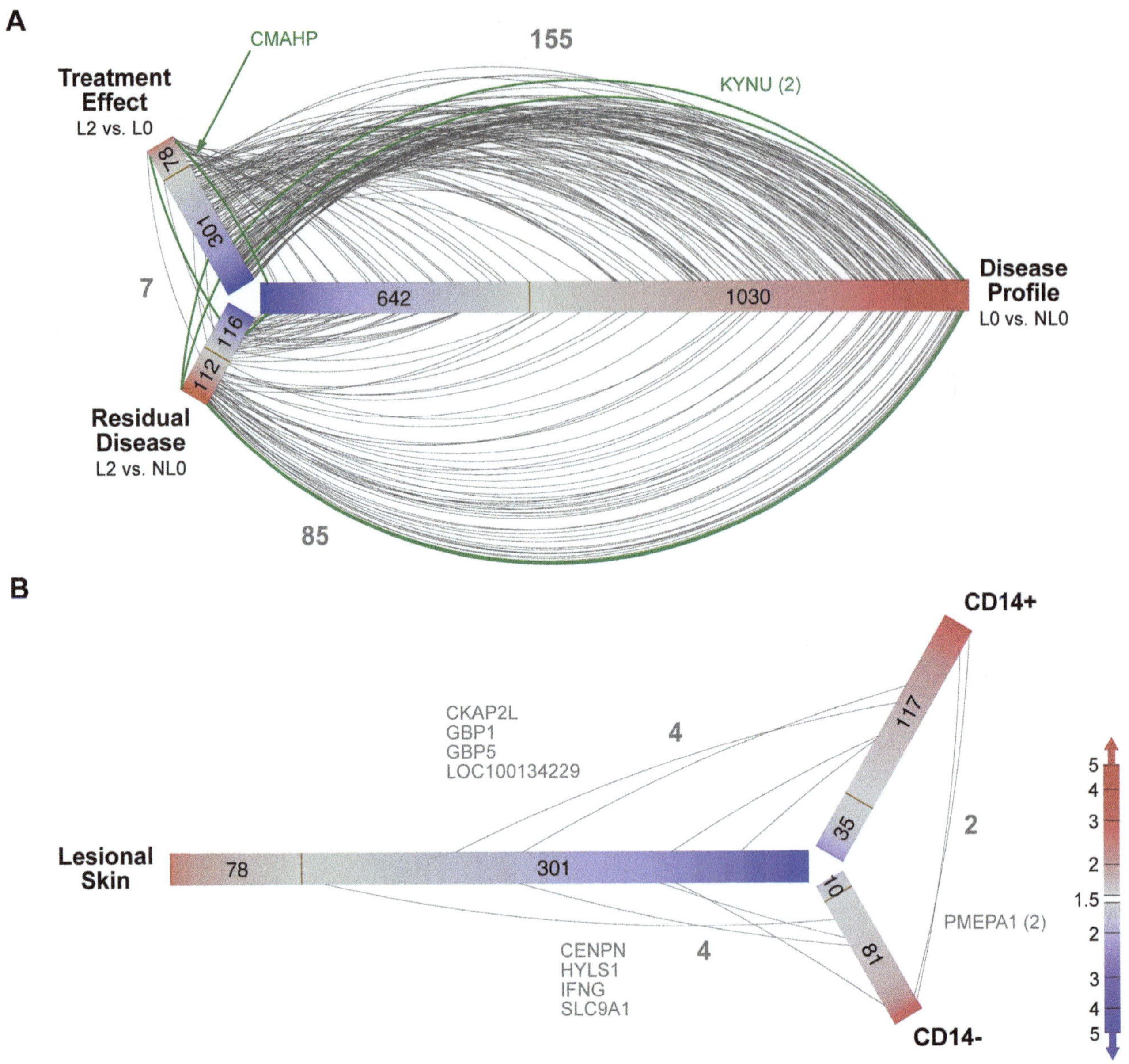

Figure 5. Venn/hive plots showing genes common in multiple lists for Ps samples. A. Comparisons of Ps gene lists based on skin biopsy samples. B. Comparisons of Ps Infliximab response gene lists from $CD14^+$, $CD14^-$ and biopsy samples. In each plot, the three shaded bars emanating from the center each represent a list of significant probe sets where their members are distributed along the bar sorted by fold-change (indicated by color). The numbers of genes up- and down-regulated are shown on the red and blue portions of the bars, respectively. Gray arcs that connect pairs of shaded bars represent genes that are common between two comparisons (in the same fashion of the intersect of two circles in a Venn diagram). Probe sets that are common to all three lists are represented by green arcs (3 in A, 0 in B). For skin biopsy comparisons, probe set lists were derived from five patients using paired t-tests based on five subjects with $p<.01$. For primary cell comparisons, a general linear model was used with $p<.05$ for ten patients. In both cases, the log_2 signal was required to be >5 for at least one of the sample groups and the absolute fold change was required to be greater than 1.5. The false discovery rates for the biopsy samples in A, starting at the top and going clockwise, are estimated to be up to approximately 27%, 5% and 35%.

excellent clinical responses was still significantly different from uninvolved skin. We also noted that the IFX response in both circulating $CD14^+$ and $CD14^-$ cells was strikingly different than the response observed in the skin or synovium of the same patients. Functional enrichment analysis revealed involvement of signaling cascades in $CD14^-$ cells (B, T lymphocytes, NK cells) in RA, $CD14^+$ cells (monocytes) in PsA and a mixture of these different cell lineages in Ps. Moreover, little overlap was noted in the 3 diseases regarding involvement of specific functional pathways in the IFX response. These data suggest that although TNF is of central importance in all three diseases based on the excellent clinical responses, the pathways modulated by TNF differ suggesting distinct disease mechanisms. Finally, a number of key transcriptional regulators were either activated or suppressed after treatment but little overlap was observed between the disorders in terms of specific regulators involved.

Overall, analysis of peripheral blood resulted in significant gene lists that were not maintained following corrections for multiple

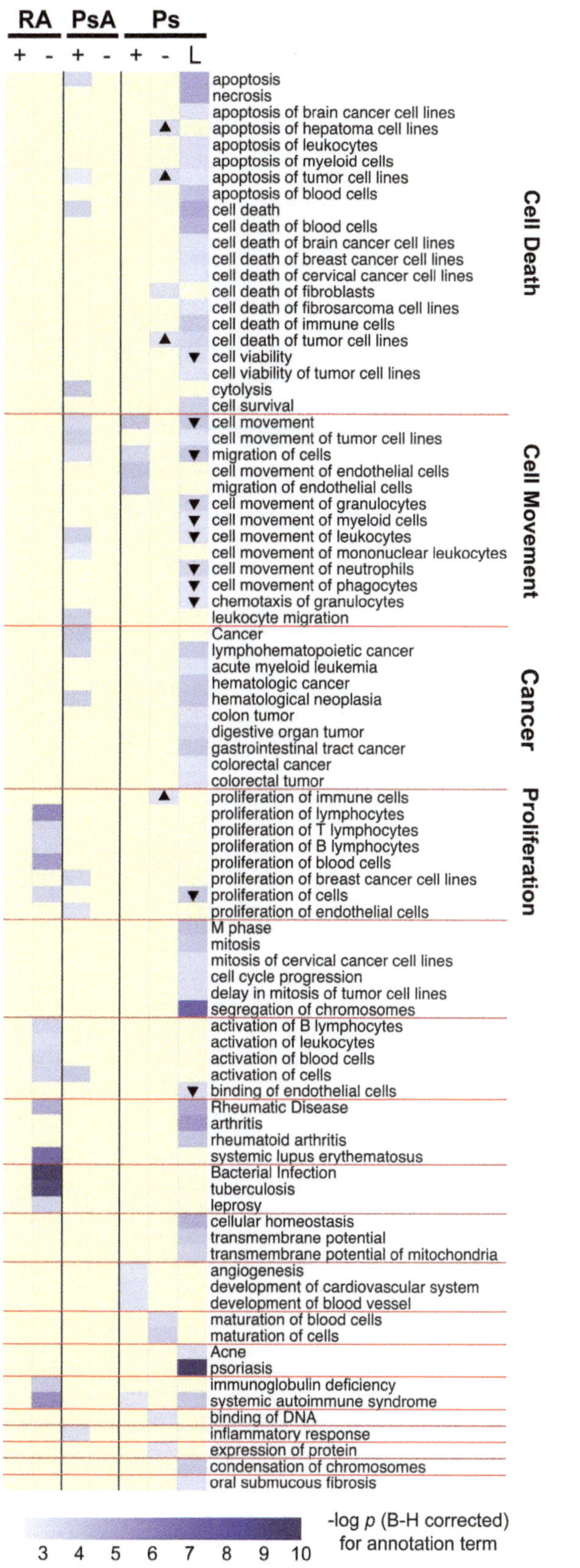

Figure 6. Summary of enriched functions for IFX responses for different tissues and diseases. For each of seven pre/post IFX gene lists, results from Ingenuity Pathway Analysis functional enrichment were retained if the Benjamini-Hochberg-corrected p value was <0.001 and if there were more than four probe sets associated with the function. The unions of these functions are listed alongside of the heat map. Color maps to $-\log_{10}$ of the corrected p-value, with blue being very significant. Functions (rows) were clustered based on their associated broader, category labels using the kappa statistic in order to group similar functions together to aid in visualization. Up and down triangles indicate functions that were increased or decreased, respectively, based on activation z-score.

comparisons. As a result, determination of specific transcription factor involvement in blood was also limited. This could be due in part either to more subtle transcriptional changes in the blood, or to the heterogeneous nature of the $CD14^+$ and, especially, $CD14^-$ subsets. Ps skin biopsy samples gave strong transcriptional responses, whereas knee biopsy samples in PsA and RA resulted in less clear-cut signatures, most likely due to the sample size. The data support the concept that PsA is more dependent on innate immune responses mediated largely by monocytes ($CD14^+$) in contrast to RA which is driven largely by an acquired immune signature ($CD14^-$) expressed by T cells, T lymphocytes and NK cells while Ps reveals involvement of both immune mechanisms ($CD14^+$ and $CD14^-$).

The high number of genes in $CD14^+$ and $CD14^-$ cells with significant changes in expression following IFX treatment in PsA compared to RA and Ps samples was unexpected. Also, the largest effect on gene expression was noted at week 10 in PsA and Ps compared to 2 weeks for most of the genes in the RA samples. This may explain why skin responses often lag behind the joint response to anti-TNF agents in PsA. In addition, changes in the number of genes altered by IFX showed greater similarity in RA and PsA compared to Ps. One potential explanation is that the majority of RA and PsA patients were on methotrexate prior to IFX therapy whereas none of the Ps patients were on this medication at baseline. Two other studies examined cross-sectional gene expression in 29 PsA patients and controls. Batliwalla et al. [46] found that 257 genes were expressed at low and 56 at elevated levels compared to controls. They found low levels of several genes that suppress innate and acquired immune responses and upregulation of 3 proinflammatory genes (S100A, S100A12) and thioredoxin. The gene signature for PsA was different than RA. In another study, Stoeckman et al. found 310 differentially expressed genes in 16 PsA patients compared to controls, most of which were upregulated [47]. The signature differed from those found in RA and SLE but interestingly showed little overlap with Batliwalla et al. [46]. We cannot directly compare our findings with these 2 studies, since we examined the change in gene expression after IFX, but we did not see overlap with our gene lists and these two data sets. The reason for the higher number of differential gene expression in PsA compared to RA and Ps after IFX may relate to the fact that inflammatory cells that transit to both the skin and joint may be triggered by an array of signals that activate numerous gene networks. Further study is required to address this finding, however.

Transcriptome analysis of Ps lesional skin showed marked differential gene expression compared to non-lesional skin at baseline. Our findings strongly correlate with the results of a Ps transcriptome meta-analysis recently published by Tian et al [28] [39](see Figure S5). In this meta-analysis of 5 microarray data sets, 1832 differentially expressed genes in Ps lesional compared to non-lesional skin were identified (1084 up and 748 down) similar to our results (1672 differentially expressed probe sets: 1030 up and 642 down). Of the top 50 differentially regulated probe sets (25 up and 25 down) reported by this group, we found 48 of the 50 probe sets in our dataset had fold changes in the same direction. For those

Table 4. Upstream regulator analysis using Ingenuity Pathway Analysis.

Regulator	Changed	z-Score	Predicted State	Bias	$-\log_{10}$ p-Value
TP53	–	3.25	activated	–	11.89
FOXO1	–	−3.29	inhibited	yes	9.7
JUN	–	−1.28	–	yes	7.07
FOXM1	–	−2.56	inhibited	yes	7.01
RELA	–	−2.62	inhibited	yes	5.34
TP63	–	−1.59	–	yes	5.2
KDM5B	–	2.99	activated	yes	4.33
STAT3	down	−0.48	–	–	4.19

Upstream regulators predicted based on genes that were significantly different for lesional skin before and after treatment with IFX ($n = 379$). Subset of "significant" transcription factors are shown that had an overlap p-value $<.0001$ (negative log of 4) and a reported activation z-score, indicating that many of the targets were enriched in the gene list. Except for STAT3 which was down-regulated, none of these were in the gene list. The further the activation z-score is from zero, the more likely that the direction of change of the target genes are consistent with the regulator being in either an "activated" or "inhibited" state. Bias terms over 25 are shown, indicating that the regulation of the targets in the data set as well as all of those for the regulator are skewed towards a particular direction [26]. Six additional upstream regulators, E2F4, E2F1, PBRM1, NFYB, MYBL2 and NFkB, had low overlap p-values, but there wasn't sufficient data about known relationships with targets to predict an activation state. Although no upstream regulator was predicted to be activated or inhibited for the IFX-response in $CD14^+$ or $CD14^-$ cells, some still had low overlap p-values.

that were up (L0 vs. NL0), 21 of the 25 probe sets were significant at $p<.01$. For those that were down, 6 of the 23 were significant at the same level. Most strikingly, we found that all of these 25 genes up-regulated at baseline were down-regulated 2 weeks after IFX treatment ($p<.05$ for 12 of those; for all the 1030 probe sets up-regulated in L0 relative to NL0 in our data set, 131 were down-regulated at L2 as depicted in Figure 5A). Despite the suppression of these genes following treatment, lesional skin showed differential up-regulation (112 genes) and down-regulation (116 genes) in treated L skin compared to NL skin. This residual disease genomic profile or 'molecular scar' was also noted in psoriatic lesions after treatment with etanercept [48]. It represents continued activation of cytokines and chemokines in skin where Ps has phenotypically resolved. Of their 20 selected, up-regulated disease genes that didn't show "improvement" following etanercept, five overlapped with our L2 vs. NL0 up-regulated list for at least one probe set (RAB31, WNT5A, SYK, IFI27 and ISG20, with IFI27 and WNT5A having the most residual response). Of their 9 selected, down-regulated disease genes, only AQP9 overlapped with our L2 vs. NL0 down-regulated list. The other important finding is that only 8 probe sets differentially expressed after IFX treatment, were shared between the lesional skin and any of the blood cells, and with fairly small fold-changes. Thus, our findings confirm those presented in the meta-analysis and demonstrate a dramatic suppression of key differentially expressed genes as early as two weeks following IFX therapy, however, residual inflammatory pathways remain active, despite apparent skin response.

Several transcription factors were predicted to be involved following treatment in the skin and blood cells of the 3 patient groups included in the study based on the significant overlap of associated gene lists and known upstream regulator [26]. In Ps plaques, transcription factor genes that promote cell differentiation and proliferation including STAT3, RELA and JUN were predicted to be inhibited. In contrast KDM5B a histone demethylase and TP53 a suppressor oncogene was predicted to be activated after treatment. The effect of treatment on the blood cells in RA was more limited and upstream-regulator involvement was noted for SMARCA4 and ILF4 in $CD14^+$ cells and CEPBE and MSC in $CD14^-$ cells. In PsA, the only enrichment was noted for CEBPA in $CD14^+$ cells. These findings indicate that the effect of IFX is far more robust at the tissue level and that changes in the blood transcriptome do not correlate well with changes in the tissue.

The enriched gene functions for IFX responses in the 3 disorders were of particular interest and likely reflect contrasting disease mechanisms and/or differing treatment responses to IFX. In reviewing the pathway differences between RA and PsA, it is apparent the response to IFX is most notable only in RA $CD14^-$ cells. Pathways affected are those related to proliferation of lymphocytes, T cells, B cells, bacterial infection, tuberculosis, SLE and systemic autoimmune syndrome among others. In the case of PsA, pathways that changed were limited to the $CD14^+$cells and included proliferation of cells and endothelial cells, apoptotic pathways, inflammatory response, cell movement and migration. In contrast, significant treatment changes were observed in pathways associated with both $CD14^+$ and $CD14^-$ cells in psoriatic peripheral blood. $CD14^+$ associated pathways noted to be affected were those associated with angiogenesis, blood vessel development, autoimmunity, cell movement and migration. $CD14^+$ pathways significantly impacted by IFX in psoriasis were proliferation of immune cells, apoptosis and cell death, and maturation. The longitudinal data in table 2 demonstrate that IFX therapy at 10 weeks was associated with a more pronounced effect on the number of genes associated with $CD14^-$ compared to $CD14^+$ cells in PsA and contrasts with the predominance of genes expressed by $CD14^+$ cells outlined in the pathway analysis outlined above. It is important to note that the numbers of differentially expressed genes do not always correspond to enriched pathways derived from gene lists which are dependent on specific genes that comprise the pathway. The results from the pathway analysis support a disease paradigm put forth by McGonagle et al. in which RA pathogenesis is mediated largely by acquired immune mechanisms, PsA primarily by the innate immune response, and Ps by a combination of acquired and innate pathways, but further studies with larger sample sizes are required to confirm this model [49].

Our study is the first examination of differential gene expression in cell populations and target tissues from different immune mediated inflammatory disorders but several limitations must be considered. First, the low number of synovial samples in diseases with heterogeneous tissue responses does not provide a comprehensive assessment of the joint response although the relationship between differential gene regulation in the joint and skin of an individual patient is informative. Second, we do not have confirmatory immunohistochemistry data on tissue expression of differentially expressed genes determined by microarray. Third, the lack of a sufficient number of non-responders to IFX (for RA there were two overall, one in the biopsy patient set) did not allow us to identify genes that may be responsible for persistent inflammation following treatment. Fourth, microarray studies are directed towards analysis of defined genes and increasing evidence points to the importance of critical regulatory elements outside the protein-coding regions which will not be captured with this approach [39].

In conclusion, these results indicate that anti-TNF treatment modulates different disease pathways in specific immune-mediated inflammatory disorders. Thus, clinical and tissue responses can be achieved with TNF inhibition by divergent mechanisms dependent on the underlying disease. Moreover, careful analysis of differential gene expression in involved tissues and possibly blood cells following treatment with biologic therapies may provide insights into disease pathogenesis and unveil new disease targets.

Supporting Information

Figure S1 Heat map of cross-sectional expression data for CD14$^+$ cells. In each heat map, columns correspond to patient samples and rows to probe sets. Color is the per-probe set z-score of $\log_2$ expression across all 50 baseline samples. Gene clustering was accomplished using Euclidean distance and complete linkage. Only genes where p<.0005 for one of the disease vs. healthy control (HC) comparisons are shown. Dots to the left of the probe set names indicate which comparison met this p-value threshold. Columns (patients) were sorted by baseline disease activity (DAS28 for RA and PsA, PASI for Ps) and are shown beneath the heat maps.

Figure S2 Heat map of cross-sectional expression data for CD14$^-$ cells. See description for Figure S1. The high number of Hb genes noted (13 probe sets for HBA1, HBB, HBG1 and HBD in the bottom third of the heat map) in RA may be related to 1) upregulation of Hb genes (previously reported in juvenile RA [50], 2) presence of erythroid precursors 3) contamination with blood. We think the latter possibility very unlikely because all samples were handled in an identical fashion and increased expression of Hb genes was not observed in the psoriasis or PsA samples.

Figure S3 Heat map of longitudinal expression data for CD14$^-$ cells. See description for Figure 3. Missing data for one 10 week PsA samples (third column, white).

Figure S4 Examples of gene expression pattern across all 255 samples for genes in call-outs of Figure 4. x-axis labels are time points. B = baseline; BN = baseline, non-lesional skin, HC = healthy control.

Figure S5 Ps lesional skin vs. non-lesional skin data for 50 genes identified in Ps meta-analysis of Tian et al. [28]. Log2 fold change values for the 50 genes in the meta-analysis compared to the values for the same genes in our study.

Table S1 Upstream regulator analysis using Ingenuity Pathway Analysis, including target molecules.

Table S2 Validation of microarray results by RT-PCR for CD14$^+$ samples in longitudinal comparisons.

Table S3 Validation of microarray results by RT-PCR for CD14$^+$ samples in cross-sectional comparisons.

Table S4 Validation of microarray results by RT-PCR for biopsy samples.

Table S5 TaqMan primers used for validation.

Author Contributions

Conceived and designed the experiments: R. Bolce DS EMS YGC CTR. Performed the experiments: R. Barrett DT DS YGC CTR. Analyzed the data: AR HF R. Bolce SM FB HL NP YGC DS. Contributed reagents/materials/analysis tools: SM FB HL NP DS YGC CTR. Wrote the paper: AR EMS CTR.

References

1. Davidovici BB, Sattar N, Prinz J, Puig L, Emery P, et al. (2010) Psoriasis and systemic inflammatory diseases: potential mechanistic links between skin disease and co-morbid conditions. J Invest Dermatol 130: 1785–1796.
2. Firestein GS, Corr M (2005) Common mechanisms in immune-mediated inflammatory disease. Journal of Rheumatology - Supplement 73: 8–13; discussion 29–30.
3. Gudjonsson JE (2007) Analysis of global gene expression and genetic variation in psoriasis. J Am Acad Dermatol 57: 365.
4. Arend WP, Firestein GS (2012) Pre-rheumatoid arthritis: predisposition and transition to clinical synovitis. Nat Rev Rheumatol 8: 573–586.
5. Nograles KE, Brasington RD, Bowcock AM (2009) New insights into the pathogenesis and genetics of psoriatic arthritis. Nat Clin Pract Rheumatol 5: 83–91.
6. Perera GK, Di Meglio P, Nestle FO (2012) Psoriasis. Annu Rev Pathol 7: 385–422.
7. Moots RJ, Naisbett-Groet B (2012) The efficacy of biologic agents in patients with rheumatoid arthritis and an inadequate response to tumour necrosis factor inhibitors: a systematic review. Rheumatology (Oxford) 51: 2252–2261.
8. Mease P, Genovese MC, Gladstein G, Kivitz AJ, Ritchlin C, et al. (2011) Abatacept in the treatment of patients with psoriatic arthritis: results of a six-month, multicenter, randomized, double-blind, placebo-controlled, phase II trial. Arthritis Rheum 63: 939–948.
9. Mease PJ (2012) Is there a role for rituximab in the treatment of spondyloarthritis and psoriatic arthritis? J Rheumatol 39: 2235–2237.
10. Kingsley GH, Kowalczyk A, Taylor H, Ibrahim F, Packham JC, et al. (2012) A randomized placebo-controlled trial of methotrexate in psoriatic arthritis. Rheumatology (Oxford) 51: 1368–1377.
11. Leonardi C, Matheson R, Zachariae C, Cameron G, Li L, et al. (2012) Anti-interleukin-17 monoclonal antibody ixekizumab in chronic plaque psoriasis. N Engl J Med 366: 1190–1199.
12. Papp KA, Leonardi C, Menter A, Ortonne JP, Krueger JG, et al. (2012) Brodalumab, an anti-interleukin-17-receptor antibody for psoriasis. N Engl J Med 366: 1181–1189.
13. McInnes IB, Kavanaugh A, Gottlieb AB, Puig L, Rahman P, et al. (2013) Efficacy and safety of ustekinumab in patients with active psoriatic arthritis: 1 year results of the phase 3, multicentre, double-blind, placebo-controlled PSUMMIT 1 trial. Lancet 382: 780–789.
14. Genovese MC, Durez P, Richards HB, Supronik J, Dokoupilova E, et al. (2012) Efficacy and safety of secukinumab in patients with rheumatoid arthritis: a phase II, dose-finding, double-blind, randomised, placebo controlled study. Ann Rheum Dis.
15. Haupl T, Stuhlmuller B, Grutzkau A, Radbruch A, Burmester GR (2010) Does gene expression analysis inform us in rheumatoid arthritis? Ann Rheum Dis 69 Suppl 1: i37–42.
16. Toonen EJ, Barrera P, Radstake TR, van Riel PL, Scheffer H, et al. (2008) Gene expression profiling in rheumatoid arthritis: current concepts and future directions. Ann Rheum Dis 67: 1663–1669.

17. Lindberg J, af Klint E, Ulfgren AK, Stark A, Andersson T, et al. (2006) Variability in synovial inflammation in rheumatoid arthritis investigated by microarray technology. Arthritis Res Ther 8: R47.
18. Julia A, Erra A, Palacio C, Tomas C, Sans X, et al. (2009) An eight-gene blood expression profile predicts the response to infliximab in rheumatoid arthritis. PLoS One 4: e7556.
19. Lindberg J, Wijbrandts CA, van Baarsen LG, Nader G, Klareskog L, et al. (2010) The gene expression profile in the synovium as a predictor of the clinical response to infliximab treatment in rheumatoid arthritis. PLoS One 5: e11310.
20. Meugnier E, Coury F, Tebib J, Ferraro-Peyret C, Rome S, et al. (2011) Gene expression profiling in peripheral blood cells of patients with rheumatoid arthritis in response to anti-TNF-alpha treatments. Physiol Genomics 43: 365–371.
21. Tuller T, Atar S, Ruppin E, Gurevich M, Achiron A (2012) Common and specific signatures of gene expression and protein-protein interactions in autoimmune diseases. Genes Immun.
22. Arnett FC, Edworthy SM, Bloch DA, McShane DJ, Fries JF, et al. (1988) The American Rheumatism Association 1987 revised criteria for the classification of rheumatoid arthritis. Arthritis Rheum 31: 315–324.
23. Taylor W, Gladman D, Helliwell P, Marchesoni A, Mease P, et al. (2006) Classification criteria for psoriatic arthritis: development of new criteria from a large international study. Arthritis Rheum 54: 2665–2673.
24. van Gestel AM, Prevoo ML, van t Hof MA, van Rijswijk MH, van de Putte LB, et al. (1996) Development and validation of the European League Against Rheumatism response criteria for rheumatoid arthritis. Comparison with the preliminary American College of Rheumatology and the World Health Organization/International League Against Rheumatism Criteria. Arthritis Rheum 39: 34–40.
25. Marks R, Barton SP, Shuttleworth D, Finlay AY (1989) Assessment of disease progress in psoriasis. Arch Dermatol 125: 235–240.
26. Systems I (2013) Ingenuity Upstream Regulator Analysis Whitepaper.
27. Edgar R, Domrachev M, Lash AE (2002) Gene Expression Omnibus: NCBI gene expression and hybridization array data repository. Nucleic Acids Res 30: 207–210.
28. Tian S, Krueger JG, Li K, Jabbari A, Brodmerkel C, et al. (2012) Meta-analysis derived (MAD) transcriptome of psoriasis defines the "core" pathogenesis of disease. PLoS One 7: e44274.
29. Huffmeier U, Bergboer JG, Becker T, Armour JA, Traupe H, et al. (2010) Replication of LCE3C-LCE3B CNV as a risk factor for psoriasis and analysis of interaction with other genetic risk factors. J Invest Dermatol 130: 979–984.
30. Jackson-Boeters L, Wen W, Hamilton DW (2009) Periostin localizes to cells in normal skin, but is associated with the extracellular matrix during wound repair. J Cell Commun Signal 3: 125–133.
31. Walsh DS, Borke JL, Singh BB, Do NN, Hsu SD, et al. (2005) Psoriasis is characterized by altered epidermal expression of caspase 14, a novel regulator of keratinocyte terminal differentiation and barrier formation. J Dermatol Sci 37: 61–63.
32. Ito M, Ogawa K, Takeuchi K, Nakada A, Heishi M, et al. (2004) Gene expression of enzymes for tryptophan degradation pathway is upregulated in the skin lesions of patients with atopic dermatitis or psoriasis. J Dermatol Sci 36: 157–164.
33. Sakamaki J, Daitoku H, Yoshimochi K, Miwa M, Fukamizu A (2009) Regulation of FOXO1-mediated transcription and cell proliferation by PARP-1. Biochem Biophys Res Commun 382: 497–502.
34. Zhao J, Xu Y, Zong Y, Zhang S, Song Y, et al. (2011) Inhibition of Stat3 expression induces apoptosis and suppresses proliferation in human leukemia HL-60 cells. Hematology 16: 232–235.
35. Bargou RC, Emmerich F, Krappmann D, Bommert K, Mapara MY, et al. (1997) Constitutive nuclear factor-kappaB-RelA activation is required for proliferation and survival of Hodgkin's disease tumor cells. J Clin Invest 100: 2961–2969.
36. Angel P, Karin M (1991) The role of Jun, Fos and the AP-1 complex in cell-proliferation and transformation. Biochim Biophys Acta 1072: 129–157.
37. Dey BK, Stalker L, Schnerch A, Bhatia M, Taylor-Papidimitriou J, et al. (2008) The histone demethylase KDM5b/JARID1b plays a role in cell fate decisions by blocking terminal differentiation. Mol Cell Biol 28: 5312–5327.
38. Yang A, Kaghad M, Wang Y, Gillett E, Fleming MD, et al. (1998) p63, a p53 homolog at 3q27-29, encodes multiple products with transactivating, death-inducing, and dominant-negative activities. Mol Cell 2: 305–316.
39. Consortium EP, Dunham I, Kundaje A, Aldred SF, Collins PJ, et al. (2012) An integrated encyclopedia of DNA elements in the human genome. Nature 489: 57–74.
40. Nakajima H, Watanabe N, Shibata F, Kitamura T, Ikeda Y, et al. (2006) N-terminal region of CCAAT/enhancer-binding protein epsilon is critical for cell cycle arrest, apoptosis, and functional maturation during myeloid differentiation. J Biol Chem 281: 14494–14502.
41. Robb L, Hartley L, Wang CC, Harvey RP, Begley CG (1998) musculin: a murine basic helix-loop-helix transcription factor gene expressed in embryonic skeletal muscle. Mech Dev 76: 197–201.
42. Pabst T, Mueller BU, Zhang P, Radomska HS, Narravula S, et al. (2001) Dominant-negative mutations of CEBPA, encoding CCAAT/enhancer binding protein-alpha (C/EBPalpha), in acute myeloid leukemia. Nat Genet 27: 263–270.
43. Ortega C, Fernandez AS, Carrillo JM, Romero P, Molina IJ, et al. (2009) IL-17-producing CD8+ T lymphocytes from psoriasis skin plaques are cytotoxic effector cells that secrete Th17-related cytokines. J Leukoc Biol 86: 435–443.
44. Manenschijn L, van den Akker EL, Lamberts SW, van Rossum EF (2009) Clinical features associated with glucocorticoid receptor polymorphisms. An overview. Ann N Y Acad Sci 1179: 179–198.
45. Allen IC, TeKippe EM, Woodford RM, Uronis JM, Holl EK, et al. (2010) The NLRP3 inflammasome functions as a negative regulator of tumorigenesis during colitis-associated cancer. J Exp Med 207: 1045–1056.
46. Batliwalla FM, Li W, Ritchlin CT, Xiao X, Brenner M, et al. (2005) Microarray analyses of peripheral blood cells identifies unique gene expression signature in psoriatic arthritis. Mol Med 11: 21–29.
47. Stoeckman AK, Baechler EC, Ortmann WA, Behrens TW, Michet CJ, et al. (2006) A distinct inflammatory gene expression profile in patients with psoriatic arthritis. Genes Immun 7: 583–591.
48. Suarez-Farinas M, Fuentes-Duculan J, Lowes MA, Krueger JG (2011) Resolved psoriasis lesions retain expression of a subset of disease-related genes. J Invest Dermatol 131: 391–400.
49. McGonagle D, Ash Z, Dickie L, McDermott M, Aydin SZ (2011) The early phase of psoriatic arthritis. Ann Rheum Dis 70 Suppl 1: i71–76.
50. Barnes MG, Grom AA, Thompson SD, Griffin TA, Pavlidis P, et al. (2009) Subtype-specific peripheral blood gene expression profiles in recent-onset juvenile idiopathic arthritis. Arthritis Rheum 60: 2102–2112.

Nimesulide Improves the Symptomatic and Disease Modifying Effects of Leflunomide in Collagen Induced Arthritis

Ahmed M. Al-Abd[1]*, Fahad A. Al-Abbasi[2], Salwa M. Nofal[3], Amani E. Khalifa[4], Richard O. Williams[5], Wafaa I. El-Eraky[3], Ayman A. Nagy[6], Ashraf B. Abdel-Naim[4]

1 Department of Pharmacology and Toxicology, Faculty of Pharmacy, King Abdulaziz University, Jeddah, Saudi Arabia, **2** Department of Biochemistry, Faculty of Science, King Abdulaziz University, Jeddah, Saudi Arabia, **3** Department of Pharmacology, Medical Division, National Research Centre, Giza, Egypt, **4** Department of Pharmacology and Toxicology, Faculty of Pharmacy, Ain Shams University, Cairo, Egypt, **5** Kennedy Institute of Rheumatology, University of Oxford, Oxford, United Kingdom, **6** Department of Forensic Medicine and Clinical Toxicology, Faculty of Medicine, Tanta University, Egypt

Abstract

Nimesulide is a COX-2 inhibitor used for symptomatic relief of rheumatoid arthritis. Leflunomide is an anti-pyrimidine used to manage the progression of rheumatoid arthritis. Herein we studied the influence of nimesulide and leflunomide combination in terms of disease symptoms and progression using collagen-induced arthritis model in mice, as a model for rheumatoid arthritis. Collagen induced arthritis was induced by immunization with type II collagen. Assessment of joint stiffness and articular hyperalgesia were evaluated using a locomotor activity cage and the Hargreaves method, respectively. Disease progression was assessed via arthritic index scoring, X-ray imaging, myeloperoxidase enzyme activity and histopathologic examination. Nimesulide induced only transient symptomatic alleviation on the top of decreased leucocytic infiltration compared to arthritis group. However, nimesulide alone failed to induce any significant improvement in the radiological or pathological disease progression. Leflunomide alone moderately alleviates the symptoms of arthritis and moderately retarded the radiological and pathological disease progression. Combination of nimesulide and leflunomide significantly improved symptomatic (analgesia and joint stiffness) and arthritic disease progression (radiological, pathological and Myeloperoxidase enzyme activity) in collagen induced arthritis animal model.

Editor: David Douglass Brand, Veterans Affairs Medical Center, United States of America

Funding: This work was funded by the Deanship of Scientific Research (DSR), King Abdulaziz University, Jeddah, under grant No (9/166/1434). The authors, therefore, acknowledge with thanks, DSR for technical and financial support. The funders had no role in study design, data collection and analysis, decision to publish, or preparation of the manuscript.

* Email: amalabd@kau.edu.sa

Introduction

Rheumatoid arthritis (RA) is a chronic progressive systemic inflammatory disorder characterized by synovial inflammation, cartilage damage, progressive bone erosion, and articular functional disability. The world wide incidence of RA ranges from 0.5% to 1.0% and it is more prevalent in women compared to men [1]. Historically, non-steroidal anti-inflammatory drugs "NSAIDs" have been considered to be the primary treatment option for RA. Yet, NSAID failed to exert any significant delay in RA disease progression. Accordingly, disease modifying anti-rheumatic drugs "DMARDs" have become the first treatment option [2]. NSAIDs can mediate short term symptomatic amelioration, but with very poor long term outcome [3]. On the other hand, DMARD based regimens mainly aim to intervene in disease progression, with limited or no short term symptomatic alleviation. Several novel treatments have been tested or suggested for managing rheumatoid arthritis symptoms and/or disease progression, such as lymphocyte co-stimulation-targeted therapy [4], TNFα blocking agents [5], B-cell targeted therapy [6] and novel anti-inflammatory drugs with antioxidant activity [7]. However, the economic burden and patient compliance to injectable drugs limited the widespread use of these agents [8,9].

Leflunomide (LEF) is a DMARD used for the treatment of several autoimmune disorders such as RA [10]. The active leflunomide metabolite, A771726LEF, is generated non-enzymatically or by hepatic microsomal enzymes (CYP 2C9) [11]. The active metabolite of leflunomide is considered to be dihydroorotate dehydrogenase (DHODH) enzyme inhibitor that decreases pyrimidine synthesis [12]. Yet, leflunomide is considered to be a selective anti- T cell agent for autoimmune disorders [13,14]. Leflunomide possesses other advantageous anti-inflammatory effects, such as COX-2 inhibition, matrix metalloproteinase inhibition and anti-chemotaxis, [15–18].

Nimesulide (NIM) is a selective potent cycloxygenase-2 (COX-2) inhibitor [19]. Besides its COX-2 inhibitory activity, nimesulide inhibits several superoxide anion generating enzymes such as myeloperoxidase (MPO) [20]. Other anti-inflammatory properties for nimesulide have been reported such as, suppression of the expression of platelet activation factor (PAF), tumor necrosis factor-α and inhibition of matrix metalloproteinase enzymes [21]. In view of these properties, nimesulide is a strong candidate for combination therapy with DMARDs for the treatment for RA.

Previously, we found that nimesulide improved the disease ameliorating effect of methotrexate in the CIA model [22]. Herein, we extended our finding by studying the influence of nimesulide and leflunomide combination in terms of clinical severity and disease progression in CIA in mice.

Results

Symptomatic assessment of arthritis

The Hargreaves's method for assessing articular hyperalgesia was used herein to monitor joint algesia and to check for the potential effect of combining nimesulide to leflunomide in mice with CIA. Before treatment, the CIA control group manifested pre-arthritic shortening in withdrawal latency (WDL) and algesic response prior to the appearance of clinical signs of arthritis. At the mid-arthritic phase, nimesulide and nimesulide+leflunomide significantly prolonged the WDL compared to CIA control group. On contrary, at the late arthritic phase, all single (LEF or NIM) and combination treatment regimens induced significant analgesic effects in terms of prolonged WDL. LEF and LEF+NIM groups induced equal prolongation in WDL with 55.3% compared to the CIA-group. Treatment with nimesulide alone resulted in weaker analgesia manifested as WDL prolongation of only 38.3% relative to CIA-group. Interestingly, WDL of animals treated with leflunomide or leflunomide/nimesulide combination was non-significantly different from normal non arthritic mice at the late arthritic phase Fig. 1-A.

Joint stiffness is one of the main symptoms of RA, leading to a reduction in mobility. As a measure of this, we recorded the number of movements each animal made within the open field instrument. Locomotor activity of CIA mice started to decline in the pre-arthritic phase with further deterioration up to the late-arthritic phase. In the mid-arthritic phase, nimesulide transiently improved joint stiffness with a significant increase in the total number of movements per minute. Nimesulide treatment did not induce any further improvement in joint stiffness at the late-arthritic phase. Leflunomide alone did not induce any significant improvement in joint stiffness at the mid-arthritic or late-arthritic phases. leflunomide+nimesulide combined treatment showed significant improvement in joint stiffness, which started from the mid-arthritic phase till the late-arthritic phase Fig. 1-B.

Assessment of disease progression

Arthritic index (AI) is a semi quantitative parameter that reflecting the severity of polyarthritis. Animals showed stable, low grade, and persistent polyarthritis after immunization with collagen. Animals treated with leflunomide+nemisulide showed the fastest onset of improvement in AI (31 days after the primary induction of arthritis). Animals treated with leflunomide or nimesulide alone started to show improvement in AI at day 35 after induction. After 40 days of induction, the reduction in AI scores was found to be 31.4%, 22.3%, and 43.8% in LEF-group, NIM-group, and (LEF+NIM)-group respectively compared to the CIA controlgroup Fig. 2-A.

After 40 days of primary immunization (arthritis induction), articular damage was assessed using diagnostic X-ray imaging. Significant periostitis, bone erosion, joint malalignment and cartilaginous deterioration was observed in CIA group indicative of severe articular damage. These radiological changes were also assessed in all other treatment groups Fig. 2-B. Nimesulide treatment alone did not show any radiological improvement. On the other hand, treatment with leflunomide improved the total radiological score by 16.5%, while treatment with leflunomide and nimesulide together provided 19.1% radiological protection Fig. 2-C.

In terms of detailed radiological assessment, leflunomide treatment significantly improved bone erosion, cartilage depth and joint alignment by 21.1%, 23.5% and 17.2%, respectively, compared to the CIA control group. However, combined leflunomide+nimesulide treatment significantly improved all radiological parameters compared to the CIA group. In addition, leflunomide+nimesulide treatment significantly improved bone erosion and periostitis compared to the LEF-group **Table 1**.

Histopathological assessment of articular damage

Articular damage was further confirmed pathologically in H&E stained sagittal sections in the joints of mice. CIA resulted in severe hyperplasia in the synovial membrane, irregularity and roughness of the articular surface, and narrowing of joint space as well as excessive leucocytic infiltration Fig. 3-A&B. Treatment with nimesulide alone resulted in decreased intra-articular leucocytic infiltration Fig. 3-D. Synovial membrane hyperplasia, articular surface roughness and narrowing of the joint space were decreased by leflunomide treatment Fig. 3-C. Of all the treatment groups, leflunomide+nimesulide showed the greatest histopathological improvement compared to the CIA group Fig. 3-E.

RA is characterized by leucocytic infiltration and the presence of neutrophils is often regarded as a marker of active disease. Herein, the activity of myeloperoxidase (MPO) was used as a marker for neutrophilic infiltration in the joints of mice with CIA. After 40 days of the primary induction of arthritis, the MPO level was elevated in the joints of mice with CIA-mice. However, all single and combination treatments significantly decreased the MPO activity compared to the CIA group (Fig. 4).

Discussion

Treatment options for RA warrants a lot of visionary decisions; it is not only confined to symptomatic alleviation [23]. NSAID's provide partial symptomatic alleviation in RA; however they do not generally induce long term joint protection. Nimesulide shows strong anti-inflammatory activity beyond COX-2 inhibition [24,25]. On the other hand DMARDS such as, leflunomide, can induce significant retardation in RA disease progression but they are relatively weak in improving key symptoms of RA such as joint stiffness and joint pain [3]. Hence, a DMARD/NSAID combination may provide long term prevention of disease progression on the top of short term symptomatic control [26]. In the current study, we have investigated the added value of combining nimesulide with leflunomide in controlling experimental arthritis.

Amelioration of the major symptoms of RA such as algesia and joint stiffness is necessary for patient compliance [27]. NSAID's are the major drug category used for this purpose [26]. Despite the huge number of existing NSAIDs, new agents with pharmacological properties and/or less toxic side effects are introduced to the field [7]. In our study, nimesulide alone alleviated joint pain at both the mid- and late arthritic phases (day 21 and day 40 after primary arthritis induction, respectively). However, nimesulide alone temporarily alleviated joint stiffness at mid-arthritic phase and failed at the late arthritic phase. Nimesulide is strong anti-inflammatory analgesic drug that possesses more than just COX-2 inhibition activity [24,25]. That might explain its ability for pain alleviation at all arthritic stages [28]; in addition, the transient improvement in joint stiffness might be partly attributed to the

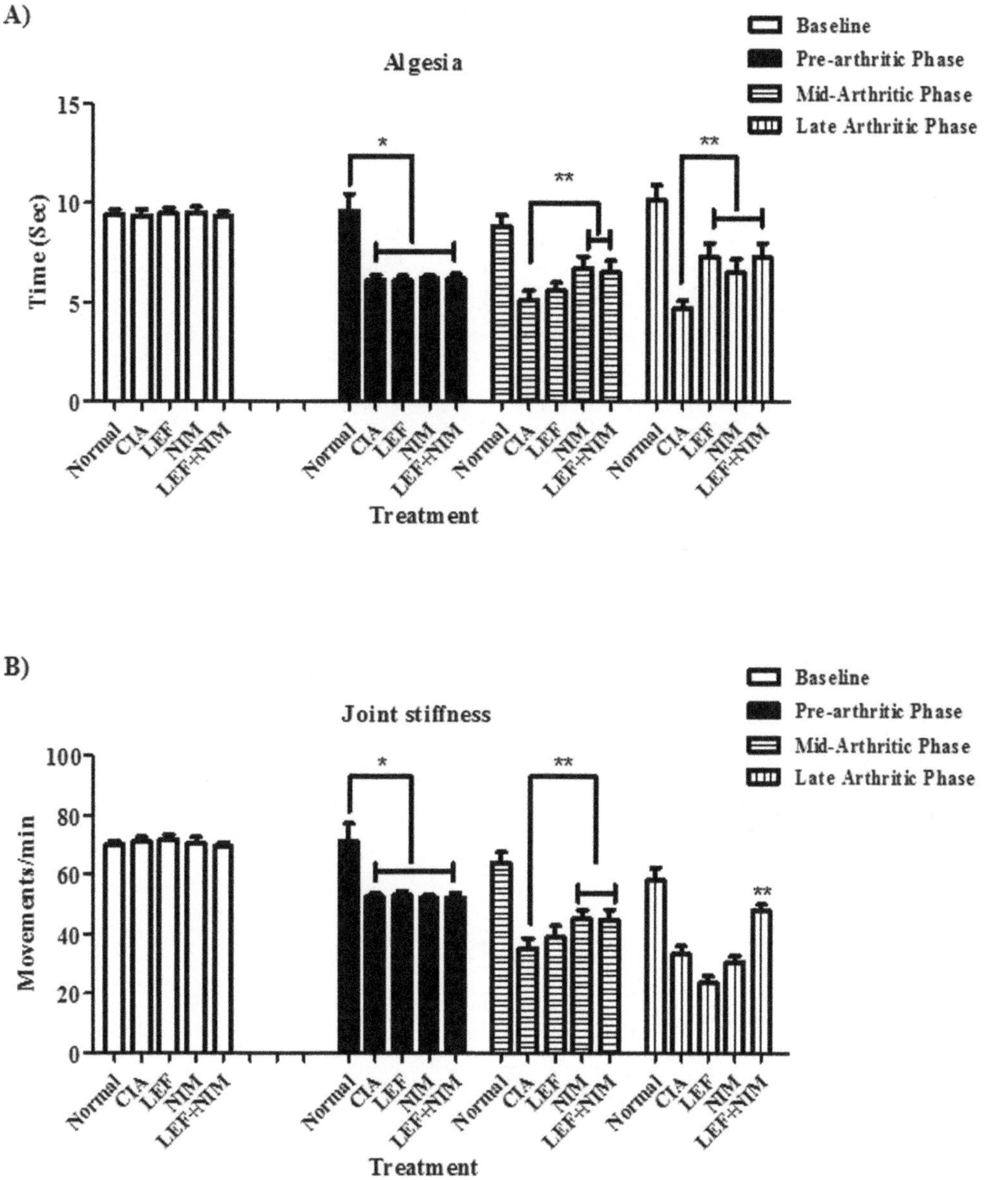

Figure 1. Symptomatic assessment of arthritis. Mice with CIA were treated with leflunomide (LEF), nimesulide (NIM), or leflunomide+ nimesulide (LEF+NIM) and compared to untreated arthritic and normal mice. Hyperalgesia (A) and joint stiffness (B) were recorded at pre-arthritic, mid-arthritic and late arthritic phases of arthritis and compared to base line readings. Data are presented as mean ± SD. * Significantly different from normal mice; ** significantly different from CIA-mice.

analgesic effect [22]. Leflunomide alone failed to induce any significant improvement in joint stiffness. This might be explained by the suboptimal dose level of leflunomide (3.75 mg/kg weekly) used in the current study compared to 10 mg/kg daily in other studies [29]. However, leflunomide at the current dose exerted some pain alleviation effect at the late arthritic phase which might be directly attributed to its moderate anti-inflammatory effects or secondary to its robust disease modifying anti-rheumatic activity [30]. The combination of nimesulide and suboptimal dose of leflunomide could be considered tentative evidence of a synergistic interaction which significantly improved both algesic and joint stiffness signs of CIA at the mid- and late arthritic stages. Symptomatic enhancement effect could be permeated partly to the shared COX-2 inhibition activity of both agents [16,19].

With respect to disease progression, leflunomide+nimesulide induced significant suppression of CIA progression in terms of time and magnitude. At day 33, the AI of LEF+NIM group was not significantly different from normal animals. In addition to the AI, the radiological evaluation showed significant protection for the leflunomide+nimesulide combination compared to either agent alone. Radiological progression is an important feature of RA, as well as CIA [31]. Despite the use of a sub-optimal dose of leflunomide in the current study, combination with nimesulide showed significant improvement in all aspects of the radiological evaluation of arthritis. Moreover, periostitis and bone erosion were significantly improved compared to the LEF-group. This strengthens the tentative synergistic interaction between leflunomide and nimesulide not only on the symptomatic level, but also on the disease modifying level [32].

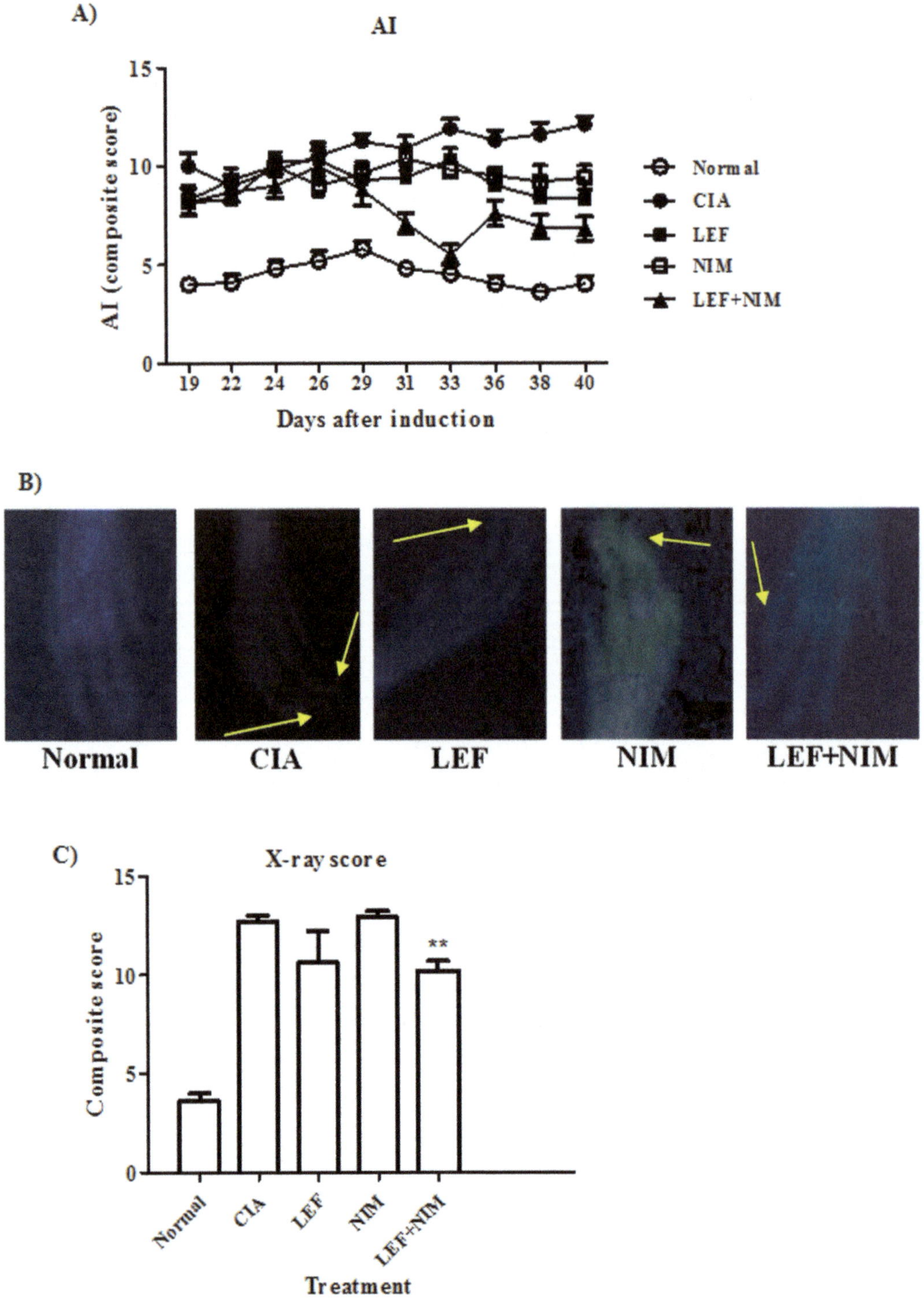

Figure 2. Assessment of disease progression. Mice with CIA were treated with leflunomide (LEF: ■), nimesulide (NIM: □), or leflunomide+ nimesulide (LEF+NIM: ▲) and compared to untreated arthritic (○) and normal mice (●). Arthritic index (AI) of mice was recorded over the duration of 40 days (A). Hind paws of mice were x-ray imaged at day 40 (B) and given a radiological score (C) as shown in the methods section. Data are presented as mean ± SD. ** Significantly different from CIA-mice.

The enhancement effect of nimesulide to leflunomide was further examined histopathologically. Nimesulide alone, significantly blunted the neutrophilic infiltration within joints of mice with CIA as shown by decreased MPO to almost normal levels. MPO is an enzyme known to be highly abundant to the azurophilic granules of neutrophils [33]. The role of neutrophil involvement in CIA and joint damage is well established. Yet, the anti-chemotaxis effect of nimesulide might partly explain the synergistic interaction with leflunomide in terms of disease progression [25,34].

Table 1. Detailed radiographic evaluation of articular damage.

Treatment group	CIA-group	LEF-group	NIM-group	LEF+NIM-group
Bone erosion	3.3 ± 0.1	$2.6^{a}\pm0.3$	3.6 ± 0.2	$2^{a,b}\pm0.2$
Cartilage distance	3.4 ± 0.1	$2.6^{a}\pm0.5$	3.1 ± 0.2	$2.9^{a}\pm0.2$
Periostitis	3.2 ± 0.2	3 ± 0.3	3.1 ± 0.2	$2.6^{a,b}\pm0.2$
Joint alignment	2.9 ± 0.1	$2.4^{a}\pm0.3$	3.1 ± 0.2	$2.9^{a}\pm0.3$

Data are presented as mean ± SEM.
n = 10.
a: significantly different from CIA-group at $p<0.05$.
b: significantly different from LEF-group at $p<0.05$.

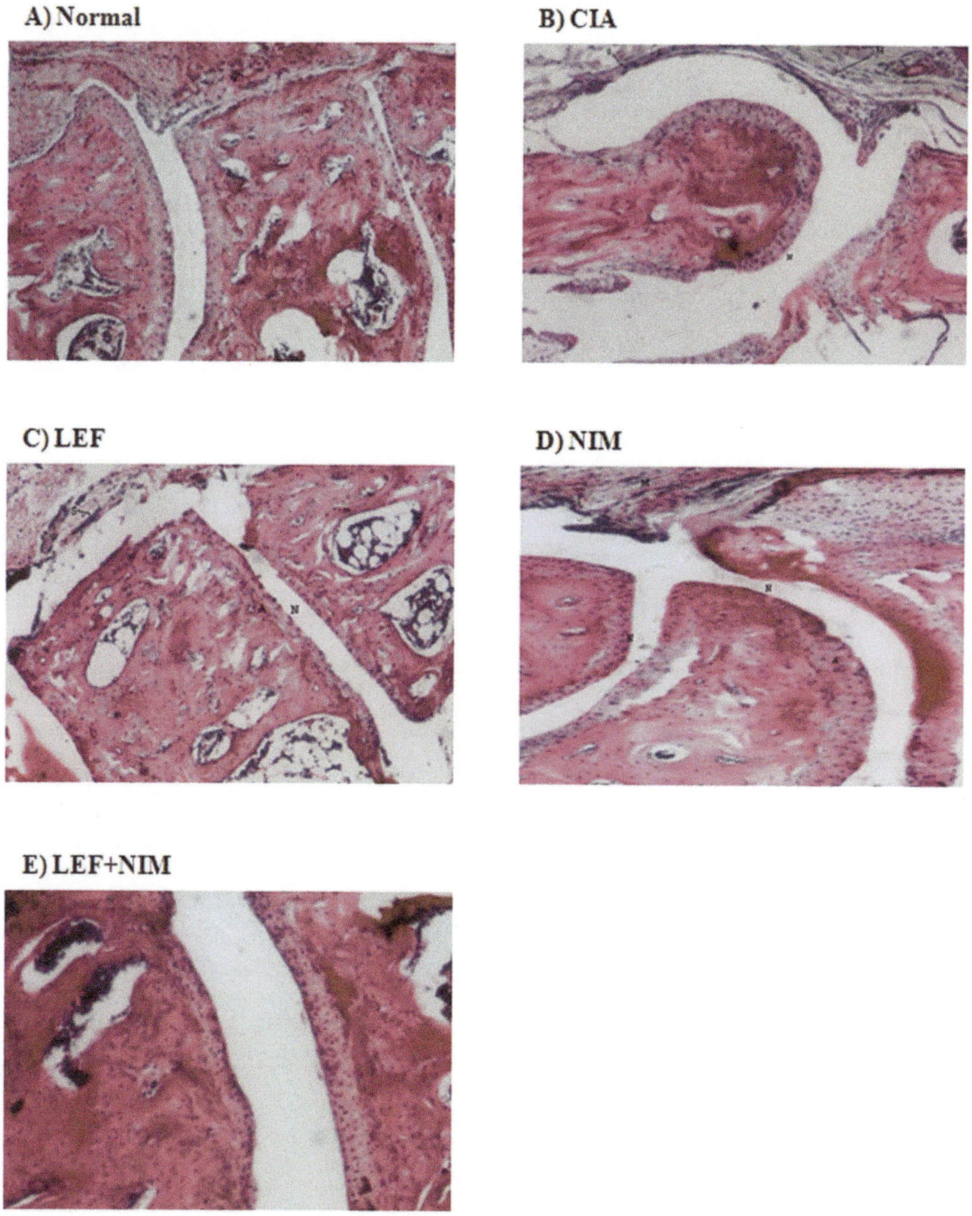

Figure 3. Histopathological assessment of articular damage. Mice with CIA were treated with leflunomide (LEF: Panel C), nimesulide (NIM: Panel D), or leflunomide+nimesulide (LEF+NIM: Panel E) for 40 days and the H&E stained joints were compared with untreated arthritic (CIA: Panel B) and normal mice (Panel A). Pathological findings were compared in terms of synovial hyperplasia (S), articular irregularity (A), narrowing of joint space (N), and lymphocytic infiltration (M).

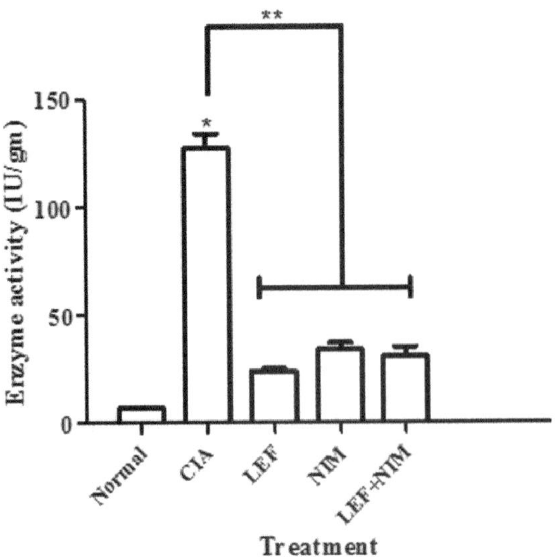

Figure 4. Intra-articular MPO activity. Mice with CIA were treated with leflunomide (LEF), nimesulide (NIM), or leflunomide+nimesulide (LEF+NIM) and compared to untreated arthritic and normal mice. Articular MPO activity was measured 40 days after treatment as a marker of leucocytic infiltration.

Conclusions

Nimesulide enhances the symptomatic, clinical and radiological anti rheumatic activity of Leflunomide in mice with CIA.

Materials and Methods

Chemicals and Drugs

Collagen Type II was prepared as previously described from bovine cartilage [35]. Complete Freund Adjuvant (CFA), leflunomide, hexadecyl trimethylammonium bromide (HTAB), and *o*-dianisidin were purchased from Sigma-Aldrich Chemical Company (St. Louis, MO, USA). Nimesulide was gifted from Alkan Pharmaceutical Co., (6th of October city, Egypt).

Arthritis induction

Male Swiss albino mice (7 weeks old, 30 g weight) were bred in the animal house of the National Research Center (Dokki, Giza, Egypt). Mice were left for one week to acclimatize in the local animal house facility of the Department of Pharmacology prior to experimentation. Animals were kept at controlled environmental conditions with 12 h day/night cycles (20±4°C and 65±10% relative humidity) during the whole experiment. Standardized food pellets and water were supplied *ad libitum*.

Collagen type II solution (4 mg/ml) was prepared by dissolution in 0.1 M acetic acid. Collagen solution was emulsified with an equal volume of CFA. A Volume of 100 µl of final emulsion was injected intradermally (day 0). Only animals with positive signs of arthritis after 2 weeks of induction (87% of animals developed arthritis) were assigned randomly into 5 treatment groups (n = 10 animals/group). After 7 days of the primary induction, another dose (100 µg collagen in CFA) was injected intradermally [36]. The LEF-group received leflunomide 3.75 mg/kg i.p every week; NIM-group received nimesulide 20 mg/kg i.p. every two day; and LEF+NIM-group received leflunomide (3.75 mg/kg i.p) every week and nimesulide (20 mg/kg i.p.) daily. All treatments started 7 days after induction. Treatment groups were compared to mice with CIA (CIA-group) that received no treatment and to a normal non-immunised group (Normal-group).

The Animal Care and Use Committee (IACUC) of the National Research Center (Animal Rights and ethics Committee) approved this complete study.

Assessment of arthritis severity

Arthritic index (AI) was recorded as previously described [37]. Briefly, mice paws were inspected every other day and AI was scored in each paw as follows: erythema and slight swelling in a single digit is given 0.5; erythema and slight swelling in two or more digits is given 1; erythend ma mild swelling in the whole limb is given 2; 3 = erythema and gross swelling in the whole limb is given 3; limb disability and massive limb deformity is given 4. Composite AI equals the sum of each animal's four paws. AI scores were assessed blindly by 2 independent observers starting 2 days before the primary induction of arthritis until the end of the experiment.

Assessment of articular hyperalgesia

Articular hyperalgesia was measured by Hargreaves method with minor in-house modifications [38]; briefly, mice were let to adapt in a designated chamber of planter test (Ugo Basile, Comerio, Italy) for 30 min. Inflamed joints were irradiated with an IR-beam from a movable bulb (Ugo Basile, Comerio, Italy) to induce algesia. The time taken for each animal to lick/withdraw IR-challenged limb was recorded and designated as withdrawal latency (WDL) [39]. The base-line for articular hyperalgesia was determined (2 days before the primary induction of arthritis) and compared to pre-arthritic phase (10 days after the primary induction of arthritis); mid-arthritic phase (25 days after the primary induction of arthritis); and late-arthritic phase (40 days after the primary induction of arthritis).

Assessment of joint stiffness

Joint stiffness was correlated to the locomotor activity of animlas and measured using open field activity cage method. As previously described [39], animals were left for five minutes in the grid floor activity cage (Ugo Basile, Comerio, Italy). The animals' movements with their paws were converted into electric signals and the number of movements per minute was recorded. The base-line for locomotor activity was recorded (2 days before the primary induction of arthritis) and compared to pre-arthritic phase (10 days after the primary induction of arthritis); mid-arthritic phase (25 days after induction); and late-arthritic phase (40 days after the primary induction of arthritis).

Determination of myeloperoxidase enzyme activity

MPO activity was determined in paws at the late-arthritic phase (40 days after the primary induction of arthritis) as previously described [40]. Briefly, mice were sacrificed; paws were immediately excised, weighed and rapidly homogenized for 15 minutes (0.5% hexadecyl trimethylammonuim bromide (HTAB) in 50 mM phosphate buffer, pH 6). Articular tissue homogenate (10% w/v) was centrifuged and 2.9 ml *o*-dianisidin (0.167 mg/ml) was added to 100 µL of the clear supernatant. Hydrogen peroxide (0.0005%) was finally added and absorbance was measured every 15 sec for 2 min (λ_{max} 460 nm). The rate of absorbance change was used to calculate the MPO activity per gram tissue (Molar absorbtivity of the color adduct is 1.13×10^4). [33].

X-rays analysis

Radiological assessment for joint damage was undertaken by X-ray imaging at the late-arthritic phase. Briefly, mice were sacrificed; anterior and hind limbs were excised and fixed in 10% buffered formalin solution. Paws were placed on an X-ray cassette (Medivance Instrument Limited, London, UK) and X-ray images were taken at 40 KV, 0.04 mA sec (Pioneer road-S-240 Salt Lake city, UT, USA). Radiological assessment for joint damage was performed as previously described [41]. Briefly, each limb's X-ray film was scored from 0–4 (4 is the worst) with respect to joint alignment, cartilage distance, bone erosion, and periostitis. The composite scores of each X-ray image represent the total radiological score. Each film was assessed blindly by 3 different observers [42].

Histopathological examination

Histological assessment for articular tissues was performed as follows. Paraformaldhyde fixed tissues were decalcified by EDTA and embedded in paraffin wax. Cross sagittal sections (5 μm) were obtained and after dewaxing and rehydration, sections were stained with H&E.

Statistical analysis

Data are presented as average ± SEM. Significance was tested using ANOVA) with LSD post hoc test was used for testing the significance of parametric data. Significance of non-parametric data was determined using the Mann-Whitney U test. All statistical calculations were carried out by SPSS software for windows, version 17.0.0.; $P<0.05$ was taken as the cut off value for significance.

Author Contributions

Conceived and designed the experiments: AMA WIE ROW ABA. Performed the experiments: AMA WIE ROW AAN. Analyzed the data: AMA FAA AEK AAN ABA. Contributed reagents/materials/analysis tools: FAA SMN AEK ROW. Wrote the paper: AMA AAN ABA. Fund raising: FAA.

References

1. Helmick CG, Felson DT, Lawrence RC, Gabriel S, Hirsch R, et al. (2008) Estimates of the prevalence of arthritis and other rheumatic conditions in the United States. Part I. Arthritis Rheum 58: 15–25.
2. Weinblatt ME (1996) Rheumatoid arthritis: treat now, not later! Ann Intern Med 124: 773–774.
3. Pincus T, O'Dell JR, Kremer JM (1999) Combination therapy with multiple disease-modifying antirheumatic drugs in rheumatoid arthritis: a preventive strategy. Ann Intern Med 131: 768–774.
4. Falgarone G, Semerano L, Rulle S, Boissier MC (2009) Targeting lymphocyte activation to treat rheumatoid arthritis. Joint Bone Spine 76: 327–332.
5. Wiens A, Correr CJ, Pontarolo R, Venson R, Quinalha JV, et al. (2009) A systematic review and meta-analysis of the efficacy and safety of etanercept for treating rheumatoid arthritis. Scand J Immunol 70: 337–344.
6. Bracewell C, Isaacs JD, Emery P, Ng WF (2009) Atacicept, a novel B cell-targeting biological therapy for the treatment of rheumatoid arthritis. Expert Opin Biol Ther 9: 909–919.
7. Khalil NA, Ahmed EM, El-Nassan HB, Ahmed OK, Al-Abd AM (2012) Synthesis and biological evaluation of novel pyrazoline derivatives as anti-inflammatory and antioxidant agents. Arch Pharm Res 35: 995–1002.
8. Schipper LG, Kievit W, den Broeder AA, van der Laar MA, Adang EM, et al. (2011) Treatment strategies aiming at remission in early rheumatoid arthritis patients: starting with methotrexate monotherapy is cost-effective. Rheumatology (Oxford) 50: 1320–1330.
9. Benucci M, Li Gobbi F, Sabadini L, Saviola G, Baiardi P, et al. (2009) The economic burden of biological therapy in rheumatoid arthritis in clinical practice: cost-effectiveness analysis of sub-cutaneous anti-TNFalpha treatment in Italian patients. Int J Immunopathol Pharmacol 22: 1147–1152.
10. Bartlett RR, Brendel S, Zielinski T, Schorlemmer HU (1996) Leflunomide, an immunorestoring drug for the therapy of autoimmune disorders, especially rheumatoid arthritis. Transplant Proc 28: 3074–3078.
11. Rozman B (2002) Clinical pharmacokinetics of leflunomide. Clin Pharmacokinet 41: 421–430.
12. Fox RI (1998) Mechanism of action of leflunomide in rheumatoid arthritis. J Rheumatol Suppl 53: 20–26.
13. Dimitrova P, Skapenko A, Herrmann ML, Schleyerbach R, Kalden JR, et al. (2002) Restriction of de novo pyrimidine biosynthesis inhibits Th1 cell activation and promotes Th2 cell differentiation. J Immunol 169: 3392–3399.
14. Fox RI, Herrmann ML, Frangou CG, Wahl GM, Morris RE, et al. (1999) Mechanism of action for leflunomide in rheumatoid arthritis. Clin Immunol 93: 198–208.
15. Kent EF Jr., Crawford J, Cohen HJ, Buckley RH (1990) Development of multiple monoclonal serum immunoglobulins (multiclonal gammopathy) following both HLA-identical unfractionated and T cell-depleted haploidentical bone marrow transplantation in severe combined immunodeficiency. J Clin Immunol 10: 106–114.
16. Hamilton LC, Vojnovic I, Warner TD (1999) A771726, the active metabolite of leflunomide, directly inhibits the activity of cyclo-oxygenase-2 in vitro and in vivo in a substrate-sensitive manner. Br J Pharmacol 127: 1589–1596.
17. Burger D, Begue-Pastor N, Benavent S, Gruaz L, Kaufmann MT, et al. (2003) The active metabolite of leflunomide, A77 1726, inhibits the production of prostaglandin E(2), matrix metalloproteinase 1 and interleukin 6 in human fibroblast-like synoviocytes. Rheumatology (Oxford) 42: 89–96.
18. Cao WW, Kao PN, Aoki Y, Xu JC, Shorthouse RA, et al. (1996) A novel mechanism of action of the immunomodulatory drug, leflunomide: augmentation of the immunosuppressive cytokine, TGF-beta 1, and suppression of the immunostimulatory cytokine, IL-2. Transplant Proc 28: 3079–3080.
19. Sengupta S (1998) Cyclooxygenase-2: a new therapeutic target. Indian J pharmacology 31: 322–332.
20. Bevilacqua M, Vago T, Baldi G, Renesto E, Dallegri F, et al. (1994) Nimesulide decreases superoxide production by inhibiting phosphodiesterase type IV. Eur J Pharmacol 268: 415–423.
21. Pelletier JP, Martel-Pelletier J (1993) Effects of nimesulide and naproxen on the degradation and metalloprotease synthesis of human osteoarthritic cartilage. Drugs 46 Suppl 1: 34–39.
22. Al-Abd AM, Inglis JJ, Nofal SM, Khalifa AE, Williams RO, et al. (2010) Nimesulide improves the disease modifying anti-rheumatic profile of methotrexate in mice with collagen-induced arthritis. Eur J Pharmacol 644: 245–250.
23. Walker-Bone K, Farrow S (2007) Rheumatoid arthritis. Clin Evid (Online) 2007.
24. Capecchi PL, Ceccatelli L, Beermann U, Laghi Pasini F, Di Perri T (1993) Inhibition of neutrophil function in vitro by nimesulide. Preliminary evidence of an adenosine-mediated mechanism. Arzneimittelforschung 43: 992–996.
25. Tool AT, Mul FP, Knol EF, Verhoeven AJ, Roos D (1996) The effect of salmeterol and nimesulide on chemotaxis and synthesis of PAF and LTC4 by human eosinophils. Eur Respir J Suppl 22: 141s–145s.
26. Ramiro S, Radner H, van der Heijde D, van Tubergen A, Buchbinder R, et al. (2011) Combination therapy for pain management in inflammatory arthritis (rheumatoid arthritis, ankylosing spondylitis, psoriatic arthritis, other spondyloarthritis). Cochrane Database Syst Rev: CD008886.
27. Inotai A, Meszaros A (2012) Determinants of NSAID choice in rheumatoid arthritis–a drug utilization study. Acta Pol Pharm 69: 773–777.
28. da Costa Araujo FA, de Santana Santos T, de Morais HH, Laureano Filho JR, de Oliveira ESED, et al. (2012) Comparative analysis of preemptive analgesic effect of tramadol chlorhydrate and nimesulide following third molar surgery. J Craniomaxillofac Surg 40: e346–349.
29. Coulthard LG, Costello J, Robinson B, Shiels IA, Taylor SM, et al. (2011) Comparative efficacy of a secretory phospholipase A2 inhibitor with conventional anti-inflammatory agents in a rat model of antigen-induced arthritis. Arthritis Res Ther 13: R42.
30. Curnock AP, Robson PA, Yea CM, Moss D, Gadher S, et al. (1997) Potencies of leflunomide and HR325 as inhibitors of prostaglandin endoperoxide H synthase-1 and -2: comparison with nonsteroidal anti-inflammatory drugs. J Pharmacol Exp Ther 282: 339–347.
31. Joosten LA, Helsen MM, Saxne T, van De Loo FA, Heinegard D, et al. (1999) IL-1 alpha beta blockade prevents cartilage and bone destruction in murine type II collagen-induced arthritis, whereas TNF-alpha blockade only ameliorates joint inflammation. J Immunol 163: 5049–5055.
32. Williams RO (1998) Combination therapy in mice: what can we learn that may be useful for understanding rheumatoid arthritis? Springer Semin Immunopathol 20: 165–180.
33. Bradley PP, Priebat DA, Christensen RD, Rothstein G (1982) Measurement of cutaneous inflammation: estimation of neutrophil content with an enzyme marker. J Invest Dermatol 78: 206–209.
34. de Mello SB, Laurindo IM, Cossermelli W (1994) Action of the 4-nitro-2-phenoximethanesulphonanilide (nimesulide) on neutrophil chemotaxis and superoxide production. Sao Paulo Med J 112: 489–494.
35. Miller EJ, Rhodes RK (1982) Preparation and characterization of the different types of collagen. Methods Enzymol 82 Pt A: 33–64.
36. Cook AD, Braine EL, Campbell IK, Rich MJ, Hamilton JA (2001) Blockade of collagen-induced arthritis post-onset by antibody to granulocyte-macrophage

colony-stimulating factor (GM-CSF): requirement for GM-CSF in the effector phase of disease. Arthritis Res 3: 293–298.
37. Urakawa K, Mihara M, Suzuki T, Kawamura A, Akamatsu K, et al. (2000) Polyglutamation of antifolates is not required for induction of extracellular release of adenosine or expression of their anti-inflammatory effects. Immunopharmacology 48: 137–144.
38. Hargreaves K, Dubner R, Brown F, Flores C, Joris J (1988) A new and sensitive method for measuring thermal nociception in cutaneous hyperalgesia. Pain 32: 77–88.
39. Chillingworth NL, Donaldson LF (2003) Characterisation of a Freund's complete adjuvant-induced model of chronic arthritis in mice. J Neurosci Methods 128: 45–52.
40. McVey DC, Vigna SR (2001) The capsaicin VR1 receptor mediates substance P release in toxin A-induced enteritis in rats. Peptides 22: 1439–1446.
41. Clark RL, Cuttino JT Jr., Anderle SK, Cromartie WJ, Schwab JH (1979) Radiologic analysis of arthritis in rats after systemic injection of streptococcal cell walls. Arthritis Rheum 22: 25–35.
42. Asanuma Y, Nagai K, Kato M, Sugiura H, Kawai S (2002) Weekly pulse therapy of methotrexate improves survival compared with its daily administration in MRL/lpr mice. Eur J Pharmacol 435: 253–258.

Fc Gamma Receptor IIb on GM-CSF Macrophages Controls Immune Complex Mediated Inhibition of Inflammatory Signals

Kim C. M. Santegoets[1,2,3], Mark H. Wenink[1,2,3], Wim B. van den Berg[3], Timothy R. D. J. Radstake[1,2,3]*

1 Department of Rheumatology & Clinical Immunology, University Medical Center Utrecht, Utrecht, the Netherlands, **2** Laboratory of Translational Immunology, Department of Immunology, University Medical Center Utrecht, Utrecht, the Netherlands, **3** Department of Rheumatology, Radboud university medical center, Nijmegen, the Netherlands

Abstract

Background: In rheumatoid arthritis (RA) macrophages play a major role in amplifying synovial inflammation. Important activating signals are those induced by Toll-like receptor (TLR) ligands and by activated T cells. The balance between activating and inhibitory Fc gamma receptors (FcγRs) on macrophages might be crucial in modulating these inflammatory responses. The purpose of this study was to determine FcγR expression on pro- and anti-inflammatory macrophages (gmMφ and mMφ, respectively) and identify functional consequences on immune complex uptake and macrophage activation.

Methods: Human monocytes were isolated and differentiated into gmMφ and mMφ. A full FcγR characterization of both macrophage subtypes was performed and uptake of fluorescent immune complexes (ICs) was determined. FcγRIIb isoforms were determined by qPCR. Macrophages were stimulated via different TLRs or cytokine activated T cells in the presence or absence of ICs and cytokine production was determined. Blocking studies were performed to look into the pathways involved.

Results: mMφ expressed high levels of the activating FcγRIIa and FcγRIII and low levels of the inhibitory FcγRIIb, while the FcγR balance on gmMφ was shifted towards the inhibitory FcγRIIb. This was accompanied by a clear increase in FcγRIIb1 mRNA expression in gmMφ. This resulted in higher IC uptake by mMφ compared to gmMφ. Furthermore, FcγR-mediated stimulation of gmMφ inhibited TLR2, 3, 4 and 7/8 mediated cytokine production via FcγRIIb and PI3K signaling. In addition, gmMφ but not mMφ produced TNFα upon co-culture with cytokine activated T cells, which was reduced by IC binding to FcγRIIb. The latter was dependent on PI3K signaling and COX2.

Conclusions: FcγR expression patterns on gmMφ and mMφ are significantly different, which translates in clear functional differences further substantiating FcγRIIb as an interesting target for inflammation control in RA and other autoimmune/inflammatory diseases.

Editor: Jagadeesh Bayry, Institut National de la Santé et de la Recherche Médicale U 872, France

Funding: This work was supported by the Dutch Arthritis Foundation (Reumafonds) [NR 09-1-3-4] and a VENI and VIDI grant (NWO, Dutch science foundation) given to TR. The funders had no role in study design, data collection and analysis, decision to publish, or preparation of the manuscript.

Competing Interests: The authors have declared that no competing interests exist.

* Email: T.R.D.J.Radstake@umcutrecht.nl

Introduction

One of the major pathways underlying the pathogenesis of rheumatoid arthritis (RA) is the aberrant production of inflammatory cytokines by macrophages. In the arthritic joint, macrophages are one of the main effector cells present and their levels correlate with disease activity and joint destruction [1,2]. Their levels are mainly associated with inflammatory cytokines such as TNFα and interleukin (IL) 1β, and could be sustained by factors like granulocyte-macrophage colony-stimulating factor (GM-CSF), present in the RA synovial joint [3–5]. Multiple pathways are proposed to play a role in macrophage activation in RA. One mechanism inducing cytokine production by RA macrophages is the triggering of Toll-like receptors (TLRs). Many endogenous TLR ligands have been found in an arthritic joint, such as GP96 and SNAPIN, which activate cells via TLR2, small heat shock protein B8 that can activate TLR4, and self-RNA from damaged cells which is likely to stimulate macrophages via TLR3 or TLR7/8 [6–10]. Blocking antibodies against these TLRs reduce spontaneous cytokine production by RA synovial tissue cultures, confirming they are not only present in the arthritic joint but also contribute to the abundant cytokine production seen in RA [10–12].

Another pathway mediating synovial macrophage activation is by direct interaction with activated T cells. Cytokine activated T cells resemble RA synovial T cells in their contact-dependent effector function and activation phenotype [13,14]. These cells can be cultured from peripheral blood lymphocytes in the presence of IL-2, IL-6 and TNFα (cytokine activated T cells, Tck) and induce an unbalanced, inflammatory cytokine response from monocytes [14].

Another component present in many RA patients are auto-antibodies. These can form immune complexes (IC) and especially when deposited in tissues they can activate macrophages. Soluble ICs can have cell activating but also inhibitory effects, as is emphasized by IVIg treatment [15]. An important deciding factor for the cellular response to ICs is the balance of activating and inhibitory Fc gamma receptors (FcγRs).

The FcγR system consists of the activating FcγRI, FcγRIIa and FcγRIII that trigger cell activation via an immunoreceptor tyrosine-based activation motif (ITAM) in their cytoplasmic domain and the inhibitory FcγRIIb that signals via an immunoreceptor tyrosine-based inhibition motif (ITIM) [16]. As the only inhibitory FcγR, FcγRIIb is an important brake on the immune system by inhibition of cell activation via the activating FcγRs on a wide array of cells and inhibition of the B cell receptor. FcγRIIb has two major isoforms, namely FcγRIIb1 and FcγRIIb2, which differ in their capabilities to mediate endocytosis and in their distribution on immune cells [17–20]. FcγRIIb1 predominates in B cells, while FcγRIIb2 is the major isoform in myeloid cells. We and others have previously shown that IC binding to FcγRIIb can also inhibit TLR4 signaling [21,22]. In our previous report, only RA patients that could control their disease activity without the need of anti-rheumatic drugs had high FcγRIIb levels on their dendritic cells (DC) and were capable of this inhibition [21]. This supports an important regulatory role for FcγRIIb in controlling inflammation in RA.

Since proinflammatory macrophages are important in the pathogenic process in RA and there is no data on the expression and function of the inhibitory FcγR on such macrophages we aimed to delineate the expression of FcγR receptors on homeostatic M-CSF macrophages (mMφ) and inflammatory GM-CSF macrophages (gmMφ). We determined the complete FcγR balance on gmMφ and mMφ and tested whether functional differences were attributed to this. We mainly focused on combined FcγR triggering with macrophage activation via a range of TLRs implicated in RA pathology or activated T cells and found that FcγRIIb was able to dampen both TLR and Tck induced TNFα production when this inhibitory FcγRIIb was highly expressed.

Materials and Methods

Ethics statement

The study protocol was approved by the medical ethical committee of the Radboud university medical center (Nijmegen, the Netherlands) and the University Medical Center Utrecht (Utrecht, the Netherlands) and all healthy volunteers gave their written informed consent. All experiments were performed in accordance with the Helsinki Declaration.

Culture of monocyte-derived gmMφ and mMφ and Tck cells

Peripheral blood mononuclear cells were isolated from venous blood of healthy volunteers using density-gradient centrifugation over Ficoll (GE Healthcare, Uppsala, Sweden). Monocytes and CD4+ T cells were obtained using CD14 and CD4 microbeads (Miltenyi Biotec, Bergisch Gladbach, Germany). gmMφ and mMφ were generated by culturing monocytes in the presence of GM-CSF (800 U/ml; R&D Minneapolis, Minnesota, USA) or macrophage colony-stimulating factor (M-CSF, 25 ng/ml; R&D) for 6 days. Macrophages were cultured in 6 well plates (Corning, New York, USA) with $1{,}0\times10^6$ cells per well in 2 ml medium (RPMI-1640 Dutch modification (Gibco Life Technologies, Grand Island, New York, USA)) supplemented with 10% FCS, antibiotic-antimycotic and L-glutamine (Gibco Life Technologies). Culture medium with the same supplements (1 ml) was added at day 3 and the cells were harvested at day 6. In parallel, autologous CD4+ T cells were cultured in complete medium with recombinant human IL-2 (25 ng/ml), IL-6 (100 ng/ml) and TNFα (25 ng/ml) at 2×10^6 cells/ml for 6 days (all from R&D).

Phenotypical analysis

Using standardized flow cytometry protocols as described previously gmMφ and mMφ were phenotyped using antibodies against CD14, CD163 (both BD Biosciences, Franklin Lakes, New Jersey, USA) and MHC-II DR/DP (clone Q1514) [23]. FcγR expression was determined with antibodies against FcγRI (CD64, PE labeled, clone 10.1; Dako, Glostrup, Denmark), FcγRIII (CD16, PE labeled, clone DJ130c; Dako), clone IV.3 which preferentially binds to FcγRIIa (StemCell Technologies, Vancouver, Canada) and the FcγRIIb specific antibody 2B6 (Alexa488 labeled; MacroGenics, Rockville, Maryland, USA). Expression of unlabeled markers was visualized via a FITC labeled goat-anti-mouse secondary antibody. Cell fluorescence was measured on a FACS Calibur (BD) and analyzed using Flowjo software for the mean fluorescence intensity (MFI) and the proportion of positive cells relative to cells stained with the appropriate IgG isotypes.

RNA isolation and qPCR

Total RNA was extracted in 0.5 ml of TRI-reagent and treated with DNase to remove genomic DNA before being reverse-transcribed into cDNA. qPCR was performed on a Quantstudio 12K Flex (Life Technologies) with SYBR Select Master Mix (Life Technologies), 7.5 ng cDNA and a primer concentration of 0.5 μM in a total volume of 15 μl. qPCR signals were quantified by comparing the cycle threshold value (Ct) of the gene of interest of each sample with the Ct value of the reference gene GAPDH (ΔCt). Results were deployed as relative expression ($2^{-\Delta Ct}$). The following primers were used: GAPDH forward ATGGG-GAAGGTGAAGGTCG, reverse GGGGTCATTGATGGCAA-CAATA; FcγRIIb1 forward GGATTTCAGCTCTCCCAG-GAT, reverse CGGTTCTGGTCATCAGGCTC; FcγRIIb2 forward AAAGCGGATTTCAGCCAATC, reverse CAAGA-CAATGGAGACTAAATACGGT.

Phagocytosis and binding assay

Phagocytosis assays were performed with fluorescently labeled ICs, prepared as previously described [24]. Macrophages were incubated with FITC-labeled ICs (50 μg/ml) for 30 min at 4°C and 37°C to determine binding and uptake, respectively. Unattached ICs were washed away before determining binding and uptake by flow cytometry. To determine IC uptake extracellular attached FITC-IC was quenched by adding trypan blue (1/40 diluted in PBS, Sigma-Aldrich) to the samples just before determining the IC uptake by flow cytometry.

Stimulation of monocyte-derived macrophages

At day 6 macrophages were harvested and plated in a concentration of 0.5×10^6 cells/ml in 96 well culture plates (100 μl). Immune complexes used in this study were prepared by heating human IgG (Sigma-Aldrich, St. Louis, Missouri, USA) in PBS at 63°C for 30 minutes (heat-aggregated immune complexes

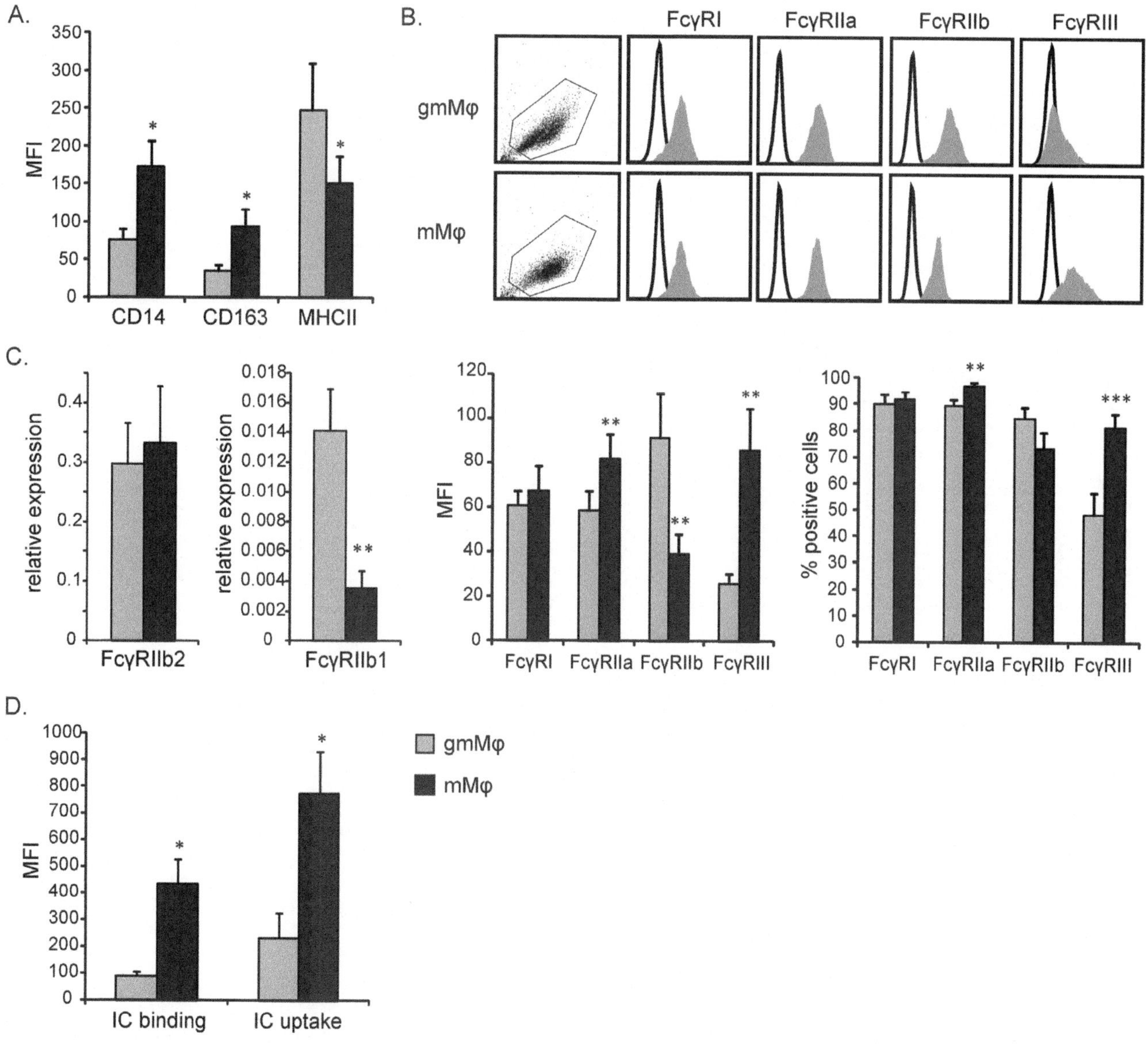

Figure 1. gmMφ express high FcγRIIb levels, while mMφ express more FcγRIIa and FcγRIII. Monocytes were cultured for 6 days with GM-CSF or M-CSF into gmMφ and mMφ respectively. Expression of CD14, CD163 and MHC-II (**A**) and all FcγRs (**B**) was determined by flow cytometry. (**B**) For FcγR expression, representative FACS plots are shown together with bar graphs showing mean (and SEM of) MFI and percentage of positive cells from 11 donors. Histograms show isotype control (thin line) and FcγR specific antibody (solid grey). (**C**) mRNA expression of FcγRIIb1 and FcγRIIb2 were determined by qPCR and plotted as relative expression compared to GAPDH. Bars are mean and SEM of 7 donors. (**D**) gmMφ and mMφ were incubated with FITC-labeled ICs (50 μg/ml) for 30 min at 4°C for binding and 37°C for uptake. IC uptake was determined in the presence of trypan blue. Bars are mean and SEM from 4 donors. *P<0.05, **P<0.01 and ***P<0.001 compared to mφ-1.

(IC)), as previously described [25] and were used in a concentration of 50 μg/ml. Macrophages were stimulated or not with ICs for 15–30 minutes before the addition of TLR agonists for 20 hours. The following concentrations of TLR agonists were used: Pam3CSK4 (5 μg/ml, EMC Microcollections, Tübingen, Germany), Poly(I:C) (25 μg/ml, Invivogen, San Diego, California, USA), LPS (100 ng/ml, E. coli 0111:B4, Sigma-Aldrich) and R848 (2 μg/ml, Invivogen) for TLR2/1, 3, 4 and 7/8 respectively. The LPS was double-purified to remove any contaminating proteins as described previously [26]. Macrophages were also co-cultured with cytokine-activated T cells for 20 hours in a 1:5 ratio in the presence or absence of IC (50 μg/ml) prestimulation for 1 h.

FcγRIIb blocking was performed by 30 min incubation of mφ-1 with 10 μg/ml 2B6 antibody (MacroGenics) or an isotype control at 4°C before stimulation with ICs and LPS or Tck. In other experiments gmMφ were treated with the PI3K inhibitors Wortmannin (0.1 μM; Calbiochem, San Diego, California, USA) or LY294002 (10 μM; Calbiochem) or COX2 inhibitor I (20 μM; Calbiochem) for 1 h at 37°C before stimulation.

Measurement of cytokines in culture supernatants

Levels of IL-10 and TNFα were measured in the supernatants using commercially available kits (Millipore, Billerica, Massachusetts, USA) according to the manufacturer's instructions. Cytokine levels were measured and analyzed with the Bio-Plex system (Bio-Rad, Hercules, California, USA).

Statistical analysis

Differences were analyzed using paired Student's t-tests. P values less than 0.05 were considered significant.

Results

gmMφ express high levels of the inhibitory FcγRIIb, while mMφ express higher levels of the activating FcγRIIa and FcγRIII

Monocytes were cultured into pro- and anti-inflammatory gmMφ and mMφ in the presence of either GM-CSF or M-CSF. To confirm the phenotype of our gmMφ and mMφ we first analyzed their expression of CD14, CD163 and MHC-II. In line with literature the expression of CD14 and CD163 was higher on mMφ, while MHC-II was increased on gmMφ (Figure 1A) [21]. We further evaluated the expression of activating and inhibitory FcγRs. The monomeric IgG receptor FcγRI was similarly expressed in gmMφ and mMφ, while FcγRIII expression was highly increased on mMφ compared to gmMφ (regarding both MFI and percentage of positive cells, Figure 1B). Investigating the activating and inhibiting subtype of FcγRII separately, we observed a marked difference between the gmMφ en mMφ. Whereas the activating FcγRIIa is expressed higher on mMφ, expression of the inhibitory FcγRIIb was increased on gmMφ (Figure 1B). More specifically, the FcγRIIb/FcγRIIa ratio was 1.56 for gmMφ and 0.48 for mMφ. Thus, gmMφ display an FcγR balance favored towards the inhibitory subtype whereas the opposite was found on mMφ. FcγR expression was also determined on gmMφ and mMφ from some RA patients, which showed a similar FcγR distribution compared to healthy controls (data not shown). In vivo in situations in which GM-CSF is produced most likely also a basal level of M-CSF will be present. To determine the effect of the combination of both growth factors on macrophage development we also cultured macrophages with GM-CSF and M-CSF. This resulted in a phenotype similar to gmMφ, suggesting GM-CSF is dominant over M-CSF, at least regarding FcγR expression (data not shown).

We further aimed to differentiate between the two major FcγRIIb isoforms, FcγRIIb1 and FcγRIIb2. Since the extracellular domain of these isoforms is the same we used qPCR to determine the expression of these variants in mMφ and gmMφ. Using isoform specific primers we found that FcγRIIb2 expression was similar in both macrophage subtypes, while FcγRIIb1 expression was significantly increased in gmMφ compared to mMφ (Figure 1C). gmMφ thus have an increased expression of the FcγRIIb variant usually more predominant in B cells which is less capable of mediating endocytosis.

The capacity to take up ICs is an important function of macrophages. To evaluate the functionality of the altered aforementioned FcγR balance, we investigated whether the gmMφ and mMφ display a different binding and uptake capacity of ICs. mMφ show a significantly increased potential for both binding and uptake of ICs compared to gmMφ (Figure 1D). This is fitting with the enhanced expression of FcγRIIa and FcγRIII on mMφ, which have a higher affinity for most IgG isotypes compared to FcγRIIb [27] and the increased expression of the non-endocytosing FcγRIIb1 on gmMφ.

ICs inhibit TLR induced cytokine production by gmMφ but not by mMφ

To further evaluate the functional consequences of the differential FcγR expression on gmMφ and mMφ and to test whether ICs can also inhibit TLR4 signaling in human macrophages that express high FcγRIIb levels, gmMφ and mMφ were stimulated with TLR ligands in combination with ICs. mMφ and gmMφ were first stimulated with ICs alone to determine the effect of differential FcγR expression on these cells on IC induced cytokine production. In mMφ ICs induced significant but low levels of TNFα and IL-10 production, while there was no clear cytokine induction observed in gmMφ (Figure 2A). Upon TLR 4 stimulation with LPS gmMφ produced high levels of TNFα and low levels of IL-10, while mMφ were marked by their relatively high IL-10 production and low production of TNFα which corroborates the literature (Figure 2B) [5,28]. After co-stimulation with ICs, gmMφ were able to significantly attenuate TNFα production compared to those stimulated with LPS alone, while IL-10 production was relatively unaffected (Figure 2B). In contrast, but in line with our observations on FcγR expression, the addition of ICs to LPS did not result in inhibition of TLR4 mediated cytokine production in mMφ. In fact, mMφ produced significantly more IL-10 after co-stimulation with ICs.

To determine if this inhibitory pathway can also affect cytokine induction by other TLR ligands, similar experiments were performed with specific ligands for TLR2/1 (Pam3CSK4), TLR3 (Poly(I:C)) and TLR7/8 (R848). These experiments learned that the inhibitory effect of ICs on TLR signaling by gmMφ is not limited to TLR4, but also extends to TLR2/1, TLR3 and TLR7/8 (Figure 2C), further substantiating the pivotal role of the FcγR balance in the regulation of cell activation. Again, IL-10 production by gmMφ was not clearly affected by the presence of ICs and the inhibitory effect on TNFα production was not present in mMφ (data not shown). To determine if ICs could also affect TLR induced cytokine production after TLR stimulation has already occurred, we performed a time course with addition of ICs from 2 hours prior to Pam3CSK4 till 2 hours after Pam3CSK stimulation. ICs were able to significantly modulate TNFα production during the whole time range, without significantly affecting IL-10 (data not shown). ICs can thus modulate TLR induced cytokine production before and after TLR triggering.

Immune complexes can inhibit gmMφ activation by activated T cells

Another important activator of RA synovial macrophages are cytokine activated T cells. We therefore evaluated cytokine production in co-cultures of Tck with gmMφ or mMφ. Tck induced a synergistic production of TNFα when co-cultured with gmMφ (Figure 3A), while IL-10 is almost absent, resulting in an unbalanced proinflammatory response. The TNFα production by mMφ after co-culture with Tck is much lower and not significantly different from mMφ alone (Figure 3A). In contrast to mMφ stimulation by TLR ligands, in co-culture with Tck also IL-10 production remained low. Thus, Tck mainly stimulate gmMφ. To determine if ICs could inhibit Tck induced TNFα production when macrophages express high FcγRIIb levels, gmMφ were stimulated with ICs and Tck. IC co-stimulation reduced the TNFα release by gmMφ with approximately 50% upon Tck stimulation (Figure 3B). ICs can thus modulate both TLR and T cell induced gmMφ activation.

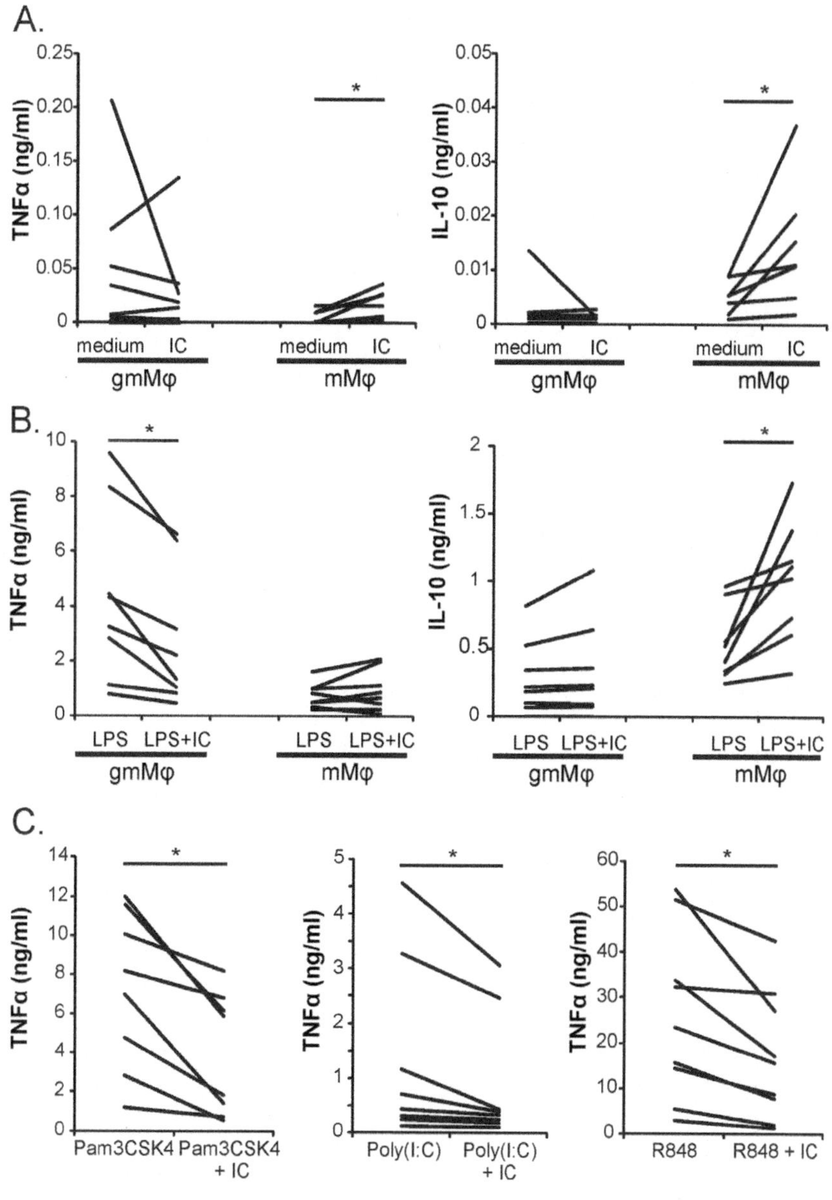

Figure 2. Immune complexes can inhibit TLR2, 3, 4 and 7/8 induced cytokine production in gmMφ. gmMφ and mMφ were stimulated with ICs (50 μg/ml) (**A**), LPS (100 ng/ml) or LPS+ICs (**B**) and TNFα and IL-10 were measured in culture supernatants after 20 hours. (**C**) gmMφ were stimulated with Pam3CSK4 (5 μg/ml), Poly(I:C) (25 μg/ml) or R848 (2 μg/ml) in the presence or absence of ICs. After 20 hours, supernatants were collected and analyzed for TNFα levels. Figure shows data of at least 7 donors for all stimulations. *$P<0.05$ difference with and without IC.

The inhibitory effect of ICs is mediated via FcγRIIb and the PI3K pathway

To confirm whether the high FcγRIIb expression on gmMφ was indeed responsible for the inhibitory effect of ICs on TLR and Tck induced signaling in these cells, we used a blocking antibody against FcγRIIb. Blocking of FcγRIIb fully abrogated the inhibitory effect of ICs on both TLR and Tck induced TNFα production (Figure 4A and B).

In DCs our group has previously shown that the PI3K/Akt pathway is involved in the crosstalk between FcγRIIb and TLR4 [21]. To determine if this pathway is also involved in the FcγRIIb effect on macrophages, we blocked PI3K signaling before stimulation of gmMφ with ICs and LPS. The IC mediated inhibition of LPS induced TNFα production was abrogated in the presence of Wortmannin or LY294002, confirming the role of the PI3K pathway in FcγRIIb mediated TLR4 signaling inhibition in gmMφ (Figure 4C and data not shown). Mice studies pointed towards an additional role for prostaglandin E2 in the inhibitory actions of FcγRIIb on TLR4 signaling [22]. To test this in the human setting we performed our experiments in the presence of a COX2 inhibitor. This did not affect the IC mediated inhibition of cytokine production by gmMφ upon TLR4 stimulation (Figure 4C). To test if the same mechanism was involved in IC mediated blocking of other TLRs we tested FcγRIIb blocking and PI3K inhibition also for ICs in combination with TLR2/1 stimulation and this gave similar results as shown for TLR4 (data not shown).

To further determine if similar pathways are involved in inhibition of Tck induced macrophage activation we performed

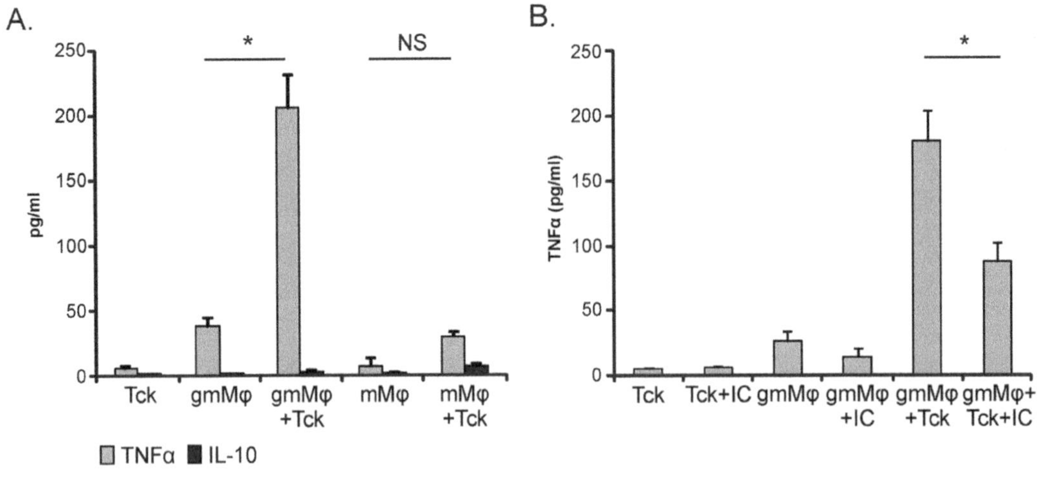

Figure 3. IC can inhibit T cell mediated macrophage activation in gmMφ. gmMφ or mMφ and Tck were cultured from the same donor. (**A**) At day 6 the macrophages and Tcks were harvested, washed and cultured together in a ratio of 1:5. TNFα and IL-10 were measured in the supernatant after 20 hours. Bars are mean and SEM from 3 independent experiments. (**B**) gmMφ were cultured alone or in a 1:5 ratio with Tck in the presence or absence of ICs (50 μg/ml) for 20 hours before collecting the supernatant. Bars are mean and SEM from 6 independent experiments. *P<0.05, NS is not significant.

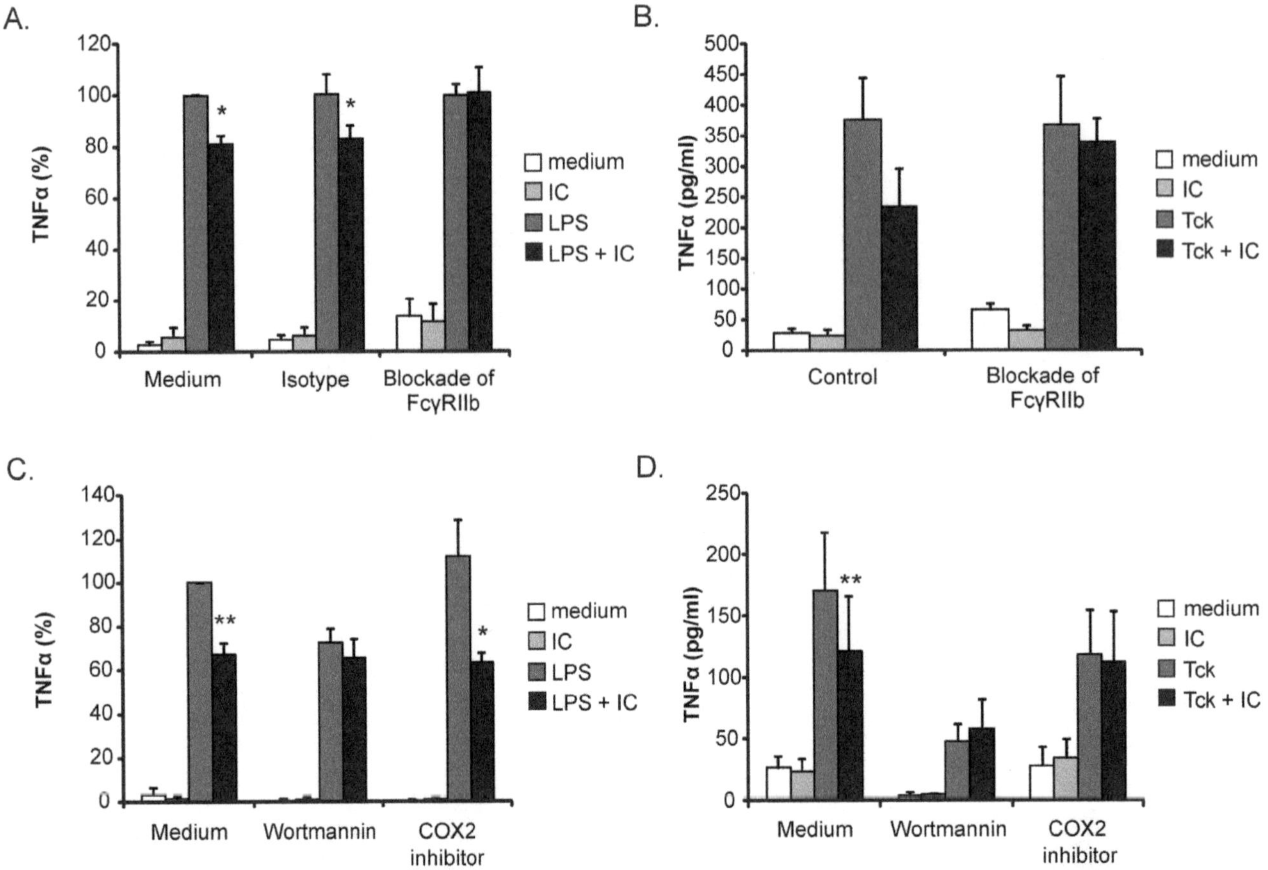

Figure 4. TLR and Tck inhibition by IC is mediated via FcγRIIb and PI3K. gmMφ were pre-incubated for 30 minutes with the FcγRIIb specific blocking antibody 2B6 (10 μg/ml) or an isotype control before stimulation with IC (50 μg/ml) and LPS (100 ng/ml) (**A**) or Tck (**B**). gmMφ were pre-incubated with Wortmannin (0.1 μM) or a Cox2 inhibitor (20 μM) for 1 hr before stimulation with IC and LPS (**C**) or Tck (**D**). 20 hour supernatants were collected to analyze TNFα levels. In the graphs showing TLR stimulation (A and C) the percentage of TNFα production is plotted with the LPS only stimulation set at 100%. In the Tck graphs (B and D) absolute values are shown. All graphs show the mean and SEM of at least 3 experiments. *P<0.05.

the Tck experiments in the presence of Wortmannin or a COX2 inhibitor. As for TLR activation a functioning PI3K pathway was necessary for the inhibitory effect of ICs, however IC mediated blocking of gmMφ activation via Tck also appeared to be dependent on prostaglandin production, as is exemplified by the lack of IC mediated inhibition in the presence of a COX2 inhibitor (Figure 4D). IC mediated inhibition of gmMφ TNFα production via both pathways is mediated via binding to FcγRIIb and involves the PI3K pathway. Prostaglandins are necessary for the effect of IC when combined with Tck, but not for TLR mediated cell activation.

Discussion

The present study shows that gmMφ have a relatively high expression of FcγRIIb compared to the activating FcγRs, while this balance is shifted towards the activating FcγRs on mMφ. gmMφ secrete large amounts of TNFα upon stimulations relevant in RA, such as TLR ligands and cytokine activated T cells. Under these conditions inhibitory immune receptors, such as FcγRIIb, are crucial to counter-regulate the induced inflammatory responses to prevent excessive tissue damage. We show that the switched balance towards the inhibitory FcγRIIb on gmMφ is functionally relevant and can inhibit TNFα secretion from these cells induced by either TLRs or Tck in the presence of soluble ICs. This way it could function as a natural brake in an attempt to prevent excessive cytokine production and inflammation in RA.

The important regulatory role of FcγRIIb is extensively shown in animal models for autoimmunity (Reviewed in [29]). In this context it was shown that the transfer of RA but not healthy control serum can induce arthritis in FcγRIIb$^{-/-}$, but not in normal B6 mice [30]. This was caused by the IgG portion supporting a pathogenic role for IgG (auto) antibodies from RA patients and an important regulatory role for FcγRIIb. This model bypasses the effect of B cells because human IgG is passively transferred and it thus shows that FcγRIIb expression on other effector cells, including macrophages and DCs, is crucial to prevent autoimmune inflammation.

We demonstrated for the first time that FcγRIIb can inhibit cytokine induction by a wide range of TLRs, of which ligands have been found in the arthritic joint, including TLR2, TLR3, TLR4 and TLR7/8. In addition, FcγRIIb can also inhibit macrophage TNFα production induced by activated T cells. This way FcγRIIb can actively control two important stimulatory pathways for macrophages in RA. Inhibitor studies taught us that normal PI3K signaling is necessary for FcγRIIb inhibition of both TLR and Tck induced cytokine release, while prostaglandins are only involved in the latter. Prostaglandins were postulated as an essential signaling molecule in FcγRIIb mediated inhibition of TLR4 in mouse macrophages [22]. However, in our human experimental setting prostaglandins are dispensable for FcγRIIb mediated inhibition of TLRs. In our cultures prestimulation of gmMφ with ICs for only 15–30 minutes or up to 2 hours after TLR stimulation was enough to get inhibition, while in mouse macrophages the dependency on prostaglandins was demonstrated after 24 hour prestimulation with ICs [22]. So prostaglandins are not necessary for the direct inhibition of TLR4 signaling by FcγRIIb in humans, but might have additional inhibitory effects at later time points. This would be in line with the dependency of Tck inhibition on prostaglandin production, since the induction of TNFα in this setting is described to be much slower (peaks at 24 hrs.) compared to TLR stimulated TNFα induction (peaks at 4–8 hrs.) [31]. However, much is still unknown about the pathways involved in macrophage activation upon interaction with Tcks. CD69, CD18 and CD49d on the Tck were shown to be involved in the induction of TNFα by monocytes upon Tck co-culture [14]. On monocytes/macrophages ICAM-1 and VCAM-1 might be involved as binding partners for CD18 and CD49d, respectively. Thus far, no direct interactions are known between these molecules and FcγR signaling. Hence, our work justifies more research focused at deciphering potential mechanisms involved in FcγRIIb inhibition on T cell mediated macrophage activation.

Interestingly, the increased membrane FcγRIIb expression on gmMφ coincides with an increased expression of FcγRIIb1 on mRNA level. This suggests that FcγRIIb1 expression on gmMφ could play a role in the inhibitory effects of ICs on these cells. Although the FcγRIIb isoforms have been repeatedly shown to have differential endocytosis potential [17–19], not much is known about possible differences in inhibitory signaling. It has been described that FcγRIIb1 is differently phosphorylated in B cells compared to FcγRIIb2 and might have additional inhibitory functions [19,32], but this has not been repeated by another group in macrophage cell lines [33]. Whether this could have functional implications for macrophage responses towards ICs needs to be further investigated.

Some groups have tried to identify the macrophage phenotype or the FcγR expression on macrophages from RA synovial tissue. FcγRII overall, FcγRIIb in particular and FcγRIII were all increased in RA synovium and correlated with the amount of macrophages present [34,35]. Looking at in vitro markers for gmMφ and mMφ it remains difficult to fully characterize the macrophages from the synovial tissue since they express markers representing both phenotypes [36,37]. Supported by our data the expression of FcγRIIb could be an additional marker for gmMφ while FcγRIII marks mMφ macrophages. The ratio between these two FcγRs could be a good discriminator between these macrophage subsets. The high expression of activating FcγRs by mMφ, which are mainly described for their controlling/homeostatic functions, and the high expression of the inhibitory FcγRIIb on the more inflammatory gmMφ might seem contradictory. However, because of the easily activated phenotype of gmMφ regulatory mechanisms including those via FcγRIIb are crucial to prevent excessive inflammation and tissue damage. In addition, the capacity of mMφ to remove IC is facilitated by the high expression of FcγRs, preventing accumulation of IC and thereby preventing unwanted inflammatory responses. Next to that we show that small ICs in combination with TLR stimulation mainly increase IL-10 production in mMφ and no major induction of TNFα was observed.

The in vivo situation is not as black and white as shown by this in vitro model, but knowledge about functional characteristics of these macrophage subsets combined with more detailed phenotyping of local macrophages, including differentiation between FcγRIIa and FcγRIIb in different diseases might give clues about the pathogenic processes going on in vivo. This could possibly give leads for therapeutic options to increase FcγRIIb expression on macrophages even further to induce a more inhibitory phenotype.

Conclusions

gmMφ and mMφ are characterized by a different FcγR balance, with high FcγRIIa and FcγRIII levels on mMφ and increased FcγRIIb expression on pro-inflammatory gmMφ. The relatively high FcγRIIb expression on gmMφ makes these cells sensitive to IC mediated inhibition of proinflammatory cytokine release upon stimulation by TLR ligands and Tck, which can be an important feedback mechanism to prevent excessive inflammation. This shows that FcγRIIb mediated cell inhibition is not restricted to ITAM containing receptors or TLR4, but can broadly regulate immune responses. Specific targeting of FcγRIIb might therefore open novel therapeutic avenues for RA and other chronic immune mediated inflammatory disorders.

Acknowledgments

We thank MacroGenics for providing us with the FcγRIIb specific antibody 2B6 for flow cytometry and blocking studies.

Author Contributions

Conceived and designed the experiments: KS MW WB TR. Performed the experiments: KS MW. Analyzed the data: KS MW. Contributed reagents/materials/analysis tools: KS MW WB TR. Contributed to the writing of the manuscript: KS MW WB TR.

References

1. Mulherin D, Fitzgerald O, Bresnihan B (1996) Synovial tissue macrophage populations and articular damage in rheumatoid arthritis. Arthritis Rheum 39: 115–124.
2. Tak PP, Smeets TJ, Daha MR, Kluin PM, Meijers KA, et al. (1997) Analysis of the synovial cell infiltrate in early rheumatoid synovial tissue in relation to local disease activity. Arthritis Rheum 40: 217–225.
3. Vandooren B, Noordenbos T, Ambarus C, Krausz S, Cantaert T, et al. (2009) Absence of a classically activated macrophage cytokine signature in peripheral spondylarthritis, including psoriatic arthritis. Arthritis Rheum 60: 966–975. 10.1002/art.24406 [doi].
4. Xu WD, Firestein GS, Taetle R, Kaushansky K, Zvaifler NJ (1989) Cytokines in chronic inflammatory arthritis. II. Granulocyte-macrophage colony-stimulating factor in rheumatoid synovial effusions. J Clin Invest 83: 876–882. 10.1172/JCI113971 [doi].
5. Verreck FA, De Boer T, Langenberg DM, Hoeve MA, Kramer M, et al. (2004) Human IL-23-producing type 1 macrophages promote but IL-10-producing type 2 macrophages subvert immunity to (myco)bacteria. Proc Natl Acad Sci U S A 101: 4560–4565.
6. Huang QQ, Sobkoviak R, Jockheck-Clark AR, Shi B, Mandelin AM, et al. (2009) Heat shock protein 96 is elevated in rheumatoid arthritis and activates macrophages primarily via TLR2 signaling. J Immunol 182: 4965–4973. 182/8/4965 [pii];10.4049/jimmunol.0801563 [doi].
7. Shi B, Huang Q, Tak PP, Vervoordeldonk MJ, Huang CC, et al. (2012) SNAPIN: an endogenous Toll-like receptor ligand in rheumatoid arthritis. Ann Rheum Dis 71: 1411–1417. annrheumdis-2011-200899 [pii];10.1136/annrheumdis-2011-200899 [doi].
8. Brentano F, Schorr O, Gay RE, Gay S, Kyburz D (2005) RNA released from necrotic synovial fluid cells activates rheumatoid arthritis synovial fibroblasts via Toll-like receptor 3. Arthritis Rheum 52: 2656–2665.
9. Roelofs MF, Boelens WC, Joosten LA, Abdollahi-Roodsaz S, Geurts J, et al. (2006) Identification of small heat shock protein B8 (HSP22) as a novel TLR4 ligand and potential involvement in the pathogenesis of rheumatoid arthritis. J Immunol 176: 7021–7027.
10. Sacre SM, Lo A, Gregory B, Simmonds RE, Williams L, et al. (2008) Inhibitors of TLR8 reduce TNF production from human rheumatoid synovial membrane cultures. J Immunol 181: 8002–8009. 181/11/8002 [pii].
11. Abdollahi-Roodsaz S, Joosten LA, Koenders MI, Devesa I, Roelofs MF, et al. (2008) Stimulation of TLR2 and TLR4 differentially skews the balance of T cells in a mouse model of arthritis. J Clin Invest 118: 205–216.
12. Ultaigh SN, Saber TP, McCormick J, Connolly M, Dellacasagrande J, et al. (2011) Blockade of Toll-like receptor 2 prevents spontaneous cytokine release from rheumatoid arthritis ex vivo synovial explant cultures. Arthritis Res Ther 13: R33. ar3261 [pii];10.1186/ar3261 [doi].
13. Brennan FM, Hayes AL, Ciesielski CJ, Green P, Foxwell BM, et al. (2002) Evidence that rheumatoid arthritis synovial T cells are similar to cytokine-activated T cells: involvement of phosphatidylinositol 3-kinase and nuclear factor kappaB pathways in tumor necrosis factor alpha production in rheumatoid arthritis. Arthritis Rheum 46: 31–41.
14. Brennan FM, Smith NM, Owen S, Li C, Amjadi P, et al. (2008) Resting CD4+ effector memory T cells are precursors of bystander-activated effectors: a surrogate model of rheumatoid arthritis synovial T-cell function. Arthritis Res Ther 10: R36.
15. Schwab I, Nimmerjahn F (2013) Intravenous immunoglobulin therapy: how does IgG modulate the immune system? Nat Rev Immunol 13: 176–189. nri3401 [pii];10.1038/nri3401 [doi].
16. Nimmerjahn F, Ravetch JV (2008) Fcgamma receptors as regulators of immune responses. Nat Rev Immunol 8: 34–47. nri2206 [pii];10.1038/nri2206 [doi].
17. Miettinen HM, Rose JK, Mellman I (1989) Fc receptor isoforms exhibit distinct abilities for coated pit localization as a result of cytoplasmic domain heterogeneity. Cell 58: 317–327. 0092-8674(89)90846-5 [pii].
18. van den Herik-Oudijk IE, Westerdaal NA, Henriquez NV, Capel PJ, van De Winkel JG (1994) Functional analysis of human Fc gamma RII (CD32) isoforms expressed in B lymphocytes. J Immunol 152: 574–585.
19. Budde P, Bewarder N, Weinrich V, Schulzeck O, Frey J (1994) Tyrosine-containing sequence motifs of the human immunoglobulin G receptors FcRIIb1 and FcRIIb2 essential for endocytosis and regulation of calcium flux in B cells. J Biol Chem 269: 30636–30644.
20. Su K, Yang H, Li X, Li X, Gibson AW, et al. (2007) Expression profile of FcgammaRIIb on leukocytes and its dysregulation in systemic lupus erythematosus. J Immunol 178: 3272–3280. 178/5/3272 [pii].
21. Wenink MH, Santegoets KC, Roelofs MF, Huijbens R, Koenen HJ, et al. (2009) The inhibitory Fc gamma IIb receptor dampens TLR4-mediated immune responses and is selectively up-regulated on dendritic cells from rheumatoid arthritis patients with quiescent disease. J Immunol 183: 4509–4520.
22. Zhang Y, Liu S, Liu J, Zhang T, Shen Q, et al. (2009) Immune complex/Ig negatively regulate TLR4-triggered inflammatory response in macrophages through Fc gamma RIIb-dependent PGE2 production. J Immunol 182: 554–562.
23. Radstake TR, Blom AB, Sloetjes AW, van Gorselen EO, Pesman GJ, et al. (2004) Increased FcgammaRII expression and aberrant tumour necrosis factor alpha production by mature dendritic cells from patients with active rheumatoid arthritis. Ann Rheum Dis 63: 1556–1563.
24. Radstake TR, Nabbe KC, Wenink MH, Roelofs MF, Oosterlaar A, et al. (2005) Dendritic cells from patients with rheumatoid arthritis lack the interleukin 13 mediated increase of Fc gamma RII expression, which has clear functional consequences. Ann Rheum Dis 64: 1737–1743.
25. Radstake TR, van Lent PL, Pesman GJ, Blom AB, Sweep FG, et al. (2004) High production of proinflammatory and Th1 cytokines by dendritic cells from patients with rheumatoid arthritis, and down regulation upon Fc{gamma}R triggering. Ann Rheum Dis 63: 696–702.
26. Abdollahi-Roodsaz S, Joosten LA, Roelofs MF, Radstake TR, Matera G, et al. (2007) Inhibition of Toll-like receptor 4 breaks the inflammatory loop in autoimmune destructive arthritis. Arthritis Rheum 56: 2957–2967.
27. Bruhns P, Iannascoli B, England P, Mancardi DA, Fernandez N, et al. (2009) Specificity and affinity of human Fcgamma receptors and their polymorphic variants for human IgG subclasses. Blood 113: 3716–3725. blood-2008-09-179754 [pii];10.1182/blood-2008-09-179754 [doi].
28. Verreck FA, De Boer T, Langenberg DM, van der ZL, Ottenhoff TH (2006) Phenotypic and functional profiling of human proinflammatory type-1 and anti-inflammatory type-2 macrophages in response to microbial antigens and IFN-gamma- and CD40L-mediated costimulation. J Leukoc Biol 79: 285–293.
29. Stefanescu RN, Olferiev M, Liu Y, Pricop L (2004) Inhibitory Fc gamma receptors: from gene to disease. J Clin Immunol 24: 315–326. 10.1023/B:JOCI.0000029105.47772.04 [doi];487184 [pii].
30. Petkova SB, Konstantinov KN, Sproule TJ, Lyons BL, Awwami MA, et al. (2006) Human antibodies induce arthritis in mice deficient in the low-affinity inhibitory IgG receptor FcgammaRIIB. J Exp Med 203: 275–280.
31. Agbanoma G, Li C, Ennis D, Palfreeman AC, Williams LM, et al. (2012) Production of TNF-alpha in macrophages activated by T cells, compared with lipopolysaccharide, uses distinct IL-10-dependent regulatory mechanism. J Immunol 188: 1307–1317.
32. Bewarder N, Weinrich V, Budde P, Hartmann D, Flaswinkel H, et al. (1996) In vivo and in vitro specificity of protein tyrosine kinases for immunoglobulin G receptor (FcgammaRII) phosphorylation. Mol Cell Biol 16: 4735–4743.
33. Joshi T, Ganesan LP, Cao X, Tridandapani S (2005) Molecular analysis of expression and function of hFcgammaRIIbl and b2 isoforms in myeloid cells. Mol Immunol 43: 839–850. S0161-5890(05)00227-0 [pii];10.1016/j.molimm.2005.06.037 [doi].
34. Blom AB, Radstake TR, Holthuysen AE, Sloetjes AW, Pesman GJ, et al. (2003) Increased expression of Fcgamma receptors II and III on macrophages of rheumatoid arthritis patients results in higher production of tumor necrosis factor alpha and matrix metalloproteinase. Arthritis Rheum 48: 1002–1014.
35. Magnusson SE, Engstrom M, Jacob U, Ulfgren AK, Kleinau S (2007) High synovial expression of the inhibitory FcgammaRIIb in rheumatoid arthritis. Arthritis Res Ther 9: R51.
36. Kennedy A, Fearon U, Veale DJ, Godson C (2011) Macrophages in synovial inflammation. Front Immunol 2: 52. 10.3389/fimmu.2011.00052 [doi].
37. Ambarus CA, Noordenbos T, de Hair MJ, Tak PP, Baeten DL (2012) Intimal lining layer macrophages but not synovial sublining macrophages display an IL-10 polarized-like phenotype in chronic synovitis. Arthritis Res Ther 14: R74. ar3796 [pii];10.1186/ar3796 [doi].

20

ClinicalTrials.gov as a Data Source for Semi-Automated Point-Of-Care Trial Eligibility Screening

Pascal B. Pfiffner[1,2], JiWon Oh[3], Timothy A. Miller[1,2], Kenneth D. Mandl[1,2,4]*

1 Boston Children's Hospital Informatics Program, Boston, Massachusetts, United States of America, **2** Department of Pediatrics, Harvard Medical School, Boston, Massachusetts, United States of America, **3** Wellesley College, Wellesley, Massachusetts, United States of America, **4** Center for Biomedical Informatics, Harvard Medical School, Boston, Massachusetts, United States of America

Abstract

Background: Implementing semi-automated processes to efficiently match patients to clinical trials at the point of care requires both detailed patient data and authoritative information about open studies.

Objective: To evaluate the utility of the ClinicalTrials.gov registry as a data source for semi-automated trial eligibility screening.

Methods: Eligibility criteria and metadata for 437 trials open for recruitment in four different clinical domains were identified in ClinicalTrials.gov. Trials were evaluated for up to date recruitment status and eligibility criteria were evaluated for obstacles to automated interpretation. Finally, phone or email outreach to coordinators at a subset of the trials was made to assess the accuracy of contact details and recruitment status.

Results: 24% (104 of 437) of trials declaring on open recruitment status list a study completion date in the past, indicating out of date records. Substantial barriers to automated eligibility interpretation in free form text are present in 81% to up to 94% of all trials. We were unable to contact coordinators at 31% (45 of 146) of the trials in the subset, either by phone or by email. Only 53% (74 of 146) would confirm that they were still recruiting patients.

Conclusion: Because ClinicalTrials.gov has entries on most US and many international trials, the registry could be repurposed as a comprehensive trial matching data source. Semi-automated point of care recruitment would be facilitated by matching the registry's eligibility criteria against clinical data from electronic health records. But the current entries fall short. Ultimately, improved techniques in natural language processing will facilitate semi-automated complex matching. As immediate next steps, we recommend augmenting ClinicalTrials.gov data entry forms to capture key eligibility criteria in a simple, structured format.

Editor: Gajendra P. S. Raghava, CSIR-Institute of Microbial Technology, India

Funding: The work was supported by the following: Strategic Health IT Advanced Research Projects Award 90TR000101 from the Office of the National Coordinator of Health Information Technology (www.healthit.gov): KM; National Institutes of Health (www.nih.gov); National Center for Advancing Translational Sciences (UL1TR001102): PP, KM; National Institute of Child Health and Human Development (1R21HD072382): KM; National Institute on Aging (R21AG043715): KM; National Library of Medicine (R01LM010090): TM, KM; and National Library of Medicine (U54LM008748): TM. The funders had no role in study design, data collection and analysis, decision to publish, or preparation of the manuscript.

Competing Interests: The authors have declared that no competing interests exist.

* Email: Kenneth_Mandl@Harvard.edu

Introduction

Recruiting patients to clinical trials is an expensive, time consuming, and increasingly difficult process [1–6]. High market penetration of electronic medical records (EMR) presents an opportunity to integrate clinical trial eligibility evaluation into clinical workflows [7]. The physician at the point of care could be productively engaged in trial recruiting [8], for example by being alerted when a patient might be suitable for a trial. Further, a clinician seeking a trial for her patient should be readily presented with an array of appropriate trials. Because the data in the EMR contains many elements of eligibility criteria (age, gender, diagnoses, laboratory data), an application that accesses EMR data could help automate screening for clinical trials [9]. However to be integrated into daily clinical workflow the process would need to be highly efficient and streamlined. There currently is no standardized workflow or toolkit to perform such automated eligibility screening.

The new focus under the Patient Affordable Care Act on a national-scale pragmatic trial infrastructure, in which patients are randomized in trials within the delivery system, heightens the importance of efficient point-of-care eligibility screening.

ClinicalTrials.gov (CTG) [10], maintained by the United States National Library of Medicine (NLM), is the largest registry of clinical trials [11]. It has achieved a high rate of prospective trial registration for interventional trials, largely attributable to the 2005 registration requirement instituted by the International Committee of Medical Journal Editors (ICMJE) [12] and the 2007 requirement to register trials for Food and Drug Administration approval [13]. The data captured in CTG includes medical information, such as the trial's purpose, interventions and eligibility criteria, organizational information such as timeframes, sponsors and participating centers as well as basic results of completed trials.

Using CTG as a source of ground truth for trial eligibility would obviate the need to maintain separate trial databases. CTG could become an engine not only of trial registration, but also enrollment. The database could be queried at the point of care and eligibility criteria compared to EMR data and physician and patient input. In fact, several academic institutions and companies are already using CTG to provide customized trial suggestions, but those solutions are primarily designed to be used directly by the patient [14] and usually limited to a specific disease domain [15–19].

However, to repurpose CTG to efficiently serve as source for trial eligibility data, new processes for collecting said data may be necessary. Reliable eligibility criteria to support eligibility screening or even automated matching must be both accurate and "readable" by a computer. We sought to evaluate the utility of CTG for trial eligibility screening. We assessed:

- accuracy of trial recruitment status, that is whether a trial is still recruiting patients when its recruitment status is set to "open". Reliable recruitment status is needed so only trials that are still open for recruitment are suggested after a first filtering step.
- semantic characteristics of patient eligibility criteria with respect to automated text interpretation through natural language processing (NLP). Structured data in CTG includes age, gender and whether healthy volunteers are being accepted and can be readily interpreted computationally. However, the remaining majority of eligibility criteria in CTG are expressed as free text and require computerized interpretation [20]. Such interpretation by means of NLP is an active area of research and several key issues are being addressed, of which we chose 3 to predict feasibility of automated criteria interpretation: defined subpopulations; laboratory values and scores [21]; and temporal constraints [21,22]. Additionally we looked at how many criteria require specific patient action or abilities and are thus unamenable to computational evaluation.
- adequacy of contact details for the trial coordinator.

We sought to define parameters that would guide further development of automated and semi-automated clinical trial eligibility screening and matching tools and approaches.

Methods

Data Retrieval

The data source is CTG, listing 160,552 clinical trials from 185 countries as of February 5, 2014. We accessed CTG data using a specialized application programming interface (API) adding location data (latitude and longitude accurate to the city level) for the individual recruitment centers of each trial [23]. Scripts to facilitate data retrieval and analysis were written in the Python programming language and made openly available on our GitHub repository [24].

Trial Set

Our goal was to create a diverse sample of trials to not limit our analysis to a certain field of study. We extracted trials open for recruitment by querying CTG for: the antineoplastic medication imatinib mesylate ("Gleevec"); "cataract"; "neuroblastoma"; and "rheumatoid arthritis".

Exploratory searches revealed approximately 100 trials for three of the clinical areas, but over 400 for rheumatoid arthritis. Hence we randomly selected 25% of the rheumatoid arthritis trials to develop comparably sized sets.

Recruitment Status

Several elements are in structured fields. Trial identification number, date first entered, date last updated, and study completion date were captured. The study completion date is defined as the final date on which data was (or is expected to be) collected. Trials listing a recruitment status of "Not yet recruiting" or "Recruiting" but specified a completion date in the past were marked as "conflicting".

Eligibility Criteria

Plain text eligibility criteria of all trials in our four sets were evaluated for the following properties:

- Do criteria adhere to the CTG recommended macro-format, in which they are formatted as a list, preceded by the words "Inclusion Criteria" and "Exclusion Criteria", in that order?
- Are subpopulations defined? In other words are there different recruitment groups for different study arms or do certain criteria apply only to specific patients (e.g. "If patients are receiving oral corticosteroids, then…"), or are there different properties or lab ranges depending on the patient's demographics or precise diagnosis.
- How many laboratory values and medical scores do the criteria require?
- Are the criteria temporally constrained? E.g. "at least 2 weeks since therapy with drug", "no more than 2 months since intervention" or "diagnosis of disease ≤3 years".
- How many criteria rely on patient behavior or abilities? E.g., criteria stating "patient must be willing to comply with radiation safety procedures" or "able to walk on treadmill or cycle on a stationary bike."

These structural elements of eligibility relate directly to the ability to use NLP techniques to parse and automatically interpret the text [25]. Where patient behavior and preferences come into play, physician or patient involvement in eligibility screening must complement automation.

Contact Information

Contact Information from CTG was validated in a sample of representatives from 40 trials in each set. One of the authors (JO) reached out by phone or email and the representative was asked whether the trial center was still recruiting patients and, if not, when recruitment had ended.

The sets were created as follows: all trials with at least one trial location in the United States, specifically marked as "recruiting" or "not yet recruiting", were collected per clinical area and ordered by date last updated. Each resulting list was divided into 4 segments. From each segment 10 trials were randomly selected using a Python script and the 4 segments were again combined into one list of 40 trials per clinical area. Individual trial locations of each trial were then ordered by distance to Boston, Massachusetts. The closest three locations with their contact data plus the trial's overall and backup contact data was stored in a spreadsheet.

A workflow for phone and email follow up was created that included a maximum of 3 phone calls and 1 email per trial location, starting with the geographically closest location, moving on to the other 2 locations and resorting to the overall contact information depending on contact information availability (Figure S1). The time window allowed for reply to our inquiry emails was 2 weeks.

Responses were classified into 4 categories: "open", "closed", "don't know" or "no answer". The "no answer" category also applied to trials that did not supply any contact information while those who refused to answer our inquiry were categorized as "don't know".

Analysis

Results are described primarily with descriptive statistics. Correlation between recruitment status and the date last updated was assessed with one-sided Mann-Whitney U-tests using R 3.0.2 [26] on Mac OS X 10.9.

Results

Figure 1 provides an overview of trial selection. Table 1 lists the number of trials for each of the clinical areas and the date data were downloaded from CTG. Our full data set of eligibility criteria evaluation consisted of 437 trials with 5,950 individual inclusion and exclusion criteria.

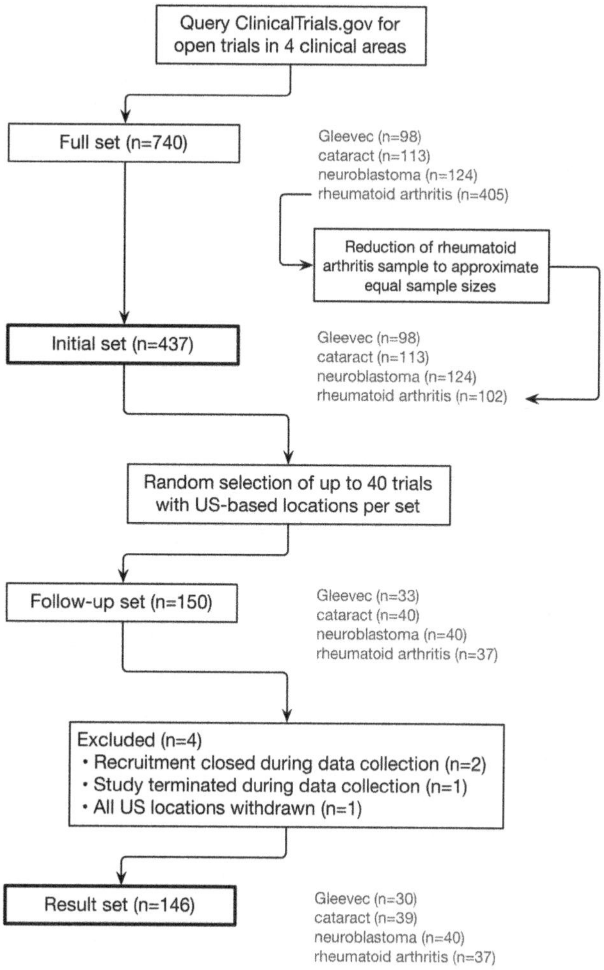

Figure 1. Trial selection workflow.

Recruitment Status

We prompted CTG to only return trials recruiting or not yet open for recruitment. A number of trials returned as "recruiting" hadn't been updated in years and some of the trials listed a completion date in the past. Thus we determined how many trials were listing an open recruitment status conflicting with a completion date in the past. Nearly half, 46% of the cataract trials, had a conflicting recruitment status, compared to 14% for the Gleevec, 15% for the neuroblastoma and 19% for the rheumatoid arthritis sets. We then compared recruitment status conflicts to the time passed since the trial was last updated on CTG. Trials with conflicting recruitment status tended to not have been updated recently (Figure 2).

Eligibility Criteria

Textual Format. A majority of trials (90%) followed the CTG-suggested macro format for inclusion and exclusion criteria. There were notable differences between the sets however, the lowest being 79% for the neuroblastoma trials, then 88% for Gleevec trials to up to 98% for cataract and rheumatoid arthritis trials (Table 2).

Notably, many of the noncompliant studies expressed eligibility criteria in an alternative format, listing only inclusion criteria – potentially negated – under the topics "disease characteristics", "patient characteristics" and "prior concurrent therapy". This alternative format could be accounted for in software and would raise the percentage of criteria suitable for automated interpretation to 97% for the Gleevec, 99% for the cataract and 97% for the neuroblastoma trials, resulting in an overall percentage of 98%.

Computational Barriers. Next we quantified occurrences of three categories of linguistic constructs difficult for NLP technologies to interpret correctly and whether criteria required patient actions or abilities (Table 3).

Subpopulations: When a trial specifies eligibility criteria that only apply to a subset of the study population, algorithms face additional challenges. We found that between 12% (cataract) and 42% (Gleevec) of trials specified at least one sub-population.

Laboratory Values and Scores: Between 45% (rheumatoid arthritis) and 73% (neuroblastoma) of trials contained at least one laboratory value or medical score.

Temporal Restrictions: Another difficulty for text interpretation is extracting information in the context of a temporal constraint. As Table 3 shows, three of our four sets had at least one temporal constraint in ⅔ or more of their trials. Only in the cataract set less than ⅓ of all trials had temporal constraints.

Patient Behavior and Abilities: Between 47% (rheumatoid arthritis) and 61% (Gleevec) of trials contained at least one criterion that a patient is able or willing to adhere to a given condition, necessitating patient input in a screening algorithm.

Overall, between 81% (Cataract) and 94% (Gleevec) of the trials contained at least one of these barriers to automated eligibility determination.

Table 1. Number of trials and eligibility criteria.

domain	date retrieved	# trials	# eligibility criteria
Gleevec	June 6, 2013	98	1641
cataract	June 12, 2013	113	1163
neuroblastoma	June 20, 2013	124	1979
rheumatoid arthritis	July 5, 2013	102	1167

Number of trials and individual eligibility criteria in our 4 data sets and the date of data retrieval from ClinicalTrials.gov.

Contact Information

We followed up with trial coordinators of 40 trials per set and asked about their recruitment status. Our selection method – trials that had at least one US location and were still marked as recruiting – resulted in 33 Gleevec, 40 cataract, 40 neuroblastoma and 37 rheumatoid arthritis trials.

We dropped 4 trials from our follow-up sets: three trials did complete recruitment or terminate the trial in the time between creation of our data sets and downloading contact data, which makes contact data unavailable via CTG. One trial withdrew all US locations while still maintaining non-US locations. Because we only regarded the overall recruitment status when creating our data set, this trial was erroneously included.

During follow-up we were unable to contact 31% (45 of 146) of all trials (Figure 3A). These follow-ups encompassed three phone calls to the closest three recruitment locations and the contact supplied as "overall contact" to CTG as well as at least one email, depending on data availability.

Three trial centers refused to give out recruitment status information and were categorized as "don't know". We were able

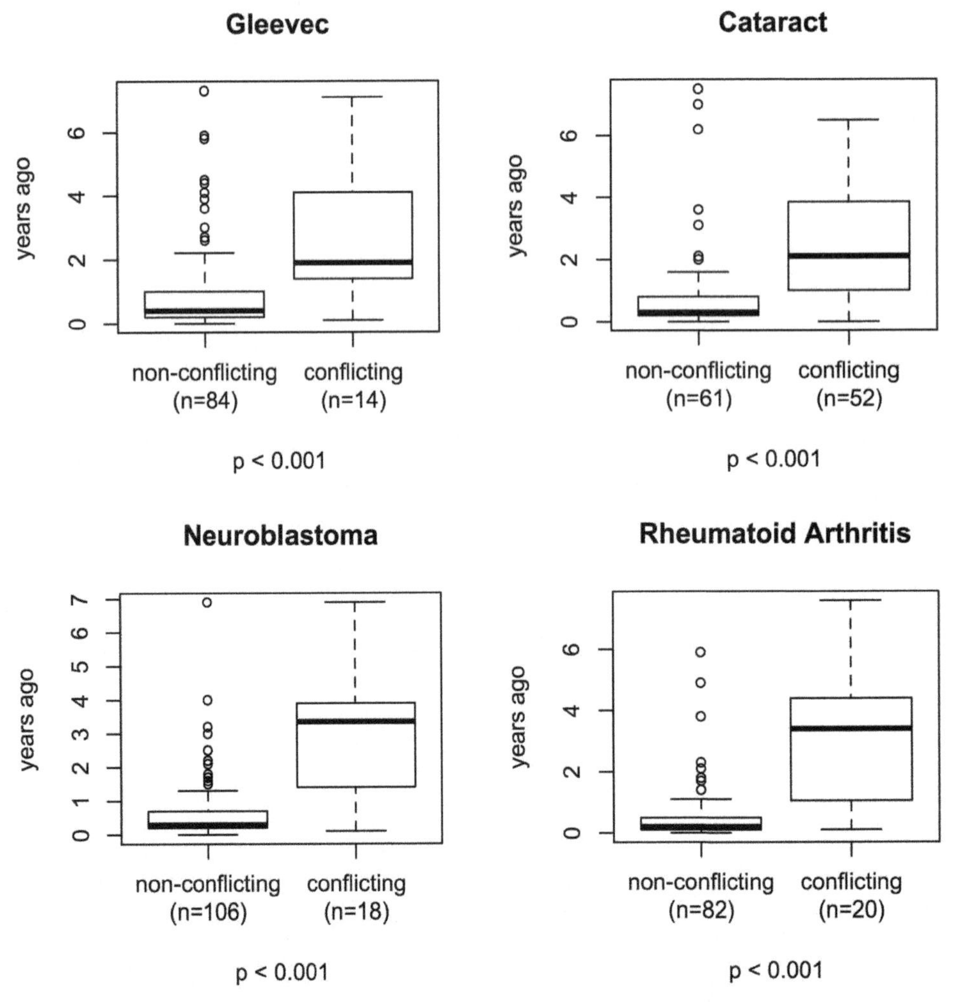

Figure 2. Comparison of the time since last update to whether the recruitment status is conflicting with the stated study completion date. Trials with a recruitment status conflicting with their stated completion date tended to not have been updated recently ($p < 0.001$).

Table 2. Eligibility text format.

domain	suggested format	with extended format
Gleevec	88%	97%
cataract	98%	99%
neuroblastoma	79%	97%
rheumatoid arthritis	98%	98%

Percentage of trials, per trial set, that adhere to the format suggested by CTG and the percentage of trials that either adhere to the suggested format or a second format, often found in cancer trials.

to confirm that 53% (74 of 146) of trials in our sample, listed as "recruiting" on CTG, were still recruiting patients. Figure 3A breaks down the recruitment status per clinical area.

While trials open for recruitment tended to have been updated more recently when compared to trials closed for recruitment ($p < 0.001$), there was no difference in the time since last update among the trials still open for recruitment, those that didn't know their recruitment status and trials at centers that couldn't be contacted (Figure 3B).

Discussion

With a goal of assessing feasibility of robust, semi-automated screening of patients' eligibility for clinical trials we evaluated sample aspects of data quality in CTG registrations. We identified several key issues.

Nearly a quarter of trial records were notably out of date, in that they listed as "open for recruitment" but stating a study completion date in the past. Out-of-date registrations are an issue previously reported in a study comparing registry data to study protocols [27].

Further, most trials adhere to one of two textual formats for eligibility criteria, represented as unstructured text. Computational processing of such data thus requires a preliminary data extraction step, which poses an obstacle to automation. A particular difficulty is extraction of laboratory values expressed as free text – which occurs in about two thirds of the trials. Matching laboratory values from CTG directly to EMR data is an important opportunity.

Another complexity is understanding temporal information in the eligibility criteria. For example, "Patients must be taking MTX [Methotrexate] for at least 3 months before randomization and have to be on a stable dose at least 4 weeks before randomization." Extracting temporal information is an active area of research in clinical NLP [28,29], but temporal relation extraction is a difficult problem and has not yet been satisfactorily solved [30]. Thus temporal relations are likely to be lost to NLP pipelines, affecting 32% of the trials in the cataract set, similar to previously reported results of 40% [21] and 38% [22], up to 78% in the Gleevec set.

A third challenge is that many of the criteria require logical inference – both semantic understanding of the text in context and real world knowledge. For example, "Have limited disease that would not normally be treated with CYC [Cyclophosphamide]" is easily understood by a clinician but context ("limited disease") and real world knowledge ("normally") is a sufficiently hard problem for automated interpretation. Similarly, understanding that a textual list of criteria, indented one level deeper than the previous list item, only applies to patients with a specific diagnosis (a sub-population) requires interpretation of textual as well as structural context. Sub-populations may be present in more than a third of the trials and invalidate automated matching for a whole trial, not only a single criterion, because requirements only intended for specific patients will be applied to all patients.

More than half of trials require, for eligibility, specific patient actions and abilities. Hence there will be residual information to obtain directly from patients and clinicians beyond EMR and CTG data even in a robust semi-automated matching process.

Finally, trial status and contact are low quality fields in CTG. Only half of our trials could be contacted and would confirm that they were still recruiting patients. No contact could be established with almost one third of the trials. Trials that hadn't been updated recently were associated with a higher probability of being closed for recruitment, however the date last updated was not a predictor of whether trial recruitment centers could successfully be contacted or not.

Conclusions and Recommendations

We suggest that a tightly integrated informatics toolkit could facilitate identification of clinical trials for which a patient might be eligible. Point-of-care apps [31], utilizing trial data sources supplemented with data from EMRs and direct clinician or

Table 3. Computationally challenging elgibility criteria.

domain	sub-populations	labs and scores	temporal	patient	any
Gleevec	42%	70%	78%	61%	94%
cataract	12%	48%	32%	54%	81%
neuroblastoma	35%	73%	65%	49%	90%
rheumatoid arthritis	17%	45%	64%	47%	84%

The percentage of trials, broken down per trial set, that include at least one criterion only applying to a sub-population (sub-population) of the targeted patient cohort, that contain at least one laboratory value or medical score (labs and scores), that have at least one criterion that is temporally constrained (temporal), that have at least one criterion describing patient behavior or abilities (patient) and that have at least one of these four criteria (any).

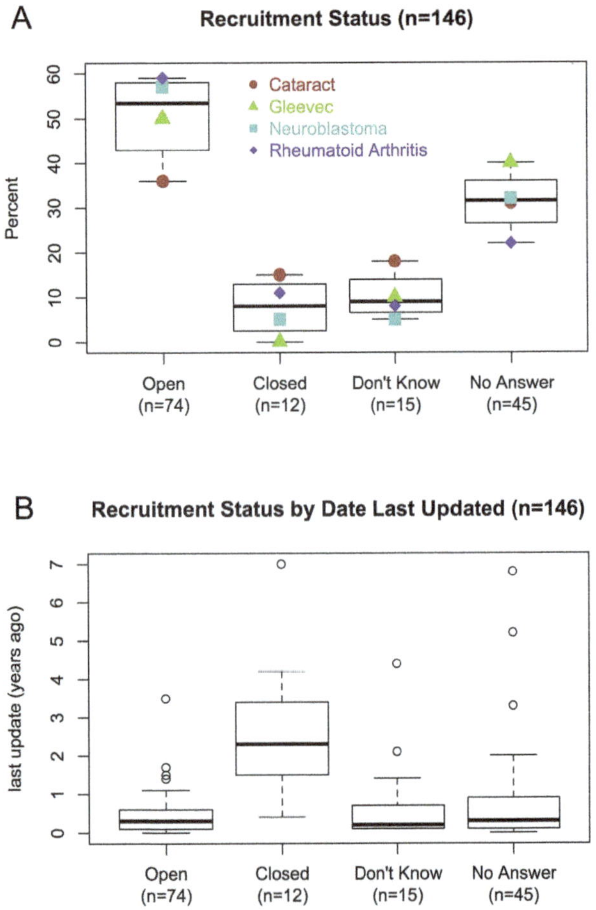

Figure 3. Effective recruitment status. A) Recruitment status (x-axis), verified by phone or email, of the trials in our 4 trial sets. B) The same recruitment status compared against how long ago the trials were last updated on ClinicalTrials.gov. Trials closed for recruitment tended not to have been updated recently when compared to trials open for recruitment (p<0.001).

patient input, can then be developed for different stakeholders such as hospitals, primary care physicians and patients. Using CTG as data source for trial eligibility evaluation is a promising approach, not least because the requirements for prospective clinical trial registration continuously increase the quantity of available trial data. However, registry data are partially out of date or inaccurate (recruitment status, contact data) and largely unstructured and therefore not readily amenable to automated data matching (eligibility criteria). Using NLP for eligibility criteria extraction from CTG holds promise but considerable obstacles must be overcome. Arriving at a formal representation of eligibility criteria that are interpretable by computer systems is an active area of research [20,21,25,32,33] and (semi-)automated systems to help translate free-text criteria into computable representations are being developed [22,34,35].

There are, broadly speaking, two approaches for automated trial matching based on CTG data:

1. Working with the data already contained in CTG, enhanced with NLP technologies and/or manual curation to arrive at computable eligibility criteria representations.
2. Extend and standardize the eligibility data contained in CTG to additionally contain structured eligibility data.

The first approach bumps up against the cutting edge of NLP technology and may create services that are not universally available. The second approach relies on an accepted standard for formal eligibility criteria representation and shifts additional burden to CTG, which needs to provide additional data fields, and data providers who need to enter and maintain additional registry data. We contend that data providers may be motivated to do so based on the value proposition of accelerated accrual in return.

However, there might be a middle ground to enable initial eligibility screening at a finer level than is currently possible. Allowing data providers to specify a handful of key eligibility criteria in structured form, in addition to age and gender, might provide data for very powerful initial trial filtering. Such key criteria would vary between clinical specialties and could include "taking Methotrexate", "no previous eye surgery" or even simple laboratory value ranges. They ideally would not require an extensive format specification but could rely on existing coding systems such as SNOMED-CT and RxNorm, coupled with boolean logic or numeric ranges.

Though an extensive modeling effort to represent all clinical trial eligibility criteria in structured form could lead to a prolonged consensus process, targeting the "low hanging fruit" first – by adapting existing data standards – would be a straight forward and cost effective approach to improving automated trial matching. Leaders of clinical trials would be presented with an attractive value proposition – keeping their CTG records accurate and up to date might promote improved and timelier accrual.

Importantly, substantial investment by the National Institutes of Health and the Patient Centered Outcomes Research Institute in infrastructure to implement pragmatic trials at the point of care may dramatically increase the utility of a high quality, computable, ClinicalTrials.gov-based trial data source.

Supporting Information

Figure S1 Phone and email follow up.

Acknowledgments

We thank Lee Nadler for his support and wisdom. We thank Deborah Zarin for her keen insights and generosity with her time in guiding our study design as well as for her comments on our manuscript drafts. The cTAKES team, especially Dmitriy Dligach and Guergana Savova, engaged with us in enlightening discussions about technical aspects and limitations of current NLP technologies.

Author Contributions

Conceived and designed the experiments: PP KM. Performed the experiments: PP JO TM. Analyzed the data: PP TM KM. Contributed reagents/materials/analysis tools: PP TM. Wrote the paper: PP TM KM.

References

1. Probstfield JL, Frye RL (2011) Strategies for recruitment and retention of participants in clinical trials. JAMA: The Journal of the American Medical Association 306: 1798–1799. doi:10.1001/jama.2011.1544.
2. Sibai T, Carlisle H, Tornetta P (2012) The darker side of randomized trials: recruitment challenges. J Bone Joint Surg Am 94 Suppl 1: 49–55. doi:10.2106/JBJS.L.00240.

3. Hawkes N (2012) UK must improve its recruitment rate in clinical trials, report says. BMJ 345: e8104. doi:10.1136/bmj.e8104.
4. Penberthy LT, Dahman BA, Petkov VI, DeShazo JP (2012) Effort required in eligibility screening for clinical trials. J Oncol Pract 8: 365–370. doi:10.1200/JOP.2012.000646.
5. Ferris M, Norwood V, Radeva M, Gassman JJ, Al-Uzri A, et al. (2012) Patient Recruitment into a Multicenter Randomized Clinical Trial for Kidney Disease: Report of the Focal Segmental Glomerulosclerosis Clinical Trial (FSGS CT). CTS 6: 13–20. doi:10.1111/cts.12003.
6. Opar A (2013) New tools automatically match patients with clinical trials. Nat Med 19: 793. doi:10.1038/nm0713-793.
7. Martin SS, Ou FS, Newby LK, Sutton V, Adams P, et al. (2013) Patient- and Trial-Specific Barriers to Participation in Cardiovascular Randomized Clinical Trials. Journal of the American College of Cardiology 61: 762–769. doi:10.1016/j.jacc.2012.10.046.
8. Siminoff L, Zhang A, Colabianchi N, Sturm CMS, Shen Q (2000) Factors that predict the referral of breast cancer patients onto clinical trials by their surgeons and medical oncologists. J Clin Oncol 18: 1203–1211.
9. Mandl KD, Mandel J, Murphy SN, Bernstam EV, Ramoni RL, et al. (2012) The SMART Platform: early experience enabling substitutable applications for electronic health records. JAMIA 19: 597–603. doi:10.1136/amiajnl-2011-000622.
10. NLM (2013) ClinicalTrials.gov: 157588. Available: http://www.clinicaltrials.gov.
11. Huser V, Cimino JJ (2013) Linking ClinicalTrials.gov and PubMed to track results of interventional human clinical trials. PLoS ONE 8: e68409. doi:10.1371/journal.pone.0068409.
12. International Committee of Medical Journal Editors (2009) Uniform requirements for manuscripts submitted to medical journals: publishing and editorial issues related to publication in biomedical journals. Available: https://www.blackwellpublishing.com/products/journals/freepdf/med339.pdf.
13. FDA (2007) Food and Drug Administration Amendments Act of 2007. Available: http://www.gpo.gov/fdsys/pkg/PLAW-110publ85/pdf/PLAW-110publ85.pdf.
14. Atkinson NL, Saperstein SL, Massett HA, Leonard CR, Grama L, et al. (2008) Using the Internet to search for cancer clinical trials: a comparative audit of clinical trial search tools. Contemp Clin Trials 29: 555–564. doi:10.1016/j.cct.2008.01.007.
15. Patients Like Me (2014) Patients Like Me. Available: http://www.patientslikeme.com/.
16. Research Match (2014) Research Match. Available: https://www.researchmatch.org/.
17. Fox Trial Finder (2014) Fox Trial Finder. Available: https://foxtrialfinder.michaeljfox.org/.
18. Trial X (2014) Trial X. Available: http://trialx.com.
19. Corengi Diabetes Research (2014) Corengi Diabetes Research. Available: https://www.corengi.com.
20. Weng C, Tu SW, Sim I, Richesson R (2010) Formal representation of eligibility criteria: a literature review. Journal of Biomedical Informatics 43: 451–467. doi:10.1016/j.jbi.2009.12.004.
21. Ross J, Tu S, Carini S, Sim I (2010) Analysis of eligibility criteria complexity in clinical trials. AMIA Summits Transl Sci Proc 2010: 46–50.
22. Tu SW, Peleg M, Carini S, Bobak M, Ross J, et al. (2011) A practical method for transforming free-text eligibility criteria into computable criteria. Journal of Biomedical Informatics 44: 239–250. doi:10.1016/j.jbi.2010.09.007.
23. Lilly (2014) Lilly Clinical Open Innovation. Available: http://portal.lillycoi.com.
24. Pfiffner P (2014) Clinical Trials Eval. Available: https://github.com/p2/clinical-trials-eval.
25. Weng C, Wu X, Luo Z, Boland MR, Theodoratos D, et al. (2011) EliXR: an approach to eligibility criteria extraction and representation. JAMIA 18 Suppl 1: i116–i124. doi:10.1136/amiajnl-2011-000321.
26. Team RDC (2009) R: A language and environment for statistical computing.
27. Zarin DA, Tse T (2013) Trust but verify: trial registration and determining fidelity to the protocol. Ann Intern Med 159: 65–67. doi:10.7326/0003-4819-159-1-201307020-00011.
28. Sun W, Rumshisky A, Uzuner O (2013) Evaluating temporal relations in clinical text: 2012 i2b2 Challenge. JAMIA 20: 806–813. doi:10.1136/amiajnl-2013-001628.
29. Miller TA, Bethard S, Dligach D, Pradhan S, Lin C (2013) Discovering Narrative Containers in Clinical Text. ACL 2013.
30. Boland MR, Tu SW, Carini S, Sim I, Weng C (2012) EliXR-TIME: A Temporal Knowledge Representation for Clinical Research Eligibility Criteria. AMIA Summits Transl Sci Proc 2012: 71–80.
31. Mandl KD, Kohane IS (2012) Escaping the EHR trap – the future of health IT. N Engl J Med 366: 2240–2242. doi:10.1056/NEJMp1203102.
32. Miotto R, Weng C (2013) Unsupervised mining of frequent tags for clinical eligibility text indexing. Journal of Biomedical Informatics 46: 1145–1151. doi:10.1016/j.jbi.2013.08.012.
33. Boland MR, Miotto R, Gao J, Weng C (2013) Feasibility of feature-based indexing, clustering, and search of clinical trials: A case study of breast cancer trials from ClinicalTrials.gov. Methods Inf Med 52: 382–394. doi:10.3414/ME12-01-0092.
34. Korkontzelos I, Mu T, Ananiadou S (2012) ASCOT: a text mining-based web-service for efficient search and assisted creation of clinical trials. BMC Med Inform Decis Mak 12 Suppl 1: S3. doi:10.1186/1472-6947-12-S1-S3.
35. Luo Z, Miotto R, Weng C (2013) A human-computer collaborative approach to identifying common data elements in clinical trial eligibility criteria. Journal of Biomedical Informatics 46: 33–39. doi:10.1016/j.jbi.2012.07.006.

21

MiR-30a-3p Negatively Regulates BAFF Synthesis in Systemic Sclerosis and Rheumatoid Arthritis Fibroblasts

Ghada Alsaleh[1*], Antoine François[1], Lucas Philippe[1], Ya-Zhuo Gong[1], Seiamak Bahram[1], Semih Cetin[2], Sébastien Pfeffer[2], Jacques-Eric Gottenberg[1], Dominique Wachsmann[1], Philippe Georgel[1], Jean Sibilia[1]

1 Immunorhumatologie moléculaire, INSERM UMR S_1109, Centre de Recherche en Immunologie et Hématologie, Faculté de Médecine, Fédération de Médecine Translationnelle de Strasbourg (FMTS), Université de Strasbourg, Strasbourg, France and Service de Rhumatologie, Centre National de Référence pour les Maladies Systémiques Autoimmunes Rares, Hôpitaux Universitaires de Strasbourg, Strasbourg, France, **2** Université de Strasbourg, UPR 9002 du CNRS Architecture et Réactivité de l'ARN, Institut de Biologie Moléculaire et Cellulaire, Strasbourg, France

Abstract

We evaluated micro (mi) RNA-mediated regulation of BAFF expression in fibroblasts using two concomitant models: (i) synovial fibroblasts (FLS) isolated from healthy controls (N) or Rheumatoid Arthritis (RA) patients; (ii) human dermal fibroblasts (HDF) isolated from healthy controls (N) or Systemic Sclerosis (SSc) patients. Using RT-qPCR and ELISA, we first showed that SScHDF synthesized and released BAFF in response to Poly(I:C) or IFN-γ treatment, as previously observed in RAFLS, whereas NHDF released BAFF preferentially in response to IFN-γ. Next, we demonstrated that miR-30a-3p expression was down regulated in RAFLS and SScHDF stimulated with Poly(I:C) or IFN-γ. Moreover, we demonstrated that transfecting miR-30a-3p mimic in Poly(I:C)- and IFN-γ-activated RAFLS and SScHDF showed a strong decrease on BAFF synthesis and release and thus B cells survival in our model. Interestingly, FLS and HDF isolated from healthy subjects express higher levels of miR-30a-3p and lower levels of BAFF than RAFLS and SScHDF. Transfection of miR-30a-3p antisense in Poly(I:C)- and IFN-γ-activated NFLS and NHDF upregulated BAFF secretion, confirming that this microRNA is a basal repressors of BAFF expression in cells from healthy donors. Our data suggest a critical role of miR-30a-3p in the regulation of BAFF expression, which could have a major impact in the regulation of the autoimmune responses occurring in RA and SSc.

Editor: Shervin Assassi, University of Texas Health Science Center at Houston, United States of America

Funding: Prof. Jean Sibilia's work was supported by grants from Bristol Myers Squibb, Roche, Pfizer, Courtin Foundation and CAMPLP. Sébastien Pfeffer's work was supported by the European Research Council (ERC-StG-260767) and Agence Nationale pour la Recherche (labex netRNA, ANR-10-LABX-36). The funders had no role in study design, data collection and analysis, decision to publish, or preparation of the manuscript.

Competing Interests: The authors have declared that no competing interests exist.

* Email: galfarhan@unistra.fr

These authors contributed equally to this work.

Introduction

TNFSF13B (also known as B cell-activating factor -BAFF, which will be the only nomenclature used thereafter in the manuscript) is a member of the TNF superfamily which plays a central role in the survival and homeostasis of transitional and naive B cells, plasmablasts and plasma cells [1]. BAFF is produced as a membrane-bound form or secreted by cells of hematopoietic origin, essentially monocytes, dendritic cells, macrophages and stimulated neutrophils [2,3]. However non-immune cells, such as astrocytes, can also constitutively produce BAFF [4].

The finding that BAFF transgenic mice develop autoimmune manifestations exhibiting similarities with systemic lupus erythematosus (SLE) and Sjögren's syndrom (SS) suggested a critical role for this cytokine in autoimmune diseases [5–7]. Consistent with this observation, auto-reactive B cells have a greater dependency for BAFF compared to naive mature B cells and elevated levels of BAFF were detected in the serum of patients with SLE, rheumatoid arthritis (RA) and SS [8]. In addition, these increased BAFF levels correlated with high auto-antibody titers and disease activity [9]. In patients with systemic sclerosis (SSc), increased levels of BAFF were associated with worsening of the skin sclerosis [10,11]. Similar results were obtained in experimental arthritis where overproduction of BAFF by dendritic cells and macrophages was demonstrated to play a crucial role in the disease [12]. Fibroblast-like synoviocytes isolated from RA patients (RAFLS) are characterized by their aggressive phenotype in response to various stimuli. In these inflammatory conditions, these cells also produce large amounts of cytokines including BAFF, thus enabling them to collaborate with autoimmune B cells [13]. Altogether, these data illustrate the central role played by BAFF in the pathogenesis of autoimmune diseases, which prompted the development of biological agents targeting BAFF. Belimumab, a humanized IgG1 monoclonal antibody which inhibits both soluble and membrane BAFF binding to BAFFR and TACI, was approved for the treatment of SLE [14–16].

However, modulation of BAFF activity for therapeutic purposes by targeting its synthesis has not yet been considered. The control of cytokine expression can occur at various levels including post-transcriptional regulation, which is now the focus of intense attention. The modulation of gene expression can take place at several levels, among which regulation by microRNAs (miRNAs) has gained increased interest in the recent years. MiRNAs are an evolutionarily conserved class of endogenous small non-coding RNAs. They are produced from long precursor molecules by the consecutive action of the RNase III enzymes DROSHA and DICER, before being loaded on an ARGONAUTE protein within the RNA-induced-silencing complex (RISC). The mature miRNA acts a guide for RISC to mediate destabilization and/or translational repression of target mRNAs. The regulation of miRNA expression is itself controlled at various levels such as transcription, processing or stability and can be influenced by various stress factors including inflammation. In addition, emerging data have identified an important contribution of miRNA to the development and control of the inflammatory response which position these small non-coding RNAs at the heart of feedback and feed-forward loops controlling the inflammation process in both immune and non immune cells. Recently, microRNAs (miRNAs) have emerged as a new class of cytokines regulators, although computational analysis indicates that the 3′UTR (Three prime untranslated region) of many cytokines lacks miRNA target sites. Indeed, miRNAs could also regulate cytokine expression by targeting ARE-binding proteins (ARE machinery components) such as TTP, AUF1 and members of the HuR family [17,18].

In this study, we found that miR-30a-3p (and miR30d-3p and e-3p, which exhibit high sequence homology) is predicted to bind the 3′UTR region of BAFF transcripts. In SSc patients, we observed concomitant up-regulation of BAFF transcripts and decreased expression of miR-30a-3p in skin fibroblasts (HDF) isolated from SSc patients after cell stimulation with Poly (I:C) or IFN-γ. Analysis of synovial fibroblasts from RA patients yielded similar results. The prediction provided by bioinformatic tools and this inverse correlation between miR-30 family members and BAFF expression prompted us to analyze their likely direct interaction. To this end, we used reporter constructs containing a luciferase gene fused to the wild type or mutated full length human BAFF 3′UTR. Co-transfection of these reporter plasmids with miRNA mimic in cultured cells confirmed direct interaction. Furthermore, transfection of miR-30a-3p mimic or inhibitor in fibroblasts isolated from the skin or the synovium of healthy donors or from patients confirmed that this miRNA modulate IFN-γ- and Poly (I:C)-dependent BAFF expression. Finally, we report that miRNA-modulated BAFF secretion by activated skin or synovial fibrocytes significantly reduces the capacity of these cells to promote B cells survival, which provides physiological significance to our findings. Altogether, our data describe a novel mechanism involved in the regulation of BAFF expression and potentially provide an additional level of intervention for future therapeutic purposes.

Materials and Methods

Reagents

Cell culture media (RPMI 1640, M199 and DMEM), fetal calf serum (FCS), L-glutamine, penicillin, streptomycin, amphotericin B, TRIzol reagent and $DiOC_6$ (3,3′-Dihexyloxacarbocyanine Iodide) were from Invitrogen (Cergy-Pontoise, France). LPS from *Salmonella abortus equi* and Propidium Iodide (PI) solution was obtained from Sigma Aldrich (Saint-Quentin-Fallavier, France). Synthetic bacterial lipopeptide Pam_3CSK_4 (BLP) was obtained from EMC Microcollections GmbH (Tuebingen, Germany). Polyinosine-Polycytidylic acid (Poly(I:C)) was obtained from InvivoGen (Toulouse, France). iScript cDNA Synthesis Kit and SsoAdvanced SYBR Green Supermix from Bio-Rad (Marnes-la-Coquette, France). The miScript System, miRNA mimc and Allstars negative control siRNA were obtained from Qiagen (Courtabeuf, France). miR-30a-3p antagonists were from Fisher scientific (Illkirch Cedex, France). Human Dermal Fibroblast Nucleofector kit was from Lonza (Cologne, Germany). The enzyme immunoassay kits for human BAFF, APRIL and IL-6 detection and recombinant IFN-γ were from R&D systems (Lille, France).

Cell culture

Human FLS were isolated from synovial tissues from five different RA patients and from five healthy subjects at the time of knee joint arthroscopic synovectomy. RA patients were 3 female and two male, the average age is 49 years, and had all FR positive but only three were antiCCP positive. Human dermal fibroblasts (HDF) were obtained by biopsy of 4 mm diameter from the affected areas (dorsal forearm) of four patients with SSc (SScHDF)and from the corresponding area of three healthy subjects (NHDF). All SSc patients were female (average age52 years) and had diffuse cutaneous systemic sclerosis and anti-Scl70-positive antibodies. The total modified Rodnan skin scores were 29, 8, 25 and 14, and that for the biopsy area were 2, 1, 2, 2.Blood B cells were isolated from 6 healthy donors. Institutional ethics committee of the Hopitaux Universitaires de Strasbourg specifically approved this study.Written informed consent was obtained by all the participants of this study (patients and healthy donors). The diagnosis of RA and SSc was conformed to the revised criteria of the American College of Rheumatology (ACR). FLS, HDF and HEK293 cultures were done as previously described [19]. Experiments were performed between the 3rd and the 9th passage. During that time, cultures were constituted of a homogeneous population of fibroblastic cells, negative for CD16 as determined by FACS analysis. HEK293 cells were purchased from the American type culture collection (ATCC) and maintained in DMEM supplemented with 10% heat-inactivated FBS, 2 mM of L-glutamine, 40 U/ml penicillin and 50 mg/ml streptomycin. Cell number and cell viability were checked by the MTT (3-(4,5 dimethylthiazol-2-yl)-2,5-diphenyltetrazolium bromide) assay. Blood mononuclear cells were isolated from healthy blood donors by Ficoll-Paque centrifugation as described in standard protocols. B cells were then selected by negative sorting using EasySep Human B Cell Enrichment Kit (Stemcell Technologies). The efficacy of B cell isolation was determined by FACS analysis using anti-CD19 antibodies. The yield of isolated B cells was composed of 99% $CD19^+/CD3^-$ B cells and 0.01% of $CD19^-/CD3^+$ T cells.

Stimulation of cells for total RNA extraction

FLS (2.10^5 cells) and HDF (2.10^5 cells) were seeded in 24-well plates and stimulated with medium alone or medium containing LPS (1 μg/mL), BLP (1 μg/mL), Poly(I:C) (10 μg/mL) and IFN-γ (0.1, 1 or 5 ng/mL). After a 6 h, 48 h and 72 h incubation period, total RNA was extracted using TRIzol according to the manufacturer's instruction.

Real-time quantitative PCR (RT-qPCR)

Total RNA was reverse transcribed using the iScript cDNA Synthesis Kit according to the manufacturer's instructions (BioRad). Real-time quantitative RT-qPCR was performed in a total volume of 20 μL using SsoAdvanced SYBR Green Supermix (BioRad) and gene-specific primers: BAFF: 5′-TGAAACAC-CAACTATACAAAAAG-3′ and 5′-TCAATTCATCCCCAAA-GACAT-3′;

April: 5′- CTCTGCTGACCCAACAAACA-3′ and 5′-CTCCTTTTCCGGGATCTCTC-3′;

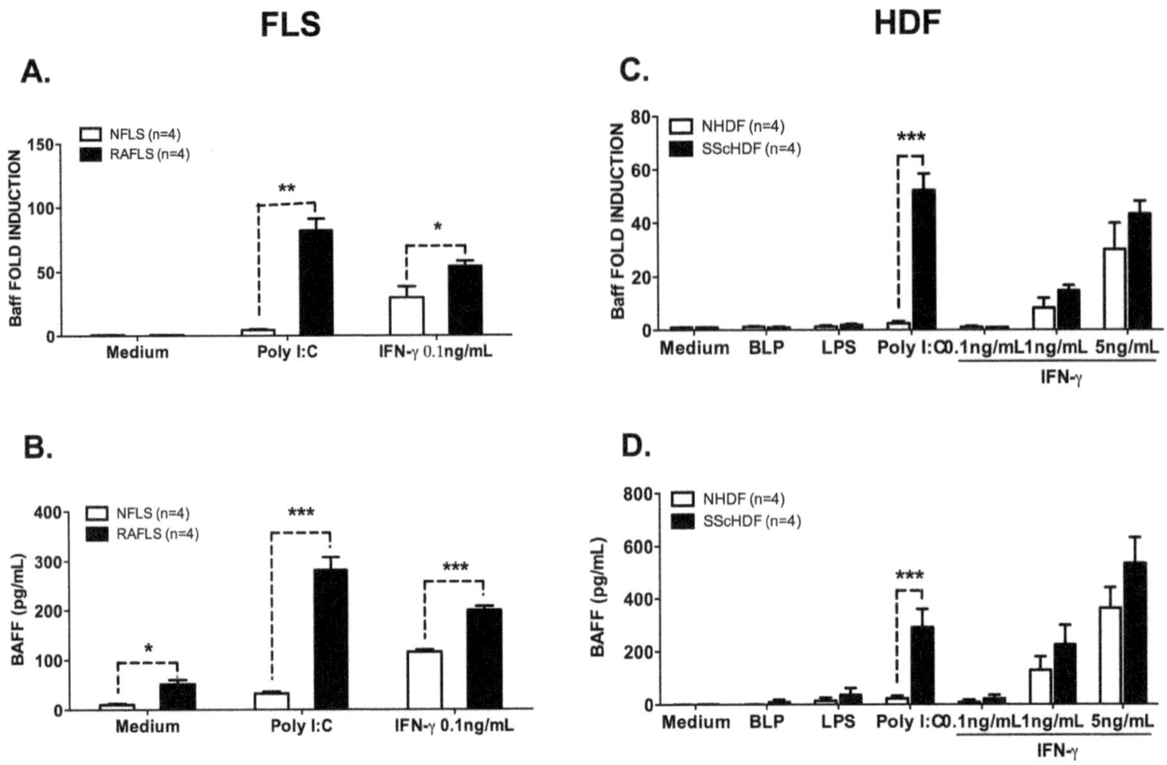

Figure 1. BAFF expression and secretion are up-regulated in Poly (I:C)- and IFN-γ-stimulated rheumatoid arthritis (RA) fibroblast-like synoviocytes (FLS) and systemic sclerosis (SSc) human dermal fibroblast (HDF). A, C. BAFF mRNA expression was determined by RT-qPCR in NFLS(n = 4) and RAFLS(n = 4) (A) or NHDF(n = 3) and SScHDF (n = 4) (C) stimulated (depending of the cell types) with BLP (1 μg/ml), LPS (1 μg/ml), Poly (I:C) (10 μg/mL) or IFN-γ (0.1, 1 or 5 ng/mL) for 72 h. Results were normalized to Gapdh and expressed as fold change compared with samples from cells incubated in medium. B, D. BAFF release was quantified by ELISA in culture supernatants of NFLS (n = 4) and RAFLS(n = 4) (B) or NHDF(n = 3) and SScHDF (n = 4) (D) in the same conditions as panels A and C. Data are expressed as the mean of triplicate samples ± SEM. *p<0.05, **p<0.01, ***p<0.001.

Gapdh: 5′-GGTGAAGGTCGGAGTCAACGGA-3′ and 5′-GAGGGATCTCGCTCCTGGAAGA-3′

After an initial denaturing at 96°C for 10 min, the temperatures used were 95°C for 10 s, 60°C for 15 s, 72°C for 25 s using a Rotor-Gene 6000 real-time PCR machine (Corbett Life Science). Amplification products were detected as an increased fluorescent signal of SYBR Green during the amplification cycles. Results were obtained using Rotor-Gene 6000 Series Software and evaluated using Excel (Microsoft). Melting-curve analysis was performed to assess the specificity of PCR products.

Real-time quantitative PCR analyses for miRNAs were performed using the miScript System and the primers (Qiagen). RNA concentrations were determined with a NanoDrop instrument (NanoDrop Technologies). 500 ng of RNA per sample was used for the assays. Reverse transcriptase reactions and RT-qPCR were performed according to the manufacturer's protocols. Expression of endogenous U6snRNA was used for normalization. Relative expression was calculated using the comparative threshold cycle (Ct) method and fold induction in cells activated by Poly(I:C) or IFN-γ was obtained by calculating $2^{-\Delta\Delta Ct}$.

Transfections and luciferase assay

Transient transfection of FLS or HDF with miR-30a-3p mimic (20 pM/sample), miR-30a-3p antagonists or with the negative controls was performed using the Human Dermal Fibroblast Nucleofector kit from Lonza as previously described [20]. Transfection of HEK293 cells was performed using Lipofectamine 2000 (Invitrogen) as previously described [19].

B cells viability assay

FLS or HDF were transfected with miR-30a-3p mimic, miR-30a-3p antagonists or with the negative controls as described above and stimulated with medium alone or medium with Poly(I:C) (10 μg/mL) or IFN-γ (5 ng/mL) for 72 h. Supernatants (800 μL) were harvested and used to culture B cells (5×10^5) for 72 h. In some experiments, anti-human BAFF antibodies or control IgG (R&D Systems) were added (10 ng/mL) to the supernatant. Then, B cells were stained with 3,3-dihexyloxacarbocyanine iodide ($DiOC_6$) to assess the mitochondrial transmembrane potential, and with Propidium Iodide (PI) to assess membrane permeability, as described [21]. Briefly, cell suspensions were incubated with 40 nmol/L $DiOC_6$ and 1 μg/ml PI for 15 min at 37°C, washed with FACS buffer and then analyzed on FACSCalibur (BD Biosciences). A lymphocyte gate was set using forward-angle and side-angle light scatter characteristics of lymphocytes. The vital B cells were brightly positive when stained with $DiOC_6$ and excluded PI.

Statistical analysis

Student's t test (two-tailed unpaired) was used to compare two independent groups using GraphPad 5 software. A probability (p) value of <0.05 was considered significant. *p<0.05; **p<0.01; ***p<0.001.

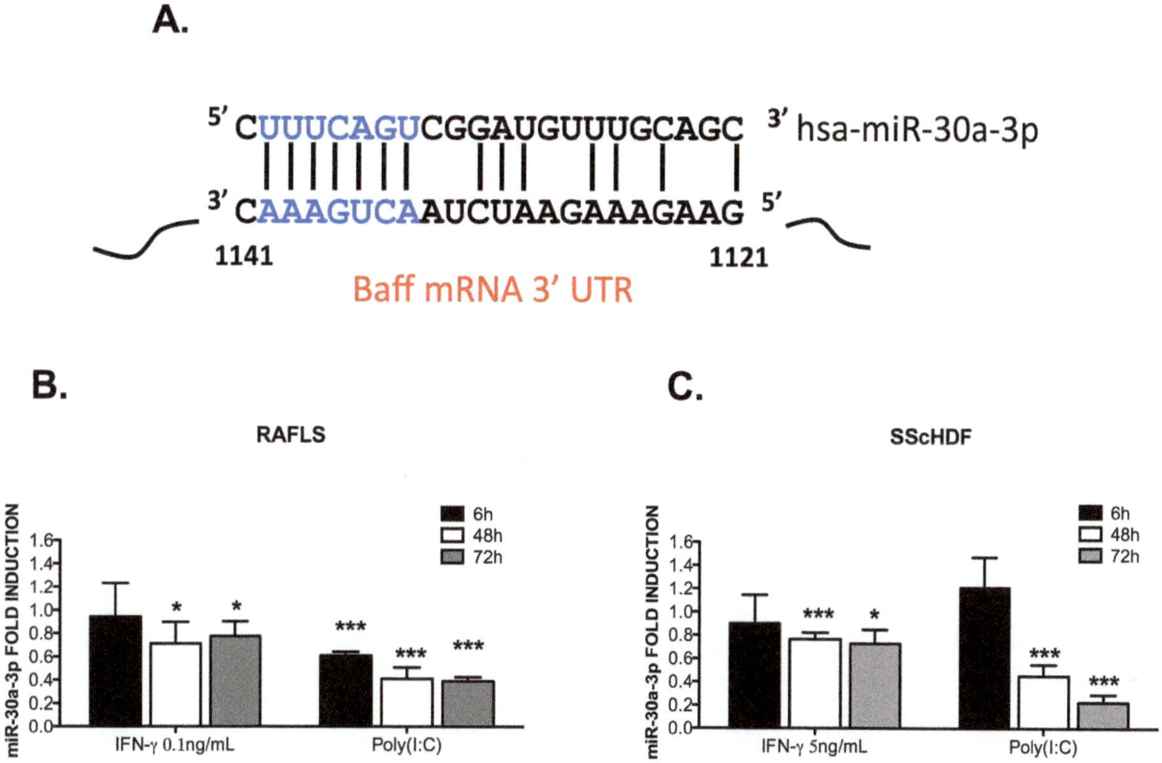

Figure 2. miR-30a-3p expression is down-regulated in Poly (I:C)- and IFN-γ-stimulated RAFLS and SScHDF. A. miR-30a-3p is predicted to target BAFF 3' UTR mRNA. B, C. miR-30a-3p expression was determined by RT-qPCR in RAFLS (n = 4) (B) and SScHDF (n = 4) (C) stimulated with Poly (I:C) (10 μg/mL) or IFN-γ (0.1 or 5 ng/mL) for 6 h, 48 h and 72 h. Results were normalized to U6snRNA and expressed as fold change compared with samples from cells incubated in medium. Data are expressed as the mean of triplicate samples ± SEM. *$p<0.05$, ***$p<0.001$.

Results

Increased BAFF secretion by SScHDF after stimulation with Poly(I:C) or IFN-γ

Upregulation of BAFF expression by Poly (I:C)- and IFN-γ-activated RAFLS, but not upon TLR2 or TLR4 activation, has been previously reported [13,22]. To gain more insights into the physiopathological consequences of this observation, we first compared BAFF expression in FLS isolated from healthy donors or RA patients. As shown in figure 1A and B, we observed that IFN-γ-dependent BAFF expression reaches maximum levels in RAFLS, whereas FLS isolated from healthy donors (NFLS) exhibit reduced cytokine expression at both mRNA and protein levels. Of note, Poly (I:C) stimulation induced very limited BAFF expression and secretion by NFLS, while RAFLS appeared extremely responsive to this stimulus. Next, we tested whether this difference between a healthy and a pathological (inflammatory) state could also be observed in another fibroblastic cell type and for this, we chose Human Dermal Fibroblasts (HDF) isolated from skin biopsies harvested from healthy donors (NHDF) or from patients suffering from systemic sclerosis (SScHDF). IFN-γ stimulation (1 and 5 ng/mL) resulted in a comparable increased expression of BAFF transcripts (figure 1C) and cytokine secretion (figure 1D) by NHDF or SScHDF. Interestingly, up-regulation of BAFF transcripts and protein release in response to TLR3 triggering by Poly (I:C) was only detectable in SScHDF and not from healthy individuals. We also investigated here the ability of Bacterial LipoProteins (BLP, Pam_3CSK4) or LipoPolysaccharide (LPS), which are respectively ligands for TLR2 and 4, to stimulate BAFF synthesis by NHDF and SScHDF. As seen in figure 1C and D, these PAMPs (Pathogen Associated Molecular Pattern) are not activators of BAFF transcription.

Thus, these results show that FLS and HDF from both healthy donors and RA or SSc patients can produce BAFF in response to IFN-γ stimulation, whereas BAFF transcription and protein secretion upon Poly (I:C) triggering occurred only in fibroblasts isolated from RA or SSc patients.

miR-30a-3p is down-regulated in Poly(I:C)- and IFN-γ-activated RAFLS and SScHDF

To understand the mechanisms underlying Poly (I:C)- and IFN-γ-dependent BAFF induction, we then focused our work on miRNA-driven post-transcriptional regulation. A computer-assisted search for miRNAs predicted to target BAFF mRNA performed using microCosm (http://www.ebi.ac.uk/enright-srv/microcosm/htdocs/targets/v5) identified several miRNAs candidates: miR-144*, miR-452, miR-340, miR-202, miR-500, miR-626, miR-330-3p, miR-302c* and miR-30 family members (miR-30a, d and e which share the same seed sequence). To evaluate the possible involvement of these miRNAs in BAFF regulation, we first performed RT-qPCR analysis to quantify their expression in RAFLS and SScHDF treated with Poly(I:C) or IFN-γ for 6 h, 48 h and 72 h. This analysis revealed that miR-144*, miR-30d-3p, miR-340, miR-626, miR-330-3p and miR-302c* could not be detected in RAFLS and SScHDF (figure 1S). miR-202 and miR-500 were expressed constitutively but their expression did not change after activation by Poly(I:C) or IFN-γ in both cell type. Finally, miR-452 was upregulated in Poly (I:C) treated RAFLS.

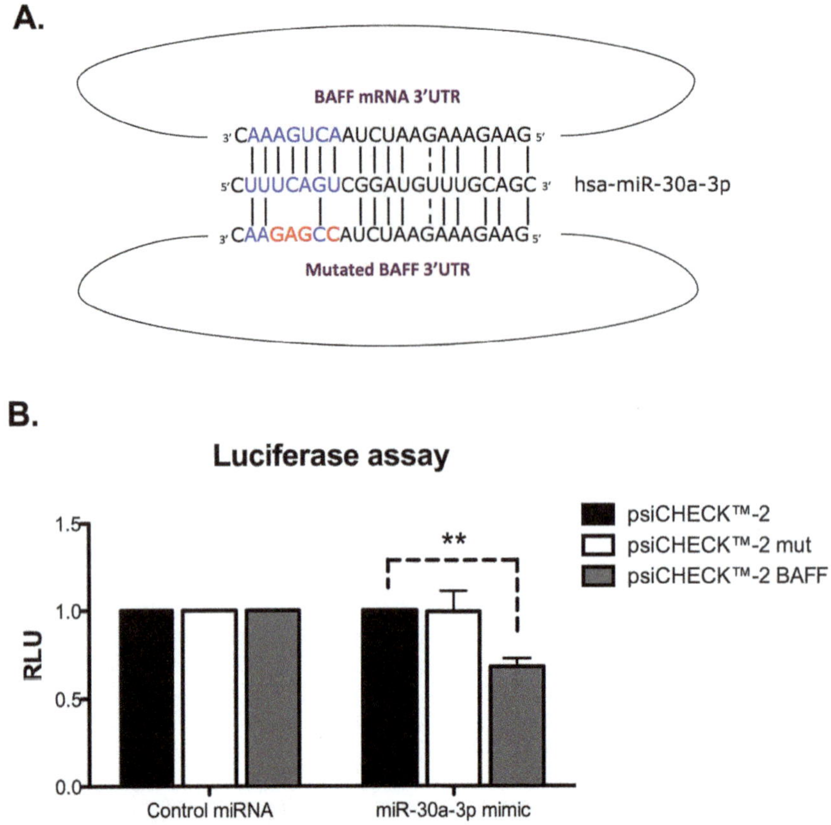

Figure 3. miR-30a-3p directly targets the 3′UTR of BAFF mRNA. A. Luciferase reporter constructs with wild-type or mutated (for miR-30-3p binding sites) BAFF 3′UTR were generated. B. HEK293 cells were transiently co-transfected with reporter constructs and with miR-30a-3p mimic (20 pM). Firefly Luciferase activities were measured 48 h after transfection and normalized to Renilla Luciferase expressed by the control psi-CHECK-2 vector devoid of 3′UTR sequences. Data are expressed as the mean of triplicate samples ± SEM and are representative of three independent experiments. $^{**}p<0.01$.

Interestingly, we noted that both miR-30a-3p and miR-30e-3p (data not shown), were significantly down-regulated in Poly (I:C)- and IFN-γ-activated, RAFLS (Figure 2B) and SScHDF (figure 2C) 48 h and 72 h after stimulation. These data, together with those illustrated in figure 1, indicate that BAFF transcripts and miR-30a-3p exhibit opposite expression patterns, therefore suggesting potential interactions. Given the strong similarities between miR-30a-3p and miR-30e-3p, we decided to focus on miR-30a-3p.

miR-30a-3p directly interacts with the 3′UTR of BAFF mRNA

To validate the involvement of miR-30a-3p in the regulation of *BAFF* expression, we generated luciferase reporter constructs (derived from the pSI-CHECK2 vector) containing the firefly luciferase gene fused to the entire human BAFF 3′UTR sequence and the renilla luciferase for normalization. We also generated a reporter construct in which a mutated version, designed to disrupt the predicted seed-match for miR-30a-3p of the human BAFF 3′UTR, was inserted (figure 3A). These plasmids were co-transfected in HEK293 cells with miR-30a-3p mimic or AllStars negative control siRNA (CT). In the presence of miR-30a-3p mimic, we observed a significant down regulation of the BAFF 3′UTR-controlled luciferase sensor, whereas luciferase expression upon transfection of the mutated form of the reporter vector remained unchanged (figure 3B). Altogether, these data suggest that BAFF transcripts can be directly targeted by miR-30a-3p for post-transcriptional regulation.

miR-30a-3p modulates BAFF expression in RAFLS and SScHDF

To assess the effect of miR-30a-3p on BAFF expression, we measured the production of BAFF mRNA by RT-qPCR in RAFLS and SScHDF transfected with miR-30a-3p mimic or with the AllStars negative siRNA control (CT). 24 h after transfection, cells were stimulated with Poly (I:C) or IFN-γ for 72 h. As seen in Figure 4, we found that overexpression of miR-30a-3p led to a global decrease in BAFF mRNA production and protein secretion by Poly (I:C)- and IFN-γ-activated RAFLS and SScHDF (panels A–D). Of note, transfection of miR-30a-3p mimic did not modulate IL-6 secretion by RAFLS and SScHDF activated with Poly (I:C) or IFN-γ (figure 4E–F), which is another major cytokine involved in B cells proliferation [23]. This indicates that miR-30a-3p does not interact with transcripts encoding factors involved in cytokine expression or inflammatory responses, but rather specifically interferes with BAFF mRNA in these cells, hence strengthening a potential role for BAFF in this process. Similar results were obtained upon transfection of miR-30e-3p and miR-30d-3p (data not shown).

These data demonstrate that miR-30a-3p is implicated in the negative regulation of BAFF synthesis in Poly (I:C)- and IFN-γ-activated FLS and HDF.

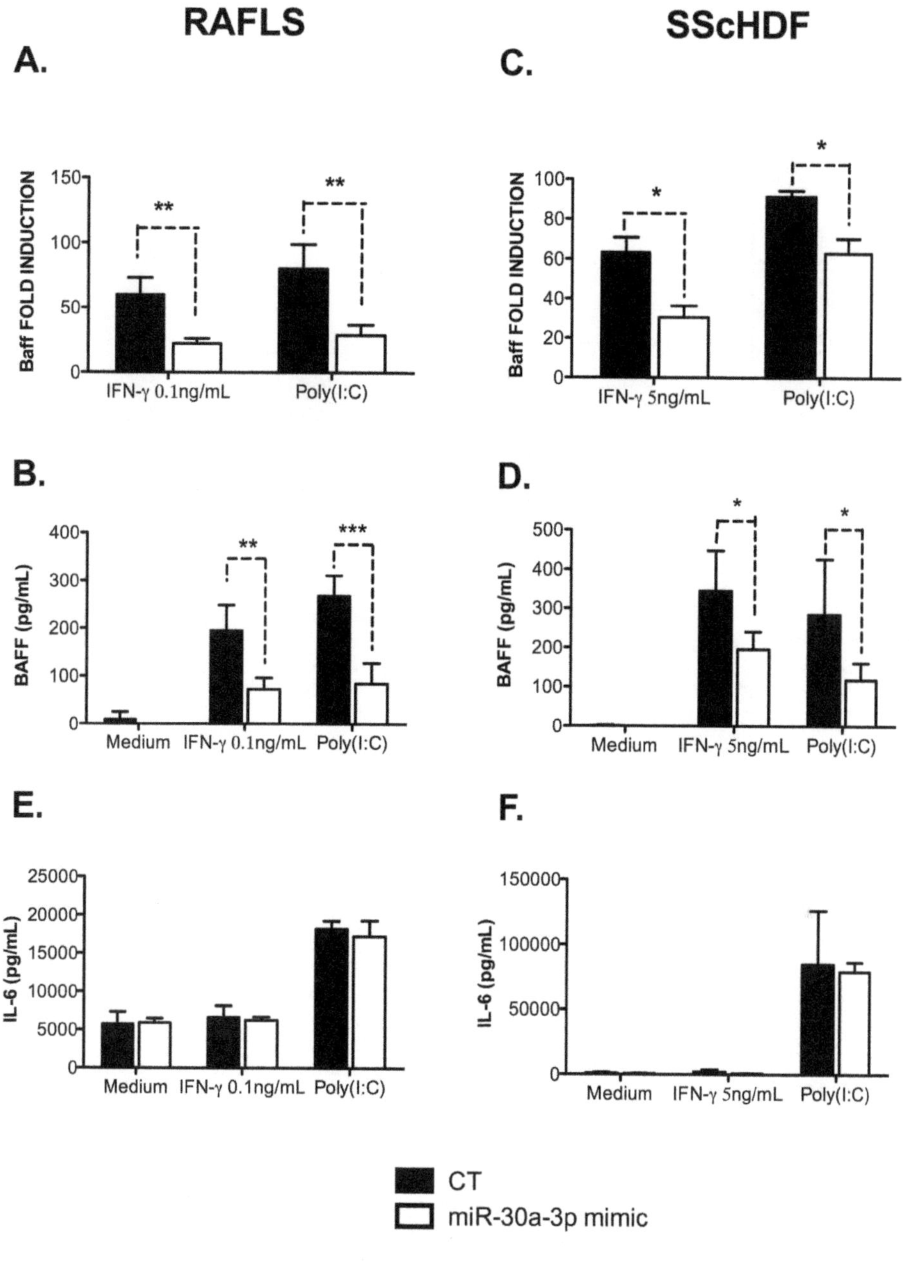

Figure 4. miR-30a-3p transfection affects BAFF mRNA expression and BAFF secretion in RAFLS and SScHDF. A, C. RAFLS (n = 5) (A) and SScHDF (n = 4) (C) were transfected with miR-30a-3p mimic (20 pM/sample) or with an AllStars negative control (CT). After 24 h, cells were activated with Poly (I:C) (10 μg/mL), IFN-γ (0.1 or 5 ng/mL, depending on cell types) or medium for 72 h. BAFF mRNA expression was determined by RT-qPCR. Results were normalized to Gapdh and expressed as fold change compared with samples from cells incubated with medium. B, D. BAFF release was determined by ELISA in culture supernatants in the same conditions as panel A and C. E, F. IL-6 release was determined by ELISA in culture supernatants in the same conditions as panel A and C. Data are expressed as the mean of triplicate samples ± SEM. *$p<0.05$; **$p<0.01$; ***$p<0.001$.

miR-30a-3p specifically represses BAFF-dependent B cells survival

Next, we checked the physiological relevance of BAFF regulation by miR-30a-3p. To this end, we measured the faculty of stimulated RAFLS and SScHDF to promote B cells survival following transfection of miR-30a-3p mimic. RAFLS and SScHDF were transfected with miR-30a-3p mimic or with the AllStars negative control siRNA (CT) for 24 h and then activated with IFN-γ for 72 h. The supernatants (conditioned medium) were harvested and added in the culture medium of B cells. After 3 days, survival of CD19-gated B cells was assessed by FACS analysis. As shown in figure 5, addition of supernatant from IFN-γ-stimulated fibroblasts significantly ($p<0.05$) increases the proportion of viable B cells, which shifts from 10 to 26% in the case of RAFLS supernatant and from 35 to 56% in the case of SScHDF. Importantly, increasing miRNA activity upon transfection of miR-30a-3p mimic in activated fibroblasts lowers B cells viability (15% and 35%, respectively. $p<0.05$). Additionally, we analyzed the supernatant of Poly (I:C)-activated RAFLS and SScHDF but we could not detect any difference in B cells survival (data not shown). Indeed, Poly (I:C), unlike IFN-γ, is also a potent inducer of IL-6 release by RAFLS and SScHDF (figure 4 E–F) which could

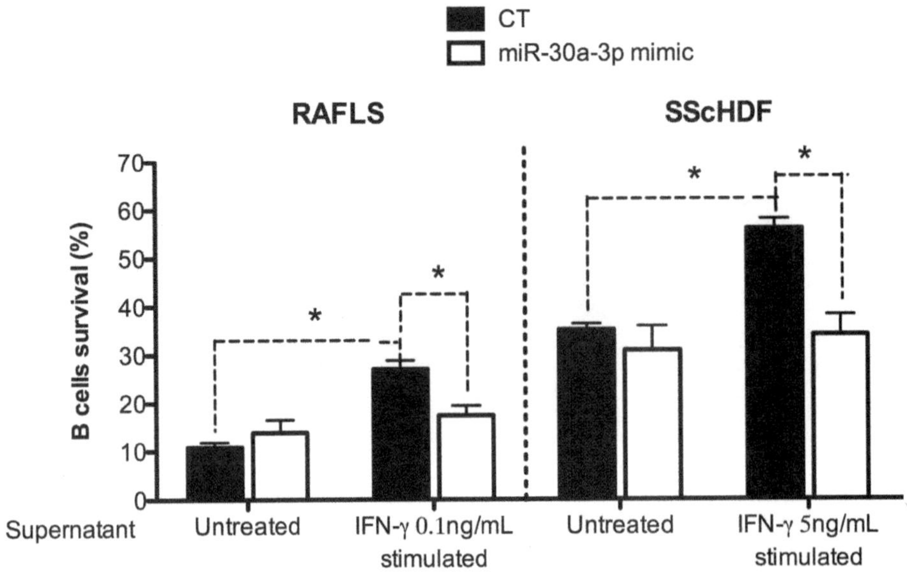

Figure 5. miR-30a-3p expression in RAFLS and SScHDF regulates BAFF-dependent B cells survival in vitro. RAFLS (n = 4) (left) and SScHDF (n = 4) (right) were transfected with miR-30a-3p mimic (20 pM/sample) or with an AllStars negative control (CT). After 24 h, cells were activated with IFN-γ (0.1 or 5 ng/mL depending on the cell type) or medium for 72 h. Then, supernatants were harvested and cultured with purified blood B cells isolated from healthy subjects. B cells viability was determined by FACS analysis; vital B cells were brightly positive when stained with DiOC6 and excluded PI. Data are expressed as the mean of triplicate samples ± SEM. *$p<0.05$.

regulate B cells survival. Similar results were obtained upon transfection of miR-30e-3p and miR-30d-3p (data not shown).

This experiment reveals that the modulation of miR-30a-3p activity induces important physiological changes with potentially relevant immune repercussions within the frame of autoimmune diseases.

miR-30a-3p is a basal repressors of BAFF expression in non-inflammatory fibroblasts (NFLS and NHDF)

Finally, we considered the possibility that miR-30a-3p family members could represent an essential mechanism to maintain BAFF expression at a very low level necessary in healthy conditions. Indeed, excessive BAFF secretion leading to increased B cells activation constitutes a major trigger promoting auto-immunity. A first insight into this model is provided by our initial observation of augmented BAFF secretion in the supernatant of RAFLS compared to NFLS in response to Poly(I:C) and IFN-γ (figure 1B). Therefore, we compared the expression of miR-30a-3p between healthy donor and patients cells in response to Poly(I:C) and IFN-γ for 48 h and 72 h. Interestingly, we showed that control NFLS as well as Poly(I:C)- and IFN-γ-stimulated cells expressed higher levels of miR-30a-3p compared to RAFLS under the same conditions (figure 6A). Moreover, NHDF which did not release BAFF in response to Poly(I:C) (figure 1D), also expressed higher levels of miR-30a-3p in the same conditions (figure 6B). These observations strongly suggest that miR-30a-3p could be a basal repressor of BAFF expression in these cells. Similar results were obtained upon transfection of miR-30e-3p (data not shown).

To test this hypothesis, we next lowered the activity of miR-30a-3p by transfecting specific antagonists (antisense 2′O methylated oligoribonucleotides) or negative controls (CT) in NFLS and NHDF. 24 h after transfection, cells were stimulated with Poly(I:C) or IFN-γ for 72 h. As illustrated in figure 6C, treatment with Poly(I:C) significantly induced higher levels of BAFF release by activated NHDF transfected with antisense oligonucleotides targeting miR-30a-3p compared to activated NHDF transfected with control (CT) (113,15±23,75 *vs* 30,75±3,25 pg/ml). A similar increase in BAFF secretion was obtained in NFLS transfected with antisense oligonucleotides targeting miR-30a-3p stimulated with Poly(I:C) (122±22 vs 38,2±5,5 pg/ml) and IFN-γ (109,45±20,85 vs 29,65±4,85 pg/ml). This experiment suggests that miR-30a-3p could represent an essential mechanism to maintain BAFF expression at a very low level necessary in healthy conditions. Moreover, we checked whether BAFF transcripts modulation upon miR-30a-3p inhibition also positively impacts on B cells survival. For this, we added anti-BAFF antibodies to poly (I:C)-stimulated NHDF treated with miR-30-3p antagomiRs. As seen in figure 6D, addition of anti-BAFF antibodies significantly ($p<0.01$ **) eradicates miR-30a-dependant-B cells survival improvement, thereby demonstrating that miR-30a-3p specifically modulates BAFF expression.

Discussion

The role of B cells in autoimmunity has undergone a major renaissance after the demonstration of the efficacy of B cells depletion in RA [24]. BAFF plays a pivotal role in B cells activation in autoimmune diseases and is secreted by resident cells of target organs such as fibroblast-like synoviocytes [22,25,26]. On the other hand, the pivotal role of innate immunity in the initiation of autoimmune diseases is now well established, which prompted our present investigation on the role of innate immune receptors ligands and interferon-γ on BAFF secretion. We performed our analysis in fibroblasts isolated either from the skin (HDF) of healthy donors or from patients suffering from SSc or from the synovium (FLS) of RA patients or controls. Our results clearly show that, while Poly (I:C) stimulation induces high levels of BAFF transcription, LPS or BLP (respectively ligands of TLR4 and TLR2) remain poor activators of BAFF expression and secretion. Likewise, Poly (I:C) as well as LPS or BLP did not induce the synthesis of APRIL (a proliferation inducing ligand), which regulates also lymphocyte survival and activation (data not shown).

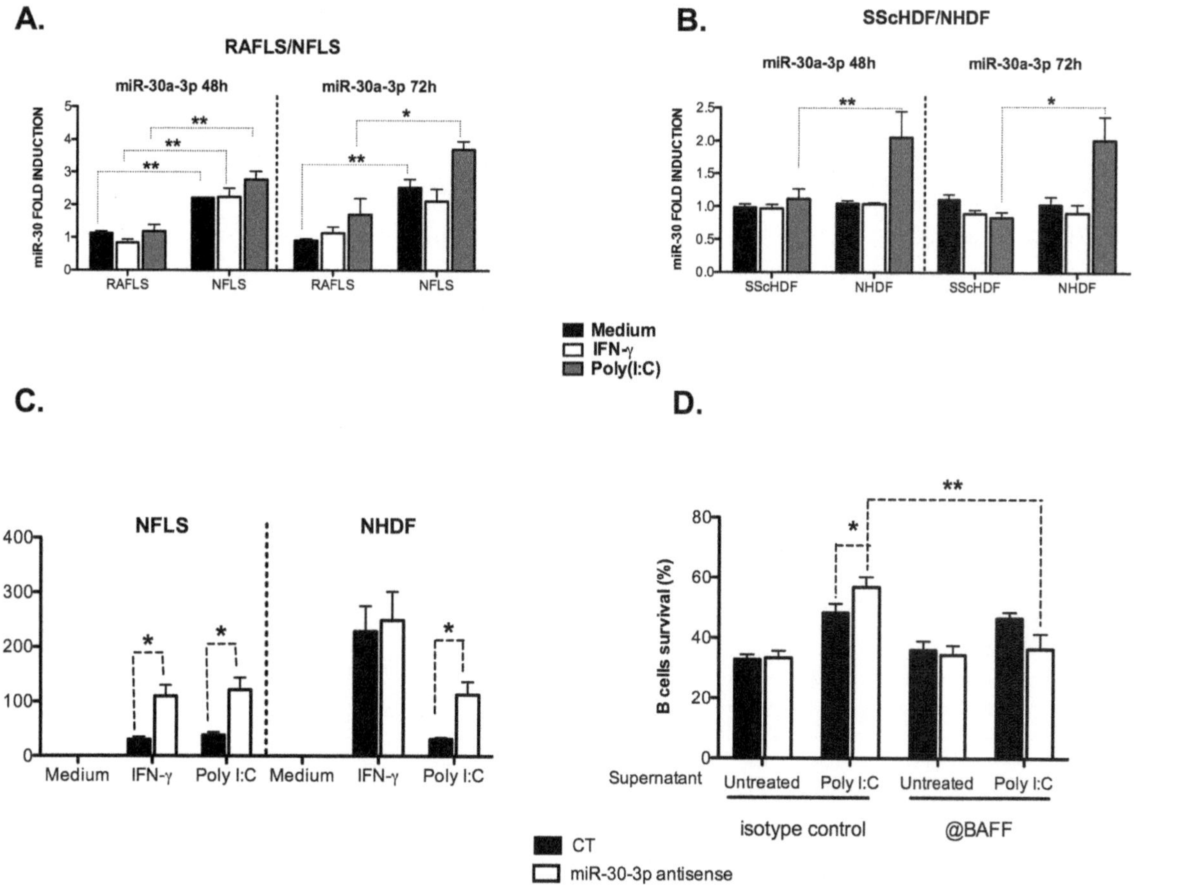

Figure 6. MiR-30a-3p represses BAFF secretion by healthy FLS and HDF. A, B. miR-30a-3p expression was determined by RT-qPCR in NFLS (n = 4)/RAFLS (n = 4) (A) and NHDF (n = 3)/SScHDF (n = 4) (B) stimulated with Poly(I:C) (10 μg/mL), IFN-γ (0.1 or 5 ng/mL) or medium for 48 h and 72 h. Results were normalized to U6snRNA and expressed as fold change compared with samples from RAFLS (A) or SScHDF (B) incubated with medium. C. NFLS (n = 3) and NHDF (n = 3) were transfected with miR-30-3p antisense oligonucleotides (20 pM/sample) or with an AllStars negative control (CT). After 24 h, cells were activated with Poly(I:C) (10 μg/mL), IFN-γ (0.1 or 5 ng/mL) or medium for 72 h. BAFF release was determined by ELISA in culture supernatants. D. NHDF (n = 3) transfected with miR-30-3p antisense, were stimulated with poly (I:C). The supernatant was then treated with control IgG or with anti-BAFF antibodies and added to purified B cells. B cells survival was next evaluated as in panel Figure 5. $^*p<0.05$; $^{**}p<0.01$.

This finding is consistent with results from our group which proposed that TLR2, 4 and 9 ligands failed to induce BAFF mRNA and protein in rheumatoid FLS [22]. Likewise, stimulation of salivary gland epithelial cells (SGEC) obtained from patients with primary Sjögren's syndrome (pSS) or bronchial epithelial cells with TLR2, 7 and 9 ligands does not induce BAFF transcription and secretion [27,28]. Therefore, a first important result of this study is our description of specific Poly (I:C)-dependent BAFF transcriptional induction and subsequent secretion by SScHDF. This observation provides a conceptual framework whereby pathogens, such as herpesviruses which are capable of triggering a TLR3-dependent response [29] and have been associated to many autoimmune diseases [30], can initiate BAFF secretion and ignite a vicious circle leading to pathogenic auto-antibodies production. In line with this hypothesis, Ittah et al. suggested that PKR is the major mediator of BAFF expression and secretion after dsRNA virus infection or Poly (I:C) stimulation by salivary epithelial cells of pSS [31].

Next, we investigated the mechanisms involved in the regulation of BAFF production by FLS and HDF. miRNAs, which are considered as efficient fine tuners of immune responses because they usually modulate gene expression by a factor 1.2 to 4 [32], exhibit abnormal expression associated with inflammatory disorders such as RA [33,34], SLE [35,36] and SSc [37,38]. In an initial attempt to identify miRNAs involved in the control of BAFF expression, we performed RT-qPCR analysis of Poly (I:C)- and IFN-γ-activated RAFLS and SScHDF to quantify the expression of 9 miRNAs that were predicted to target BAFF transcripts. Among these candidates, miR-30a-3p was selected for further analysis because its expression was down regulated in Poly (I:C)- and IFN-γ-activated RAFLS and SScHDF; such inverse correlation with the expression of BAFF transcripts in the same cells and the same conditions indicated that miR-30-3p family members might have a role in the regulation of BAFF expression. We next demonstrated by several complementary approaches that miR-30a-3p actually bind specifically to the 3′UTR of BAFF transcripts and modulate cytokine expression. Importantly, additional results (data not shown) indicate that additional members (and closely related) of the miR-30a-3p family (miR30-d-3p and -e-3p) also regulate BAFF expression in RAFLS and SScHDF stimulated with Poly (I:C) or IFN-γ. Therefore, our study additionally suggests a novel mechanism for the regulation of BAFF expression at the posttranslational level in response to inflammatory stimuli but the transcriptional regulation of BAFF expression must also be considered. Usually, miRNAs can function together with RNA-binding proteins to regulate mRNA expression through the AU-rich elements (AREs) that are found in numerous cytokine-encoding mRNAs. For example, TNF-α and IL-10 mRNAs both contain long AREs that are targeted by the RNA-binding protein tristetraprolin (TTP) [39]. Our group previously showed that blocking miR-346 decreases TTP expression and re-established mature TNF-α intracellular expression in LPS-activated RAFLS [40,41]. Although evidence for the direct targeting of cytokine mRNAs by miRNAs is limited [39], we demonstrated in this study that miR 30a-3p directly regulates BAFF mRNA.

Importantly, we also analyzed in our study the functional outcome of miRNA-dependent BAFF regulation. We demonstrated that IFN-γ stimulation of fibroblasts favors an extracellular milieu that promotes B cells survival. Importantly, our experiments (illustrated in Figure 5) demonstrated that specifically altering BAFF secretion (with miR-30a mimic or upon anti-BAFF antibodies addition following antagomiRs transfection) reduces the B cells survival capacity of supernatant from IFN-γ stimulated RAFLS or SScHDF back to normal (as observed in control cells). This indicates that BAFF (and not IL-6) is the major B cells survival factor expressed by these fibrocytes upon IFN-γ stimulation. Similar to our findings, Ohata et al reported that FLS treated with IFN-γ and/or TNF-α had a greater capacity to support B cells survival than did untreated FLS [26]. B cells survival could be inhibited by BAFF-R:Fc, indicating that BAFF/BAFF-R interactions were involved in B cells survival [26]. Altogether, this work provides a mechanistic explanation to the control of BAFF transcripts expression and demonstrates that cytokine secretion by resident cells of target organs of autoimmune diseases can be negatively regulated at the post-transcriptional level by miRNAs. A tentative model describing these interactions is depicted in Figure 2S. The understanding of these complex pathways has important implications for the development of future therapeutic applications. Indeed, the success of Belimumab in the treatment of patients with RA and ongoing clinical trials in SSc (NCT01670565) suggest that therapeutic targeting of BAFF could be of interest [42]. Our present study suggests that miR-30a-3p (and others family members) mimic could be used to target BAFF mRNA in autoimmune diseases. Recently, patients chronically infected with hepatitis C virus (HCV) treated with locked nucleic acid (modified antisense oligonucleotides) against miR-122 showed a prolonged dose-dependent reductions in HCV RNA levels without evidence of viral resistance [43], which suggests that miRNA modulation in patients could become a new therapeutic option in the future.

Supporting Information

Figure S1 miRNAs expression in RAFLS and SScHDF. MiR-144*, miR-30d-3p, miR-452, miR-340, miR-202, miR-500, miR-626, miR-330-3p and miR-302c* expression was determined by RT-qPCR in RAFLS (n = 3) and SScHDF (n = 3) stimulated with Poly (I:C) (10 µg/mL) or IFN-γ (0.1 or 5 ng/mL) for 72 h. Results were normalized to U6snRNA and expressed as fold change compared with samples from RAFLS or SScHDF incubated with medium.

Figure S2 Model describing the role of miR-30a-3p in BAFF secretion by FLS (A) and HDF (B) from RA or SSc patients and healthy subjects.

Acknowledgments

The authors are grateful to Angélique Pichot for technical help and to Prof. François Bonnomet, (Service de chirurgie orthopédique, Strasbourg Hospital) Dr. Emmanuel Chatelus and Dr. Christelle Sordet (service de rheumatology, Strasbourg hospital) for patients' biopsies.

Author Contributions

Conceived and designed the experiments: GA AF SP DW PG. Performed the experiments: GA AF LP YZG SC. Analyzed the data: GA AF SP PG. Contributed reagents/materials/analysis tools: SP SB JS. Wrote the paper: GA AF SP PG JEG JS.

References

1. Mackay F, Schneider P, Rennert P, Browning J (2003) BAFF AND APRIL: a tutorial on B cell survival. Annu Rev Immunol 21: 231–264. doi:10.1146/annurev.immunol.21.120601.141152.
2. Nardelli B, Belvedere O, Roschke V, Moore PA, Olsen HS, et al. (2001) Synthesis and release of B-lymphocyte stimulator from myeloid cells. Blood 97: 198–204.
3. Scapini P, Nardelli B, Nadali G, Calzetti F, Pizzolo G, et al. (2003) G-CSF-stimulated neutrophils are a prominent source of functional BLyS. J Exp Med 197: 297–302.
4. Krumbholz M, Theil D, Derfuss T, Rosenwald A, Schrader F, et al. (2005) BAFF is produced by astrocytes and up-regulated in multiple sclerosis lesions and primary central nervous system lymphoma. J Exp Med 201: 195–200. doi:10.1084/jem.20041674.
5. Kalled SL (2005) The role of BAFF in immune function and implications for autoimmunity. Immunol Rev 204: 43–54. doi:10.1111/j.0105-2896.2005.00219.x.
6. Mackay F, Woodcock SA, Lawton P, Ambrose C, Baetscher M, et al. (1999) Mice Transgenic for Baff Develop Lymphocytic Disorders along with Autoimmune Manifestations. Journal of Experimental Medicine 190: 1697–1710. doi:10.1084/jem.190.11.1697.
7. Seyler TM, Park YW, Takemura S, Bram RJ, Kurtin PJ, et al. (2005) BLyS and APRIL in rheumatoid arthritis. J Clin Invest 115: 3083–3092. doi:10.1172/JCI25265.
8. Mackay F, Schneider P (2009) Cracking the BAFF code. Nat Rev Immunol 9: 491–502. doi:10.1038/nri2572.
9. Pers J-O, Daridon C, Devauchelle V, Jousse S, Saraux A, et al. (2005) BAFF overexpression is associated with autoantibody production in autoimmune diseases. Ann N Y Acad Sci 1050: 34–39. doi:10.1196/annals.1313.004.
10. Matsushita T, Hasegawa M, Matsushita Y, Echigo T, Wayaku T, et al. (2007) Elevated serum BAFF levels in patients with localized scleroderma in contrast to other organ-specific autoimmune diseases. Exp Dermatol 16: 87–93. doi:10.1111/j.1600-0625.2006.00485.x.
11. Matsushita T, Fujimoto M, Hasegawa M, Tanaka C, Kumada S, et al. (2007) Elevated serum APRIL levels in patients with systemic sclerosis: distinct profiles of systemic sclerosis categorized by APRIL and BAFF. J Rheumatol 34: 2056–2062.
12. Zhang M, Ko K-H, Lam QLK, Lo CKC, Srivastava G, et al. (2005) Expression and function of TNF family member B cell-activating factor in the development of autoimmune arthritis. Int Immunol 17: 1081–1092. doi:10.1093/intimm/dxh287.
13. Alsaleh G, François A, Knapp A-M, Schickel J-N, Sibilia J, et al. (2011) Synovial fibroblasts promote immunoglobulin class switching by a mechanism involving BAFF. Eur J Immunol 41: 2113–2122. doi:10.1002/eji.201041194.
14. Baker KP, Edwards BM, Main SH, Choi GH, Wager RE, et al. (2003) Generation and characterization of LymphoStat-B, a human monoclonal antibody that antagonizes the bioactivities of B lymphocyte stimulator. Arthritis Rheum 48: 3253–3265. doi:10.1002/art.11299.
15. Chan AC (2011) B cell immunotherapy in autoimmunity–2010 update. Mol Immunol 48: 1344–1347. doi:10.1016/j.molimm.2010.11.021.
16. Chugh PK, Kalra BS (2013) Belimumab: targeted therapy for lupus. Int J Rheum Dis 16: 4–13. doi:10.1111/1756-185x.12002.
17. Jing Q, Huang S, Guth S, Zarubin T, Motoyama A, et al. (2005) Involvement of microRNA in AU-rich element-mediated mRNA instability. Cell 120: 623–634. doi:10.1016/j.cell.2004.12.038.
18. Asirvatham AJ, Magner WJ, Tomasi TB (2009) miRNA regulation of cytokine genes. Cytokine 45: 58–69. doi:10.1016/j.cyto.2008.11.010.
19. Philippe L, Alsaleh G, Pichot A, Ostermann E, Zuber G, et al. (2013) MiR-20a regulates ASK1 expression and TLR4-dependent cytokine release in rheumatoid fibroblast-like synoviocytes. Ann Rheum Dis 72: 1071–1079. doi:10.1136/annrheumdis-2012-201654.
20. Alsaleh G, Suffert G, Semaan N, Juncker T, Frenzel L, et al. (2009) Bruton's tyrosine kinase is involved in miR-346-related regulation of IL-18 release by lipopolysaccharide-activated rheumatoid fibroblast-like synoviocytes. J Immunol 182: 5088–5097. doi:10.4049/jimmunol.0801613.

21. Zamzami N, Marchetti P, Castedo M, Zanin C, Vayssière JL, et al. (1995) Reduction in mitochondrial potential constitutes an early irreversible step of programmed lymphocyte death in vivo. J Exp Med 181: 1661–1672.
22. Alsaleh G, Messer L, Semaan N, Boulanger N, Gottenberg J-E, et al. (2007) BAFF synthesis by rheumatoid synoviocytes is positively controlled by alpha5beta1 integrin stimulation and is negatively regulated by tumor necrosis factor alpha and Toll-like receptor ligands. Arthritis Rheum 56: 3202–3214. doi:10.1002/art.22915.
23. Kishimoto T (2005) Interleukin-6: from basic science to medicine–40 years in immunology. Annu Rev Immunol 23: 1–21. doi:10.1146/annurev.immunol.23.021704.115806.
24. Finnegan A, Ashaye S, Hamel KM (2012) B effector cells in rheumatoid arthritis and experimental arthritis. Autoimmunity 45: 353–363. doi:10.3109/08916934.2012.665526.
25. Moisini I, Davidson A (2009) BAFF: a local and systemic target in autoimmune diseases. Clin Exp Immunol 158: 155–163. doi:10.1111/j.1365-2249.2009.04007.x.
26. Ohata J, Zvaifler NJ, Nishio M, Boyle DL, Kalled SL, et al. (2005) Fibroblast-like synoviocytes of mesenchymal origin express functional B cell-activating factor of the TNF family in response to proinflammatory cytokines. J Immunol 174: 864–870.
27. Ittah M, Miceli-Richard C, Gottenberg J-E, Sellam J, Eid P, et al. (2008) Viruses induce high expression of BAFF by salivary gland epithelial cells through TLR- and type-I IFN-dependent and -independent pathways. Eur J Immunol 38: 1058–1064. doi:10.1002/eji.200738013.
28. Kato A, Truong-Tran AQ, Scott AL, Matsumoto K, Schleimer RP (2006) Airway epithelial cells produce B cell-activating factor of TNF family by an IFN-beta-dependent mechanism. J Immunol 177: 7164–7172.
29. Zhang S-Y, Jouanguy E, Sancho-Shimizu V, Von Bernuth H, Yang K, et al. (2007) Human Toll-like receptor-dependent induction of interferons in protective immunity to viruses. Immunol Rev 220: 225–236. doi:10.1111/j.1600-065X.2007.00564.x.
30. Ferraccioli G, Tolusso B (2007) Infections, B cell receptor activation and autoimmunity: different check-point impairments lead to autoimmunity, clonal B cell expansion and fibrosis in different immunological settings. Autoimmun Rev 7: 109–113. doi:10.1016/j.autrev.2007.02.013.
31. Ittah M, Miceli-Richard C, Gottenberg J-E, Sellam J, Lepajolec C, et al. (2009) B-cell-activating factor expressions in salivary epithelial cells after dsRNA virus infection depends on RNA-activated protein kinase activation. Eur J Immunol 39: 1271–1279. doi:10.1002/eji.200839086.
32. Mukherji S, Ebert MS, Zheng GXY, Tsang JS, Sharp PA, et al. (2011) MicroRNAs can generate thresholds in target gene expression. Nat Genet 43: 854–859. doi:10.1038/ng.905.
33. Stanczyk J, Pedrioli DML, Brentano F, Sanchez-Pernaute O, Kolling C, et al. (2008) Altered expression of MicroRNA in synovial fibroblasts and synovial tissue in rheumatoid arthritis. Arthritis Rheum 58: 1001–1009. doi:10.1002/art.23386.
34. Ceribelli A, Nahid MA, Satoh M, Chan EKL (2011) MicroRNAs in rheumatoid arthritis. FEBS Lett 585: 3667–3674. doi:10.1016/j.febslet.2011.05.020.
35. Dai Y, Huang Y-S, Tang M, Lv T-Y, Hu C-X, et al. (2007) Microarray analysis of microRNA expression in peripheral blood cells of systemic lupus erythematosus patients. Lupus 16: 939–946. doi:10.1177/0961203307084158.
36. Tang Y, Luo X, Cui H, Ni X, Yuan M, et al. (2009) MicroRNA-146A contributes to abnormal activation of the type I interferon pathway in human lupus by targeting the key signaling proteins. Arthritis Rheum 60: 1065–1075. doi:10.1002/art.24436.
37. Li H, Yang R, Fan X, Gu T, Zhao Z, et al. (2012) MicroRNA array analysis of microRNAs related to systemic scleroderma. Rheumatol Int 32: 307–313. doi:10.1007/s00296-010-1615-y.
38. Maurer B, Stanczyk J, Jüngel A, Akhmetshina A, Trenkmann M, et al. (2010) MicroRNA-29, a key regulator of collagen expression in systemic sclerosis. Arthritis Rheum 62: 1733–1743. doi:10.1002/art.27443.
39. O'Neill LA, Sheedy FJ, McCoy CE (2011) MicroRNAs: the fine-tuners of Toll-like receptor signalling. Nat Rev Immunol 11: 163–175. doi:10.1038/nri2957.
40. Alsaleh G, Suffert G, Semaan N, Juncker T, Frenzel L, et al. (2009) Bruton's tyrosine kinase is involved in miR-346-related regulation of IL-18 release by lipopolysaccharide-activated rheumatoid fibroblast-like synoviocytes. J Immunol 182: 5088–5097. doi:10.4049/jimmunol.0801613.
41. Semaan N, Frenzel L, Alsaleh G, Suffert G, Gottenberg J-E, et al. (2011) miR-346 controls release of TNF-α protein and stability of its mRNA in rheumatoid arthritis via tristetraprolin stabilization. PLoS ONE 6: e19827. doi:10.1371/journal.pone.0019827.
42. Stohl W, Merrill JT, McKay JD, Lisse JR, Zhong ZJ, et al. (2013) Efficacy and safety of belimumab in patients with rheumatoid arthritis: a phase II, randomized, double-blind, placebo-controlled, dose-ranging Study. J Rheumatol 40: 579–589. doi:10.3899/jrheum.120886.
43. Janssen HLA, Reesink HW, Lawitz EJ, Zeuzem S, Rodriguez-Torres M, et al. (2013) Treatment of HCV Infection by Targeting MicroRNA. N Engl J Med. doi:10.1056/NEJMoa1209026.

22

Rheumatoid Arthritis Increases the Risk of Nontuberculosis Mycobacterial Disease and Active Pulmonary Tuberculosis

Jun-Jun Yeh[1,2,3], Yu-Chiao Wang[4,5], Fung-Chang Sung[5,6], Chia-Hung Kao[6,7]*

1 Department of Internal Medicine and Family Medicine, Ditmanson Medical Foundation Chia-Yi Christian Hospital, Chiayi, Taiwan, **2** Chia Nan University of Pharmacy and Science, Tainan, Taiwan, **3** Meiho University, Pingtung, Taiwan, **4** Management Office for Health Data, China Medical University Hospital, Taichung, Taiwan, **5** College of Medicine, China Medical University, Taichung, Taiwan, **6** Graduate Institute of Clinical Medical Science, China Medical University College of Medicine, Taichung, Taiwan, **7** Department of Nuclear Medicine and PET Center, China Medical University Hospital, Taichung, Taiwan

Abstract

Background: Few studies have examined the association of rheumatoid arthritis (RA) with nontuberculosis mycobacterium (NTM) disease and pulmonary tuberculosis (PTB).

Methods: We identified 29 131 patients with RA from the catastrophic illness registry who were diagnosed from 1998–2008; 116 524 patients without RA from inpatient data files were randomly frequency matched according to sex, age, and index year and used as a comparison group. Both groups were followed-up until the end of 2010 to measure the incidence of NTM disease and active PTB. We analyzed the risk of NTM disease and active PTB using the Cox proportional hazards regression models, controlling for sex, age, and Charlson comorbidity index (CCI).

Results: The incidence of NTM disease was 4.22 times greater in the RA group than in the non-RA group (1.91 vs 0.45 per 10,000 person-years). The incidence of PTB was 2.99 times greater in the RA group than in the non-RA group (25.3 vs 8.46 per 10,000 person-years). After adjusting for age, sex, and CCI, the adjusted hazard ratios (HRs) of NTM disease and active PTB for the RA group were 4.17 (95% CI = 2.61–6.65) and 2.87 (95% CI = 2.55–3.23), respectively, compared with the non-RA group. In the first 2 years of follow-up, the RA group yielded corresponding adjusted HRs of 4.98 and 3.39 compared with the non-RA group. The follow-up time-specific RA group to the non-RA group HR of both the NTM disease and active PTB varied.

Conclusion: This study can serve as a reference for clinical physicians to increase awareness regarding the detection of NTM disease and active PTB in RA patients among the any stage of the clinical course even without CCI.

Editor: Andres R. Floto, Cambridge University, United Kingdom

Funding: This study was supported in part by the study projects DMR-103-018 and DMR-103-020 in our hospital. This study is supported in part by Taiwan Ministry of Health and Welfare Clinical Trial and Research Center of Excellence (MOHW103-TDU-B-212-113002), Health and welfare surcharge of tobacco products, China Medical University Hospital Cancer Research Center of Excellence (MOHW103-TD-B-111-03, Taiwan). The funders had no role in the study design, data collection and analysis, the decision to publish, or preparation of the manuscript.

Competing Interests: The authors have declared that no competing interests exist.

* Email: d10040@mail.cmuh.org.tw

Introduction

Rheumatoid arthritis (RA) is the most common connective tissue disease (CTD) and exerts an increasing burden on health resources globally [1,2]. Pulmonary infection is related to RA [3]. The reactivation of mycobacterium tuberculosis (MTB) infection is a major complication in patients treated with antitumor necrosis factor (anti-TNF) agents in RA [4]. Treating opportunistic infections emerging in RA is crucial, as is providing therapy for the original disease. MTB is a pathogen among the main opportunistic infections [5], but no study has observed that RA increases the risk of active pulmonary tuberculosis (PTB).

The chronic use of methotrexate (MTX) to treat RA can result in opportunistic infections such as pulmonary nontuberculosis mycobacterium (NTM) disease [6]. One study observed NTM disease in immunosuppressed RA patients using anti-TNF-alpha therapy [7]. Yamakawa et al showed disease deterioration because of an antirheumatic drug received during NTM disease follow-up [8]. However, no study has focused on whether RA increases the risk of NTM disease.

The Charlson comorbidity index (CCI) was originally developed to create a single-value summary for several comorbid conditions for breast cancer patients in 1984, and is suitable for assessing general medical inpatient populations [9,10]. Among the comorbidity scales developed for general medical patients, CCI is the most popular and the easiest to apply [11]. Tiippana-Kinnunen et al observed that comorbidities increased during 15 years of RA, and patients with a high baseline CCI showed high disease activity, both in early disease and at the end-point [12].

PTB appears to increase in RA patients, independent of treatment [13,14], although a U.S. study differed in this regard [15]. Furthermore, no research has discussed conditions comorbid with RA that are associated with NTM disease and active PTB. Therefore, we conducted a nationwide RA-cohort study to investigate whether RA increases the risk of NTM disease and active PTB. This is the first study to examine the association of RA and CCI with the development of NTM disease and active PTB among the clinical course by using time-dependent covariates in a general Asian population.

Materials and Methods

Data Source

The Taiwan National Health Insurance (NHI) is a universal insurance program established by the Taiwan Department of Health in March 1995 by consolidating 13 insurance programs. The insurance system has a coverage rate of 99% for 23.74 million people. The Taiwan NHI Research Database (NHIRD) (http://nhird.nhri.org.tw/en/index.htm) is authorized to provide insured registration files and original reimbursement claims data in the 1996–2010 periods.

In this study, we used two datasets included the all of the hospitalization clams data and the Registry for Catastrophic Illness Patient Database (RCIPD) of Taiwan, in which the International Classification of Diseases, 9th Revision, Clinical Modification (ICD-9-CM) was used to define diseases. To protect patient privacy, all personal identification numbers are encrypted before electronic files are released. Both datasets were scrambled with surrogate identifications of the insured and analyzed anonymously.

Data Availability Statement

All data and related metadata are deposited in an appropriate public repository. The study population's data which were from Taiwan NHIRD (http://w3.nhri.org.tw/nhird//date_01.html) are maintained by Taiwan NHIRD (http://nhird.nhri.org.tw/). The National Health Research Institutes (NHRI) is a non-profit foundation established by the government.

Ethics Statement

The NHIRD encrypts patient personal information to protect privacy and provides researchers with anonymous identification numbers associated with relevant claim information, including patients' sex, dates of birth, medical services utilized, and prescriptions. Patient consent is not required for accessing the NHIRD. This study was approved by the Institutional Review Board of China Medical University (CMU-REC-101-012). Our IRB specifically waived the consent requirement.

Study Population

This study is a retrospective population-based cohort study. In Taiwan, the rheumatologists can apply for the catastrophic illness card for any patient with RA, who fulfils the presence of 4 or more diagnostic criteria based on the 1987 ACR criteria [16]. The application of the catastrophic illness card should be scrutinized by peer review. The patients with RA with a catastrophic illness card can be exempt from paying a copayment. We used the Registry for Catastrophic Illness Patient Database (RCIPD) to identify RA (ICD-9-CM 714) patients in the claims data, and the first-time RA diagnosis served as the index date from 1998 to 2008. Meanwhile, these consensuses of chest physician, infection specialist and personnel working in the coding room confirmed the new diagnosis of NTM disease and active PTB. The definition of NTM disease [17] and active PTB based on World Health Organization (W.H.O) report [18] and the American Thoracic Society (A.T.S) [17,19,20]. Furthermore, the Center for Disease Control (C.D.C) is the supervisor of the infection control of active PTB.These procedure may avoid bias such as misclassification.

The comparison group was 4 times the size of the RA group and consisted of patients without RA, selected randomly from the inpatient data files, frequency matched by age, sex, and diagnosis year. Patients with a history of NTM disease (ICD-9-CM 031.0, 031.2, 031.8, 0.31.9) or active PTB (ICD-9-CM 011) at the baseline, and those with incomplete age or sex information, were excluded. The follow-up person-years were calculated for each participant since index date until the diagnosis of new event (NTM disease or active PTB), the end of 2010, or withdrawal from the insurance system. Patients who had experienced NTM disease or active PTB prior to the baseline year (1996–1997) were excluded.

According to each participant's inpatient diagnosis, we calculated the CCI scores as the comorbidity measure. A weight was assigned in each indicated diagnosis and added together to provide a total CCI score. In CCI score, sixteen kinds of different comorbidities were classified in different categories. Participants with the comorbidity was calculated weighted 1, such as myocardial infarction, congestive heart failure, peripheral vascular disease, cerebrovascular accident, dementia, chronic obstructive pulmonary disease (COPD), connective tissue disease, peptic ulcer disease, mild liver disease and diabetes mellitus. Moderate to severe chronic kidney disease, hemiplegia, diabetes with end-organ damage, leukemia, tumor of any type and malignant lymphoma were weighted 2. Participants with moderate to severe liver disease were weighted 3. Acquired immune deficiency syndrome (AIDS) and metastatic solid tumor were weighted 6 [9].

Statistical Analysis

Data analysis compared distributions of demographic variables and the CCI score between the RA and comparison groups. The chi-square test was used to determine the differences between the 2 groups regarding the distribution of categorical demographic variables. Mean ages and mean CCI scores between the 2 groups were examined using Student's t-test. Incidence rates of NTM disease and active PTB were calculated for both groups (per 10,000 person-years) stratified by demographic variables and CCI scores. The incidence density of outcome (NTM disease or active PTB) was calculated by using the number of incident NTM disease or active PTB dividing by person-years at risk in both groups. We used the Poisson regression model to test the different incidence density of outcome (NTM disease or active PTB) between RA and non-RA groups and present with the incidence rate ratio (IRR) and 95% confidence interval (95% CI). We also used multivariable Cox proportional hazards regression analysis to measure the adjusted hazard ratio (aHR) of NTM disease and active PTB with 95% CI for the RA group compared with the comparison group, while manual controlling for sex, age, and CCI score. We assessed changes in the risk and aHR of NTM disease and active PTB during the follow-up years by using time-dependent covariates ($<$ 2 y, 2–4 y, 4–6 y, $\geq$6 y after RA diagnosis). The Kaplan-Meier method was used to plot the cumulative proportions of the studied subjects free of active PTB and NTM disease during the follow-up period, and the log-rank test was used to assess the differences between these curves.

All statistical analyses were performed using the SAS 9.1 statistical package (SAS Institute Inc., NC, USA). R software (R

Foundation for Statistical Computing, Vienna, Austria) was used to prepare the Kaplan–Meier survival curves. A $P<.05$ in 2-tailed tests was considered significant.

Results

Characteristics of the Study Participants

In this study, we identified 29 131 patients for the RA group and selected 116 524 patients for the comparison group (Table 1). Both groups were similar in sex and age distribution and women (77.2%) and younger participants (78% <65 y of age) were dominant. The comorbidities were more prevalent in the RA group than non-RA group at the baseline (0.43±0.89 vs 019±0.67, $P<.0001$).

Incidence Rate Ratios of NTM Disease and active PTB

The incidence of NTM disease was 4.22 times greater in the RA group than in the non-RA group (1.91 vs 0.45 per 10,000 person-years), with an adjusted HR of 4.17 (95% CI = 2.61–6.65) (Table 2). However, the incidence of PTB was 2.99 times greater in the RA group than in the non-RA group (25.3 vs 8.46 per 10,000 person-years), with an adjusted HR of 2.87 (95% CI = 2.55–3.23). The risks of developing NTM disease and active PTB were greater for men than for women in both cohorts, although the incidence of both was much greater in the RA group. Patients with comorbidities had higher incidences of NTM disease and active PTB in both groups, rates of which were also higher in the RA group than in the non-RA group.

Trend in Follow-up Times

Table 3 shows the incidence of NTM disease and active PTB according to follow-up time. In the first 2 years of follow-up, the RA group had a higher incidence than the non-RA group for both NTM disease (2.10 vs 0.39 per 10,000 person-years) and PTB (29.5 vs 8.02 per 10,000 person-years). The corresponding adjusted HRs were 4.98 and 3.39 for the RA group compared with the non-RA group.

Cumulative Incidence of NTM disease and active PTB Between the RA Group and Non-RA Group

With 13 years of follow-up, Kaplan-Meier analysis showed that the cumulative incidence of NTM disease was 0.175% higher in the RA group than in the non-RA group. The incident number declined steadily in the RA group. The cumulative incidence of active PTB was 2.0% greater in the RA group than in the non-RA group. However, the event number declined faster in the RA group than in the non-RA group (Figures 1 and 2).

Discussion

The first crucial result of our study as those RA patients' risks of developing NTM disease and active PTB were increased 4.17-fold and 2.87-fold compared with the general population. The age-stratified effects of the RA cohort on NTM disease and active PTB development were high in patients between 50–65 years of age (yielding HRs of 4.94 and 3.89, respectively) and >65 years of age (yielding HRs of 3.49 and 2.26, respectively). The risks of developing NTM disease and active PTB increased with age in both groups with a much greater gradient in the RA group. Our results were similar to those of Winthrop et al, who observed that among anti-TNF users (n = 8418, 60% with RA; 18 with NTM disease, 12/18 with pulmonary NTM; 16 with active TB, 11/16 with active PTB), NTM case-patients with a median age of 68 years active TB case-patients with a median age of 57.5 years were both more likely to have RA [21]. Our study concurs with the results of numerous other reports regarding the frequency among older people (>50 years) of mycobacterial infections such as NTM disease [22] and active PTB [23].

The second crucial result is that the risk of NTM disease significantly increased in the first 2 years (rate = 2.10) and ≥6 years (rate = 2.44) of RA diagnosis, whereas the rate of active PTB was higher in the first 2 years of diagnosis (rate = 29.47). Winthrop et al found that, among anti-TNF users (60% with RA), active TB case-patients exhibited a median time to onset after drug start of 670 days (<2 y), which was similar to that indicated in our study.

Table 1. Demographic status and Charlson comorbidity index score in cohorts with and without rheumatoid arthritis.

	Rheumatoid arthritis				
	No (N = 116524)		Yes (N = 29131)		
	n	%	n	%	*p*-value
Sex†					0.98
Women	89896	77.2	22474	77.2	
Men	26628	22.8	6657	22.8	
Age, year†					0.98
<50	48856	41.9	12214	41.9	
50–65	42052	36.1	10513	36.1	
≥65	25616	22.0	6404	22.0	
Mean (SD)#	52.3 (15.7)	52.4 (15.6)	0.4325		
Charlson comorbidity index, classification†					<.0001
None	104101	89.3	21111	72.5	
1–2	10010	8.6	6945	23.8	
≥3	2413	2.1	1075	3.7	
Mean of score (SD)#	0.19(0.67)		0.43(0.89)		<.0001

†Chi-square test;
#Two sample t-test.

Table 2. Risks of non-TB mycobacterial disease and active pulmonary tuberculosis measure by sex, age and Charlson index score for study cohorts.

	Rheumatoid arthritis							
	No			Yes			Compared to non-Rheumatoid arthritis	
Variables	**Event**	**PY**	**Rate#**	**Event**	**PY**	**Rate#**	**IRR* (95% CI)**	**Adjusted HR† (95% CI)**
Non-TB mycobacterial disease	36	796901	0.45	37	193934	1.91	4.22(4.05–4.40)***	4.17(2.61–6.65)***
Sex								
Women	18	623372	0.29	18	152377	1.18	4.09(3.90–4.29)***	3.80(1.95–7.38)***
Men	18	173530	1.04	19	41557	4.57	4.41(4.06–4.79)***	4.58(2.38–8.83)***
Age, years†								
<50	6	347795	0.17	7	87315	0.80	4.65(4.35–4.97)***	3.77(1.24–11.49)*
50–65	12	347795	0.41	16	70999	2.25	5.49(5.12–5.88)***	4.94(2.30–10.61)***
≥65	18	156982	1.15	14	35621	3.93	3.43(3.15–3.73)***	3.49(1.71–7.11)***
Charlson comorbidity index								
No	27	726318	0.37	18	143213	1.26	3.38(3.23–3.54)***	3.82(2.10–6.94)***
Yes	9	70585	1.28	19	50721	3.75	2.94(2.63–3.28)***	3.62(1.61–8.15)**
Active Pulmonary Tuberculosis	673	795227	8.46	487	192585	25.29	2.99(2.89–3.09)***	2.87(2.55–3.23)***
Sex								
Women	353	622385	5.67	269	151563	17.75	3.13(3.00–3.26)***	2.92(2.48–3.42)***
Men	320	172842	18.51	218	41022	53.14	2.87(2.68–3.07)***	2.81(2.36–3.35)***
Age, years†								
<50	74	347526	2.13	66	87068	7.58	3.56(3.36–3.77)***	2.95(2.10–4.14)***
50–65	164	291652	5.62	179	70451	25.41	4.52(4.27–4.79)***	3.89(3.13–4.83)***
≥65	435	156049	27.88	242	35065	69.01	2.48(2.31–2.65)***	2.26(1.93–2.65)***
Charlson comorbidity index								
No	406	725228	5.60	243	142548	17.05	3.05(2.93–3.17)***	3.43(2.93–4.03)***
Yes	267	69999	38.14	244	50037	48.76	1.28(1.18–1.39)***	1.82(1.52–2.17)***

Rate#, incidence rate, per 10,000 person-years; IRR*, incidence rate ratio; Adjusted HR†: model manual adjusted for sex, age, and CCI score; p<0.05, **p<0.01, ***p<0.001.

Table 3. Trends of non-TB mycobacterial disease and active pulmonary tuberculosis risk by follow-up years.

	Rheumatoid arthritis						Compared to non-Rheumatoid arthritis	
	No			Yes				
Follow time, years	Event	PY	Rate#	Event	PY	Rate#	IRR* (95% CI)	Adjusted HR† (95% CI)
Non-TB mycobacterial disease								
<2	9	229578	0.39	12	57145	2.10	5.36(5.12–5.60)***	4.98(2.08–11.92)***
2–4	7	202095	0.35	6	49851	1.20	3.47(3.32–3.64)***	3.55(1.17–10.74)*
4–6	4	155564	0.26	7	37788	1.85	7.20(6.82–7.61)***	6.75(1.94–23.55)**
≥6	16	209665	0.76	12	49150	2.44	3.20(3.02–3.39)***	3.34(1.55–7.21)**
Active Pulmonary Tuberculosis								
<2	184	229455	8.02	168	57008	29.47	3.68(3.54–3.82)***	3.39(2.74–4.18)***
2–4	177	201765	8.77	113	49598	22.78	2.60(2.50–2.70)***	2.53(1.99–3.21)***
4–6	153	155132	9.86	99	37466	26.42	2.70(2.58–2.82)***	2.59(2.00–3.35)***
≥6	159	208874	7.61	107	48514	22.06	2.90(2.76–3.05)***	2.89(2.25–3.72)***

Rate#, incidence rate, per 10,000 person-years; IRR*, incidence rate ratio; Adjusted HR†: model manual adjusted for sex, age, and CCI score; *p<0.05, **p<0.01, ***p<0.001.

The NTM case-patients exhibited a median time to onset after drug start of 1024 days. This result slightly differed with that in our study [21]. In our study, the risk of NTM significantly increased in the first 2 years and ≥6 years of RA diagnosis. After adjusting for HRs, both NTM disease (HR: 4.98) and PTB (HR: 3.39) in the first 2 years of follow-up had higher incidents in the RA group compared with the non-RA group. NTM disease (HR: 3.34) during ≥6 years of RA diagnosis was also more prevalent in the RA group than in the non-RA group. In a previous study, active PTB was found to be a predisposing factor [24] for the development of pulmonary NTM disease, which might explain this discrepancy. Additionally, the risk of developing NTM disease progressively increased with follow-up period; this may be associated with RA [25] and the aging process [26].

Disorders of the immune system can result in autoimmune diseases, inflammatory diseases, and cancer [27]. In certain instances, a primary immunodeficiency disease (PIDD) is associated with autoimmune disorders such as rheumatoid arthritis [28]. Having both cellular and antibody deficiencies carries an increased risk for juvenile RA [29]. RA increases the risk of infections [13]. Whether opportunistic infections resulting from mycobacteria occur more frequently in patients with RA, independent of immunosuppressive therapy, is uncertain [13,14,15]. Previous studies have proposed that an altered lymphocyte homeostasis in RA that may contribute to the autoimmune response as well as to the immunodeficiency in these patients [30].

A relationship between active TB and RA is currently recognized, and is primarily attributable to the immunosuppressive therapies used to treat RA. TNF is essential for controlling mycobacterium tuberculosis infection and cannot be replaced by other proinflammatory cytokines. The overproduction of TNF may cause immunopathology, whereas defective TNF production results in uncontrolled infection. The critical role of TNF in controlling tuberculosis has been recently illustrated by primary reactivation of latent infection in certain patients under pharmacological anti-TNF therapy for RA [31]. Therefore, RA patients treated with TNF-alpha inhibitors exhibit an increased incidence of active TB [32] compared with RA patients who are not being treated with TNF-alpha inhibitors [15]. NTM disease is also frequently found in patients being treated for RA by using anti-TNF therapy [21]. Whereas active TB can complicate the successful management of RA, NTM disease has perhaps become as challenging as (if not more so than) active TB in the RA setting, and represents an even greater challenge to rheumatologists that wish to use immunosuppressive therapies [33]. In the RA cohort without CCI displayed a 3.82-fold higher risk of developing NTM disease and the 3.43-fold higher risk of developing PTB compared with the comparison cohort (all $P<.05$) supported that RA cohort play a critical role for development of NTM disease and active PTB even without CCI (Table 2). Meanwhile Seong et al. study, active PTB event in RA cohort without immunosuppressive therapies imply that RA cohort itself is a risk factor of mycobactereial infection [14].

In this study, we found that CCI score was a strong predictor of the increased risk of both NTM disease (HR: 2.87) and active PTB (HR: 1.82) in the RA cohort (Table 2). The CCI score in the RA cohort was also higher than that in the non-RA cohort (0.19±0.67 vs 0.43±0.89, $P<.001$) (Table 1). In Crowson et al, RA disease characteristics and comorbidities were used to accurately assess the risk of serious infection in patients with RA in accordance with this finding [2]. Therefore, providing adequate RA care based on CCI scores is a crucial step in preventing the further development of NTM disease and active PTB [12]. Thus, a multidisciplinary team

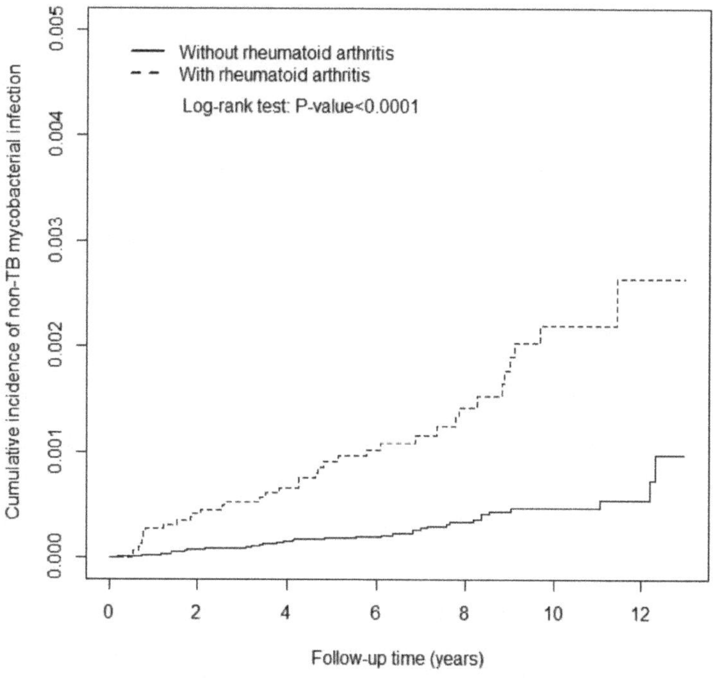

Variables	Follow-up time (year)						
	0	2	4	6	8	10	12
Non-Rheumatoid arthritis, n							
At risk	116524	113007	89386	66301	43862	23689	6242
Event	0	9	7	4	8	5	1
Rheumatoid arthritis, n							
At risk	29131	28035	21916	15957	10341	5501	1391
Event	0	12	6	7	5	6	1

Figure 1. Cumulative incidence of non-TB mycobacterial disease for patients with rheumatoid arthritis (dashed line) and comparison subjects (solid line).

should guide the assessment, treatment, and holistic care of RA patients [34].

The greatest risk of developing NTM disease and active PTB was observed within 2 years of RA diagnosis. This phenomenon may be associated with RA identification at a later stage, strictly based on the 1987 American College of Rheumatology (ACR) diagnostic criteria [16] used in Taiwan. The ACR and European League Against Rheumatism (EULAR) posited revised classification criteria to focus on features at earlier stages of RA in 2010 [35], which may be helpful in identifying patients who may benefit from early effective intervention. Preventing active PTB development may also reduce the risk of NTM disease [24].

The primary (80%–85%) NTM disease is pulmonary NTM disease [36,37], which may develop into acute respiratory failure (ARF) and burden hospitals [38]. Active PTB disease also presents as ARF and admission to the intensive care unit [39]. We suggest that RA is a critical factor for developing NTM disease and active PTB, irrespective of CCI score. Among RA patients, the therapeutic outcomes of pulmonary diseases caused by NTM diseases in a biological therapy setting were favorable [40].

With 13 years of follow-up, Kaplan-Meier analysis showed that the cumulative incidence of NTM disease and active PTB were higher in the RA group than in the non-RA group (0.175% for NTM disease, 2.0% for active PTB). The incidence of NTM disease and active PTB declined in the RA group. Therefore, it is necessary for physicians to detect NTM disease and active PTB patients at any stage of RA diagnosis among the clinical course. This study can serve to increase awareness of clinical physicians of the necessity of the early detect of pulmonary NTM disease and active PTB in RA patients, even those without CCI scores that are cause for concern. Because anti-RA therapy as this factor was not controlled in the study, therefore anyone on anti-TNF therapy will show increased NTM and PTB regardless of their RA status also.

Finally, bias in cohort studies include: diagnosis bias and loss to follow-up [41]. In this study, the cohort based on Registry for Catastrophic Illness Patient Database (RCIPD) and in-hospital patients. Meanwhile, the healthcare system of diagnosis of NTM disease and active PTB is relatively well established as compared to that in previous reported areas [43]. These policies avoid the diagnostic bias. Furthermore, we assess changes in the risk and adjusted hazard ratio of NTM disease and active PTB disease during the follow-up years by using time-dependent covariates for avoiding the follow-up bias.

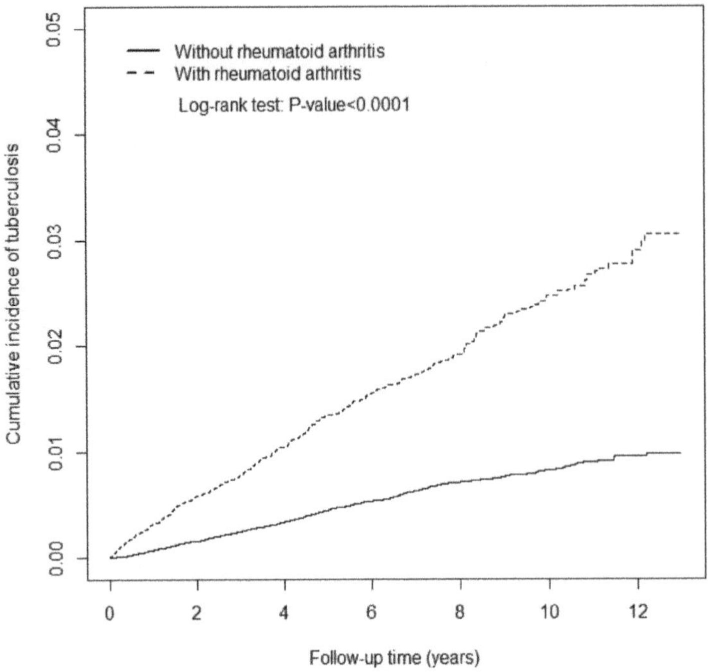

Variables	Follow-up time (year)						
	0	2	4	6	8	10	12
Non-Rheumatoid arthritis, n							
At risk	116524	112884	89187	66091	43707	23587	6212
Event	0	184	178	152	99	38	21
Rheumatoid arthritis, n							
At risk	29131	27916	21771	15787	10219	5416	1367
Event	0	168	113	99	47	45	13

Figure 2. Cumulative incidence of active pulmonary tuberculosis for patients with rheumatoid arthritis (dashed line) and comparison subjects (solid line).

Limitations

Several limitations must be considered when interpreting these findings. The NHIRD does not provide detailed lifestyle information, such as information regarding smoking, body mass index, or physical activity, all of which are potential confounding factors in this study. However, RA patients undergo RA treatment and must modify their lifestyles; these may be implicated as factors for pulmonary infection in RA patients. Additionally, information on the RA severity scale, such as disease activity, functional impairment, and physical damage was unavailable in our data. The lack of drug data, such as data regarding treatment with anti-TNF drugs, MTX, and glucocorticosteroids, could be another limitation, as treatment with these drugs was not adjusted for in determining the outcomes under study. The incidence of NTM disease and active PTB in RA cohorts that are and are not receiving drug treatment requires further comparison. Despite the meticulous study design, which was employed to control for confounding factors, a key limitation of this study was its potential for bias caused by possible unmeasured or unknown confounders.

Strengths

The strength of this study is that it is a nationwide population-based cohort longitudinal analysis of the risk of NTM disease and active PTB development in Asian people with RA. This cohort study is representative of the general population [42], and our findings can be generalized to the general population.

Conclusion

This study raises awareness among clinical physicians regarding the necessity of the detection of NTM disease and active PTB in RA patients among the any stage of the clinical course even without CCI.

Author Contributions

Conceived and designed the experiments: J-JY C-HK. Performed the experiments: J-JY Y-CW C-HK. Analyzed the data: J-JY Y-CW C-HK. Contributed reagents/materials/analysis tools: F-CS C-HK. Wrote the paper: J-JY Y-CW F-CS C-HK. Approved the manuscript: J-JY Y-CW F-CS C-HK.

References

1. Mutru O, Laakso M, Isomaki H, Koota K (1985) Ten year mortality and causes of death in patients with rheumatoid arthritis. Br Med J (Clin Res Ed) 290: 1797–1799.
2. Crowson CS, Hoganson DD, Fitz-Gibbon PD, Matteson EL (2012) Development and validation of a risk score for serious infection in patients with rheumatoid arthritis. Arthritis Rheum 64: 2847–2855.
3. Listing J, Gerhold K, Zink A (2013) The risk of infections associated with rheumatoid arthritis, with its comorbidity and treatment. Rheumatology (Oxford) 52: 53–61.
4. Hsia EC, Cush JJ, Matteson EL, Beutler A, Doyle MK, et al. (2013) Comprehensive tuberculosis screening program in patients with inflammatory arthritides treated with golimumab, a human anti-tumor necrosis factor antibody, in Phase III clinical trials. Arthritis Care Res (Hoboken) 65: 309–313.
5. Takabayashi K, Hanaoka H (2004) [Collagen diseases with opportunistic infections]. Nihon Rinsho Meneki Gakkai Kaishi 27: 156–163.
6. Park JS, Jung ES, Choi W, Park SY, Rim MY, et al. (2013) Mycobacterium intracellulare Pulmonary Disease with Endobronchial Caseation in a Patient Treated with Methotrexate. Tuberc Respir Dis (Seoul) 75: 28–31.
7. Collins CS, Terrell C, Mueller P (2013) Disseminated Mycobacterium haemophilum infection in a 72-year-old patient with rheumatoid arthritis on infliximab. BMJ Case Rep 2013.
8. Yamakawa H, Takayanagi N, Miyahara Y, Ishiguro T, Kanauchi T, et al. (2013) Prognostic factors and radiographic outcomes of nontuberculous mycobacterial lung disease in rheumatoid arthritis. J Rheumatol 40: 1307–1315.
9. Charlson ME, Pompei P, Ales KL, MacKenzie CR (1987) A new method of classifying prognostic comorbidity in longitudinal studies: development and validation. J Chronic Dis 40: 373–383.
10. Charlson M, Szatrowski TP, Peterson J, Gold J (1994) Validation of a combined comorbidity index. J Clin Epidemiol 47: 1245–1251.
11. Hall SF (2006) A user's guide to selecting a comorbidity index for clinical research. J Clin Epidemiol 59: 849–855.
12. Tiippana-Kinnunen T, Kautiainen H, Paimela L, Leirisalo-Repo M (2013) Comorbidities in Finnish patients with rheumatoid arthritis: 15-year follow-up. Scand J Rheumatol.
13. Newton SM, Mackie SL, Martineau AR, Wilkinson KA, Kampmann B, et al. (2008) Reduction of chemokine secretion in response to mycobacteria in infliximab-treated patients. Clin Vaccine Immunol 15: 506–512.
14. Seong SS, Choi CB, Woo JH, Bae KW, Joung CL, et al. (2007) Incidence of tuberculosis in Korean patients with rheumatoid arthritis (RA): effects of RA itself and of tumor necrosis factor blockers. J Rheumatol 34: 706–711.
15. Wolfe F, Michaud K, Anderson J, Urbansky K (2004) Tuberculosis infection in patients with rheumatoid arthritis and the effect of infliximab therapy. Arthritis Rheum 50: 372–379.
16. Arnett FC, Edworthy SM, Bloch DA, McShane DJ, Fries JF, et al. (1988) The American Rheumatism Association 1987 revised criteria for the classification of rheumatoid arthritis. Arthritis Rheum 31: 315–324.
17. (1997) Diagnosis and treatment of disease caused by nontuberculous mycobacteria. This official statement of the American Thoracic Society was approved by the Board of Directors, March 1997. Medical Section of the American Lung Association. Am J Respir Crit Care Med 156: S1–25.
18. WHO (1994) WHO tuberculosis programme-Framework for effective tuberculosis control. In. Geneva, Switzerland.
19. Yeh JJ, Neoh CA, Chen CR, Chou CY, Wu MT (2014) A high resolution computer tomography scoring system to predict culture-positive pulmonary tuberculosis in the emergency department. PLoS ONE 9: e93847.
20. Yeh JJ, Chen SC, Chen CR, Yeh TC, Lin HK, et al. (2014) A high-resolution computed tomography-based scoring system to differentiate the most infectious active pulmonary tuberculosis from community-acquired pneumonia in elderly and non-elderly patients. Eur Radiol.
21. Winthrop KL, Baxter R, Liu L, Varley CD, Curtis JR, et al. (2013) Mycobacterial diseases and antitumour necrosis factor therapy in USA. Ann Rheum Dis 72: 37–42.
22. Menzies D, Nahid P (2013) Update in tuberculosis and nontuberculous mycobacterial disease 2012. Am J Respir Crit Care Med 188: 923–927.
23. Perez-Guzman C, Vargas MH (2010) Mycobacterial infections in the elderly. Semin Respir Crit Care Med 31: 575–586.
24. Griffith DE, Aksamit T, Brown-Elliott BA, Catanzaro A, Daley C, et al. (2007) An official ATS/IDSA statement: diagnosis, treatment, and prevention of nontuberculous mycobacterial diseases. Am J Respir Crit Care Med 175: 367–416.
25. Swart RM, van Ingen J, van Soolingen D, Slingerland R, Hendriks WD, et al. (2009) Nontuberculous mycobacteria infection and tumor necrosis factor-alpha antagonists. Emerg Infect Dis 15: 1700–1701.
26. Chan ED, Iseman MD (2010) Slender, older women appear to be more susceptible to nontuberculous mycobacterial lung disease. Gend Med 7: 5–18.
27. Seve P, Broussolle C, Pavic M (2013) [Primary immunodeficiencies presenting with autoimmune cytopenias in adults]. Rev Med Interne 34: 148–153.
28. Notarangelo L, Casanova JL, Conley ME, Chapel H, Fischer A, et al. (2006) Primary immunodeficiency diseases: an update from the International Union of Immunological Societies Primary Immunodeficiency Diseases Classification Committee Meeting in Budapest, 2005. J Allergy Clin Immunol 117: 883–896.
29. Sleasman JW (1996) The association between immunodeficiency and the development of autoimmune disease. Adv Dent Res 10: 57–61.
30. Wagner UG, Koetz K, Weyand CM, Goronzy JJ (1998) Perturbation of the T cell repertoire in rheumatoid arthritis. Proc Natl Acad Sci U S A 95: 14447–14452.
31. Solovic I, Sester M, Gomez-Reino JJ, Rieder HL, Ehlers S, et al. (2010) The risk of tuberculosis related to tumour necrosis factor antagonist therapies: a TBNET consensus statement. Eur Respir J 36: 1185–1206.
32. Harboe E, Damas JK, Omdal R, Froland SS, Sjursen H (2012) [Risk of infection through use of selective immunomodulating drugs for rheumatoid arthritis]. Tidsskr Nor Laegeforen 132: 1867–1871.
33. Winthrop KL, Iseman M (2013) Bedfellows: mycobacteria and rheumatoid arthritis in the era of biologic therapy. Nat Rev Rheumatol 9: 524–531.
34. Petersson IF, Strombeck B, Andersen L, Cimmino M, Greiff R, et al. (2013) Development of healthcare quality indicators for rheumatoid arthritis in Europe: the eumusc.net project. Ann Rheum Dis.
35. Aletaha D, Neogi T, Silman AJ, Funovits J, Felson DT, et al. (2010) 2010 rheumatoid arthritis classification criteria: an American College of Rheumatology/European League Against Rheumatism collaborative initiative. Ann Rheum Dis 69: 1580–1588.
36. Winthrop KL, McNelley E, Kendall B, Marshall-Olson A, Morris C, et al. (2010) Pulmonary nontuberculous mycobacterial disease prevalence and clinical features: an emerging public health disease. Am J Respir Crit Care Med 182: 977–982.
37. Yeh JJ, Wang YC, Sung FC, Chou CY, Kao CH (2014) Nontuberculosis mycobacterium disease is a risk factor for chronic obstructive pulmonary disease: a nationwide cohort study. Lung 192: 403–411.
38. Yeh JJ, Wang YC, Lin CL, Chou CY, Yeh TC, et al. (2014) Nontuberculous mycobacterial infection is associated with increased respiratory failure: a nationwide cohort study. PLoS ONE 9: e99260.
39. Erbes R, Oettel K, Raffenberg M, Mauch H, Schmidt-Ioanas M, et al. (2006) Characteristics and outcome of patients with active pulmonary tuberculosis requiring intensive care. Eur Respir J 27: 1223–1228.
40. Mori S, Tokuda H, Sakai F, Johkoh T, Mimori A, et al. (2012) Radiological features and therapeutic responses of pulmonary nontuberculous mycobacterial disease in rheumatoid arthritis patients receiving biological agents: a retrospective multicenter study in Japan. Mod Rheumatol 22: 727–737.
41. Lash TL, Fox MP, MacLehose RF, Maldonado G, McCandless LC, et al. (2014) Good practices for quantitative bias analysis. Int J Epidemiol.
42. Chen YY, Chang JR, Huang WF, Kuo SC, Yeh JJ, et al. (2014) Molecular epidemiology of Mycobacterium tuberculosis in aboriginal peoples of Taiwan, 2006–2011. J Infect 68: 332–337.
43. Booth CM, Rapoport B (2011) Uptake of novel medical therapies in the general population. Curr Oncol 18: 105–108.

23

Lymphotoxin-LIGHT Pathway Regulates the Interferon Signature in Rheumatoid Arthritis

Jadwiga Bienkowska[1], Norm Allaire[1], Alice Thai[1], Jaya Goyal[1], Tatiana Plavina[1], Ajay Nirula[2], Megan Weaver[3], Charlotte Newman[3], Michelle Petri[4], Evan Beckman[2], Jeffrey L. Browning[2*¤]

1 Translational Medicine, Biogen Idec, Cambridge, Massachusetts, United States of America, **2** Immunobiology, Biogen Idec, Cambridge, Massachusetts, United States of America, **3** Global Clinical Operations, Biogen Idec, Cambridge, Massachusetts, United States of America, **4** Johns Hopkins University School of Medicine, Baltimore, Maryland, United States of America

Abstract

A subset of patients with autoimmune diseases including rheumatoid arthritis (RA) and lupus appear to be exposed continually to interferon (IFN) as evidenced by elevated expression of IFN induced genes in blood cells. In lupus, detection of endogenous chromatin complexes by the innate sensing machinery is the suspected driver for the IFN, but the actual mechanisms remain unknown in all of these diseases. We investigated in two randomized clinical trials the effects on RA patients of baminercept, a lymphotoxin-beta receptor-immunoglobulin fusion protein that blocks the lymphotoxin-αβ/LIGHT axis. Administration of baminercept led to a reduced RNA IFN signature in the blood of patients with elevated baseline signatures. Both RA and SLE patients with a high IFN signature were lymphopenic and lymphocyte counts increased following baminercept treatment of RA patients. These data demonstrate a coupling between the lymphotoxin-LIGHT system and IFN production in rheumatoid arthritis. IFN induced retention of lymphocytes within lymphoid tissues is a likely component of the lymphopenia observed in many autoimmune diseases.

ClinicalTrials.gov NCT00664716.

Editor: Sylvie Bisser, INSERM U1094, University of Limoges School of Medicine, France

Funding: Biogen Idec conducted, funded and provided infrastructure for these studies and had a role in study design, data collection and analysis, decision to publish, or preparation of the manuscript. The specific roles of the authors are listed in the authors contributions section.

Competing Interests: All authors except MP were salaried employees of Biogen Idec during the conduct of these trials. JB, NA, AT, JG, TP, JO, MW and CN report being current employees of Biogen Idec with an equity interest in the company. AN, EB and JLB are former Biogen Idec employees without equity stakes. MP has received consulting fees from Biogen Idec. There are no patents or marketed products to declare and the drug remains in use in a NIH sponsored clinical study in Sjogren's disease.

* Email: browninj@bu.edu

¤ Current address: Department of Microbiology and Section of Rheumatology, Boston University School of Medicine, Boston, Massachusetts, United States of America

Introduction

Systemic lupus erythematosus (SLE), rheumatoid arthritis (RA), Sjogren's syndrome, systemic sclerosis, myositis and multiple sclerosis patients have circulating blood cells with elevated levels of RNA from IFN-induced genes, i.e. an 'IFN signature' [1–3]. A number of observations point towards a role for IFN in some autoimmune diseases. Notably, risk alleles for SLE include several genes involved in IFN responses. Multiple immunological activities are enhanced by IFN and rodent models of lupus can be accelerated by exogenous IFN. Several rare diseases with lupus-like aspects have mutations in components of the IFN response and are termed 'interferonopathies' [4]. Thus, there is very active interest in whether inhibition of IFN signaling has therapeutic benefit [5]. However, the questions of whether the IFN signature is tightly coupled to the pathology in human disease, which immunological detection systems are engaged and what are the actual cellular sources of the IFN, remain unanswered. Moreover, type I (IFN-α, β, ε, τ and ω), type II (IFN-γ) and type III (IFN-λ) IFNs can induce similar patterns of gene expression despite being produced by different spectra of cell types and being under fundamentally different regulation. The varying distribution of receptors for each IFN type also dictates responsive populations and these aspects further confound the problem.

We have investigated the effects of inhibition of the lymphotoxin-LIGHT system in RA using a soluble lymphotoxin-beta receptor (LTBR, TNFRSF3) immunoglobulin fusion protein called baminercept. LTBR is a central component of a signaling system whereby lymphocytes instruct stromal cells to differentiate into specialized vasculature and certain reticular networks [6–9]. These components form the gateways for lymphocyte entry into organized lymphoid tissues and the reticular scaffolds that guide and position cells for optimal encounters with antigen. As such, adaptive immune responses within the lymphoid organs are impaired to varying degrees in the absence of LTBR signaling. Additionally, the differentiation of critical sentinel macrophages in the subcapsular sinus of the lymph node (LN) and the splenic marginal zone depend on LTBR signaling [10]. More recently, it has become clear that LTBR signaling is interwoven with aspects of myeloid cell homeostasis as well as more innate elements of the immune system such as communication between dendritic cells, innate lymphoid cells and epithelial surfaces especially in mucosal environments [11–15]. Baminercept binds to both LTBR ligands, namely, a membrane bound heterotrimeric lymphotoxin (LT) form LTα1β2 and the ligand called LIGHT (TNFSF14). LIGHT interacts with both LTBR and an additional receptor called HVEM (TNFRSF14) and it has pro-inflammatory roles as well being implicated in aspects of T cell survival [16]. Therefore, baminercept is a dual pathway inhibitor blocking signaling triggered by both membrane LT and LIGHT ligands.

Unexpectedly, we found that baminercept reduced the IFN signature in RA patients. The reduced IFN signature in RA patients following baminercept treatment is the first time outside of high dose steroid therapy that an IFN signature was decreased by a pharmacological treatment not targeting IFN itself. Taken together with the known effects of LTBR inhibition, these studies not only link the LTBR axis to IFN production in man, but also provide potential insight into the nature of the IFN signature.

Results

Baminercept reduces the IFN signature in RA patients

Two randomized phase IIb controlled studies of the effects of baminercept in rheumatoid arthritis were conducted. One study enrolled patients with an inadequate response to disease-modifying antirheumatic drug therapy (DMARD-IR) and the other involved patients with an inadequate response to tumor necrosis factor inhibition (TNF-IR) (flow diagrams Figure 1, patient demographics defined in Supplemental Table 1 in File S1). To examine whether baminercept treatment had an impact on the immune system, the transcriptional profiles of whole blood RNA from all RA patients at 0 and 14 weeks were assessed using Affymetrix microarrays. An unsupervised analysis revealed multiple drug-induced changes that fell into three major clusters. First baminercept treatment led to an increased B cell signature. Second, patients with elevated expression at baseline of a collection of IFN response genes had the signature decreased by baminercept treatment and, third, expression of some genes associated with NK cells were decreased following treatment.

At baseline, roughly 25% of the RA patients in both the DMARD-IR and TNF-IR groups had a high IFN signature (Figure 2) and a 15-gene IFN score was calculated from the genes shown in Figure 2 (Supplemental Table 2 in File S1). Many IFN response gene sets and scores have been utilized in the literature including other sets reported by our group [17]. In general, we found similar results regardless of the selected genes. The IFN signature has been best characterized in SLE and for comparison a control cohort of 292 SLE patients from the Johns Hopkins clinic was analyzed using an identical platform. As expected about 50% of the SLE patients had an elevated IFN signature and the IFN signature in RA patients was slightly weaker than in SLE consistent with a previous study (Supplemental Figure 1 in File S1) [1,3]. Therefore, in terms of the IFN signature, the RA patients in these studies compare favorably to previous analyses.

We divided the patients from the TNF-IR study into four groups- placebo and baminercept treated with baseline low or high IFN signature scores. Figure 3 shows a heat map of the expression changes after 14 weeks for all the genes identified in the unsupervised analysis. There was a general increase in a wide range of B cell associated genes, yet interestingly, IgA1 and IgG3 expression decreased. Baminercept can disrupt follicular dendritic cell networks and germinal center reactions and perhaps this decrease reflects impaired class switching and reduced numbers of circulating B cells or plasma cells expressing these immunoglobulins. The second cluster of genes is comprised of genes induced by IFN. Patients with a baseline high IFN score displayed substantial decreases in the IFN score following treatment. The third cluster contains multiple NK related genes and these often decreased following baminercept treatment.

To further document the IFN signature, the expression of three IFN stimulated genes, Ly6E, ISG15 and OAS1 was determined by quantitative PCR (qPCR) and an IFN score calculated (Supplemental Table 2 in File S1). The qPCR and microarray scores correlated well (Figure 4a). Figure 4b shows the change in the TNF-IR study following 14 weeks of placebo or baminercept treatment in the 3-gene PCR based IFN score as a function of the pre-treatment IFN score. This analysis revealed a significant interaction between the pre-treatment IFN and treatment, interaction p value $= 2\times10^{-7}$. A substantial reduction in the IFN signature was also observed at 6 weeks. To extend this observation, the 3-gene qPCR IFN signature was determined for patients in DMARD-IR study. Patients were binned into baseline IFN^{high} and IFN^{low} groups based on the 3-gene qPCR IFN score of greater or less than one. The DMARD-IR study had 6 treatment cohorts and only the 70 and 200 mg q2w cohorts were analyzed by qPCR. Baminercept treatment led to a trend towards a reduced IFN signature in both cohorts and combining the two cohorts showed significant reduction (Figure 4c). The biomarker data indicated approximate saturation of the pharmacodynamic response in both these cohorts justifying combining the data (see below and serum LIGHT measurements Supplemental Figure 2 in File S1). We questioned whether the incidence of infectious events could impact the observation and there was little indication that infection rates were substantially increased or decreased following baminercept treatment (Supplemental Table 3 in File S1). Since baminercept potentially dampens the immune system, an increased rate of infection was possible and therefore treatment could have increased the IFN signature. As an increased IFN signature was not observed, infection is not a likely confounder for this result.

To validate further the ability of baminercept treatment to affect an IFN signature, we examined by qPCR the expression of SIGLEC1, another IFN induced gene. In contrast to the genes in the 3-gene panel, it is expressed exclusively in monocytes and, moreover, it is a potential marker of SLE disease severity [18]. Analysis of the SIGLEC1 RNA expression using the qPCR data showed that SIGLEC1 expression was elevated in the IFN high group and baminercept treatment reduced its expression confirming the 3-gene signature analysis (Figure 5a,b). Expression (qPCR) of genes specific for monocytes (SLAMF7, SPARC), DC (CD1E) and plasmacytoid DC (pDC) (CLEC4C and LILRA4) was independent of IFN status.

There is considerable overlap in the expression profiles resulting from type 1 (IFNs α, β and ω) and type II IFN (IFNγ) and, furthermore, each IFN is capable in many contexts of inducing the expression of the other IFN class [19]. An 8 gene IFNγ signature was defined based on genes preferentially induced in blood cells by IFNγ [20]. In our data, there was no significant correlation between the basic IFN and IFNγ signatures suggesting that type I IFNs are dominating in RA (Supplemental Figure 3 in File S1). Two genes, GBP1 and GBP2, were induced selectively by IFNγ in salivary gland epithelial cells, yet in our blood data the GBP1/2 score correlated very well with the basic IFN signature (Supplemental Figure 3 in File S1). In other studies, the GBP1/2 genes are induced by type I IFN in blood cells both in vitro and in vivo in IFN treated hepatitis C and melanoma patients. Our data are consistent with exposure to type I IFN in RA.

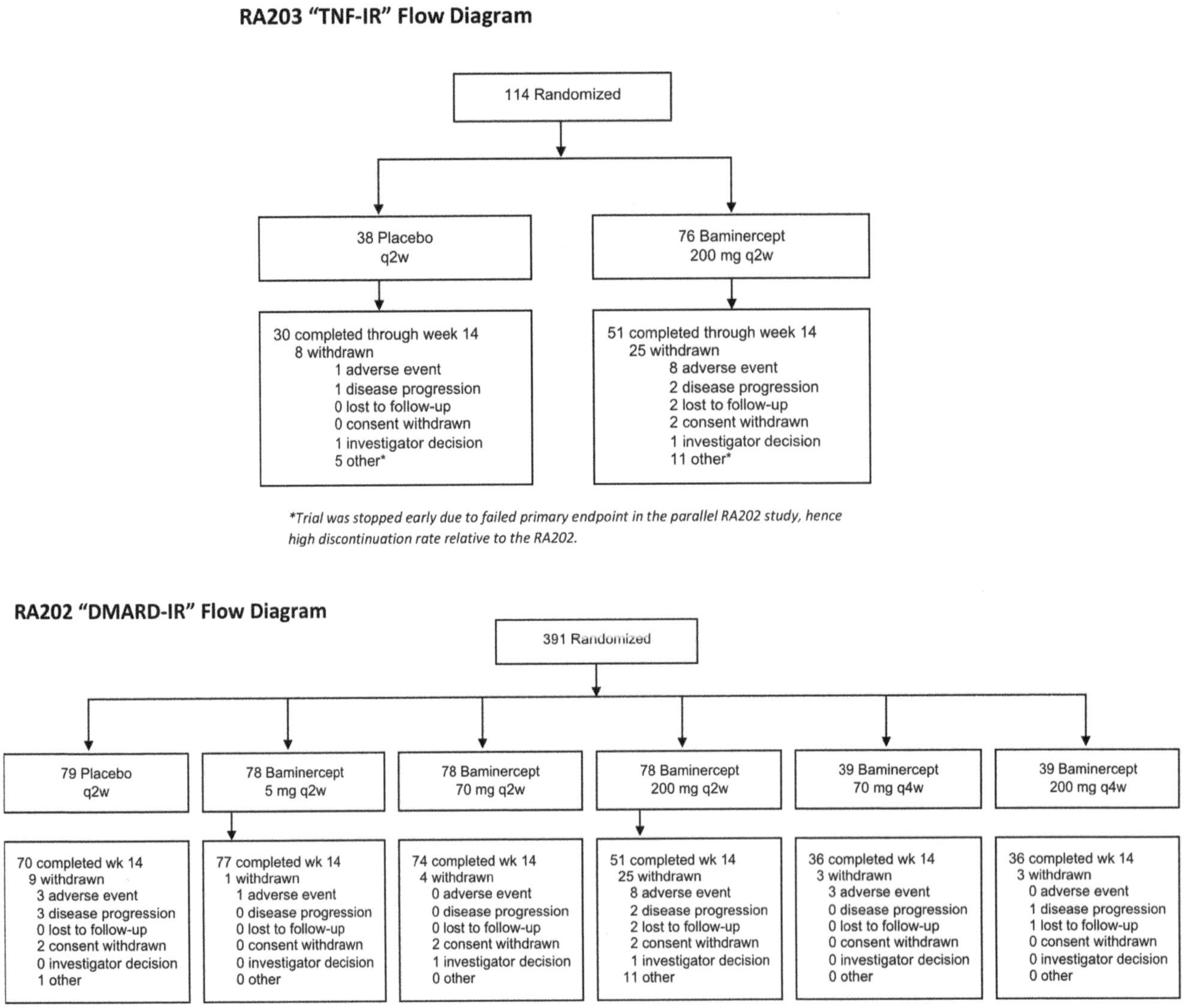

Figure 1. Flow diagrams for the two clinical trials assessing the effects of baminercept treatment on rheumatoid arthritis patients.

Elevated levels of type I IFN or an IFN-like inducing activity can be found in the sera of a subset of the SLE patients with a transcriptional IFN signature; however, in RA the results range from not detectable to low levels relative to SLE sera [21,22]. We examined serum IFN levels using highly sensitive A549 (more type I IFN selective) or WISH (similar sensitivity to type I and II IFN) cell based reporter assays with an ELISA-based Mx1 protein readout. Analysis of 64 baseline sera from the TNF-IR study including all of the patients with elevated baseline IFN signatures did not reveal IFN activity, whereas substantial activity was readily found in the sera from some SLE patients. Therefore, the blood RNA IFN signature in RA is likely derived from local exposure in organs to IFN.

IFN signature is associated with lymphopenia in both RA and SLE

SLE patients with a high IFN signature tend to be lymphopenic [23]. Using the 15 gene microarray-based IFN signature to group patients at baseline into a high or low IFN status, we observed that both IFN high RA and SLE patients were lymphopenic (Figure 6a). The degree of lymphopenia in IFN high RA patients was not as pronounced as in the comparable SLE group possibly paralleling the relative intensities of the IFN signatures in these two diseases.

In rodents, blockade of the LTBR system leads to lymphocytosis within several weeks most likely due to loss of high endothelial venule addressin expression and reduced entry into the lymph nodes and mucosal environments [24]. Treatment with baminercept led to increased lymphocyte and monocyte counts in the blood of patients with full effect observed within 2–5 weeks (Figure 6b and Supplemental Figures 4 and 5 in File S1). The 5 mg q2w dose was partially active and similar results were seen with both the 70 and 200 mg q2w doses indicating approximate saturation. It is believed that one driver for lymphopenia in SLE may be chronic IFN exposure and prolonged lymphocyte retention within the lymph nodes [25]. To assess whether reduced IFN exposure could contribute to the baminercept induced lymphocytosis, we compared the change in lymphocyte counts in the IFN low and high subsets. Lymphocyte counts increased in both groups following baminercept treatment; however, the magnitude of the change was greater in much of the IFN high subset in the TNF-IR study and trended higher in DMARD-IR

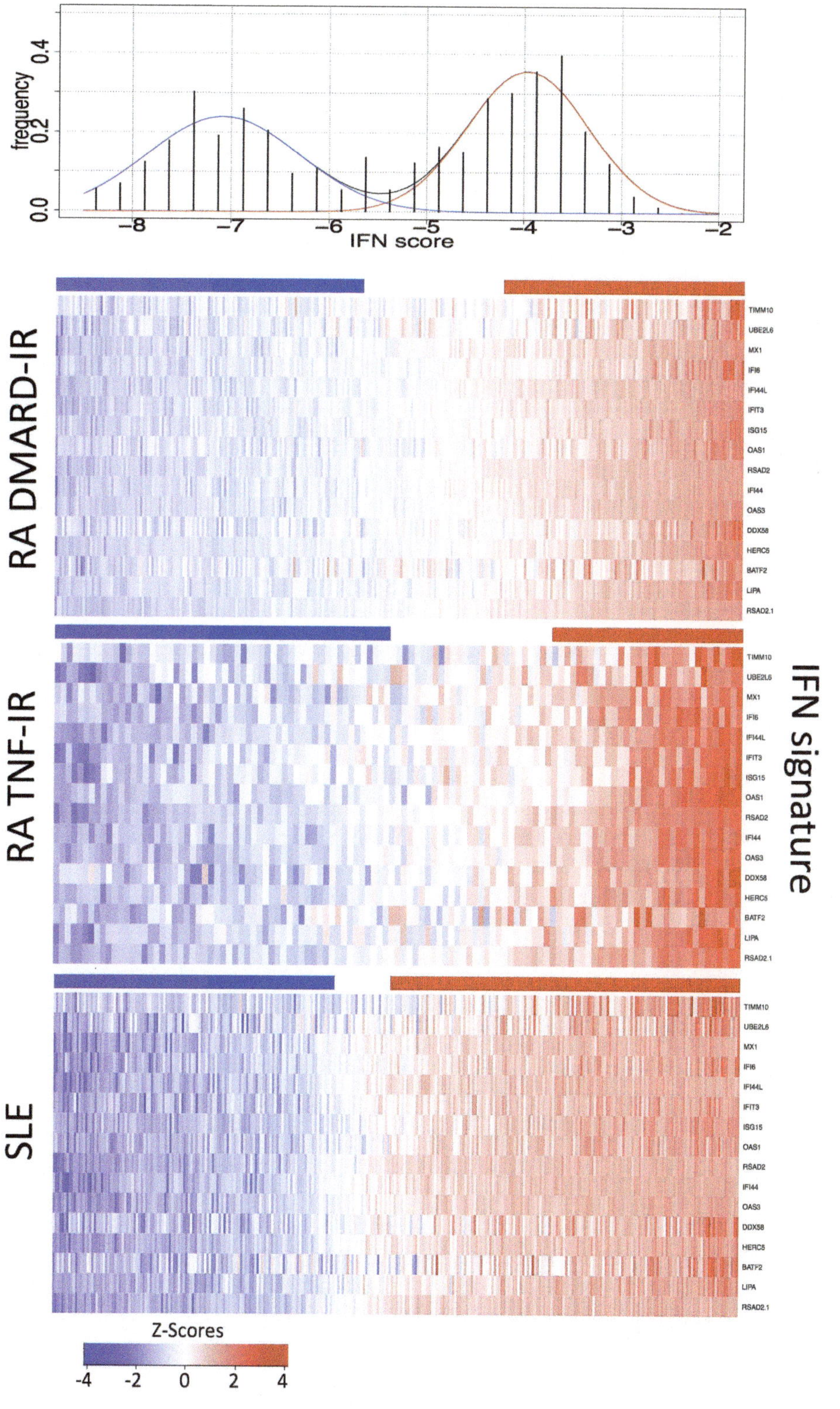

Figure 2. Comparison of the IFN signature in DMARD-IR and TNF-IR RA patients. Baseline heat maps of the RA DMARD-IR, TNF-IR and the SLE cohorts studied in this work. Red indicates increased expression of a panel of 15 IFN inducible genes showing similar percentages of IFN signature positive patients in each RA subgroup (the gene RSAD2 is represented twice). Bars above each map show the clustering as IFN positive (red) or negative (blue) based on assignment to two normal distributions as shown in the top panel with $p<0.05$. Color bar ranges are as stated for SLE and DMARD-IR, but -3 to 3 for TNF-IR (as per figure 3).

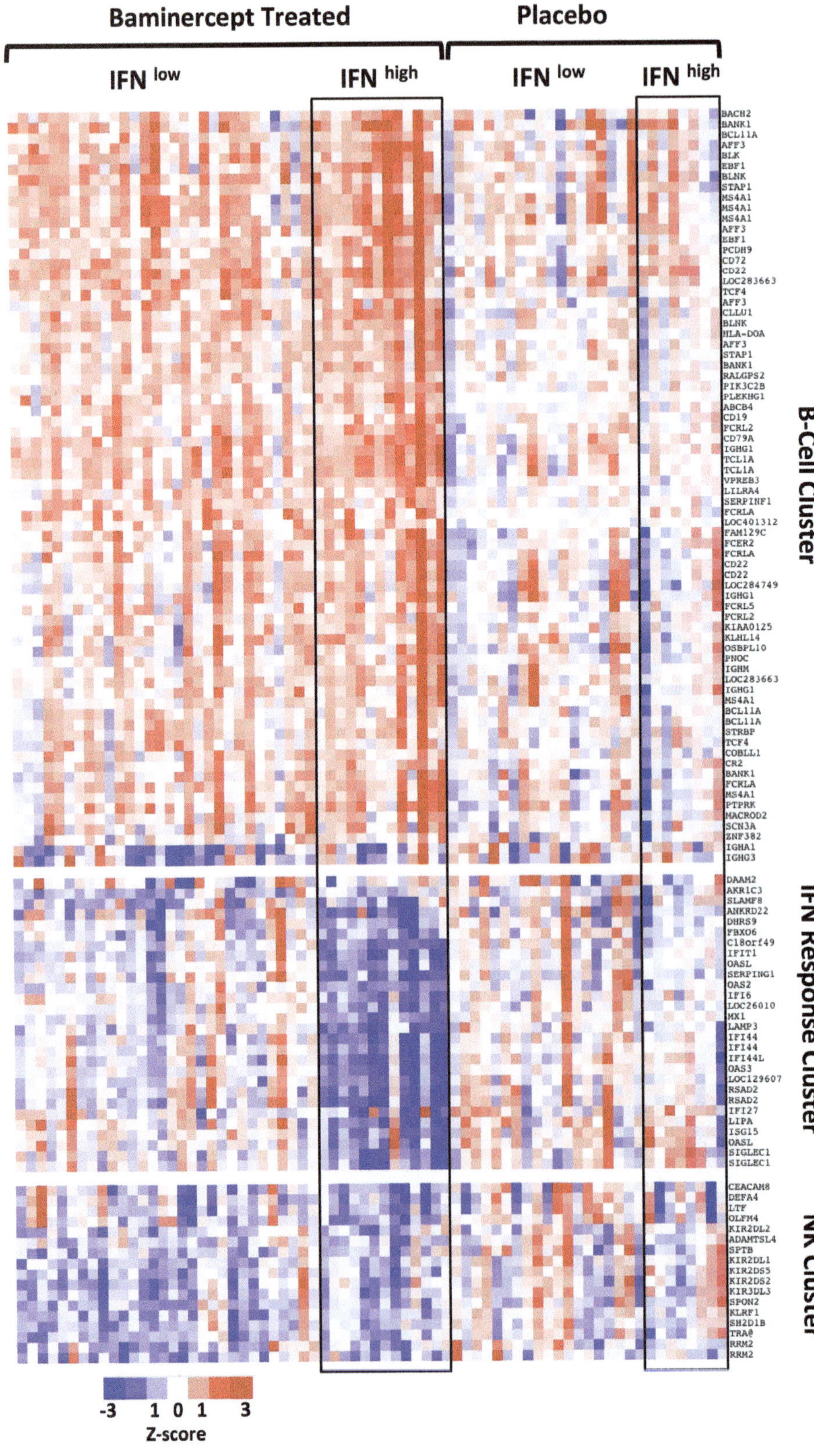

Figure 3. Baminercept induced changes in total blood RNA expression. Heat map showing the change in gene expression after 14 week of either placebo or baminercept treatment. Patients were forced into 4 groups based on treatment and baseline IFN signature. Each of the three gene clusters defined from initial unsupervised clustering are presented separately. The three clusters are characterized by genes associated with B cells, IFN response or NK cells, although some other genes are also present within each category. List only includes genes whose changes were significant ($p<0.05$), passed FDR and had greater than a 1.5 fold difference in a separate paired sample analysis.

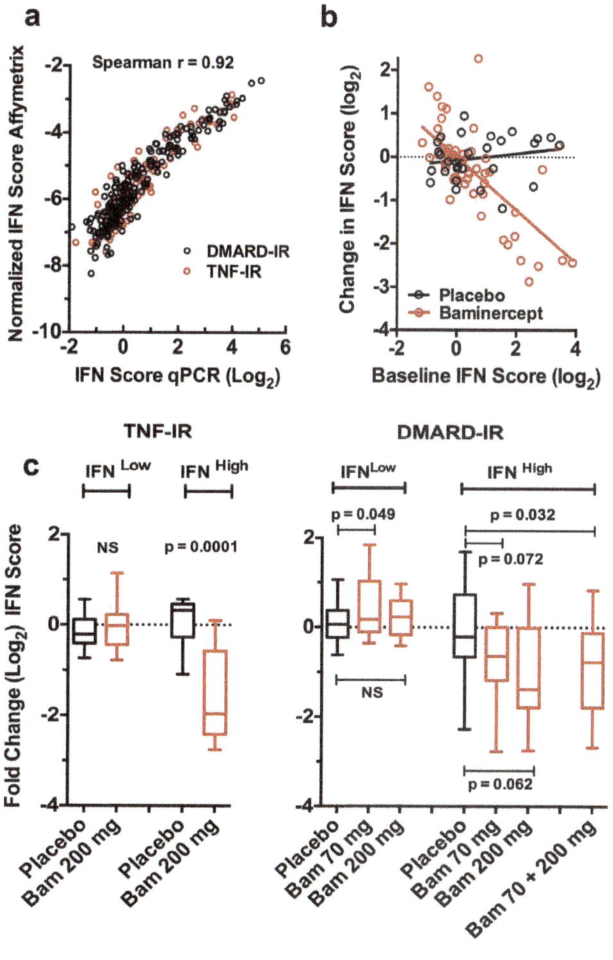

Figure 4. Blockade of the lymphotoxin-LIGHT pathway with baminercept reduces the blood RNA IFN signature in RA patients. a). Analysis of the individual baseline IFN scores as determined using the 15 gene microarray data and a three-gene qPCR score showing excellent correlation. b). Analysis of the change in the 3-gene qPCR IFN score as a function of baseline IFN score following 14 weeks of treatment with 200 mg baminercept q2w in TNF-IR patients, significance is calculated using a linear model of change in IFN score as an interaction of baseline IFN score and treatment (placebo or baminercept). The significance for baseline IFN is $p = 2\times10^{-7}$ and for the interaction term $p = 2.3\times10^{-7}$. Treatment alone is marginally significant $p = 0.0506$. c). Change in the qPCR-based IFN score at 14 weeks in patients with low vs. high baseline IFN scores (low <1, high > 1). Red boxes represent baminercept (Bam) treated patients receiving either 70 or 200 mg q2w (DMARD-IR) or 200 mg q2w (TNF-IR) while black boxes indicate placebo treated patients; n = 20, 50, 11 and 12 (TNF-IR) and 49, 44, 50, 20, 28, 18 and 38 (DMARD-IR) patients in each category in the order listed. P values are from a Mann-Whitney test of placebo vs. baminercept treated patients.

(Figure 6c). These results are consistent with contributions to baminercept induced lymphocytosis from both altered addressin expression and reduced IFN exposure.

In mice, lymphocytosis following LTBR blockade results from elevated T and B cells counts [24]. In these clinical studies, FACS analysis of a small subset of the patients (TNF-IR) showed that B cell numbers were increased roughly 70% over baseline compared to a 24% increase in T cells (Supplemental Figure 6 in File S1). The elevated B cell signature based on the data in figure 3 correlated roughly with the extent of lymphocytosis ($r = 0.338$, $p < 0.0001$,) and therefore it is likely that the B cell signature reflects differential lymphocytosis in the baminercept treated cohorts. Furthermore, PCR quantitation of the levels of genes uniquely expressed in lymphocyte subsets revealed some interesting details (Figure 7). RNA levels of CD20 (B cells) increased consistent with the general lymphocytosis, but TCRδ and some natural killer cell specific genes, KLRF1 as well as KLRD1, KIR2DS1 and KIR3DL1 decreased substantially (only a subset of genes identified from the transcriptional profiling were included in the qPCR array). Thus the qPCR data confirmed the decreased NK signature shown in figure 3. Comparison of the change in absolute lymphocyte counts with the change in RNA levels showed a positive correlation with the expression of CD20, TCRα and CD8B RNA (Spearman r values of 0.56, 0.47 and 0.49 respectively), but little correlation with TCRδ (γδ T cells), KLRF1 (NK) and Defensin 3A (immature neutrophils) ($r = 0.14$, 0.02 and 0.01 respectively). The change in KLRF1 was not coupled to baseline IFN status. In a FACS analysis, B cells and CD4 cell numbers increased, while NK cell numbers trended towards a decrease (Supplemental Figure 6 in File S1). Therefore baminercept appeared to reduce the numbers of immature neutrophils, TCRγδ and NK cells in the blood by a mechanism distinct from the lymphocytosis effects and prior studies in rodents have implicated LTBR in the biology of both TCRγδ and NK cells [26–31]. The decrease in immature neutrophils is intriguing given their propensity to generate chromatin nets and the recent suggestion that nets are a source of citrullinated antigens in RA [32,33].

Given the emphasis on plasmacytoid DC as the source of the IFN signature in SLE, we examined RNA levels in the blood of two known pDC markers, CLEC4C (BDCA2) and LILRA4 (ILT7). LILRA4 levels increased following baminercept treatment, yet CLEC4C levels were unchanged (Supplemental Figure 7 in File S1). CLEC4C appears to be a relatively specific pDC marker, whereas LILRA4 is highly expressed by both pDCs and memory B cells (Immunological Genome). Therefore these data suggest that baminercept does not affect pDC trafficking and increased LILRA4 expression is consistent with the increased numbers of B cells in the blood.

Relationship between IFN status and clinical parameters

After 3 months of treatment, changes in disease status were assessed using the American College of Rheumatology (ACR) scoring system. Overall, baminercept was well tolerated (Supplemental Table 3 in File S1); yet, in neither trial did baminercept treatment substantially increase the ACR scores (Supplemental Table 4 in File S1). Baminercept treatment resulted in a trend towards reduced swollen joint counts (SJC28) in both studies (Supplemental Figure 8 in File S1). Inhibition of TNF or IL-6 significantly decreases ESR and serum CRP levels; however, baminercept did not appreciably lower either serum parameter (Supplemental Figure 9 in File S1).

When patients were grouped based on baseline qPCR IFN status, there was no obvious trend towards a greater reduction in SJC28 in either IFN subgroup in the DMARD-IR study (Supplemental Figure 8 in file S1). The TNF-IR study was too small for such subgrouping. As these studies examined almost 800 patients, an analysis of gender effects was possible and baseline IFN scores were slightly lower in RA males ($p = 0.04$) and trended slightly lower in males in SLE. No correlation was observed between the IFN high and low groups with baseline swollen joint counts (SJC28), the Disease Activity Score 28 ESR (DAS28 ESR), C-reactive protein, erythrocyte sedimentation rates (ESR), rheumatoid factor titer or anti-CCP positivity (Supplemental Figure 10

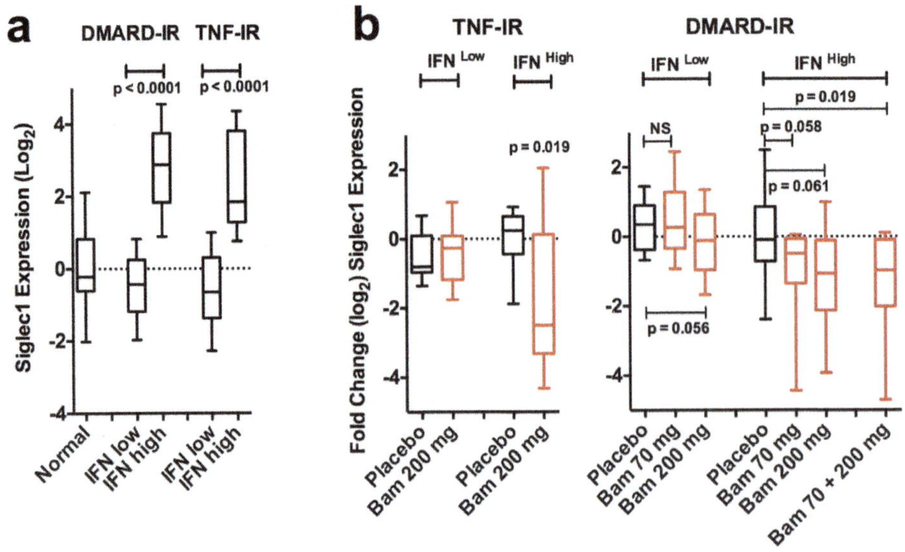

Figure 5. Baminercept treatment lowered RNA expression of the monocyte-associated gene SIGLEC1 in the blood. a). Expression of the monocyte associated gene SIGLEC1 (qPCR determination) is elevated in patients with an elevated IFN signature (qPCR IFN score cut point of 1). b.) SIGLEC1 expression (log_2) was reduced by treatment with baminercept (n's and boxes as per figure 4). P values are from a Mann-Whitney test of placebo vs. baminercept treated patients.

in File S1). Baminercept treatment did not affect total serum IgG, IgM and IgA levels nor were preexisting tetanus toxoid titers altered.

Discussion

We show here that inhibition of the LT/LIGHT pathway reduced not only the global IFN signature, but also RNA levels of SIGLEC1, an IFN-regulated gene expressed only in monocytes. RA and SLE patients with an IFN signature were more lymphopenic and baminercept treatment reversed the lymphopenia. These results demonstrate at the clinical level a fundamental linkage between the LT/LIGHT axis and IFN responses as well as between IFN and lymphopenia. To date, only high dose steroids and anti-interferon-α antibodies have been shown to reduce the signature and the inhibition by anti-IFNα antibodies appears to be partial [34–39]. Neither therapy informs on the nature of the underlying IFN biology. Importantly, a reduction in the IFN signature did not result in diminished arthritis suggesting that the pathology driving the IFN signature is not tightly coupled to the local joint disease. This conclusion needs to be qualified because the trials were insufficiently powered for the IFN positive subset, the treatment duration was relatively short and the levels of inflammatory disease were modest as indicated by the low baseline CRP levels.

The question of what biology is being reflected by the blood IFN signature in RA as well as in other autoimmune diseases remains unanswered. In SLE, the IFN signature is correlated in general with a distinct serological profile, renal disease, and progression to atherosclerosis and disease severity, yet its presence is not obviously linked to any particular immunology [23,40]. Our RA studies and those of others did not reveal obvious differences based on IFN status between the DMARD-IR and TNF-IR cohorts or their clinical or serological features [41,42]. A positive IFN signature in RA has been linked to a poor response to rituximab [43] and a weak or variable correlation with response to TNF inhibition [22,44,45]. In both systemic onset juvenile idiopathic arthritis patients and in Sjogren's syndrome, TNF inhibition led to an increased IFN signature supporting the hypothesis that TNF- and IFN-driven pathologies may lie at opposite poles of the autoimmune disease spectrum [46,47]. The ability of baminercept to dampen an IFN signature may have been a liability in a TNF dominated setting such as RA.

SLE patients are often lymphopenic and lymphopenia correlated with an elevated IFN signature in both SLE and systemic sclerosis patients [23,48]. Here, we confirmed this association in our SLE cohort and extended it to include RA patients. Lymphopenia could reflect perturbed bone marrow hematopoiesis accompanying systemic inflammation and/or increased retention of lymphocytes in the lymph nodes [49,50]. In the latter mechanism, IFN triggers complex formation between CD69 and sphingosine-1-phosphate receptors thereby inhibiting cell egress into the cortical sinuses [25]. Indeed, administration of IFNβ to multiple sclerosis patients or mice results in lymphopenia [51,52]. Increased retention of lymphocytes in the IFN-rich lymphoid microenvironments would allow more dwell time for productive encounters. Baminercept-induced lymphocytosis most likely has a contribution from restricted entry into the LN and mucosal compartments due to loss of addressin positive high endothelial venules. Baminercept could also reduce lymphopenia by shortening retention times in the LN following reduced IFN exposure. Our data are consistent with contributions from both trafficking and retention components and support the hypothesis that IFN-driven lymphocyte retention in the lymphoid tissues is a substantial component of lymphopenia in autoimmune disease.

The effect of baminercept on the blood IFN signature was largely unanticipated; however, observations from several experimental systems demonstrate that the LT/LIGHT network is entwined with IFN responses to infection [53]. First, murine CMV infection of the spleen induces an early IFN response derived from reticular stromal cells in the marginal zone [31,54,55]. Various aspects of lymphoid reticular stroma are critically dependent upon LTBR signaling and loss of LTBR signaling ablated the initial IFN response to murine CMV infection. Second, SIGLEC1-positive sentinel macrophages in both the LN and splenic environments

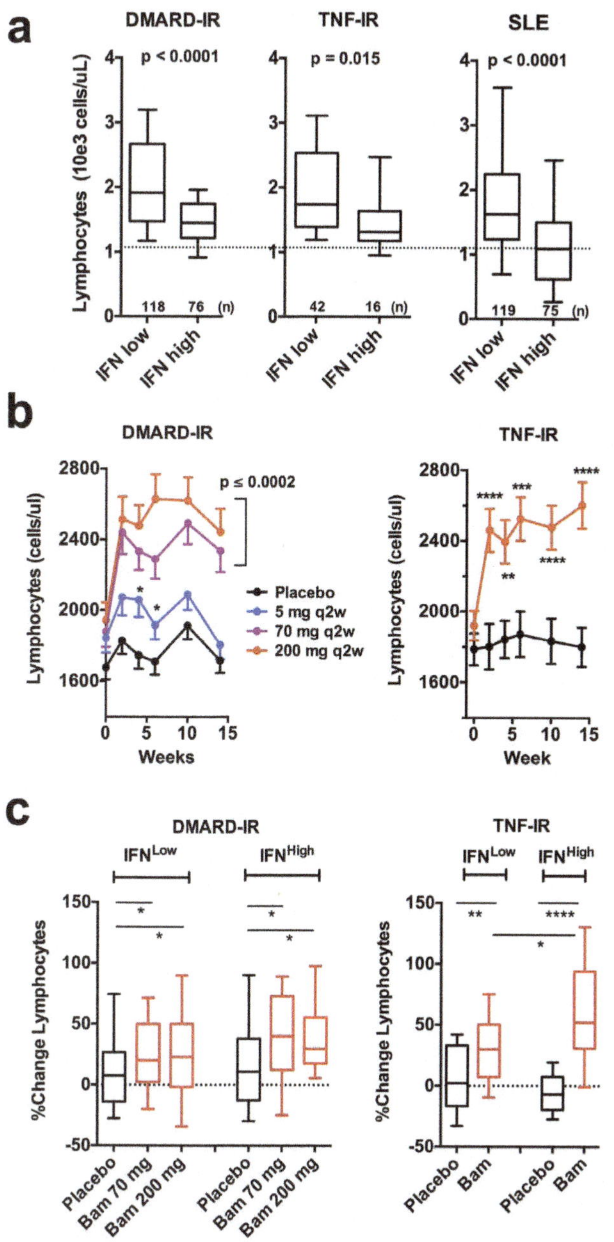

Figure 6. IFN signature positive RA patients are lymphopenic and baminercept treatment resulted in lymphocytosis. a). Patients were segregated based on low and high microarray IFN scores (<−6.5 and>−4.5) and baseline blood lymphocyte counts are plotted. b). Time course of the effects on absolute lymphocyte counts during 14 weeks of baminercept or placebo treatment (means, +/− SEM). All time points in two highest dosed cohorts in DMARD-IR were significant ($p<0.0002$), otherwise, significance is indicated by p-values * <0.05, ** < 0.01, *** <0.001 and **** <0.0001. c). Patients were grouped into baseline qPCR IFN signature low or high as in Fig. 1c. Percent change in lymphocyte counts following 14 weeks of treatment with placebo or baminercept is plotted (significance Mann-Whitney in all cases).

survey lymph or blood for immune complexes, lipids, particulates, viruses and sialylated antigens [56–58]. In the case of immune complexes or complement tagged antigens, they capture these elements and route them into the follicle for presentation to B cells. The differentiation state of these sentinel macrophages is LTBR-dependent [59,60]. Following VSV infection, virus replicates within the LN subcapsular macrophages and the splenic marginal zone metallophilic macrophages triggering IFN production and an effective host response [60–62]. Within the spleen, marginal zone metallophilic macrophages are the major local producers of type I IFN in response to an intravenous HSV challenge [63] and they also generate IFN in response to *Campylobacter jejuni* infection [64]. In a related observation, listeria infection of LTBR-deficient mice failed to generate an IFN response in the spleen [65]. Other LT-dependent sources could include both dendritic cells [11,66–68] as well as follicular dendritic cells where TLRs could be activated following internalization and recycling of antigen [69].

Why is this linkage between the LT and IFN systems manifesting itself in RA? In SLE, a subset of IFN signature high patients has measureable IFN circulating in the blood [21,70]. However, IFN was not detected in the blood of our RA patients and therefore the exposure to IFN must occur while leucocytes traffic through the organs. In RA, robust evidence for a substantial IFN signal in the joints is lacking [3,71,72]. One hypothesis is that lymphocytes become "imprinted" by IFN while trafficking through organized lymphoid microenvironments. Many if not all autoimmune diseases have undercurrents of systemic disease as evidenced by the involvement of additional organ systems, e.g. the lungs in RA, the CNS in SLE, Sjogren's and sarcoidosis, etc. We speculate that LNs draining organs with articular or extra-articular disease, as in lung or glandular involvement in RA, produce IFN as a consequence of sensing signals such as dead cell debris, chromatin complexes, neutrophil nets or antigens as complement tagged or immunoglobulin complexes [69,73]. In this scenario, the amount of IFN exposure would reflect the magnitude of the systemic involvement and may coincide with LN reactivity or even gross lymphadenopathy. Indeed, some association was noted in SLE between lymphoadenopathy and an increased IFN signature [23]. We speculate that baminercept's effects on the IFN signature are due to alteration of the sentinel functions of the lymphoid microenvironments albeit via myeloid or stromal elements.

In conclusion, inhibition of the LTR signaling in RA patients reduced IFN imprinting. The IFN signature is linked to the lymphopenia in RA and SLE supporting a role for IFN in lymphocyte retention in lymphoid organs. Experimentally, the use of viral challenges has revealed much of the linkage between LTBR and IFN responses and, while autoimmune diseases do not have obvious ongoing viral infections, parallels have been drawn between immune responses to virus and chromatin in SLE [74]. Thus, these observations may be highlighting a potential coupling mechanism between tissue damage, debris recognition and an overactive self-reactive immune response. Disruption of LTBR signaling could be a new tool for the investigation and potentially the treatment of certain subgroups in autoimmune diseases.

Experimental Procedures

Patients and Trials

Baminercept is a fusion protein of the extracellular domain of human LTBR coupled to the hinge and Fc domain of human IgG1 [75]. DMARD-IR (104RA202, NCT00664716, EUdraCT 2006-005466-39) was a multicenter, phase IIb, randomized, double-blinded placebo-controlled study of RA patients who had had an inadequate response (IR) to a disease modifying anti-rheumatic drug. In this study 391 RA patients were treated for 14 weeks with subcutaneous injections of placebo q2w (79 patients), 5 mg baminercept (BG9948) q2w (78), 70 mg q2w (78), 70 mg q4w (39), 200 mg q2w (78) or 200 mg q4w (39). 365 patients

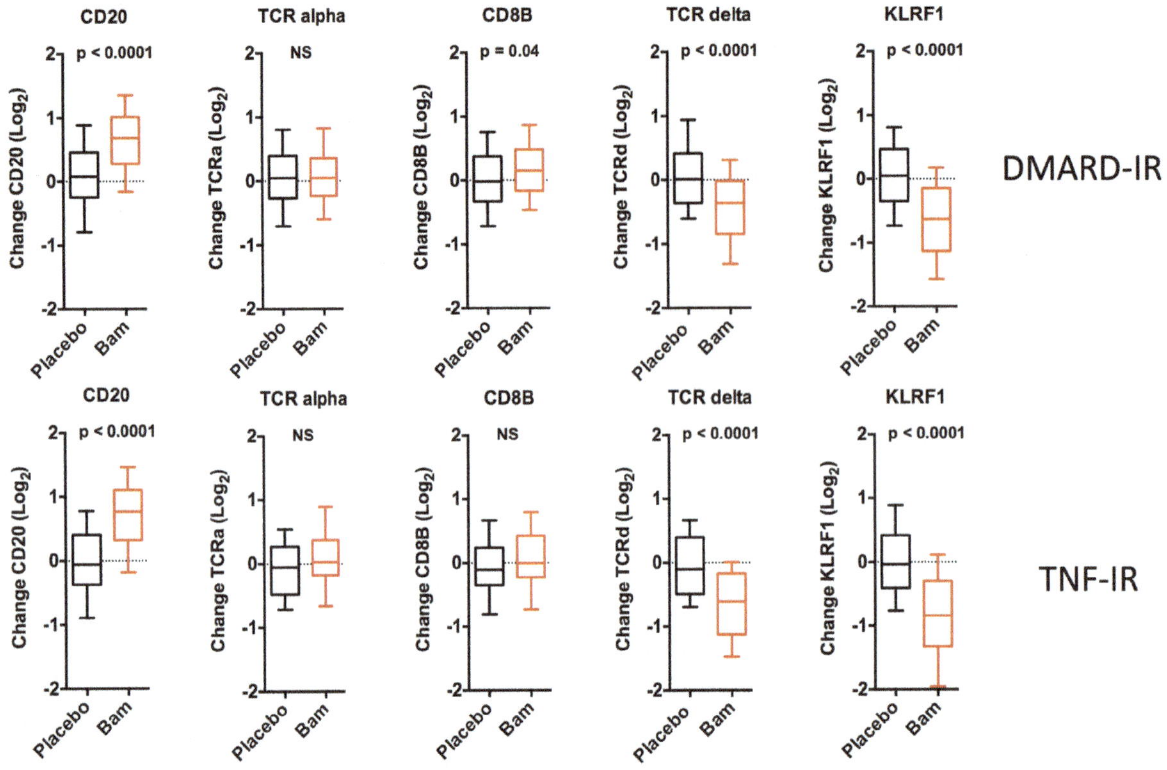

Figure 7. Baminercept alters the levels of RNAs representative of lymphocyte subsets in the blood. Baminercept treatment increased the blood RNA expression (qPCR determination) of genes representing B cells (CD20), T cells (TCRA, CD8B), whereas expression of markers for $\gamma\delta$-T cells (TCRD) and NK cells (KLRF1) decreased. In the DMARD-IR study, data from both 70 and 200 mg 2qw cohorts are pooled.

completed the study. Study was conducted between July 2007 and October 2008 at 58 sites in Argentina, Brazil, Hungary, Mexico, Poland, Romania, Russia and United Kingdom and investigators are listed in the supplemental materials.

TNF-IR (104RA203, NCT00458861, EUdraCT 2006-005467-26) was a multicenter, phase IIb, double-blinded, placebo-controlled study of RA patients who lacked an adequate response to TNF-blocking therapy and had discontinued TNF blocking treatment for at least 90 days. The study dosed 114 patients with subcutaneous injections q2w of either placebo (38) or baminercept 200 mg (76). This study was terminated early due to poor efficacy in the DMARD-IR study; however, 81 patients completed the 3 months of dosing and another 15 patients received at least 2 months of treatment. Study was conducted between March 2007 and October 2008 at 40 sites in the United States, Canada, Belgium and United Kingdom.

Investigators for both baminercept studies are listed in the supplemental materials in File S1. RA patients in both studies were eligible if they met the American College of Rheumatology (ACR) criteria for rheumatoid arthritis and had active RA for at least 6 months. Patients had to have been receiving 10–25 mg methotrexate per week for at least 3 months with a stable dose for the last 4 weeks before entry. Methotrexate therapy was maintained for the duration of the studies. Patients had to have more than 8 swollen and tender joints (66/68 joint count) and either a CRP≥ 1.5 ULN or ESR ≥28 mm/hr at screening. The protocols for these trials re available as supporting information; see Protocol S1 and S2. There is no intent to publish further clinical data from these studies and the ACR scores (primary trial endpoint) are presented within the supplemental data.

SLE data were from registry (called SPARE) representing a collection of 292 SLE patients from the Hopkins Lupus Center in the US. Patients were eligible if they were aged 18–75 years and met the American College of Rheumatology Revised Criteria for Classification of Systemic Lupus Erythematous. Baseline data were used in this study and patients were under standard clinical practice. Normal controls for RNA analyses were composed of healthy volunteer donors from Biogen Idec. Control group had equal numbers of males and females and was not exactly gender balanced with the predominantly female composition of both the RA and SLE cohorts.

Ethics Statement

The RA studies were approved by the appropriate institutional review boards or ethics committees and all patients provided written informed consent (see supplementary materials in File S1 for a complete listing). All patients from the Hopkins Lupus Center (Johns Hopkins University School of Medicine) provided written informed consent to participate in the SPARE registry and the Johns Hopkins institutional review board approved the study.

Analyses of whole blood RNA

Patient whole blood was collected into PaxGene tubes and analyzed using conventional Affymetrix microarrays and qPCR was performed on the RNA samples using the Fluidigm analyzer. Details for RNA analyses as well as the IFN reporter assays are provided in the Supplemental Materials in File S1. Baseline transcriptional profiling datasets are deposited at GEO, GSE45291.

Supporting Information

File S1 Supporting files. Supplemental Methods and Investigator Listing. Supplemental Table 1, Demographics of the Patients in the RA studies and the SLE registry. Supplemental Table 2, Measurement of IFN signatures. Supplemental Table 3, Incidence of adverse events by preferred term for the combined placebo-controlled studies. Supplemental Table 4, Lack of an appreciable effect of baminercept treatment on ACR scores as assessed at 14 weeks. Supplemental Figure 1, Comparison of IFN signatures in RA and SLE. Supplemental Figure 2, Elevation of serum LIGHT levels in RA patients following baminercept treatment. Supplemental Figure 3, Characteristics of the IFN signatures observed in this study. Elevation of serum LIGHT levels in RA patients following baminercept treatment. Supplemental Figure 4, Characteristics of baminercept induced lymphocytosis in RA patients. Supplemental Figure 5, Relationship between IFN signature and baminercept treatment on blood neutrophil and monocyte counts. Supplemental Figure 6, FACS analysis of the effects of baminercept treatment on peripheral blood lymphocyte subsets. Supplemental Figure 7, Quantitative PCR analysis on whole blood RNA of the effects of baminercept treatment on gene markers of myeloid subsets. Supplemental Figure 8, Effects of baminercept treatment on the Swollen Joint Count 28 (SJC28) scores in the DMARD-IR and TNF-IR studies. Supplemental Figure 9, Little effect of baminercept treatment on CRP levels and Erythrocyte Sedimentation Rates (ESR) in the DMARD-IR and TNF-IR studies. Supplemental Figure 10, The IFN signature status in RA patients does not correlate with clinical or serological parameters.

Checklist S1 CONSORT Checklist.

Protocol S1 Trial Protocol.

Protocol S2 Trial Protocol.

Acknowledgments

We thank the patients who participated in the studies; the investigators and personnel at the study sites, and the members of the baminercept project team, including Paul Chen, Niki Cox, Patrick Cullen, Fred D'Amato, Susan Gawlak, Janet Griffiths, Evangelia Hatzis, Bina Keshaven, Megan Lo, Helena Madden, Nick Messinese, Werner Meier, John O'Gorman, Suezanne Parker, Jitesh Rana, Ann Ranger, Joyce Sobolewski, Cynthia Theodos, Miranda Tighe, Melissa Wojcik and Jim Woodworth. We also thank Larrisa Miller for help with the IFN reporter assay, Susan Kalled and Ronenn Rubinoff for major contributions to the SPARE SLE registry and Ian Rifkin, Carl Ware, Jen Gommerman, Peter Lipsky and Peggy Crow for critique of the manuscript.

Author Contributions

Conceived and designed the experiments: JB JG TP AN MW CN MP EB JLB. Performed the experiments: JB NA AT JG TP AN MW CN MP EB JLB. Analyzed the data: JB JG TP JLB. Contributed to the writing of the manuscript: JB JG TP EB JLB.

References

1. Ronnblom L, Eloranta ML (2013) The interferon signature in autoimmune diseases. Current opinion in rheumatology 25: 248–253.
2. Elkon KB, Wiedeman A (2012) Type I IFN system in the development and manifestations of SLE. Current opinion in rheumatology 24: 499–505.
3. Higgs BW, Liu Z, White B, Zhu W, White WI, et al. (2011) Patients with systemic lupus erythematosus, myositis, rheumatoid arthritis and scleroderma share activation of a common type I interferon pathway. Annals of the rheumatic diseases 70: 2029–2036.
4. Crow YJ (2011) Type I interferonopathies: a novel set of inborn errors of immunity. Annals of the New York Academy of Sciences 1238: 91–98.
5. Kirou KA, Gkrouzman E (2013) Anti-interferon alpha treatment in SLE. Clinical immunology 148: 303–312.
6. Browning JL (2008) Inhibition of the lymphotoxin pathway as a therapy for autoimmune disease. Immunological reviews 223: 202–220.
7. Ware CF (2008) Targeting lymphocyte activation through the lymphotoxin and LIGHT pathways. Immunological reviews 223: 186–201.
8. Remouchamps C, Boutaffala L, Ganeff C, Dejardin E (2011) Biology and signal transduction pathways of the Lymphotoxin-alphabeta/LTbetaR system. Cytokine & growth factor reviews 22: 301–310.
9. Lu TT, Browning JL (2014) Role of the Lymphotoxin/LIGHT System in the Development and Maintenance of Reticular Networks and Vasculature in Lymphoid Tissues. Frontiers in immunology 5: 47.
10. Gray EE, Cyster JG (2012) Lymph node macrophages. Journal of innate immunity 4: 424–436.
11. Summers deLuca L, Gommerman JL (2012) Fine-tuning of dendritic cell biology by the TNF superfamily. Nature reviews Immunology 12: 339–351.
12. De Trez C (2012) Lymphotoxin-beta receptor expression and its related signaling pathways govern dendritic cell homeostasis and function. Immunobiology 217: 1250–1258.
13. Upadhyay V, Fu YX (2013) Lymphotoxin signalling in immune homeostasis and the control of microorganisms. Nature reviews Immunology 13: 270–279.
14. Satpathy AT, Briseno CG, Lee JS, Ng D, Manieri NA, et al. (2013) Notch2-dependent classical dendritic cells orchestrate intestinal immunity to attaching-and-effacing bacterial pathogens. Nature immunology 14: 937–948.
15. Wege AK, Huber B, Wimmer N, Mannel DN, Hehlgans T (2013) LTbetaR expression on hematopoietic cells regulates acute inflammation and influences maturation of myeloid subpopulations. Innate immunity ePub.
16. Steinberg MW, Cheung TC, Ware CF (2011) The signaling networks of the herpesvirus entry mediator (TNFRSF14) in immune regulation. Immunological reviews 244: 169–187.
17. Allaire NE, Bushnell SE, Bienkowska J, Brock G, Carulli J (2013) Optimization of a high-throughput whole blood expression profiling methodology and its application to assess the pharmacodynamics of interferon (IFN) beta-1a or polyethylene glycol-conjugated IFN beta-1a in healthy clinical trial subjects. BMC research notes 6: 8.
18. Rose T, Grutzkau A, Hirseland H, Huscher D, Dahnrich C, et al. (2013) IFNalpha and its response proteins, IP-10 and SIGLEC-1, are biomarkers of disease activity in systemic lupus erythematosus. Annals of the rheumatic diseases 72: 1639–1645.
19. Hall JC, Casciola-Rosen L, Berger AE, Kapsogeorgou EK, Cheadle C, et al. (2012) Precise probes of type II interferon activity define the origin of interferon signatures in target tissues in rheumatic diseases. Proceedings of the National Academy of Sciences of the United States of America 109: 17609–17614.
20. Waddell SJ, Popper SJ, Rubins KH, Griffiths MJ, Brown PO, et al. (2010) Dissecting interferon-induced transcriptional programs in human peripheral blood cells. PloS one 5: e9753.
21. Hua J, Kirou K, Lee C, Crow MK (2006) Functional assay of type I interferon in systemic lupus erythematosus plasma and association with anti-RNA binding protein autoantibodies. Arthritis and rheumatism 54: 1906–1916.
22. Mavragani CP, La DT, Stohl W, Crow MK (2010) Association of the response to tumor necrosis factor antagonists with plasma type I interferon activity and interferon-beta/alpha ratios in rheumatoid arthritis patients: a post hoc analysis of a predominantly Hispanic cohort. Arthritis and rheumatism 62: 392–401.
23. Kirou KA, Lee C, George S, Louca K, Peterson MG, et al. (2005) Activation of the interferon-alpha pathway identifies a subgroup of systemic lupus erythematosus patients with distinct serologic features and active disease. Arthritis and rheumatism 52: 1491–1503.
24. Browning JL, Allaire N, Ngam-Ek A, Notidis E, Hunt J, et al. (2005) Lymphotoxin-beta receptor signaling is required for the homeostatic control of HEV differentiation and function. Immunity 23: 539–550.
25. Cyster JG, Schwab SR (2012) Sphingosine-1-phosphate and lymphocyte egress from lymphoid organs. Annual review of immunology 30: 69–94.
26. Silva-Santos B, Pennington DJ, Hayday AC (2005) Lymphotoxin-mediated regulation of gammadelta cell differentiation by alphabeta T cell progenitors. Science 307: 925–928.
27. Elewaut D, Ware CF (2007) The unconventional role of LT alpha beta in T cell differentiation. Trends in immunology 28: 169–175.
28. Vallabhapurapu S, Powolny-Budnicka I, Riemann M, Schmid RM, Paxian S, et al. (2008) Rel/NF-kappaB family member RelA regulates NK1.1- to NK1.1+

transition as well as IL-15-induced expansion of NKT cells. European journal of immunology 38: 3508–3519.
29. Powolny-Budnicka I, Riemann M, Tanzer S, Schmid RM, Hehlgans T, et al. (2011) RelA and RelB transcription factors in distinct thymocyte populations control lymphotoxin-dependent interleukin-17 production in gammadelta T cells. Immunity 34: 364–374.
30. Van Den Broeck T, Van Ammel E, Delforche M, Taveirne S, Kerre T, et al. (2013) Differential Ly49e expression pathways in resting versus TCR-activated intraepithelial gammadelta T cells. Journal of immunology 190: 1982–1990.
31. Verma S, Wang Q, Chodaczek G, Benedict CA (2013) Lymphoid-tissue stromal cells coordinate innate defense to cytomegalovirus. Journal of virology 87: 6201–6210.
32. Knight JS, Kaplan MJ (2012) Lupus neutrophils: 'NET' gain in understanding lupus pathogenesis. Current opinion in rheumatology 24: 441–450.
33. Khandpur R, Carmona-Rivera C, Vivekanandan-Giri A, Gizinski A, Yalavarthi S, et al. (2013) NETs are a source of citrullinated autoantigens and stimulate inflammatory responses in rheumatoid arthritis. Science translational medicine 5: 178ra140.
34. Lepelletier Y, Zollinger R, Ghirelli C, Raynaud F, Hadj-Slimane R, et al. (2010) Toll-like receptor control of glucocorticoid-induced apoptosis in human plasmacytoid predendritic cells (pDCs). Blood 116: 3389–3397.
35. Guiducci C, Gong M, Xu Z, Gill M, Chaussabel D, et al. (2010) TLR recognition of self nucleic acids hampers glucocorticoid activity in lupus. Nature 465: 937–941.
36. Yao Y, Richman L, Higgs BW, Morehouse CA, de los Reyes M, et al. (2009) Neutralization of interferon-alpha/beta-inducible genes and downstream effect in a phase I trial of an anti-interferon-alpha monoclonal antibody in systemic lupus erythematosus. Arthritis and rheumatism 60: 1785–1796.
37. McBride JM, Jiang J, Abbas AR, Morimoto A, Li J, et al. (2012) Safety and pharmacodynamics of rontalizumab in patients with systemic lupus erythematosus: results of a phase I, placebo-controlled, double-blind, dose-escalation study. Arthritis and rheumatism 64: 3666–3676.
38. Petri M, Wallace DJ, Spindler A, Chindalore V, Kalunian K, et al. (2013) Sifalimumab, a Human Anti-Interferon-alpha Monoclonal Antibody, in Systemic Lupus Erythematosus: A Phase I Randomized, Controlled, Dose-Escalation Study. Arthritis and rheumatism 65: 1011–1021.
39. Higgs BW, Zhu W, Morehouse C, White WI, Brohawn P, et al. (2013) A phase 1b clinical trial evaluating sifalimumab, an anti-IFN-alpha monoclonal antibody, shows target neutralisation of a type I IFN signature in blood of dermatomyositis and polymyositis patients. Annals of the rheumatic diseases 78: 256–262.
40. Huang YL, Chung HT, Chang CJ, Yeh KW, Chen LC, et al. (2009) Lymphopenia is a risk factor in the progression of carotid intima-media thickness in juvenile-onset systemic lupus erythematosus. Arthritis and rheumatism 60: 3766–3775.
41. Cantaert T, van Baarsen LG, Wijbrandts CA, Thurlings RM, van de Sande MG, et al. (2010) Type I interferons have no major influence on humoral autoimmunity in rheumatoid arthritis. Rheumatology 49: 156–166.
42. Thurlings RM, Boumans M, Tekstra J, van Roon JA, Vos K, et al. (2010) Relationship between the type I interferon signature and the response to rituximab in rheumatoid arthritis patients. Arthritis and rheumatism 62: 3607–3614.
43. Raterman HG, Vosslamber S, de Ridder S, Nurmohamed MT, Lems WF, et al. (2012) The interferon type I signature towards prediction of non-response to rituximab in rheumatoid arthritis patients. Arthritis research & therapy 14: R95.
44. Reynier F, Petit F, Paye M, Turrel-Davin F, Imbert PE, et al. (2011) Importance of correlation between gene expression levels: application to the type I interferon signature in rheumatoid arthritis. PloS one 6: e24828.
45. van Baarsen LG, Wijbrandts CA, Rustenburg F, Cantaert T, van der Pouw Kraan TC, et al. (2010) Regulation of IFN response gene activity during infliximab treatment in rheumatoid arthritis is associated with clinical response to treatment. Arthritis research & therapy 12: R11.
46. Palucka AK, Blanck JP, Bennett L, Pascual V, Banchereau J (2005) Cross-regulation of TNF and IFN-alpha in autoimmune diseases. Proceedings of the National Academy of Sciences of the United States of America 102: 3372–3377.
47. Mavragani CP, Niewold TB, Moutsopoulos NM, Pillemer SR, Wahl SM, et al. (2007) Augmented interferon-alpha pathway activation in patients with Sjogren's syndrome treated with etanercept. Arthritis and rheumatism 56: 3995–4004.
48. Assassi S, Mayes MD, Arnett FC, Gourh P, Agarwal SK, et al. (2010) Systemic sclerosis and lupus: points in an interferon-mediated continuum. Arthritis and rheumatism 62: 589–598.
49. de Bruin AM, Libregts SF, Valkhof M, Boon L, Touw IP, et al. (2012) IFNgamma induces monopoiesis and inhibits neutrophil development during inflammation. Blood 119: 1543–1554.
50. Cain DW, Snowden PB, Sempowski GD, Kelsoe G (2011) Inflammation triggers emergency granulopoiesis through a density-dependent feedback mechanism. PloS one 6: e19957.
51. Hartrich L, Weinstock-Guttman B, Hall D, Badgett D, Baier M, et al. (2003) Dynamics of immune cell trafficking in interferon-beta treated multiple sclerosis patients. Journal of neuroimmunology 139: 84–92.
52. Gao Y, Majchrzak-Kita B, Fish EN, Gommerman JL (2009) Dynamic accumulation of plasmacytoid dendritic cells in lymph nodes is regulated by interferon-beta. Blood 114: 2623–2631.
53. Gommerman JL, J.L B, C.F W (2014) The Lymphotoxin Network: Orchestrating a Type I Interferon response to optimize adaptive immunity. Cytokine & growth factor reviews in press.
54. Schneider K, Loewendorf A, De Trez C, Fulton J, Rhode A, et al. (2008) Lymphotoxin-mediated crosstalk between B cells and splenic stroma promotes the initial type I interferon response to cytomegalovirus. Cell host & microbe 3: 67–76.
55. Hsu KM, Pratt JR, Akers WJ, Achilefu SI, Yokoyama WM (2009) Murine cytomegalovirus displays selective infection of cells within hours after systemic administration. The Journal of general virology 90: 33–43.
56. Barral P, Polzella P, Bruckbauer A, van Rooijen N, Besra GS, et al. (2010) CD169(+) macrophages present lipid antigens to mediate early activation of iNKT cells in lymph nodes. Nature immunology 11: 303–312.
57. Cyster JG (2010) B cell follicles and antigen encounters of the third kind. Nature immunology 11: 989–996.
58. Klaas M, Crocker PR (2012) Sialoadhesin in recognition of self and non-self. Seminars in immunopathology 34: 353–364.
59. Phan TG, Grigorova I, Okada T, Cyster JG (2007) Subcapsular encounter and complement-dependent transport of immune complexes by lymph node B cells. Nature immunology 8: 992–1000.
60. Moseman EA, Iannacone M, Bosurgi L, Tonti E, Chevrier N, et al. (2012) B cell maintenance of subcapsular sinus macrophages protects against a fatal viral infection independent of adaptive immunity. Immunity 36: 415–426.
61. Honke N, Shaabani N, Cadeddu G, Sorg UR, Zhang DE, et al. (2012) Enforced viral replication activates adaptive immunity and is essential for the control of a cytopathic virus. Nature immunology 13: 51–57.
62. Iannacone M, Moseman EA, Tonti E, Bosurgi L, Junt T, et al. (2010) Subcapsular sinus macrophages prevent CNS invasion on peripheral infection with a neurotropic virus. Nature 465: 1079–1083.
63. Eloranta ML, Alm GV (1999) Splenic marginal metallophilic macrophages and marginal zone macrophages are the major interferon-alpha/beta producers in mice upon intravenous challenge with herpes simplex virus. Scandinavian journal of immunology 49: 391–394.
64. Klaas M, Oetke C, Lewis LE, Erwig LP, Heikema AP, et al. (2012) Sialoadhesin promotes rapid proinflammatory and type I IFN responses to a sialylated pathogen, Campylobacter jejuni. Journal of immunology 189: 2414–2422.
65. Kutsch S, Degrandi D, Pfeffer K (2008) Immediate lymphotoxin beta receptor-mediated transcriptional response in host defense against L. monocytogenes. Immunobiology 213: 353–366.
66. Summers deLuca L, Ng D, Gao Y, Wortzman ME, Watts TH, et al. (2011) LTbetaR signaling in dendritic cells induces a type I IFN response that is required for optimal clonal expansion of CD8+ T cells. Proceedings of the National Academy of Sciences of the United States of America 108: 2046–2051.
67. Lorenzi S, Mattei F, Sistigu A, Bracci L, Spadaro F, et al. (2011) Type I IFNs control antigen retention and survival of CD8alpha(+) dendritic cells after uptake of tumor apoptotic cells leading to cross-priming. Journal of immunology 186: 5142–5150.
68. Spadaro F, Lapenta C, Donati S, Abalsamo L, Barnaba V, et al. (2012) IFN-alpha enhances cross-presentation in human dendritic cells by modulating antigen survival, endocytic routing, and processing. Blood 119: 1407–1417.
69. Heesters BA, Das A, Chatterjee P, Carroll MC (2014) Do follicular dendritic cells regulate lupus-specific B cells? Mol Immunol epub.
70. Yao Y, Liu Z, Jallal B, Shen N, Ronnblom L (2013) Type I interferons in Sjogren's syndrome. Autoimmunity reviews 12: 558–566.
71. Nzeusseu Toukap A, Galant C, Theate I, Maudoux AL, Lories RJ, et al. (2007) Identification of distinct gene expression profiles in the synovium of patients with systemic lupus erythematosus. Arthritis and rheumatism 56: 1579–1588.
72. Yoshida S, Arakawa F, Higuchi F, Ishibashi Y, Goto M, et al. (2012) Gene expression analysis of rheumatoid arthritis synovial lining regions by cDNA microarray combined with laser microdissection: up-regulation of inflammation-associated STAT1, IRF1, CXCL9, CXCL10, and CCL5. Scandinavian journal of rheumatology 41: 170–179.
73. Elkon KB, Santer DM (2012) Complement, interferon and lupus. Curr Opin Immunol 24: 665–670.
74. Migliorini A, Anders HJ (2012) A novel pathogenetic concept-antiviral immunity in lupus nephritis. Nature reviews Nephrology 8: 183–189.
75. Browning JL, Dougas I, Ngam-ek A, Bourdon PR, Ehrenfels BN, et al. (1995) Characterization of surface lymphotoxin forms. Use of specific monoclonal antibodies and soluble receptors. Journal of immunology 154: 33–46.

24

Functional Improvement of Regulatory T Cells from Rheumatoid Arthritis Subjects Induced by Capsular Polysaccharide Glucuronoxylomannogalactan

Eva Pericolini[1¶], Elena Gabrielli[1¶], Alessia Alunno[2], Elena Bartoloni Bocci[2], Stefano Perito[1], Siu-Kei Chow[3], Elio Cenci[1], Arturo Casadevall[3], Roberto Gerli[2], Anna Vecchiarelli[1]*

1 Microbiology Section, Department of Experimental Medicine, University of Perugia, Perugia, Italy, **2** Rheumatology Unit, Department of Medicine, University of Perugia, Perugia, Italy, **3** Department of Microbiology and Immunology, Albert Einstein College of Medicine, New York, New York, United States of America

Abstract

Objective: Regulatory T cells (Treg) play a critical role in the prevention of autoimmunity, and the suppressive activity of these cells is impaired in rheumatoid arthritis (RA). The aim of the present study was to investigate function and properties of Treg of RA patients in response to purified polysaccharide glucuronoxylomannogalactan (GXMGal).

Methods: Flow cytometry and western blot analysis were used to investigate the frequency, function and properties of Treg cells.

Results: GXMGal was able to: i) induce strong increase of FOXP3 on CD4$^+$ T cells without affecting the number of CD4$^+$CD25$^+$FOXP3$^+$ Treg cells with parallel increase in the percentage of non-conventional CD4$^+$CD25$^-$FOXP3$^+$ Treg cells; ii) increase intracellular levels of TGF-β1 in CD4$^+$CD25$^-$FOXP3$^+$ Treg cells and of IL-10 in both CD4$^+$CD25$^+$FOXP3$^+$ and CD4$^+$CD25$^-$FOXP3$^+$ Treg cells; iii) enhance the suppressive activity of CD4$^+$CD25$^+$FOXP3$^+$ and CD4$^+$CD25$^-$FOXP3$^+$ Treg cells in terms of inhibition of effector T cell activity and increased secretion of IL-10; iv) decrease Th1 response as demonstrated by inhibition of T-bet activation and down-regulation of IFN-γ and IL-12p70 production; v) decrease Th17 differentiation by down-regulating pSTAT3 activation and IL-17A, IL-23, IL-21, IL-22 and IL-6 production.

Conclusion: These data show that GXMGal improves Treg functions and increases the number and function of CD4$^+$CD25$^-$FOXP3$^+$ Treg cells of RA patients. It is suggested that GXMGal may be potentially useful for restoring impaired Treg functions in autoimmune disorders and for developing Treg cell-based strategies for the treatment of these diseases.

Editor: Maurizio Del Poeta, Stony Brook University, United States of America

Funding: This work was supported by "Fondazione Cassa di Risparmio 2012.0128.021." The funders had no role in study design, data collection and analysis, decision to publish, or preparation of the manuscript.

Competing Interests: The authors have declared that no competing interests exist.

* Email: anna.vecchiarelli@unipg.it

¶ These authors contributed equally to this work.

Introduction

Rheumatoid arthritis (RA) is an autoimmune disease characterized by destructive joint inflammation. The synovial inflammation is characterized by non-specific infiltration of both lymphocytes and innate immune cells, such as synoviocytes, macrophages and neutrophils [1]. RA is generally considered to be an autoimmune disease in which pathogenic T cells such as T helper (Th)1 and Th17 cells play an important role [2]. An exciting aspect of Th17 cell homeostasis is the reciprocal relationship with regulatory T cells (Treg), whose imbalance is believed to play a major role in the development of autoimmune disease [3–6]. Treg were originally identified by high surface expression of CD25 [7,8] and subsequently by the forkhead box protein P3 (FOXP3) transcriptional factor, which controls their development and suppressive function [9,10]. Interestingly, it was suggested that activated FOXP3$^+$ non-Treg cells may be a reservoir of silent Treg that regain their function following activation [11]. The data on the effective number of Treg cells in RA patients are inconsistent. Some studies report a decreased number of Treg cells in the blood of RA [12], while others report increased numbers of Treg cells [13], however it is clear that Treg cells appear unable to suppress inflammation in the rheumatoid joints [14]. Thus, paradoxically, CD4$^+$CD25$^+$ T cells, including CD4$^+$CD25$^+$FOXP3$^+$ Treg cells, circulate in RA patients despite the still ongoing inflammation [13,14]. The capacity of Treg cells to suppress several arthritic responses both in humans and animal models makes them potential therapeutic targets in arthritic conditions such as RA [15]. A prior study suggested that the therapeutic efficacy of methotrexate (MTX), the current "gold standard" treatment in experimental RA, was partly attributed to the increased development of CD4$^+$CD25$^+$ Treg cells [16]. Furthermore, anti-rheumatic biotechnological therapies may offer a means of restoring the Th17/Treg cell balance in favor of Treg, thereby re-establishing immune tolerance [6]. It has been demonstrated that some fungal products, such as those from *Cryptococcus neoformans* (*C. neoformans*), directly induce lymphocytes apoptosis [17]. Accordingly, we demonstrated that glucuronoxylomannogalactan (GXMGal), a purified capsular polysaccharide from the opportunistic fungus *C. neoformans* [18], directly induce apoptosis of activated lymphocytes [19]. This was recently evidenced also using activated RA T cells producing IL-17A suggesting the potential role of GXMGal in fighting deleterious Th17 cells [20]. In light of this finding, the aim of this study was to understand whether GXMGal could restore the Th17/Treg balance, both by dampening Th17 response [20] and modulating Treg cell suppressive capacity.

Methods

Cryptococcal polysaccharide and other reagents

RPMI-1640 with L-glutamine, FCS and penicillin streptomycin solution were obtained from EuroClone S.p.A. (Milan, Italy). Brefeldin A, PHA, dexametasone (DEX), MTX, the inhibitor of pSTAT3 (FLLL31) and hypotonic propidium iodide solution (PI) were obtained from Sigma-Aldrich (St. Louis, MO, USA). Monoclonal antibodies (mAbs) to human CD3 and CD28 were obtained from ImmunoTools GmbH (Friesoythe, Germany).

GXMGal [21], known until recently as galactoxylomannan, was purified as described elsewhere [22,23]. The dose of GXMGal was chosen on the basis of our previous published data [24]. All reagent and media were negative for endotoxin, as assessed by *Limulus* amebocyte lysate assay (QCL-1000, BioWhittaker, VWR International p.b.i., Milan, Italy).

Subjects

Thirty patients with established RA according to the American College of Rheumatology classification criteria [25] and followed up at the Rheumatology Unit of the Perugia University, were included in the study. This cohort included 20 women and 10 men with a mean age of 54±8 years (mean ± SD) and disease duration of 12±6 years. The mean Disease Activity Score, as evaluated including 28 swollen and tender joint count (DAS28), was 3±1.2 at the time of sample collection. All patients were MTX naïve and were receiving other synthetic or biologic disease-modifying anti-rheumatic drugs in monotherapy (leflunomide: n° 11, hydroxy-chloroquine: n° 16, tocilizumab: n° 3). Fourteen patients were also receiving low doses of corticosteroids (5 mg/day of prednisone or equivalent). Fifteen healthy subjects matched for age and sex acted as normal control (Control). Written informed consent was obtained from all subjects prior to sample collection in accordance with the Declaration of Helsinki. Local Ethical Committee CEAS (Comitato Etico delle Aziende Sanitarie, Umbria, Italy) approval was received for the whole study (AR-2 n. 1874/12).

Isolation of cells and culture condition

Heparinized venous blood was obtained from Control and RA patients. Peripheral blood mononuclear cells (PBMC) were separated by density gradient centrifugation on Ficoll-Hypaque (EuroClone). PBMC were incubated with mAb-conjugated MicroBeads to human CD4 (Miltenyi Biotec) and $CD4^+$ T lymphocytes were purified by magnetic separation. Purity of separated $CD4^+$ T cells was >90% as detected by cytofluorimetric analysis. $CD4^+CD25^+$ and $CD4^+CD25^-$ cells were purified from $CD4^+$ T lymphocytes using the $CD4^+CD25^+$ Treg cell isolation kit (Miltenyi Biotec) according to manufacturer's instructions. Unless otherwise specified, cells were seeded in 48 or 96-well culture plates pre-coated with mAbs to CD3 plus CD28 (both 2 μg/ml) and activated for 30 min with soluble mAbs to CD3 plus CD28 (both 3 μg/ml) (ImmunoTools) in RPMI-1640+10% FCS (complete medium) at 37°C plus 5% CO_2. After activation cells were washed and stimulated as described below.

Cytokine Production

Activated PBMC (5×10^6/ml) were incubated for 2, 18 and 72 h in the presence or absence of GXMGal (10 μg/ml), MTX (10 ng/ml) [26], DEX (10 nM) [27] or FLLL31 (5 μM) [20]. The supernatants were collected and cytokines were tested by specific ELISA assays (all from eBioscience, San Diego, CA). Cytokine titers were calculated relative to standard curves.

Western Blot Analysis

Activated PBMC or $CD4^+$ T cells (both 5×10^6/ml) were incubated for different times in the presence or absence of GXMGal (10 μg/ml), MTX (10 ng/ml), DEX (10 nM) or FLLL31 (5 μM). After incubation, proteins were extracted and subjected to western blotting as previously described [20]. The membranes were incubated overnight with polyclonal Abs to pSTAT3 (goat; Tyr 705), STAT3 (rabbit), FOXP3 (rabbit), T-bet (rabbit) (all dilution 1/200; all Santa Cruz Biotechnology, Delaware Avenue, Santa Cruz, CA) in blocking buffer. Immuno-reactive bands were visualized and quantified by Chemidoc Instrument (Bio-Rad Laboratories, Hercules, CA) [28].

Flow Cytometry Analysis

Activated PBMC (1×10^6/ml) were incubated for 2 or 18 h in the presence or absence of GXMGal (10 μg/ml) or MTX (10 ng/ml). After incubation, cells were fixed with 1.5% formalin for 10 min at room temperature (RT), washed and incubated with FITC-labelled mAb to human CD4, APC-labelled mAb to human CD25 (both mouse IgG1 isotype; 2 μl/tube; ImmunoTools) or PerCP-Cy5.5 labelled mAb to human CD127 (mouse IgG1, 5 μl/tube; eBioscience) for 20 min at RT. After incubation, cells were treated as previously described [29] and incubated with PE-labelled mAb to human FOXP3 (mouse IgG1 isotype; 20 μl/tube) (BD Biosciences, San Jose, CA). In selected experiments, activated purified Treg (1×10^6/ml) from RA were treated or not with GXMGal (10 μg/ml) for 18 h and then incubated with PE-labelled mAb to human FOXP3 (mouse IgG1 isotype; 20 μl/tube) (BD Biosciences) for 20 min on ice. After incubation, cells were analyzed by flow cytometry using FACSCalibur (BD Biosciences). Data are expressed as percentage of positive cells or as mean of fluorescence intensity (MFI). Autofluorescence and control staining were evaluated as previously described [29].

Intracellular staining

Activated purified $CD4^+$ T cells (1×10^6/ml) were incubated for 18 or 96 h in the presence or absence of GXMGal (10 μg/ml) or MTX (10 ng/ml). Brefeldin A (10 μg/ml) was added 2 h after GXMGal or MTX stimulation [30]. After incubation, cells were fixed with 1.5% formalin for 10 min at RT, washed and incubated with APC-labelled mAb to human CD25 (mouse IgG1 isotype; 2 μl/tube; ImmunoTools) for 20 min at RT. After incubation, cells were treated as previously described [29] and incubated with PE-labelled mAb to human FOXP3 (mouse IgG1 isotype; 20 μl/tube) (BD Biosciences), with purified mAbs to human IL-10 (mouse IgG2b isotype, 2 μg/ml) or TGF-β1 (mouse IgG1 isotype, 25 μg/ml) (both Sigma-Aldrich) [29] or in selected experiments with FITC-labelled mAb to human IFN-γ (mouse IgG_{2b} isotype; 10 μl/tube) (Sigma-Aldrich) and with Ab to T-bet (rabbit) (1/50;

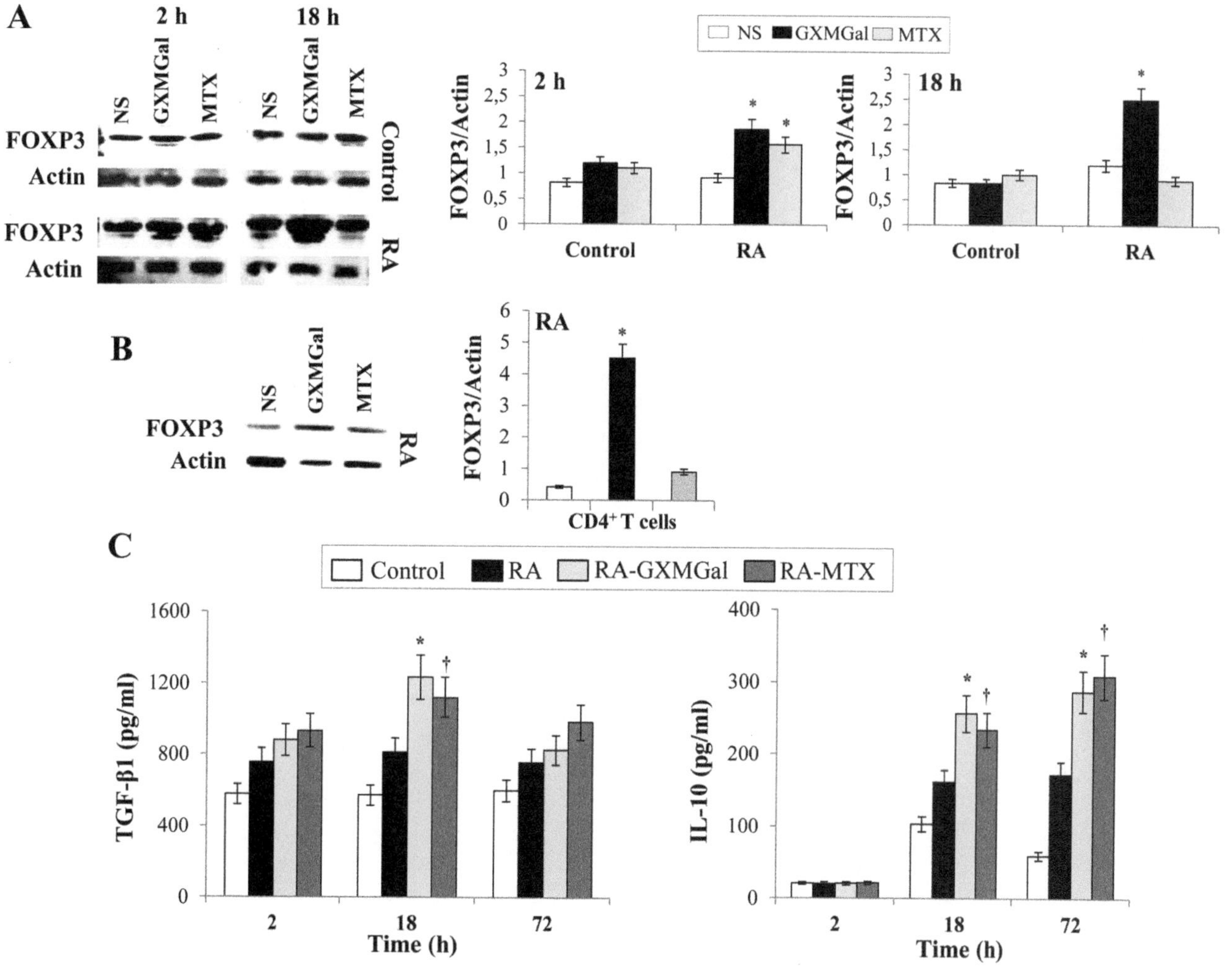

Figure 1. GXMGal effect on Treg cell response. Activated PBMC (**A** and **C**) or purified CD4$^+$ T cells (**B**) (both 5×10^6/ml) from Control and RA were incubated for 2, 18 and 72 h in the presence or absence (NS) of GXMGal (10 µg/ml) or MTX (10 ng/ml). After 2 and 18 h (**A**) or 18 h (**B**) of incubation, cell lysates were analyzed by western blotting. Membranes were incubated with Ab to FOXP3. Actin was used as an internal loading control. Normalization was shown as mean ± SEM of five independent experiments (**A** and **B**). *, $p<0.05$ (triplicate samples of 5 different Control and RA; RA treated *vs* untreated cells). Culture supernatants were collected after 2, 18 and 72 h to test TGF-β1 and IL-10 levels by specific ELISA assays. *, $p<0.05$ (triplicate samples of 7 different Control and RA; RA GXMGal-treated *vs* untreated cells); †, $p<0.05$ (triplicate samples of 7 different Control and RA; RA MTX-treated *vs* untreated cells) (**C**).

Santa Cruz) for 20 min on ice followed by Cy3 labelled conjugated affinity purified secondary antibody (dil. 1/250; Chemicon Int.). Autofluorescence and control staining were evaluated as previously described [29].

Apoptosis

Naïve or activated CD4$^+$CD25$^+$ Treg cells were stimulated in the presence or absence of GXMGal (10 µg/ml) or MTX (10 ng/ml). The percentage of cells undergoing apoptosis was evaluated by flow cytometry analysis as previously described [29].

CFSE-based suppression assays

CD4$^+$ responder T cells (Tresp) (1×10^6/ml) were stained with CFSE (1 µM) (Sigma-Aldrich) according to the manufacturer's instructions [31] and then seeded in 96-well culture plates precoated with mAbs to CD3 plus CD28 (both 2 µg/ml) and activated for 30 min with PHA (10 µg/ml) (Sigma-Aldrich) at 37°C plus 5% CO_2 in complete medium. Cells were then washed and co-cultured for 96 h in the presence or absence of autologous CD4$^+$CD25$^+$ Treg cells (Tresp/Treg: 16/1) that have been pretreated for 18 h in the presence or absence of GXMGal (10 µg/ml) or MTX (10 ng/ml). After 96 h the suppressive activity of CD4$^+$CD25$^+$ Treg cells was evaluated by measuring the percentage of inhibition of proliferation of CD4$^+$ Tresp cells by flow cytometry analysis [32]. After 96 h the percentage of CFSE-stained CD4$^+$CD25$^+$ Treg cells proliferation was determined as above described.

Statistical analysis

The results reported in the bar graphs are the mean ± SEM from triplicate samples of 5–10 different RA patients or Controls. Mann-Whitney U test was used for statistical analysis, except for the determination of CD25$^+$FOXP3$^+$ and CD25$^-$FOXP3$^+$ cells in which the statistic was calculated according to Student's t test.

A value of $p<0.05$ was considered significant.

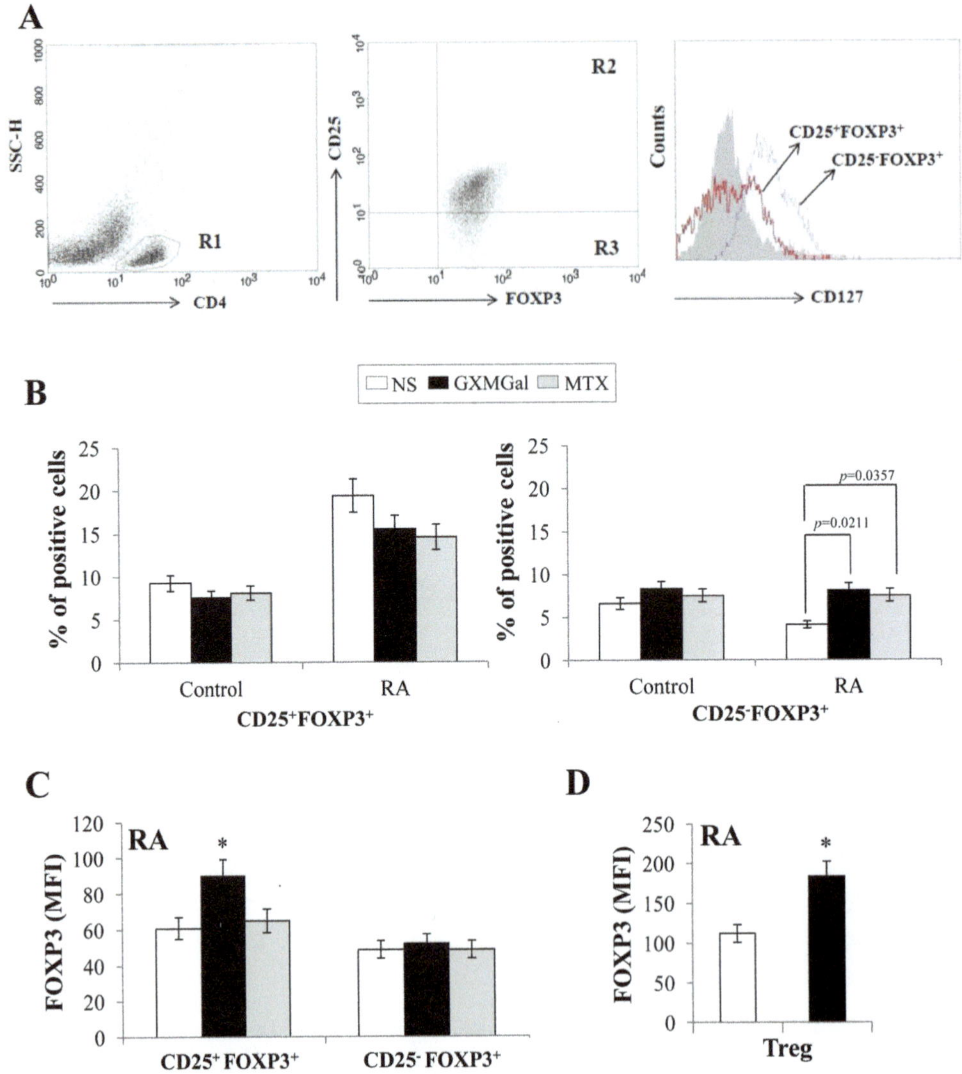

Figure 2. GXMGal effect on different subsets of Treg cells. Activated PBMC (1×10^6/ml) from Control and RA were incubated for 2 h in the presence or absence (NS) of GXMGal (10 μg/ml) or MTX (10 ng/ml). After incubation, cells were stained for cell surface expression of CD4, CD25 and CD127 and then intracellular stained for FOXP3. During the acquisition step a population of PBMC enriched of $CD4^+$ T cells was obtained. For analysis, the $CD4^+$ lymphocytes were gated on PBMC (based on side light scatter and CD4 staining: R1) and analyzed for CD25 and FOXP3 expression ($CD25^+FOXP3^+$: R2 and $CD25^-FOXP3^+$: R3). The expression of CD127 was shown as FACS histograms in R2 and R3 cells. The gating strategy was shown (**A**). The percentage of $CD25^+FOXP3^+$ and $CD25^-FOXP3^+$ cells are shown as mean ± SEM of ten independent experiments. $p = 0.0211$ (triplicate samples of 10 different Control and RA; RA GXMGal-treated *vs* untreated cells); $p = 0.0357$ (triplicate samples of 10 different Control and RA; RA MTX-treated *vs* untreated cells (**B**). The mean of fluorescence intensity (MFI) of FOXP3 in $CD25^+FOXP3^+$ and $CD25^-FOXP3^+$ cells (**C**) or magnetically purified Treg (**D**) from RA after 18 h of GXMGal or MTX treatment was shown as mean ± SEM of five independent experiments. *, $p <$ 0.05 (triplicate samples of 5 different RA; RA GXMGal-treated *vs* untreated cells).

Results

Firstly, we analyzed the effect of GXMGal on FOXP3 expression in PBMC and $CD4^+$ T cells from RA patients. PBMC from RA patients and from healthy donors (Control) were treated with GXMGal or MTX for 2 and 18 h and the expression of FOXP3 was evaluated. The results showed that GXMGal markedly induced FOXP3 activation after 2 and 18 h of incubation, while MTX only after 2 h (Fig. 1A). GXMGal and MTX treatment did not produce any modulation on PBMC from Control. GXMGal-induced FOXP3 activation at 18 h was also confirmed by using purified $CD4^+$ T cells from RA (Fig. 1B). Furthermore, we analyzed key cytokines such as TGF-β1 and IL-10 involved in Treg activation [33]. To this purpose PBMC were treated with GXMGal for 2, 18 and 72 h and the possible modulation of TGF-β1 and IL-10 production was tested. Both cytokines were produced at higher levels in culture supernatants of PBMC from RA patients with respect to Control. The production of TGF-β1 and IL-10 was further enhanced by GXMGal treatment after 18 h or 18 and 72 h of incubation respectively (Fig. 1C). The lack of the increased production of TGF-β1 after 72 h of incubation could be due to the reutilization of this cytokine by the cells during the incubation period. MTX produced similar effects.

The proportion of conventional Treg, identified by the expression of CD25 molecule and FOXP3 ($CD25^+FOXP3^+$), and non-conventional Treg $CD25^-FOXP3^+$ was tested after

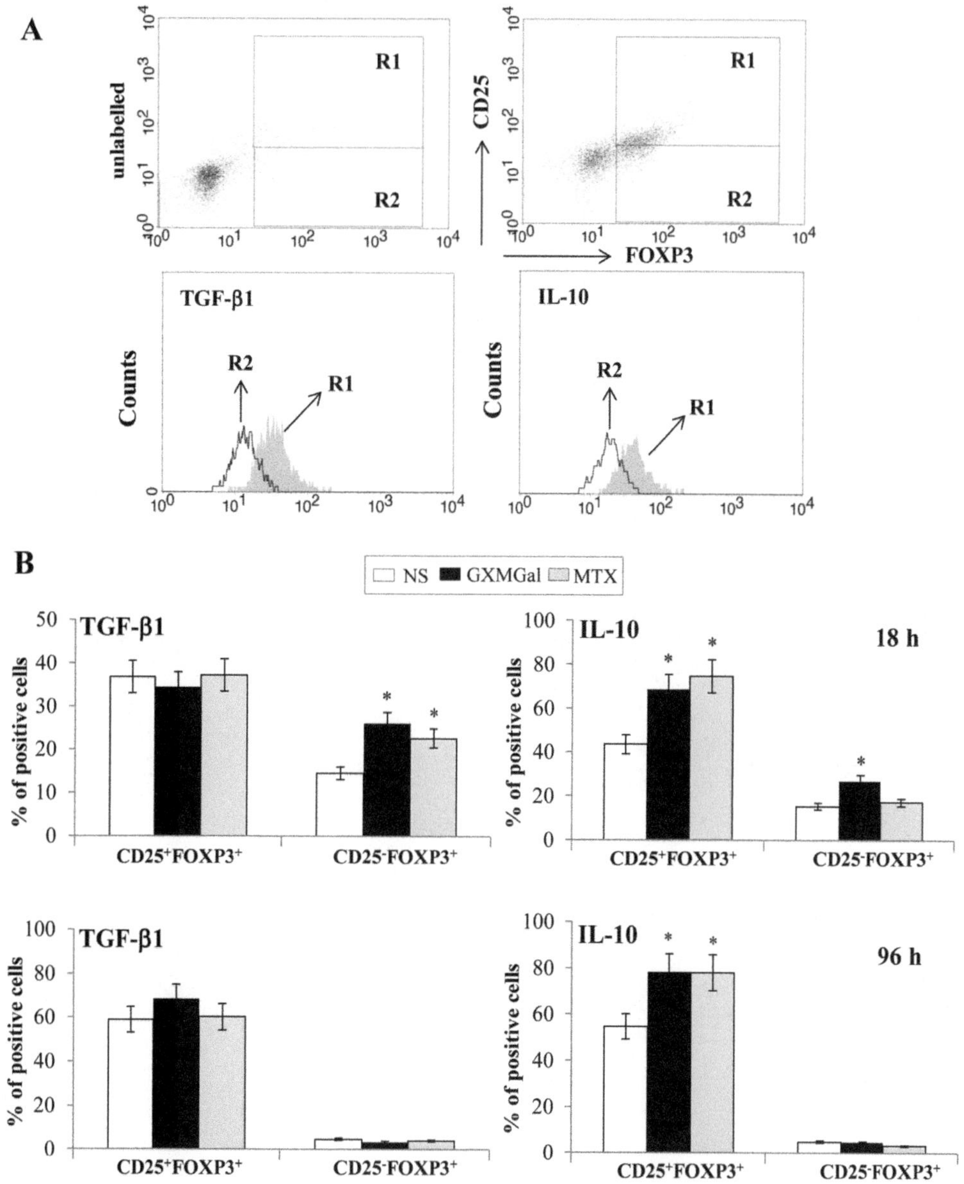

Figure 3. GXMGal effect on Treg cell intracellular cytokines production. Activated purified CD4$^+$ T cells (1×10^6/ml) from RA were incubated for 18 or 96 h in the presence or absence (NS) of GXMGal (10 µg/ml) or MTX (10 ng/ml). After incubation, cells were stained for cell surface expression of CD25 then intracellular stained for FOXP3 and TGF-β1 or IL-10. For the analysis of intracellular cytokines, CD25$^+$FOXP3$^+$ (R1) and CD25$^-$FOXP3$^+$ (R2) cells were gated on purified CD4$^+$ T cells. The gating strategy was shown (**A**). The percentage of intracellular TGF-β1 and IL-10 on CD25$^+$FOXP3$^+$ and CD25$^-$FOXP3 positive cells were shown after 18 h or 96 h (**B**) as mean ± SEM of ten independent experiments. *, $p<0.05$ (triplicate samples of 10 different RA; treated *vs* untreated cells).

GXMGal treatment in PBMC from RA patients and Control. CD4$^+$ T cells were gated on PBMC and analyzed for CD25, FOXP3 and CD127 [33] expression (Fig. 2A). It is known that Treg CD25$^+$FOXP3$^+$ are CD127^{low} [34]. As shown in Figure 2B the treatment with GXMGal for 2 h did not modulate the percentage of CD25$^+$FOXP3$^+$ Treg; however, GXMGal increased the percentage of non-conventional CD25$^-$FOXP3$^+$ Treg. The prolonged treatment with GXMGal (18 h) did not modulate the percentage of CD25$^+$FOXP3$^+$ or CD25$^-$FOXP3$^+$ Treg (not shown). Similar effect was observed by using MTX (Fig. 2B). GXMGal-induced FOXP3 expression at 18 h was evidenced in CD25$^+$FOXP3$^+$ but not in CD25$^-$FOXP3$^+$ Treg from RA (Fig. 2C). This was confirmed by using magnetically purified Treg from RA (Fig. 2D). Given that we previously demonstrated that GXMGal is able to induce apoptosis of activated T cells [19,29], we evaluated whether GXMGal affects apoptosis of Treg. Our results showed that treatment with GXMGal or MTX did not modulate neither apoptosis of naïve and activated RA Treg nor their proliferation (data not shown).

Given that TGF-β1 and IL-10 production was determined in PBMC supernatants (Fig. 1C), we analyzed the level of these cytokines in both CD25$^+$FOXP3$^+$ and CD25$^-$FOXP3$^+$ cells. For the analysis of intracellular cytokines, CD25$^+$FOXP3$^+$ (R1) and CD25$^-$FOXP3$^+$ (R2) were gated on magnetically purified CD4$^+$ T cells (Fig. 3A). After 18 h of incubation, both GXMGal and MTX induced a significant increase of intracellular TGF-β1

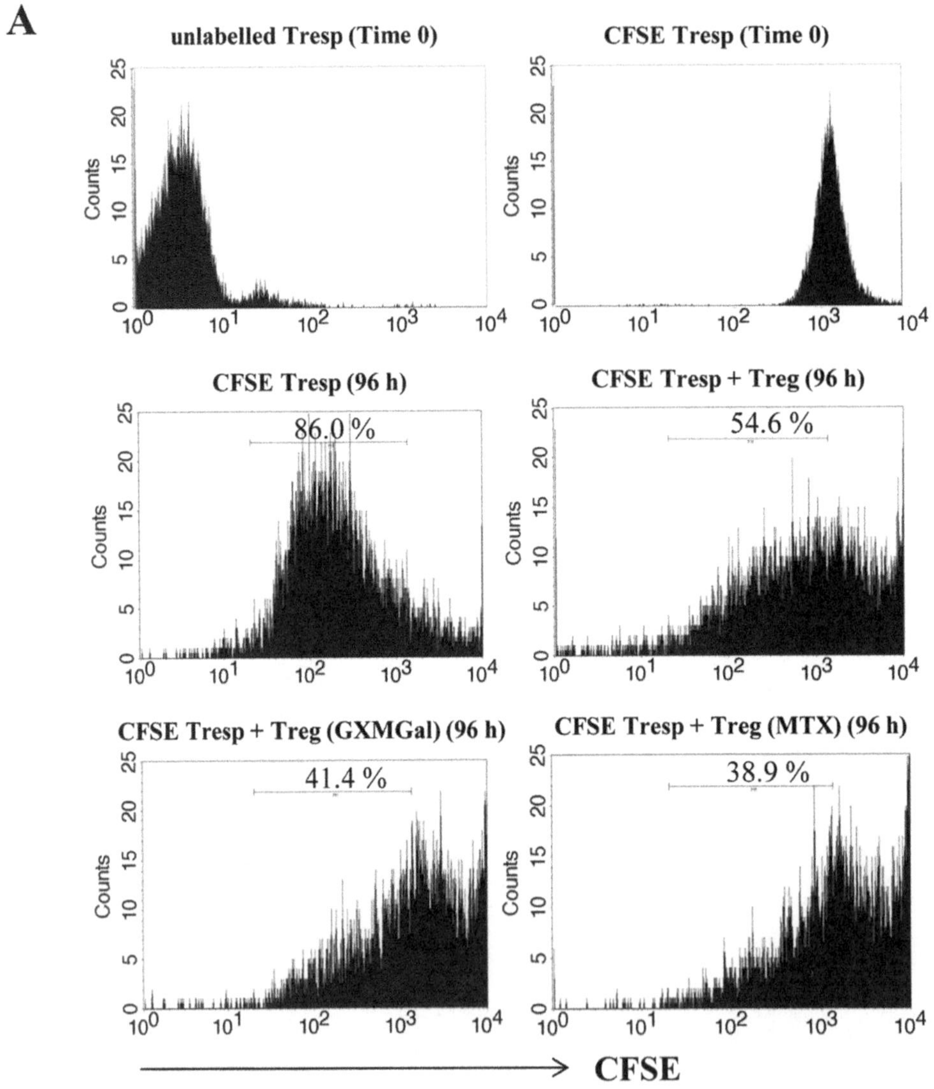

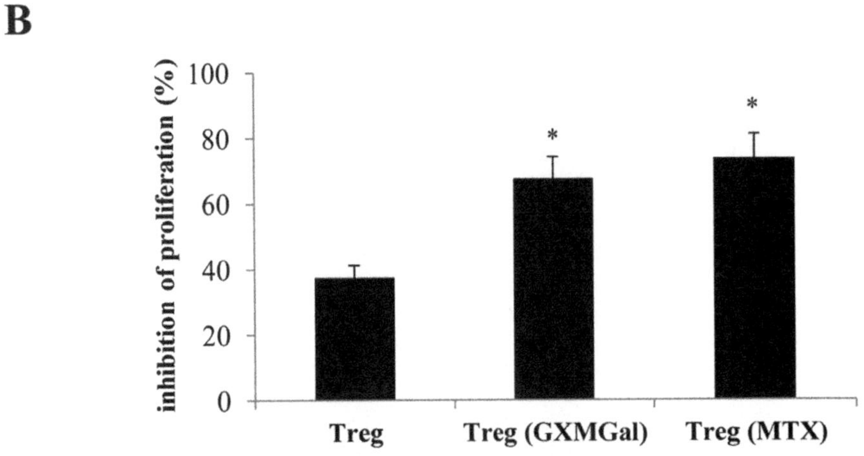

Figure 4. GXMGal effect on Treg cell suppressive activity. Activated RA purified CD4$^+$ T cells (1×10^6/ml) were stained with CFSE (1 μM) and then co-cultured for 96 h in the presence or absence of magnetically purified autologous RA Treg cells (Tresp/Treg: 16/1) that have been pre-treated for 18 h in the presence or absence of GXMGal (10 μg/ml) or MTX (10 ng/ml). After 96 h the suppressive activity of Treg cells was evaluated by measuring the percentage of inhibition of proliferation of CD4$^+$ responder T cells (Tresp). Representative CFSE histograms show the distribution of proliferating CFSE-labelled Tresp according to the intensity of the CFSE label from the start of the experiment (Time 0) until 96 h. Given that the initial cell labelling is fairly homogeneous, each CFSE peak represents a cohort of cells that proceed synchronously through the division rounds. The areas within each histograms delimitated by the marker represent the percentage of divided CFSE-labeled cells (**A**). Mean ± SEM of percentage of proliferation inhibition is shown as bar graph (**B**). *, $p<0.05$ (triplicate samples of 10 different RA; treated *vs* untreated cells).

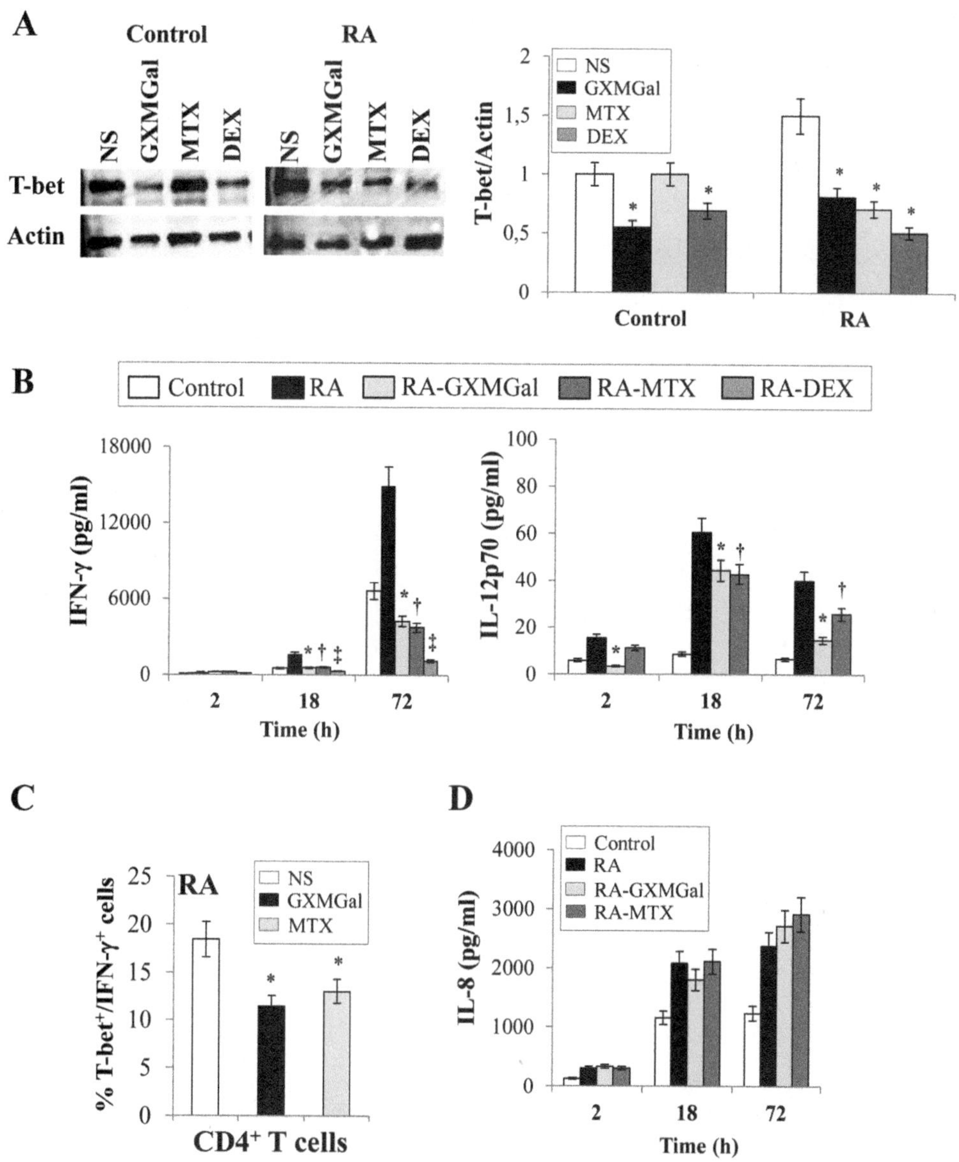

Figure 5. GXMGal effect on Th1 response. Activated PBMC (**A**, **B** and **D**) (5×10^6/ml) from Control and RA were incubated for 20 min, 2, 18 and 72 h in the presence or absence (NS) of GXMGal (10 μg/ml), MTX (10 ng/ml) or DEX (10 nM). After 20 min of incubation, cell lysates were analyzed by western blotting. Membranes were incubated with Ab to T-bet. Actin was used as an internal loading control. Normalization was shown as mean ± SEM of five independent experiments. *, $p<0.05$ (triplicate samples of 5 different Control and RA; treated *vs* untreated cells) (**A**). Culture supernatants were collected after 2, 18 and 72 h to test IFN-γ, IL-12p70 (**B**) and IL-8 (**D**) levels by specific ELISA assays. *, $p<0.05$ (triplicate samples of 7 different Control and RA; RA GXMGal-treated *vs* untreated cells); †, $p<0.05$ (triplicate samples of 7 different Control and RA; RA MTX-treated *vs* untreated cells); ‡, $p<0.05$ (triplicate samples of 7 different Control and RA; RA DEX-treated *vs* untreated cells). Activated purified $CD4^+$ T cells (1×10^6/ml) (**C**) from RA were stimulated as above described and intracellular stained for T-bet and IFN-γ. The percentage of T-bet$^+$/IFN-γ$^+$ $CD4^+$ T cells from RA after 18 h of GXMGal or MTX treatment was shown as mean ± SEM of five independent experiments. *, $p<0.05$ (triplicate samples of five different RA; treated *vs* untreated cells).

production in purified $CD25^-FOXP3^+$ cells, but they did not modulate this cytokine in purified $CD25^+FOXP3^+$ cells (Fig 3B). Moreover, intracellular IL-10 was significantly increased by GXMGal stimulation in both $CD25^+FOXP3^+$ and $CD25^-FOXP3^+$ cells. MTX induced a significant increase of intracellular IL-10 only in $CD25^+FOXP3^+$ cells (Fig. 3B). Moreover, when the treatment with GXMGal or MTX was prolonged till 96 h, a persistence of intracellular increase of IL-10 was detected only in $CD25^+FOXP3^+$ cells. At this time, no modulation of TGF-β1 was observed in both $CD25^+FOXP3^+$ and $CD25^-FOXP3^+$ cells (Fig. 3B). Moreover, we verified the *in vitro* functional activity of Treg towards autologous responder T cells (Tresp). RA activated CFSE-labelled Tresp were cultured for 96 h in the presence or absence of autologous Treg pre-treated for 18 h with or without GXMGal or MTX. Our data demonstrated that proliferation of RA Tresp cells was suppressed by Treg and this effect was significantly potentiated when Treg cells were pre-treated with GXMGal or MTX (Fig. 4A and B). Since it is recognized that Th1 cells play an important pro-inflammatory role in the pathogenesis of RA, the effect of GXMGal on Th1

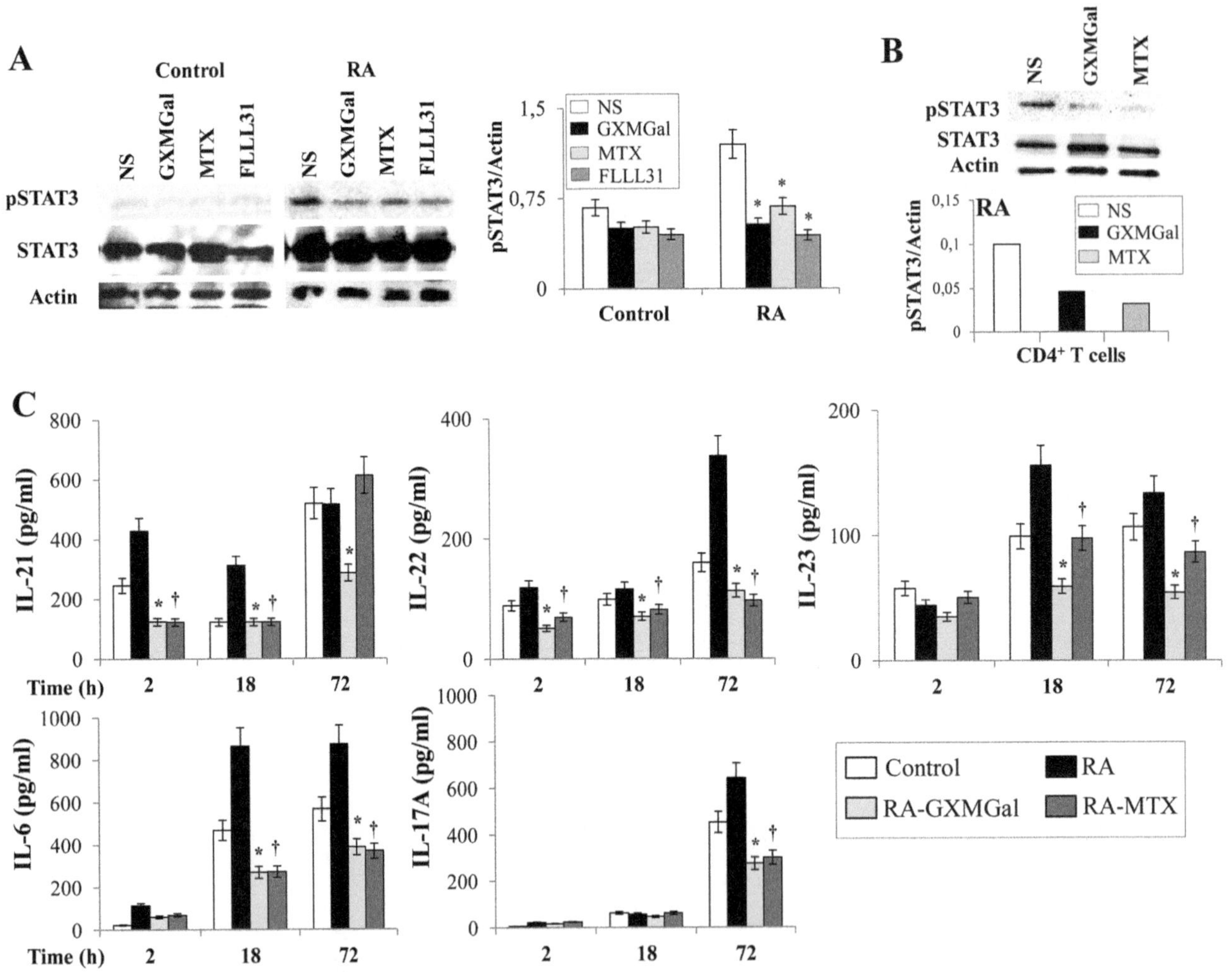

Figure 6. GXMGal effect on Th17 response. Activated PBMC (**A** and **C**) or purified $CD4^+$ T cells (**B**) (both 5×10^6/ml) from Control and RA were incubated for 2, 18 and 72 h in the presence or absence (NS) of GXMGal (10 µg/ml), MTX (10 ng/ml) or FLLL31 (5 µM). After 18 h of incubation, cell lysates were analyzed by western blotting. Membranes were incubated with Abs to pSTAT3 and STAT3. Actin was used as an internal loading control. Normalization was shown as mean ± SEM of five independent experiments (**A**) or as one representative experiment of three with similar results (**B**). *, $p<0.05$ (triplicate samples of 5 different Control and RA; RA treated *vs* untreated cells). Culture supernatants were collected after 2, 18 and 72 h to test IL-21, IL-22, IL-23, IL-6 and IL-17A levels by specific ELISA assays. *, $p<0.05$ (triplicate samples of 7 different Control and RA; RA GXMGal-treated *vs* untreated cells); †, $p<0.05$ (triplicate samples of 7 different Control and RA; RA MTX-treated *vs* untreated cells) (**C**).

differentiation was also evaluated. PBMC from RA patients and Control were treated with GXMGal, MTX and DEX for 20 min. It is well established that DEX can inhibit Th1 activation [27] and therefore DEX was used as inhibitor of T-box-containing protein expressed in T cells (T-bet) activation, exclusively expressed in Th1 cells. The results showed that GXMGal treatment was able to significantly suppress T-bet activation in PBMC from RA and Control. A similar effect was observed with DEX, whereas MTX produced inhibitory effects only in PBMC from RA patients (Fig. 5A). To further investigate the role of GXMGal in Th1 response, we analyzed the production of IFN-γ and IL-12p70, that were produced at higher levels in PBMC culture supernatants from RA compared to Control, after 18 and 72 h or 2, 18 and 72 h, respectively (Fig. 5B). A significant inhibition of IFN-γ production was observed after treatment with GXMGal or MTX after 18 and 72 h of incubation. As expected, DEX significantly reduced IFN-γ production (Fig. 5B). IL-12p70 was significantly inhibited by GXMGal at all times tested and by MTX after 18 and 72 h of incubation (Fig. 5B). GXMGal and MTX were also able to significantly reduce the percentage of T-bet$^+$/IFN-γ^+ $CD4^+$ T cells from RA after 18 h of incubation (Fig. 5C). We also tested IL-8 production by PBMC from RA patients and Control after GXMGal stimulation. Although IL-8 production was higher in RA than Control PBMC, the levels of this cytokine were not modulated neither by GXMGal nor MTX treatment at all times tested (Fig. 5D).

In addition to Th1 activation, Th17 cell activation plays a key role in the pathogenesis of arthritis [35]. To verify whether a down-regulation of Th17 occurs in our experimental condition after GXMGal treatment, we analyzed pSTAT3 activation, a master regulator of Th17 cells, by using PBMC from RA patients. FLLL31, a well-known inhibitor of STAT3 activation [36], was used as negative control. PBMC were stimulated with GXMGal and the pSTAT3 activator and Th17-related cytokines were tested. The results showed that pSTAT3 expression was down-regulated by GXMGal only in PBMC from RA patients, while no modulation was observed in PBMC from Control (Fig. 6A). Similar effects were observed after stimulation with FLLL31 or

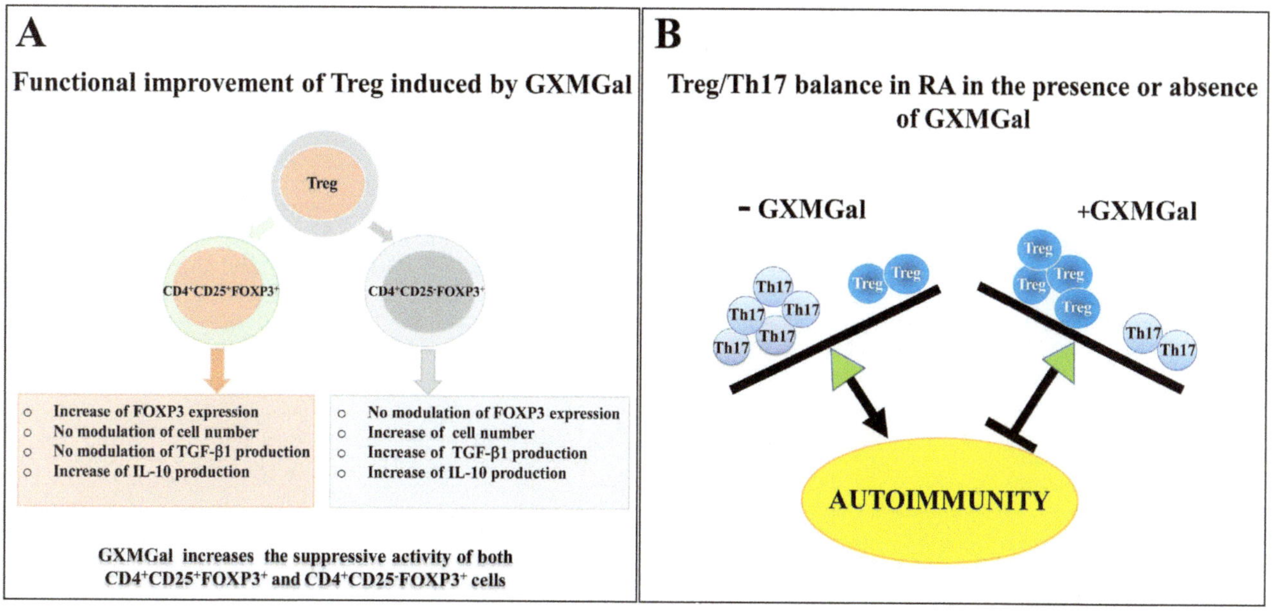

Figure 7. Schematic representation of GXMGal effects on Treg (A) and on Treg/Th17 balance (B).

MTX (Fig. 6A). GXMGal-induced pSTAT3 inactivation at 18 h was also confirmed by using purified $CD4^+$ T cells from RA (Fig. 6B). Subsequently, the production of cytokines involved in Th17 differentiation and activity were analyzed in PBMC from RA patients. Higher levels of IL-21 were produced by RA PBMC after 2 and 18 h with respect to Control; higher levels of IL-23 and IL-6 were produced by PBMC from RA patients after 18 and 72 h as compared to Control, while a significant increase of IL-22 and IL-17A was evidenced only after 72 h (Fig. 6C).

We observed an early inhibition (after 2 h) of IL-21 and IL-22 induced by GXMGal in PBMC from RA that persisted for 18 and 72 h. Moreover, the production of IL-6 and IL-23 was significantly inhibited after 18 and 72 h, while suppression of IL-17A was evidenced only after 72 h of GXMGal treatment (Fig. 6C). MTX showed the same kinetics of IL-22, IL-23, IL-6 and IL-17A inhibition than that observed for GXMGal, except for IL-21 after 72 h of incubation (Fig. 6C).

Discussion

FOXP3 is thought to be the main marker of Treg, since it plays a critical role in their development and maturation [37]. Compelling evidence show that FOXP3-deficient mice develop autoimmune disease [38,39]. The role of Treg in RA has been partially elucidated and different results have been reported. In particular, a decreased number of Treg in the blood of RA patients has been observed [12]; however, other reports show high levels of circulating conventional $CD4^+CD25^+FOXP3^+$ Treg cells in RA [13,14], while additional studies reported an unaltered number [40]. Because of these controversial results about the number of circulating Treg cells, the interpretation of the data is problematic. Nevertheless, compelling evidence has emerged about the impaired function of these cells in RA patients [6]. Recent investigations revealed that a potentiation of Treg cells is beneficial in RA [40,41]. In this study we report that the treatment with GXMGal induces strong and long-lasting increase of FOXP3 expression in RA Treg cells still evident 18 h after stimulation. This was accompanied by early and transient enhancement of TGF-β1 production and long-lasting production of IL-10. The major source of early production of TGF-β1 appeared to be the $CD4^+CD25^-FOXP3^+$ T cell subset. On the contrary, the early production of IL-10 seems to be due to both $CD4^+CD25^+FOXP3^+$ and $CD4^+CD25^-FOXP3^+$ cells, although only $CD4^+CD25^+FOXP3^+$ cells seemed to be responsible of its long-lasting production. We previously demonstrated that GXMGal inhibits pro-inflammatory cytokine secretion. Since the suppressive activity of Treg cells could be counteracted by inflammatory mediators [42,43], particularly by TNF-α [44], it is possible that the increased activity of Treg cells induced by GXMGal could also include the previously described inhibition of TNF-α [1]. Accordingly, the treatment of RA subjects with an anti-TNF-α specific antibody was shown to restore Treg cell function via increased expression of FOXP3 phosphorylation [45]. Similarly, GXMGal could retain beneficial effects similar to those of anti-TNF-α treatment by influencing Treg cell activity. GXMGal did not modulate the percentage of $CD4^+CD25^+FOXP3^+$ cells, while atypical $CD4^+CD25^-FOXP3^+$ cells appeared to be numerically increased after GXMGal addition. The percentage of both cells was calculated on $CD4^+$ T cells gated on PBMC, suggesting that the small and not statistically significant decline of $CD4^+CD25^+FOXP3^+$, observed after GXMGal treatment, could at least in part account for the increased number of $CD4^+CD25^-FOXP3^+$; however it is likely that besides the shift of $CD4^+CD25^+FOXP3^+$ into $CD4^+CD25^-FOXP3^+$, there is also an increase of the $CD4^+CD25^-FOXP3^+$ cell number *per se*. Moreover, the significant increased expression of FOXP3 observed in conventional RA Treg cells after 18 h of GXMGal treatment clearly demonstrated that the associated increase of suppressive activity of all Treg is ascribed to $CD4^+CD25^+FOXP3^+$ cells. GXMGal effects on different Treg subsets have been summarized in Figure 7.

MTX, widely accepted as the "gold standard" treatment in RA, can affect Treg cells [46] by promoting immunotolerance, despite the mechanisms are not yet fully elucidated. To our knowledge this is the first demonstration that MTX treatment increases the

$CD4^+CD25^-FOXP3^+$ fraction of the Treg cell population. Indeed, we found that the anti-inflammatory effects of GXMGal on T cells from RA were quite similar to that observed for MTX. GXMGal differed from MTX just in a few effects, such as increased production of IL-10 in atypical Treg. The fact that GXMGal retains multiple regulatory effects similar to that of MTX and anti-TNF-α agents suggests that GXMGal treatment may provide the combined beneficial effects of MTX and anti-TNF-α. Recently, we demonstrated that GXMGal inhibits Th17 activation [20] from RA patients and in the present study we confirm and extend our previously published data by demonstrating that the inhibition of Th17 was related to the inhibition of cytokines such as IL-21, IL-22 and IL-23. Moreover, we also provide evidence that in peripheral T cells from RA, GXMGal inhibits Th1 differentiation in terms of T-bet expression and IL-12p70 and IFN-γ production. Therefore, the demonstration of a Th1-cell suppression combined with a Th17-cell down-regulation reinforces the idea of a possible therapeutic use of GXMGal in RA and other inflammatory chronic disorders. GXMGal-treated Treg cells showed increased suppressive activity manifested by marked inhibition of effector T-cell proliferation. It is known that the total Treg cell pool contains a population of $CD45RA^+$ and $CD45RO^+$ Treg cells. $CD45RA^+$ Treg cells were found to be less proliferative than their $CD45RO^+$ counterparts [47]. In multiple sclerosis an impairment of suppressive activity of naïve $CD45RA^+$ Treg cells was reported, thereby suggesting that this population may be involved in the pathogenesis of autoimmune disorders [48,49]. GXMGal is able to bind to CD45RA and CD45RO isoforms and we recently suggested that activated T cells expressing the CD45RO molecule could be the main target of GXMGal-induced apoptosis [20]. Since the Treg population circulating in RA belongs to (naïve) resting CD45RA phenotype [50], it is conceivable that GXMGal binds to these cells and increases their function without inducing apoptosis. Therefore these results suggest that in RA patients GXMGal affects Treg function in a two ways: indirectly by inhibition of inflammatory T cells differentiation such as Th1 and Th17 and directly by binding to CD45RA improving activity of Treg. In this study the effect of GXMGal was specifically observed on Treg population as demonstrated by: i) enhanced production of TGF-β1, ii) increased expression of FOXP3 and iii) improved suppression activity on effector T cells. Future studies will be devoted to evaluate the effect of GXMGal in an *in vivo* experimental model of rheumatoid arthritis. Collectively these data highlight the potential for using GXMGal to enhance Treg activity, inactivate pathogenic T cells and halt the disease process in autoimmunity.

Author Contributions

Conceived and designed the experiments: EP EG AV RG EC SP EB AC. Performed the experiments: EP EG AA EB SC EC SP. Analyzed the data: EP EG AA EC SP AV AC RG EB SC. Contributed reagents/materials/analysis tools: AV AC RG SC. Wrote the paper: EP EG AV RG AC AA.

References

1. Wehrens EJ, van Wijk F, Roord ST, Albani S, Prakken BJ (2010) Treating arthritis by immunomodulation: is there a role for regulatory T cells? Rheumatology (Oxford) 49: 1632–1644.
2. Chen G, Zhang X, Li R, Fang L, Niu X, et al. (2010) Role of osteopontin in synovial Th17 differentiation in rheumatoid arthritis. Arthritis Rheum 62: 2900–2908.
3. Alunno A, Bartoloni E, Bistoni O, Nocentini G, Ronchetti S, et al. (2012) Balance between regulatory T and Th17 cells in systemic lupus erythematosus: the old and the new. Clin Dev Immunol 2012: 823085.
4. Yang J, Yang X, Zou H, Chu Y, Li M (2011) Recovery of the immune balance between Th17 and regulatory T cells as a treatment for systemic lupus erythematosus. Rheumatology (Oxford) 50: 1366–1372.
5. Yang J, Chu Y, Yang X, Gao D, Zhu L, et al. (2009) Th17 and natural Treg cell population dynamics in systemic lupus erythematosus. Arthritis Rheum 60: 1472–1483.
6. Nistala K, Wedderburn LR (2009) Th17 and regulatory T cells: rebalancing pro- and anti-inflammatory forces in autoimmune arthritis. Rheumatology (Oxford) 48: 602–606.
7. de Goer de Herve MG, Gonzales E, Hendel-Chavez H, Decline JL, Mourier O, et al. (2010) CD25 appears non essential for human peripheral T(reg) maintenance in vivo. PLoS One 5: e11784.
8. Sakaguchi S, Sakaguchi N, Asano M, Itoh M, Toda M (1995) Immunologic self-tolerance maintained by activated T cells expressing IL-2 receptor alpha-chains (CD25). Breakdown of a single mechanism of self-tolerance causes various autoimmune diseases. J Immunol 155: 1151–1164.
9. Geiger TL, Tauro S (2012) Nature and nurture in Foxp3(+) regulatory T cell development, stability, and function. Hum Immunol 73: 232–239.
10. Sakaguchi S, Miyara M, Costantino CM, Hafler DA (2010) FOXP3+ regulatory T cells in the human immune system. Nat Rev Immunol 10: 490–500.
11. Zelenay S, Lopes-Carvalho T, Caramalho I, Moraes-Fontes MF, Rebelo M, et al. (2005) Foxp3+ CD25- CD4 T cells constitute a reservoir of committed regulatory cells that regain CD25 expression upon homeostatic expansion. Proc Natl Acad Sci U S A 102: 4091–4096.
12. Cao D, van Vollenhoven R, Klareskog L, Trollmo C, Malmstrom V (2004) CD25brightCD4+ regulatory T cells are enriched in inflamed joints of patients with chronic rheumatic disease. Arthritis Res Ther 6: R335–346.
13. Xinqiang S, Fei L, Nan L, Yuan L, Fang Y, et al. (2010) Therapeutic efficacy of experimental rheumatoid arthritis with low-dose methotrexate by increasing partially CD4+CD25+ Treg cells and inducing Th1 to Th2 shift in both cells and cytokines. Biomed Pharmacother 64: 463–471.
14. Han GM, O'Neil-Andersen NJ, Zurier RB, Lawrence DA (2008) CD4+ CD25high T cell numbers are enriched in the peripheral blood of patients with rheumatoid arthritis. Cell Immunol 253: 92–101.
15. Anderson AE, Isaacs JD (2008) Tregs and rheumatoid arthritis. Acta Reumatol Port 33: 17–33.
16. Herman S, Zurgil N, Langevitz P, Ehrenfeld M, Deutsch M (2008) Methotrexate selectively modulates TH1/TH2 balance in active rheumatoid arthritis patients. Clin Exp Rheumatol 26: 317–323.
17. Fites JS, Ramsey JP, Holden WM, Collier SP, Sutherland DM, et al. (2013) The invasive chytrid fungus of amphibians paralyzes lymphocyte responses. Science 342: 366–369.
18. Vecchiarelli A, Pericolini E, Gabrielli E, Kenno S, Perito S, et al. (2013) Elucidating the immunological function of the Cryptococcus neoformans capsule. Future Microbiol 8: 1107–1116.
19. Pericolini E, Gabrielli E, Cenci E, De Jesus M, Bistoni F, et al. (2009) Involvement of glycoreceptors in galactoxylomannan-induced T cell death. J Immunol 182: 6003–6010.
20. Pericolini E, Alunno A, Gabrielli E, Bartoloni E, Cenci E, et al. (2013) The microbial capsular polysaccharide galactoxylomannan inhibits IL-17A production in circulating T cells from rheumatoid arthritis patients. PLoS One 8: e53336.
21. Heiss C, Klutts JS, Wang Z, Doering TL, Azadi P (2009) The structure of Cryptococcus neoformans galactoxylomannan contains beta-D-glucuronic acid. Carbohydr Res 344: 915–920.
22. De Jesus M, Nicola AM, Frases S, Lee IR, Mieses S, et al. (2009) Galactoxylomannan-mediated immunological paralysis results from specific B cell depletion in the context of widespread immune system damage. J Immunol 183: 3885–3894.
23. James PG, Cherniak R (1992) Galactoxylomannans of Cryptococcus neoformans. Infect Immun 60: 1084–1088.
24. Pericolini E, Cenci E, Monari C, De Jesus M, Bistoni F, et al. (2006) Cryptococcus neoformans capsular polysaccharide component galactoxylomannan induces apoptosis of human T-cells through activation of caspase-8. Cell Microbiol 8: 267–275.
25. Arnett FC, Edworthy SM, Bloch DA, McShane DJ, Fries JF, et al. (1988) The American Rheumatism Association 1987 revised criteria for the classification of rheumatoid arthritis. Arthritis Rheum 31: 315–324.
26. Seitz M, Dayer JM (2000) Enhanced production of tissue inhibitor of metalloproteinases by peripheral blood mononuclear cells of rheumatoid arthritis patients responding to methotrexate treatment. Rheumatology (Oxford) 39: 637–645.
27. Liberman AC, Refojo D, Druker J, Toscano M, Rein T, et al. (2007) The activated glucocorticoid receptor inhibits the transcription factor T-bet by direct protein-protein interaction. FASEB J 21: 1177–1188.
28. Gabrielli E, Pericolini E, Cenci E, Ortelli F, Magliani W, et al. (2009) Antibody complementarity-determining regions (CDRs): a bridge between adaptive and innate immunity. PLoS One 4: e8187.
29. Pericolini E, Gabrielli E, Bistoni G, Cenci E, Perito S, et al. (2010) Role of CD45 signaling pathway in galactoxylomannan-induced T cell damage. PLoS One 5: e12720.

30. Jandus C, Bioley G, Rivals JP, Dudler J, Speiser D, et al. (2008) Increased numbers of circulating polyfunctional Th17 memory cells in patients with seronegative spondylarthritides. Arthritis Rheum 58: 2307–2317.
31. Quah BJ, Warren HS, Parish CR (2007) Monitoring lymphocyte proliferation in vitro and in vivo with the intracellular fluorescent dye carboxyfluorescein diacetate succinimidyl ester. Nat Protoc 2: 2049–2056.
32. Bianchini R, Bistoni O, Alunno A, Petrillo MG, Ronchetti S, et al. (2011) CD4(+) CD25(low) GITR(+) cells: a novel human CD4(+) T-cell population with regulatory activity. Eur J Immunol 41: 2269–2278.
33. Gol-Ara M, Jadidi-Niaragh F, Sadria R, Azizi G, Mirshafiey A (2012) The role of different subsets of regulatory T cells in immunopathogenesis of rheumatoid arthritis. Arthritis 2012: 805875.
34. Liu W, Putnam AL, Xu-Yu Z, Szot GL, Lee MR, et al. (2006) CD127 expression inversely correlates with FoxP3 and suppressive function of human CD4+ T reg cells. J Exp Med 203: 1701–1711.
35. Volin MV, Shahrara S (2011) Role of TH-17 cells in rheumatic and other autoimmune diseases. Rheumatology (Sunnyvale) 1.
36. Lin L, Hutzen B, Zuo M, Ball S, Deangelis S, et al. (2010) Novel STAT3 phosphorylation inhibitors exhibit potent growth-suppressive activity in pancreatic and breast cancer cells. Cancer Res 70: 2445–2454.
37. Yagi H, Nomura T, Nakamura K, Yamazaki S, Kitawaki T, et al. (2004) Crucial role of FOXP3 in the development and function of human CD25+CD4+ regulatory T cells. Int Immunol 16: 1643–1656.
38. Sakaguchi S, Yamaguchi T, Nomura T, Ono M (2008) Regulatory T cells and immune tolerance. Cell 133: 775–787.
39. Morgan ME, Sutmuller RP, Witteveen HJ, van Duivenvoorde LM, Zanelli E, et al. (2003) CD25+ cell depletion hastens the onset of severe disease in collagen-induced arthritis. Arthritis Rheum 48: 1452–1460.
40. Ehrenstein MR, Evans JG, Singh A, Moore S, Warnes G, et al. (2004) Compromised function of regulatory T cells in rheumatoid arthritis and reversal by anti-TNFalpha therapy. J Exp Med 200: 277–285.
41. Huang Z, Yang B, Shi Y, Cai B, Li Y, et al. (2012) Anti-TNF-alpha therapy improves Treg and suppresses Teff in patients with rheumatoid arthritis. Cell Immunol 279: 25–29.
42. Kavanaugh A (2010) Biologic agents in rheumatology: act II. Clin Exp Rheumatol 28: S2–4.
43. Chan ES, Cronstein BN (2010) Methotrexate–how does it really work? Nat Rev Rheumatol 6: 175–178.
44. Valencia X, Stephens G, Goldbach-Mansky R, Wilson M, Shevach EM, et al. (2006) TNF downmodulates the function of human CD4+CD25hi T-regulatory cells. Blood 108: 253–261.
45. Nie H, Zheng Y, Li R, Guo TB, He D, et al. (2013) Phosphorylation of FOXP3 controls regulatory T cell function and is inhibited by TNF-alpha in rheumatoid arthritis. Nat Med 19: 322–328.
46. Ohta A, Kini R, Ohta A, Subramanian M, Madasu M, et al. (2012) The development and immunosuppressive functions of CD4(+) CD25(+) FoxP3(+) regulatory T cells are under influence of the adenosine-A2A adenosine receptor pathway. Front Immunol 3: 190.
47. Booth NJ, McQuaid AJ, Sobande T, Kissane S, Agius E, et al. (2010) Different proliferative potential and migratory characteristics of human CD4+ regulatory T cells that express either CD45RA or CD45RO. J Immunol 184: 4317–4326.
48. Haas J, Fritzsching B, Trubswetter P, Korporal M, Milkova L, et al. (2007) Prevalence of newly generated naive regulatory T cells (Treg) is critical for Treg suppressive function and determines Treg dysfunction in multiple sclerosis. J Immunol 179: 1322–1330.
49. Venken K, Hellings N, Broekmans T, Hensen K, Rummens JL, et al. (2008) Natural naive CD4+CD25+CD127low regulatory T cell (Treg) development and function are disturbed in multiple sclerosis patients: recovery of memory Treg homeostasis during disease progression. J Immunol 180: 6411–6420.
50. Kim JR, Chae JN, Kim SH, Ha JS (2012) Subpopulations of regulatory T cells in rheumatoid arthritis, systemic lupus erythematosus, and Behcet's disease. J Korean Med Sci 27: 1009–1013.

Construction and Application of a Korean Reference Panel for Imputing Classical Alleles and Amino Acids of Human Leukocyte Antigen Genes

Kwangwoo Kim[1,2,3,4], So-Young Bang[1], Hye-Soon Lee[1], Sang-Cheol Bae[1]*

1 Department of Rheumatology, Hanyang University Hospital for Rheumatic Diseases, Seoul, Republic of Korea, **2** Division of Rheumatology, Immunology and Allergy, Brigham and Women's Hospital, Harvard Medical School, Boston, Massachusetts, United States of America, **3** Division of Genetics, Brigham and Women's Hospital, Harvard Medical School, Boston, Massachusetts, United States of America, **4** Program in Medical and Population Genetics, Broad Institute, Cambridge, Massachusetts, United States of America

Abstract

Genetic variations of human leukocyte antigen (HLA) genes within the major histocompatibility complex (MHC) locus are strongly associated with disease susceptibility and prognosis for many diseases, including many autoimmune diseases. In this study, we developed a Korean HLA reference panel for imputing classical alleles and amino acid residues of several HLA genes. An HLA reference panel has potential for use in identifying and fine-mapping disease associations with the MHC locus in East Asian populations, including Koreans. A total of 413 unrelated Korean subjects were analyzed for single nucleotide polymorphisms (SNPs) at the MHC locus and six HLA genes, including *HLA-A*, *-B*, *-C*, *-DRB1*, *-DPB1*, and *-DQB1*. The HLA reference panel was constructed by phasing the 5,858 MHC SNPs, 233 classical HLA alleles, and 1,387 amino acid residue markers from 1,025 amino acid positions as binary variables. The imputation accuracy of the HLA reference panel was assessed by measuring concordance rates between imputed and genotyped alleles of the HLA genes from a subset of the study subjects and East Asian HapMap individuals. Average concordance rates were 95.6% and 91.1% at 2-digit and 4-digit allele resolutions, respectively. The imputation accuracy was minimally affected by SNP density of a test dataset for imputation. In conclusion, the Korean HLA reference panel we developed was highly suitable for imputing HLA alleles and amino acids from MHC SNPs in East Asians, including Koreans.

Editor: Valli De Re, Centro di Riferimento Oncologico, IRCCS National Cancer Institute, Italy

Funding: This work was supported by grants from the Korea Healthcare Technology R&D project of the Ministry for Health & Welfare (HI13C2124). The funders had no role in study design, data collection and analysis, decision to publish, or preparation of the manuscript.

Competing Interests: The authors have declared that no competing interests exist.

* Email: scbae@hanyang.ac.kr

Introduction

There is a well-characterized high degree of genetic variability in human leukocyte antigen (HLA) genes located at the major histocompatibility complex (MHC) locus on chromosome 6 [1]. Although diverse genetic variations and heterozygosity of HLA molecules allow the immune system to defend against a wide range of foreign molecules and pathogens [2], various classical alleles of HLA genes have been found to be associated with susceptibility to or prognosis of multiple inflammatory disorders and other complex traits [3,4].

Despite the clinical importance of the locus, the decision to genotype HLA alleles for a large number of subjects is limited by the high cost of genotyping and low throughput genotyping methods. Currently, it is possible to infer HLA alleles from SNPs in the MHC locus using several HLA imputation methods, such as SNP2HLA and HLA*IMP [5,6]. SNP2HLA has the advantage of being able to identify the most likely causal variants in complex diseases like HIV infection, rheumatoid arthritis, multiple sclerosis, and follicular lymphoma, because this method can impute amino acid residues in HLA genes as well as classical HLA alleles [7-11]. SNP2HLA uses a specialized HLA reference panel that encodes SNPs within the MHC region along with HLA classical alleles and amino acid residues [5]. However, this method has not been used in HLA association studies in non-European populations because the HLA reference panel was generated from European genetic information. To overcome this limitation, the first Asian HLA reference panel was very recently constructed mostly from Southeast Asian subjects [11,12].

In this study, we developed an HLA reference panel for East Asians, including Koreans, for use with SNP2HLA.

Materials and Methods

The genetic data of 413 unrelated Korean subjects were included in our new HLA reference panel. The subjects were examined for their SNPs by Illumina's HumanOmniExpress array at SNPgenetics Inc. (Seoul, South Korea). We applied general quality control criteria for minor allele frequency (MAF; MAF $>0.5\%$), Hardy-Weinberg equilibrium (HWE; p value of HWE $>5\times10^{-7}$), call rate per SNP ($>98\%$), call rate per individual ($>98\%$), heterozygosity rate, population stratification, sex consistency between subject-reported and genetic

Table 1. Number of classical HLA alleles and polymorphic amino acid positions in the HLA reference panel.

Gene	HLA allele markers (2-digit/4-digit)	Amino acid positions
HLA-A	11/23	144
HLA-B	25/44	139
HLA-C	11/25	216
HLA-DRB1	13/34	208
HLA-DPB1	11/13	192
HLA-DQB1	5/18	126
Total	76/157	1,025

sex, and cryptic relatedness (duplicate and cryptic 1st degree relatives). SNPs within the MHC from 25 Mb to 33 Mb on chromosome 6 (in hg18) were extracted to construct the HLA reference panel.

Classical HLA alleles of *HLA-A*, *-B*, *-C*, *-DRB1*, *-DPB1* and *-DQB1* were genotyped using Roche's GS 454 sequencing at the Institute for Immunology and Infectious Diseases (Murdoch WA, Australia). The institutional calling algorithms for HLA alleles were accredited by the American Society for Histocompatibility and Immunogenetics (ASHI). To examine sequencing and calling accuracy for the HLA allele, we independently genotyped the classical allele *HLA-DRB1* at 4-digit resolution for all subjects by a conventional sequencing method using a WAKFlow HLA typing kit (Hiroshima, Japan) at Labgenomics Clinical Laboratories (Seongnam, Korea).

All genotyped data of the MHC SNPs, HLA alleles, and HLA amino acid residues were phased by Beagle 3.0.4 in SNP2HLA with some modifications. HLA amino acid residues were assigned from the amino acid sequence information of each 4-digit HLA-allele.

Imputation accuracy of the reference panel was examined by comparing the imputed and genotyped results of classical HLA alleles. To this end, test subjects (n = 83) and reference subjects (n = 330) were randomly selected from the 413 Korean subjects 100 times at a 1:4 ratio. Using each pair of test and reference subsets, we imputed HLA alleles from MHC SNPs in the test subjects by using SNP2HLA and the reference panel from the matched reference subjects. We then calculated 100 concordance rates between imputed and genotyped classical alleles of each HLA gene and obtained an average concordance rate for each gene.

In addition, we imputed HLA alleles from the HapMap3 r2 SNP dataset of East Asian HapMap population [Han Chinese from Beijing, China (CHB) and Japanese from Tokyo, Japan (JPT)] using the reference panel, including all Korean 413 reference samples. To compare the imputed HLA alleles with actual HLA alleles, the HLA data of CHB + JPT HapMap population for *HLA-A*, *-B*, *-C*, *-DRB1* and *-DQB1* was obtained from two independent studies [13,14]. Individuals with discordant results between the two studies were excluded from this analysis. *HLA-A*, -B, -C, and *-DRB1* were genotyped in the two studies. Of 89 CHB + JPT subjects in the HapMap3 r2 dataset, 61 subjects were exactly matched for all 4-digit alleles of the HLA genes in the two studies.

To evaluate the imputation accuracy of an ethnicity-mismatched HLA reference panel, a European reference panel (constructed from data collected by the Type 1 Diabetes Genetics Consortium; T1DGC) was used to impute for the East Asian HapMap3 r2 dataset [5,13]. To ensure panel size consistency, we created subsets of the European reference panel by randomly selecting 413 individuals and independently repeated this process

Table 2. Concordance rates between imputed and genotyped alleles.

Reference panel	Test dataset	Allelic resolution	HLA gene						
			A	B	C	DRB1	DPB1	DQB1	Total
Korean* (n = 330)	Korean* (n = 83)	2-digit	0.979	0.913	0.965	0.931	0.970	0.970	0.954
		4-digit	0.908	0.859	0.928	0.868	0.950	0.937	0.908
Korean (n = 413)	CHB + JPT (n = 61)	2-digit	0.934	0.934	0.992	0.959	NA	0.967	0.957
		4-digit	0.910	0.893	0.984	0.893	NA	0.893	0.915
European** (n = 413)	Korean (n = 413)	2-digit	0.920	0.510	0.770	0.622	0.886	0.740	0.712
		4-digit	0.766	0.455	0.687	0.400	0.863	0.650	0.592
European** (n = 413)	CHB + JPT (n = 61)	2-digit	0.911	0.283	0.668	0.754	NA	0.794	0.682
		4-digit	0.829	0.233	0.602	0.591	NA	0.659	0.583

* Reference panel and test datasets were randomly assigned 100 times from all 413 Korean subjects and the mean concordance rate was calculated by 100 independent imputations using each of the 100 reference panel and test dataset pairs.
** For consistency of panel size between Korean and European panels, the mean concordance rate was calculated by 100 independent imputations using 100 different subsets (n = 413) of the European reference panel.

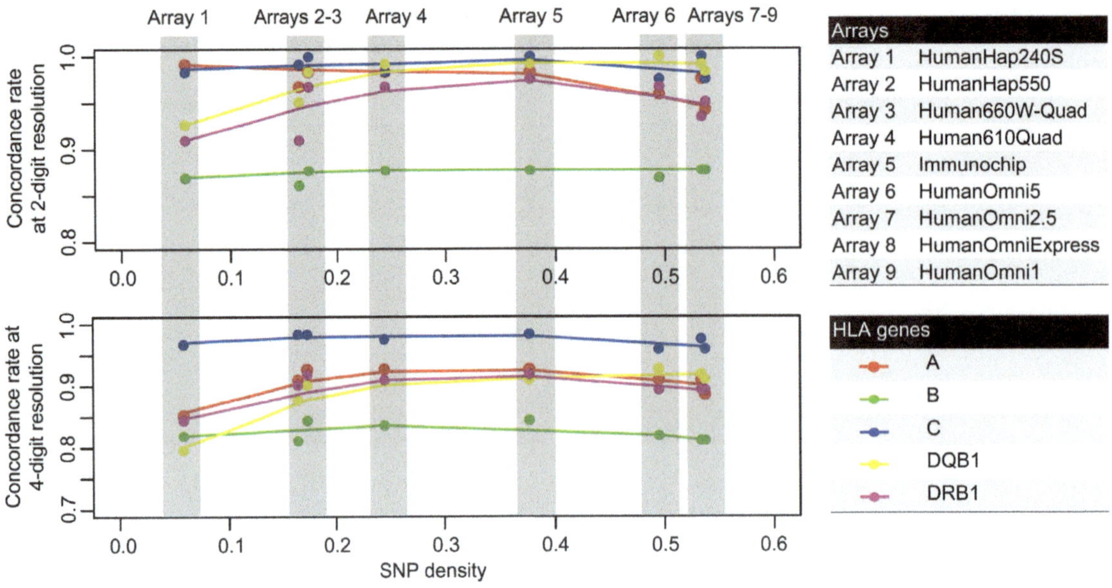

Figure 1. Concordance rates using various reference panels. SNPs present in 9 different commercial arrays were extracted for imputing the HLA alleles from the HapMap3 r2 dataset of East Asian (CHB + JPT) individuals. Each subset was imputed for *HLA-A*, *-B*, *-C*, *-DQB1* and *-DRB1* using the Korean reference panel. Concordance rates (y-axis) were plotted against the proportion of reference-panel SNPs that were present in each subset (x-axis).

100 times. Imputation accuracy was evaluated using the mean of the 100 independent concordance rates for each HLA gene.

The study was approved by the Institutional Review Board of Hanyang University (IRB file No. HYUH 2001-06-001), and written consent was obtained from study participants.

Results and Discussion

A total of 5,858 polymorphic MHC SNPs in the 413 study subjects passed our quality control criteria. The 4-digit alleles of the 6 HLA genes (*HLA-A*, *-B*, *-C*, *-DRB1*, *-DPB1* and *-DQB1*) typed using NGS methods were assigned to 233 HLA alleles, which results in 1,025 polymorphic amino acid positions in the

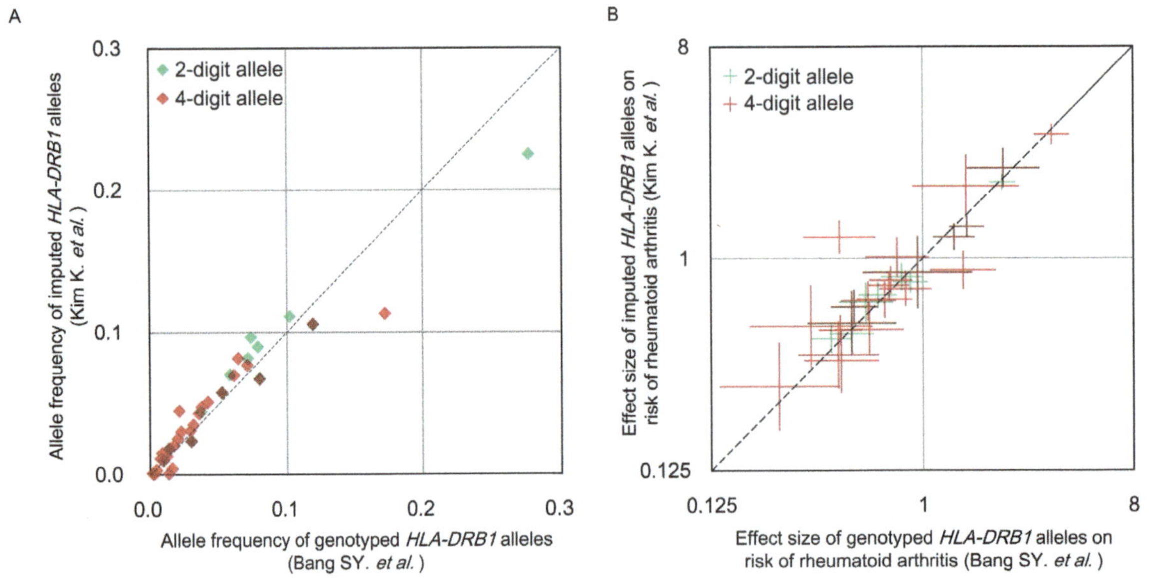

Figure 2. Frequencies and disease effect sizes of imputed and genotyped *HLA-DRB1* alleles. We revisited our previous rheumatoid arthritis association studies using either typed SNPs [16] or HLA alleles [17]. After imputing HLA variants from the SNP-based dataset, (A) frequencies and (B) disease effect sizes of the imputed classical alleles of *HLA-DRB1* were compared with those of genotyped classical alleles in the HLA-based dataset.

study subjects (**Table 1**). The frequencies of HLA alleles in the Korean subjects are shown in **Table S1 in File S1**. Given our sample size (826 haplotypes), we expected to detect at least 4.1 times the HLA alleles with frequency ≥0.5% in the general Korean population.

The reliability of the calling algorithm in the NGS-based genotyping method was evaluated by comparing *HLA-DRB1* alleles with conventionally genotyped results for all of the study subjects. A concordance rate of 99.52% was observed at 4-digit resolution of *HLA-DRB1* alleles.

The HLA reference panel encoded all information about each of the MHC SNPs, HLA-alleles, and amino acid residues as binary codes, such as absence/presence or allele1/allele2, as previously described [5]. We evaluated the newly constructed reference panel by assessing imputation accuracy using the MHC SNPs in a test subset among the subjects (n = 83; 20%) and the reference panel from the reference subset comprised of all remaining subjects (n = 330; 80%). The test subset and the reference subset were randomly selected 100 times and each pair of test and reference subsets was used in an imputation analysis by SNP2HLA. When we surveyed all imputed data and compared the data with actual genotype data, the average genotype concordance rates were 95.4% and 90.8% at 2-digit and 4-digit allele resolution, respectively. For each HLA gene, concordance ranged from 91.3% (for *HLA-B*) to 97.9% (for *HLA-A*) at 2-digit allele resolution and from 85.9% (for *HLA-B*) to 95.0% (for *HLA-DPB1*) at 4-digit allele resolution (**Table 2**).

In addition, we imputed the HLA alleles from MHC SNPs of East Asian HapMap individuals (CHB + JPT) using the Korean reference panel (n = 413) to assess imputation accuracy from an independent Asian dataset. The average concordance rates between genotyped and imputed alleles were 95.7% (93.4 - 99.2%) at the 2-digit allele resolution and 91.5% (89.3 - 98.4%) at the 4-digit allele resolution, which are similar to those in the cross-tested Korean subjects. Pearson's correlation coefficients between actual and imputed dosage of classical HLA alleles were calculated to evaluate the imputation accuracy at the allele level. The new reference panel showed a high correlation between imputed and actual dosage (average correlation coefficient r = 0.887 for alleles with frequency ≥0.01 and r = 0.735 for alleles with frequency < 0.01; **Figure S1 in File S1**).

In contrast, when we used a European reference panel for imputing HLA alleles of the East Asian HapMap subjects, imputation accuracy from the ethnicity-mismatched reference panel was much worse than that from the Korean reference panel, especially for *HLA-B*, *-C*, *-DRB1* and *-DQB1* (**Table 2**). The observed ethnicity effect in imputation has been consistently reported in previous studies [5,11,12,15].

We further investigated the effect of SNP density in test datasets on imputation accuracy in the Korean HLA reference panel. From the CHB + JPT HapMap dataset, we extracted nine sets of SNPs that were present in each of nine commercial genome-wide SNP arrays instead of using all SNPs in the HapMap3 r2 datasets. Using a low-density test dataset dramatically decreased the number of SNPs that were present in both the reference panel and the array-based test dataset. However, SNP density had little effect on imputation accuracy (**Figure 1**). Accuracy was slightly decreased only by use of very low-density genotyping arrays, which are no longer commercially available.

To illustrate the advantage of the new Korean reference panel in an association study, we applied the reference panel to our previous SNP-based case-control association study [16] on rheumatoid arthritis (RA) that shows the strongest association at *HLA-DRB1* within the extended MHC region [11]. After imputing HLA variants from the SNP-based dataset [16], we compared disease effect sizes of the imputed *HLA-DRB1* alleles with those of the genotyped *HLA-DRB1* alleles that were obtained in our previous HLA-allele-based case-control association study [17]. We note that there is a some portion of overlapping subjects (n = 2,355) between the SNP-based (n = 9,299) and HLA-based datasets (n = 3,034) [16,17], and that we already fully dissected and reported HLA-RA associations down to the amino acid level in our another recent paper [11].

We found highly correlated allele frequencies between imputed and genotyped *HLA-DRB1* alleles (correlation coefficient r = 0.976 at 2-digit resolution and r = 0.932 at 4-digit resolution; **Figure 2A**), although a large portion of subjects was not examined in the both studies. The effect sizes of each HLA allele were also highly concordant between the two datasets (r = 0.984 at 2-digit resolution and r = 0.938 at 4-digit resolution; **Figure 2B**), which demonstrating reliability, validity and usefulness of the Korean reference panel in MHC-disease association studies.

Conclusion

The Korean HLA reference panel constructed in our study was found to be highly applicable and suitable for various genome-wide array data from East Asians, including Han Chinese, Japanese, and Korean populations. The Korean reference panel is publicly available from **File S2** and https://sites.google om/site/scbaehanyang/hla_panel/.

Supporting Information

File S1 Tables S1; Figures S1.

File S2 Korean HLA reference panel.

Author Contributions

Conceived and designed the experiments: KK SCB. Performed the experiments: KK. Analyzed the data: KK. Contributed reagents/materials/analysis tools: KK SYB HYL SCB. Wrote the paper: KK SCB.

References

1. Horton R, Wilming L, Rand V, Lovering RC, Bruford EA, et al. (2004) Gene map of the extended human MHC. Nat Rev Genet 5: 889-899.
2. Apanius V, Penn D, Slev PR, Ruff LR, Potts WK (1997) The nature of selection on the major histocompatibility complex. Crit Rev Immunol 17: 179-224.
3. Ahn S, Choi HB, Kim TG (2011) HLA and Disease Associations in Koreans. Immune Netw 11: 324-335.
4. Shiina T, Hosomichi K, Inoko H, Kulski JK (2009) The HLA genomic loci map: expression, interaction, diversity and disease. J Hum Genet 54: 15-39.
5. Jia X, Han B, Onengut-Gumuscu S, Chen WM, Concannon PJ, et al. (2013) Imputing amino acid polymorphisms in human leukocyte antigens. PLoS One 8: e64683.
6. Dilthey AT, Moutsianas L, Leslie S, McVean G (2011) HLA*IMP—an integrated framework for imputing classical HLA alleles from SNP genotypes. Bioinformatics 27: 968-972.
7. International HIVCS, Pereyra F, Jia X, McLaren PJ, Telenti A, et al. (2010) The major genetic determinants of HIV-1 control affect HLA class I peptide presentation. Science 330: 1551-1557.
8. Raychaudhuri S, Sandor C, Stahl EA, Freudenberg J, Lee HS, et al. (2012) Five amino acids in three HLA proteins explain most of the association between MHC and seropositive rheumatoid arthritis. Nat Genet 44: 291-296.
9. Patsopoulos NA, Barcellos LF, Hintzen RQ, Schaefer C, van Duijn CM, et al. (2013) Fine-mapping the genetic association of the major histocompatibility

complex in multiple sclerosis: HLA and non-HLA effects. PLoS Genet 9: e1003926.

10. Foo JN, Smedby KE, Akers NK, Berglund M, Irwan ID, et al. (2013) Coding variants at hexa-allelic amino acid 13 of HLA-DRB1 explain independent SNP associations with follicular lymphoma risk. Am J Hum Genet 93: 167-172.
11. Okada Y, Kim K, Han B, Pillai NE, Ong RT, et al. (2014) Risk for ACPA-positive rheumatoid arthritis is driven by shared HLA amino acid polymorphisms in Asian and European populations. Hum Mol Genet. doi: 10.1093/hmg/ddu387
12. Pillai NE, Okada Y, Saw WY, Ong RT, Wang X, et al. (2014) Predicting HLA alleles from high-resolution SNP data in three Southeast Asian populations. Hum Mol Genet 23: 4443-4451.
13. de Bakker PI, McVean G, Sabeti PC, Miretti MM, Green T, et al. (2006) A high-resolution HLA and SNP haplotype map for disease association studies in the extended human MHC. Nat Genet 38: 1166-1172.
14. Yamamura T, Hikita J, Bleakley M, Hirosawa T, Sato-Otsubo A, et al. (2012) HapMap SNP Scanner: an online program to mine SNPs responsible for cell phenotype. Tissue Antigens 80: 119-125.
15. Marchini J, Howie B (2010) Genotype imputation for genome-wide association studies. Nat Rev Genet 11: 499-511.
16. Kim K, Bang SY, Lee HS, Cho SK, Choi CB, et al. (2014) High-density genotyping of immune loci in Koreans and Europeans identifies eight new rheumatoid arthritis risk loci. Ann Rheum Dis. doi: 10.1136/annrheumdis-2013-204749
17. Bang SY, Lee HS, Lee KW, Bae SC (2013) Interaction of HLA-DRB1*09:01 and *04:05 with smoking suggests distinctive mechanisms of rheumatoid arthritis susceptibility beyond the shared epitope. J Rheumatol 40: 1054-1062.

Permissions

All chapters in this book were first published in PLOS ONE, by The Public Library of Science; hereby published with permission under the Creative Commons Attribution License or equivalent. Every chapter published in this book has been scrutinized by our experts. Their significance has been extensively debated. The topics covered herein carry significant findings which will fuel the growth of the discipline. They may even be implemented as practical applications or may be referred to as a beginning point for another development.

The contributors of this book come from diverse backgrounds, making this book a truly international effort. This book will bring forth new frontiers with its revolutionizing research information and detailed analysis of the nascent developments around the world.

We would like to thank all the contributing authors for lending their expertise to make the book truly unique. They have played a crucial role in the development of this book. Without their invaluable contributions this book wouldn't have been possible. They have made vital efforts to compile up to date information on the varied aspects of this subject to make this book a valuable addition to the collection of many professionals and students.

This book was conceptualized with the vision of imparting up-to-date information and advanced data in this field. To ensure the same, a matchless editorial board was set up. Every individual on the board went through rigorous rounds of assessment to prove their worth. After which they invested a large part of their time researching and compiling the most relevant data for our readers.

The editorial board has been involved in producing this book since its inception. They have spent rigorous hours researching and exploring the diverse topics which have resulted in the successful publishing of this book. They have passed on their knowledge of decades through this book. To expedite this challenging task, the publisher supported the team at every step. A small team of assistant editors was also appointed to further simplify the editing procedure and attain best results for the readers.

Apart from the editorial board, the designing team has also invested a significant amount of their time in understanding the subject and creating the most relevant covers. They scrutinized every image to scout for the most suitable representation of the subject and create an appropriate cover for the book.

The publishing team has been an ardent support to the editorial, designing and production team. Their endless efforts to recruit the best for this project, has resulted in the accomplishment of this book. They are a veteran in the field of academics and their pool of knowledge is as vast as their experience in printing. Their expertise and guidance has proved useful at every step. Their uncompromising quality standards have made this book an exceptional effort. Their encouragement from time to time has been an inspiration for everyone.

The publisher and the editorial board hope that this book will prove to be a valuable piece of knowledge for researchers, students, practitioners and scholars across the globe.

List of Contributors

John W. Peabody
Departments of Epidemiology & Biostatistics and Medicine, University of California San Francisco, San Francisco, California, United States of America
QURE Healthcare, San Rafael, California, United States of America

Rachel Lee
QURE Healthcare, San Rafael, California, United States of America

Vibeke Strand
Division of Immunology/Rheumatology, Stanford University, Stanford, California, United States of America

Riti Shimkhada
QURE Healthcare, San Rafael, California, United States of America
Department of Health Policy and Management, University of California Los Angeles, Los Angeles, California, United States of America

David Chernoff
Crescendo Bioscience, South San Francisco, California, United States of America

Catherine Swales and Helen J. Knowles
Botnar Research Centre, Nuffield Department of Orthopaedics Rheumatology and Musculoskeletal Sciences, University of Oxford, Oxford, United Kingdom

Nicholas A. Athanasou
Pathology Department, Nuffield Orthopaedic Centre, University of Oxford, Oxford, United Kingdom

Chih-Chao Hsu and Ti Lu
Department of Psychiatry, Kaohsiung Veterans General Hospital, Kaohsiung, Taiwan

Li-Yu Hu
Department of Psychiatry, Kaohsiung Veterans General Hospital, Kaohsiung, Taiwan
Institute of Public Health & School of Medicine, National Yang-Ming University, Taipei, Taiwan

San-Chi Chen
Division of Hematology and Oncology, Department of Medicine, Taipei Veterans General Hospital, Taipei, Taiwan

Chia-Jen Liu
Division of Hematology and Oncology, Department of Medicine, Taipei Veterans General Hospital, Taipei, Taiwan
Institute of Public Health & School of Medicine, National Yang-Ming University, Taipei, Taiwan

Cheng-Che Shen
Department of Psychiatry, Chiayi Branch, Taichung Veterans General Hospital, Chiayi, Taiwan

Yu-Wen Hu
Institute of Public Health & School of Medicine, National Yang-Ming University, Taipei, Taiwan
Cancer Center, Taipei Veterans General Hospital, Taipei, Taiwan

Chiu-Mei Yeh
Department of Family Medicine, Taipei Veterans General Hospital, Taipei, Taiwan

Tzeng-Ji Chen
Department of Family Medicine, Taipei Veterans General Hospital, Taipei, Taiwan
School of Medicine, National Yang-Ming University, Taipei, Taiwan

Pan-Ming Chen
Department of Psychiatry, Yuanshan Branch, Taipei Veterans General Hospital, Yilan, Taiwan

Cheng-Ho Chang and Li-Yu Hu
Department of Psychiatry, Kaohsiung Veterans General Hospital, Kaohsiung, Taiwan

Shu-Li Wang
Department of Dental Laboratory Technology, Central Taiwan University of Science and Technology, Taichung, Taiwan

Shih-Jen Tsai
Department of Psychiatry, Taipei Veterans General Hospital, Taipei, Taiwan
School of Medicine, National Yang-Ming University, Taipei, Taiwan

Albert C. Yang
Department of Psychiatry, Taipei Veterans General Hospital, Taipei, Taiwan
School of Medicine, National Yang-Ming University, Taipei, Taiwan
Center for Dynamical Biomarkers and Translational Medicine, National Central University, Chungli, Taiwan

Zi-Hong You
Division of Nephrology, Department of Internal Medicine, Taichung Veterans General Hospital, Chia-Yi Branch, Chia-Yi, Taiwan
Institute of Medicine, Chung Shan Medical University, Taichung, Taiwan

Han-Ching Lin, Tzu-Hung Lin, Ming-Yueh Wu, Houng-Chi Liou, Huang-Ju Tu and Wen-Mei Fu
Department of Pharmacology, College of Medicine, National Taiwan University and Hospital, Taipei, Taiwan

Yung-Cheng Chiu
Department of Orthopaedics, Taichung Veterans General Hospital, Taichung, Taiwan

Chih-Hsin Tang
Department of Pharmacology, College of Medicine, China Medical University, Taichung, Taiwan

Mann-Jen Hour
School of Pharmacy, College of Medicine, China Medical University, Taichung, Taiwan

Rong-Sen Yang
Department of Orthopedics, College of Medicine, National Taiwan University and Hospital, Taipei, Taiwan

Jonathan C. Packham
Haywood Rheumatology Centre, Haywood Hospital, High Lane, Burslem, Stoke-on-Trent, Staffordshire, United Kingdom

Ying Chen and Derek L. Mattey
Haywood Rheumatology Centre, Haywood Hospital, High Lane, Burslem, Stoke-on-Trent, Staffordshire, United Kingdom
Institute of Science and Technology in Medicine, Keele University, Staffordshire, United Kingdom

Zanzhe Yu
Institute of Science and Technology in Medicine, Keele University, Staffordshire, United Kingdom

Bo Ruem Yoon and Yeon-Ho Chung
Department of Microbiology and Immunology, Seoul National University College of Medicine, Seoul, Korea

Yeon ho Choi
Department of Microbiology and Immunology, Seoul National University College of Medicine, Seoul, Korea
Cancer Research Institute, Seoul National University, Seoul, Korea

Seong Wook Kang, Su-Jin Yoo, Jinhyun Kim and In Seol Yoo
Department of Internal Medicine, Chungnam National University School of Medicine, Daejon, Korea

Won-Woo Lee
Department of Microbiology and Immunology, Seoul National University College of Medicine, Seoul, Korea
Department of Biomedical Sciences, Seoul National University College of Medicine, Seoul, Korea
Cancer Research Institute, Seoul National University, Seoul, Korea
Ischemic/Hypoxic Disease Institute, and Institute of Infectious Diseases, Seoul National University College of Medicine, Seoul, Korea

Ivan Caiello, Gaetana Minnone, Giusi Prencipe and Fabrizio De Benedetti
Division of Rheumatology, Bambino Gesù Children's Hospital, Rome, Italy

Thomas Vogl
Department of Paediatric Rheumatology and Immunology, University Children's Hospital Muenster, Muenster, Germany

Dirk Holzinger
Department of Paediatric Rheumatology and Immunology, University Children's Hospital Muenster, Muenster, Germany
Institute of Immunology, University Hospital Muenster, Muenster, Germany

Antonio Manzo
Rheumatology and Translational Immunology Research Laboratories (LaRIT), Division of Rheumatology, IRCCS Policlinico S. Matteo Foundation/University of Pavia, Pavia, Italy

Raffaele Strippoli
Division of Rheumatology, Bambino Gesù Children's Hospital, Rome, Italy
Department of Cellular Biotechnologies and Haematology, Sapienza University of Rome, Rome, Italy

Claire Le Jeunne
National Referral Center for Rare Systemic Autoimmune Diseases, Department of Internal Medicine, Hôpital Cochin, Assistance Publique-Hôpitaux de Paris, Université Paris Descartes, Paris, France

Xavier Puéchal
National Referral Center for Rare Systemic Autoimmune Diseases, Department of Internal Medicine, Hôpital Cochin, Assistance Publique-Hôpitaux de Paris, Université Paris Descartes, Paris, France
INSERM U1016, CNRS UMR 8104, Institut Cochin, Paris, France

Emmanuelle Génin
INSERM UMR-1078, Centre Hospitalier Universitaire, Brest, France

Thierry Bienvenu
Biochemistry and Molecular Biology Laboratory, Hôpital Cochin, Assistance Publique-Hôpitaux de Paris, Université Paris Descartes, Paris, France

Daniel J. Dusser
Department of Respiratory Diseases, Hôpital Cochin, Assistance Publique-Hôpitaux de Paris, Université Paris Descartes, Paris, France

Geraldine Cambridge and Maria J. Leandro
Centre for Rheumatology, University College London, London, United Kingdom

Rita A. Moura
Centre for Rheumatology, University College London, London, United Kingdom
Rheumatology Research Unit, Instituto de Medicina Molecular, Faculdade de Medicina da Universidade de Lisboa, Lisbon, Portugal

Akif A. Khawaja
Centre for Rheumatology, University College London, London, United Kingdom
Centre for Inflammation and Tissue Repair, University College London, London, United Kingdom

Tania Santos
Rheumatology Research Unit, Instituto de Medicina Molecular, Faculdade de Medicina da Universidade de Lisboa, Lisbon, Portugal

Joaquim Polido-Pereira, Helena Canhão and João E. Fonseca
Rheumatology Research Unit, Instituto de Medicina Molecular, Faculdade de Medicina da Universidade de Lisboa, Lisbon, Portugal
Rheumatology Department, Centro Hospitalar de Lisboa Norte, EPE, Hospital de Santa Maria, Lisbon, Portugal

Evangelia Zampeli and Petros P. Sfikakis
First Department of Propedeutic and Internal Medicine, Athens University Medical School, Athens, Greece

Ioannis Raftakis and Antonia Elezoglou
Rheumatology Department, Asklepion General Hospital, Athens, Greece

Archontoula Michelongona, Chara Nikolaou and Konstantinos Toutouzas
First Department of Cardiology, Athens University Medical School, Athens, Greece

Elias Siores
Institute for Materials Research and Innovation, University of Bolton, Bolton, United Kingdom

Nicolás Molano-González, Monica Rodríguez-Jiménez and Yeny Acosta-Ampudia
Center for Autoimmune Diseases Research (CREA), School of Medicine and Health Sciences, Universidad del Rosario, Bogotá, Colombia

Juan-Sebastian Franco, Rubén D. Mantilla, Jenny Amaya-Amaya, Adriana Rojas-Villarraga and Juan-Manuel Anaya
Center for Autoimmune Diseases Research (CREA), School of Medicine and Health Sciences, Universidad del Rosario, Bogotá, Colombia
Mederi, Hospital Universitario Mayor, Bogotá, Colombia

Mandy Sowa, Kai Grossmann and Ilka Knütter
Research and Development Department, GA Generic Assays GmbH, Dahlewitz/Berlin, Germany

Dirk Roggenbuck
Research and Development Department, GA Generic Assays GmbH, Dahlewitz/Berlin, Germany

Faculty of Science, Brandenburg University of Technology Cottbus- Senftenberg, Senftenberg, Germany

Peter Schierack, Rico Hiemann and Ursula Anderer
Faculty of Science, Brandenburg University of Technology Cottbus- Senftenberg, Senftenberg, Germany

Nadja Röber and Karsten Conrad
Institute of Immunology, Technical University of Dresden, Dresden, Germany

Elena Csernok
Department of Rheumatology, University of Schleswig-Holstein Campus Lübeck and Rheumaklinik Bad Bramstedt, Bad Bramstedt, Germany

Dimitrios P. Bogdanos
Division of Transplantation, Immunology and Mucosal Biology, King's University College, London, United Kingdom

Maria Orietta Borghi and Pier Luigi Meroni
Department of Rheumatology, University of Milan, Milan, Italy

Dirk Reinhold
Institute of Molecular and Clinical Immunology, Otto-von-Guericke University Magdeburg, Magdeburg, Germany

Xavier Janssens and Filip De Keyser
Department of Rheumatology, Ghent University Hospital, Ghent, Belgium

Saskia Decuman
Department of Rheumatology, Ghent University Hospital, Ghent, Belgium
Department of Internal Medicine, Ghent University, Ghent, Belgium

Vítor Seabra
CESPU, Institute of Research and Advanced Training in Health Sciences and Technologies, Department of Pharmaceutical Sciences, Higher Institute of Health Sciences-North (ISCS-N), Gandra PRD, Portugal

Aurea Lima
CESPU, Institute of Research and Advanced Training in Health Sciences and Technologies, Department of Pharmaceutical Sciences, Higher Institute of Health Sciences-North (ISCS-N), Gandra PRD, Portugal
Molecular Oncology Group CI, Portuguese Institute of Oncology of Porto (IPO-Porto), Porto, Portugal
Abel Salazar Institute for the Biomedical Sciences (ICBAS) of University of Porto, Porto, Portugal

Rui Medeiros
Molecular Oncology Group CI, Portuguese Institute of Oncology of Porto (IPO-Porto), Porto, Portugal
Abel Salazar Institute for the Biomedical Sciences (ICBAS) of University of Porto, Porto, Portugal
Virology Service, Portuguese Institute of Oncology of Porto (IPO-Porto), Porto, Portugal
Research Department-Portuguese League Against Cancer (LPCC-NRNorte), Porto, Portugal

Hugo Sousa
Molecular Oncology Group CI, Portuguese Institute of Oncology of Porto (IPO-Porto), Porto, Portugal
Faculty of Medicine of University of Porto (FMUP), Porto, Portugal
Virology Service, Portuguese Institute of Oncology of Porto (IPO-Porto), Porto, Portugal

Rita Azevedo
Molecular Oncology Group CI, Portuguese Institute of Oncology of Porto (IPO-Porto), Porto, Portugal
Faculty of Medicine of University of Porto (FMUP), Porto, Portugal

Miguel Bernardes
Faculty of Medicine of University of Porto (FMUP), Porto, Portugal
Rheumatology Department of São João Hospital Center, Porto, Portugal

Fernanda Genre, Raquel López-Mejías, Ricardo Blanco, Alfonso Corrales, Begoña Ubilla, Trinitario Pina and Miguel A. González-Gay
Epidemiology, Genetics and Atherosclerosis Research Group on Systemic Inflammatory Diseases, Rheumatology Division, IDIVAL, Santander, Spain

Mercedes García-Bermúdez and Javier Martín
Instituto de Parasitología y Biomedicina López-Neyra, IPBLN-CSIC, Granada, Spain

Santos Castañeda and Isidoro González-Álvaro
Department of Rheumatology, Hospital Universitario la Princesa, IIS-Princesa, Madrid, Spain

Carlos González-Juanatey
Cardiology Division, Hospital Universitario Lucus Augusti, Lugo, Spain

Javier Llorca
Department of Epidemiology and Computational Biology, School of Medicine, University of Cantabria, and CIBER Epidemiología y Salud Pública (CIBERESP), IDIVAL, Santander, Spain

José A. Miranda-Filloy
Division of Rheumatology, Hospital Universitario Lucus Augusti, Lugo, Spain

Carmen Gómez-Vaquero
Department of Rheumatology, Hospital Universitario Bellvitge, Barcelona, Spain

Luis Rodríguez-Rodríguez and Benjamín Fernández-Gutiérrez
Department of Rheumatology, Hospital Clínico San Carlos, Madrid, Spain

Alejandro Balsa and Dora Pascual-Salcedo
Department of Rheumatology, Hospital Universitario La Paz, Madrid, Spain

Francisco J. López-Longo
Department of Rheumatology, Hospital General Universitario Gregorio Marañón, Madrid, Spain

Patricia Carreira
Department of Rheumatology, Hospital Universitario 12 de Octubre, Madrid, Spain

Alexander Rosenberg, Yahui G. Chiu, Darren Tabechian, Rick Barrett and Sharon Moorehead
Division of Allergy, Immunology and Rheumatology, University of Rochester Medical Center, Rochester, NY, United States of America

Christopher T. Ritchlin
Division of Allergy, Immunology and Rheumatology, University of Rochester Medical Center, Rochester, NY, United States of America
The Center for Musculoskeletal Research, University of Rochester Medical Center, Rochester, NY, United States of America

Edward M. Schwarz
The Center for Musculoskeletal Research, University of Rochester Medical Center, Rochester, NY, United States of America

Hongtao Fan, Rebecca Bolce, Frédéric Baribaud, Hao Liu, Nancy Peffer and David Shealy
Janssen Research and Development LLC, Spring House, PA, United States of America

Ahmed M. Al-Abd
Department of Pharmacology and Toxicology, Faculty of Pharmacy, King Abdulaziz University, Jeddah, Saudi Arabia

Fahad A. Al-Abbasi
Department of Biochemistry, Faculty of Science, King Abdulaziz University, Jeddah, Saudi Arabia

Wafaa I. El-Eraky and Salwa M. Nofal
Department of Pharmacology, Medical Division, National Research Centre, Giza, Egypt

Amani E. Khalifa and Ashraf B. Abdel-Naim
Department of Pharmacology and Toxicology, Faculty of Pharmacy, Ain Shams University, Cairo, Egypt

Richard O. Williams
Kennedy Institute of Rheumatology, University of Oxford, Oxford, United Kingdom

Ayman A. Nagy
Department of Forensic Medicine and Clinical Toxicology, Faculty of Medicine, Tanta University, Egypt

Kim C. M. Santegoets, Mark H. Wenink and Timothy R. D. J. Radstake
Department of Rheumatology & Clinical Immunology, University Medical Center Utrecht, Utrecht, the Netherlands
Laboratory of Translational Immunology, Department of Immunology, University Medical Center Utrecht, Utrecht, the Netherlands
Department of Rheumatology, Radboud university medical center, Nijmegen, the Netherlands

Wim B. van den Berg
Department of Rheumatology, Radboud university medical center, Nijmegen, the Netherlands

Pascal B. Pfiffner and Timothy A. Miller
Boston Children's Hospital Informatics Program, Boston, Massachusetts, United States of America
Department of Pediatrics, Harvard Medical School, Boston, Massachusetts, United States of America

JiWon Oh
Wellesley College, Wellesley, Massachusetts, United States of America

Kenneth D. Mandl
Boston Children's Hospital Informatics Program, Boston, Massachusetts, United States of America

Department of Pediatrics, Harvard Medical School, Boston, Massachusetts, United States of America
Center for Biomedical Informatics, Harvard Medical School, Boston, Massachusetts, United States of America
Ghada Alsaleh, Antoine François, Lucas Philippe, Ya-Zhuo Gong, Seiamak Bahram, Jacques-Eric Gottenberg, Dominique Wachsmann, Philippe Georgel and Jean Sibilia
Immunorhumatologie moléculaire, INSERM UMR S_1109, Centre de Recherche en Immunologie et Hématologie, Faculté de Médecine, Fédération de Médecine Translationnelle de Strasbourg (FMTS), Université de Strasbourg, Strasbourg, France and Service de Rhumatologie, Centre National de Référence pour les Maladies Systémiques Autoimmunes Rares, Hôpitaux Universitaires de Strasbourg, Strasbourg, France

Semih Cetin and Sébastien Pfeffer
Université de Strasbourg, UPR 9002 du CNRS Architecture et Réactivité de l'ARN, Institut de Biologie Moléculaire et Cellulaire, Strasbourg, France

Jun-Jun Yeh
Department of Internal Medicine and Family Medicine, Ditmanson Medical Foundation Chia-Yi Christian Hospital, Chiayi, Taiwan
Chia Nan University of Pharmacy and Science, Tainan, Taiwan
Meiho University, Pingtung, Taiwan

Yu-Chiao Wang
Management Office for Health Data, China Medical University Hospital, Taichung, Taiwan
College of Medicine, China Medical University, Taichung, Taiwan

Fung-Chang Sung
College of Medicine, China Medical University, Taichung, Taiwan
Graduate Institute of Clinical Medical Science, China Medical University College of Medicine, Taichung, Taiwan

Chia-Hung Kao
Department of Nuclear Medicine and PET Center, China Medical University Hospital, Taichung, Taiwan

Jadwiga Bienkowska, Norm Allaire, Alice Thai, Jaya Goyal and Tatiana Plavina
Translational Medicine, Biogen Idec, Cambridge, Massachusetts, United States of America

Evan Beckman and Ajay Nirula
Immunobiology, Biogen Idec, Cambridge, Massachusetts, United States of America

Jeffrey L. Browning
Immunobiology, Biogen Idec, Cambridge, Massachusetts, United States of America
Department of Microbiology and Section of Rheumatology, Boston University School of Medicine, Boston, Massachusetts, United States of America

Megan Weaver and Charlotte Newman
Global Clinical Operations, Biogen Idec, Cambridge, Massachusetts, United States of America

Michelle Petri
Johns Hopkins University School of Medicine, Baltimore, Maryland, United States of America

Eva Pericolini, Elena Gabrielli, Stefano Perito, Elio Cenci and Anna Vecchiarelli
Microbiology Section, Department of Experimental Medicine, University of Perugia, Perugia, Italy

Alessia Alunno, Elena Bartoloni Bocci and Roberto Gerli
Rheumatology Unit, Department of Medicine, University of Perugia, Perugia, Italy

Siu-Kei Chow and Arturo Casadevall
Department of Microbiology and Immunology, Albert Einstein College of Medicine, New York, New York, United States of America

So-Young Bang, Hye-Soon Lee and Sang-Cheol Bae
Department of Rheumatology, Hanyang University Hospital for Rheumatic Diseases, Seoul, Republic of Korea

Kwangwoo Kim
Department of Rheumatology, Hanyang University Hospital for Rheumatic Diseases, Seoul, Republic of Korea
Division of Rheumatology, Immunology and Allergy, Brigham and Women's Hospital, Harvard Medical School, Boston, Massachusetts, United States of America

Division of Genetics, Brigham and Women's Hospital, Harvard Medical School, Boston, Massachusetts, United States of America
Program in Medical and Population Genetics, Broad Institute, Cambridge, Massachusetts, United States of America

Index